# MEDICAL
# EMERGENCIES
## in the
# DENTAL OFFICE

FIFTH EDITION

# MEDICAL EMERGENCIES in the DENTAL OFFICE

**Stanley F. Malamed, DDS**
*Professor of Anesthesia and Medicine*
*University of Southern California School of Dentistry*
*Los Angeles, California*

*Chapter 4, Medicolegal Considerations, by*
**Kenneth S. Robbins, BA, JD**
*Attorney in private practice*
*Law Offices of Kenneth S. Robbins*
*Honolulu, Hawaii*

with **230** illustrations

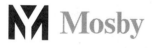
Mosby

St. Louis  Baltimore  Boston  Carlsbad  Chicago  Minneapolis  New York  Philadelphia  Portland
London  Milan  Sydney  Tokyo  Toronto

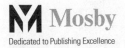

*Publisher:* John A. Schrefer
*Editor:* Penny Rudolph
*Developmental Editor:* Angela Reiner
*Project Manager:* Linda McKinley
*Designer:* Renée Duenow
*Cover Art:* © PhotoDisc, Inc.

**FIFTH EDITION**

NOTICE
Pharmacology is an ever-changing field. Standard safety precautions must be followed, but as new research and clinical experience broaden our knowledge, changes in treatment and drug therapy may become necessary or appropriate. Readers are advised to check the most current product information provided by the manufacturer of each drug to be administered to verify the recommended dose, the method and duration of administration, and contraindications. It is the responsibility of the treating physician, relying on experience and knowledge of the patient, to determine dosages and the best treatment for each individual patient. Neither the publisher nor the editor assume any liability for any injury and/or damage to persons or property arising from this publication.

Mosby, Inc.
*A Harcourt Health Sciences Company*
11830 Westline Industrial Drive
St. Louis, Missouri 63146

Printed in the United States of America
Composition by Top Graphics
Lithography/color film by Top Graphics
Printing/binding by Maple-Vail Book Manufacturing Group, Binghamton

**International Standard Book Number: 1-5566-4420-5**

99  00  01  02  /  9  8  7  6  5  4  3  2  1

*To my mother and father,*
*who made it all possible,*
*and to my wife Beverly and children,*
*Heather, Jennifer, and Jeremy,*
*who make it all so worthwhile,*
*I dedicate this book.*

# Foreword

IN the past 25 years, dental physicians have truly joined the ranks of health professionals by developing competence in internal medicine, psychosedation, physical evaluation, and emergency medicine. Although technical excellence must never be sacrificed, the role of dentistry is broadening to include adequate pain and anxiety control, significant health screening, and emergency preparedness.

Is there anything more noble than the saving of a life? It is just as noble to avoid mortality or serious morbidity by proper pretreatment physical evaluation and by appropriate modification of dental therapy. It is equally as noble to discover undiagnosed disease and to refer the patient for proper care, thus adding significantly to longevity

In a time when the credibility and motives of health professionals are under constant scrutiny, dentistry has added immeasurably to its public and professional image by extending its treatment scope in the public interest. This book on medical emergencies will be a valued addition to the library of the dental physician who has extended his or her horizons to include the broad health picture and has made the transition from the oral cavity to the complete patient. It is an excellent contribution to our literature.

**Frank M. McCarthy, MD, DDS**

# Preface

N December of 1975, I began writing the manuscript for *Medical Emergencies in the Dental Office*. The book was completed and published in April of 1978. As was mentioned in the preface to that first edition, my primary aim in writing the book was, and still remains, to stimulate the members of the dental profession—the doctor, dental hygienist, dental assistant, and all other office personnel—to improve and maintain their skill in the prevention of medical emergencies and in the recognition and management of emergencies that inevitably occur. This aim is ever more focused in my mind as this, the fifth edition of *Emergencies*, is written in 1999.

It is acknowledged that with proper patient management most medical emergency situations in the dental office can be prevented. What then is the need for a textbook on the management of medical emergencies? This thought has occurred to me on several occasions over the years. Do life-threatening situations really happen? The answer, unfortunately, is yes, they definitely do. I have received numerous letters, telephone calls, and e-mail messages and have met with many doctors and other dental personnel who have had real-life experiences with life-threatening medical problems. Virtually all of these situations have occurred in the dental office, but a significant number happened outside: on family outings, driving in a car, or at home.

There is a significant need for increased awareness by the dental profession in the area of emergency medicine. Although many states and provinces currently mandate continued certification in basic life support (cardiopulmonary resuscitation, or CPR) for dental relicensure, all too many states and provinces have not yet addressed this important issue.

As a person with a long-term commitment in the teaching of basic life support and advanced cardiac life support, I see the immense value in training all adults in the simple procedures collectively known as *basic life support*. Local and state dental societies, as well as specialty groups, should continue to present courses in basic life support or should initiate them posthaste.

Progress has been made, yet much more remains to be done. The awareness of our profession has been elevated, and laudable achievements continue. Yet, because of the very nature of the problem, what we require in dentistry is a continued maintenance of our high level of skill in the prevention, recognition, and management of medical emergencies. To do so we must all participate in ongoing programs designed by individual doctors to meet the needs of their offices. These programs should include attendance at continuing education seminars in emergency medicine, constant access to up-to-date information on this subject (through journals, texts, and the Internet), semiannual or annual recertification in basic life support or advanced cardiac life support, and in-office practice sessions in emergency procedures for the entire office staff. Such a program is discussed more completely in Chapter 3. The ultimate goal in preparation of a dental office for emergencies should be for you, the reader, to be able to put yourself into the position of a victim of a serious medical emergency in your dental office, and for you to be confident that your office staff would be able to react promptly and effectively in the recognition and management of your problem.

Emergency medicine is a constantly evolving medical specialty, and because of this many changes have occurred since publication of the first edition of this text. My goal now, as it was then, is to enable you to manage a given emergency situation in an effective yet uncomplicated manner. Alternative treatments and alternative drugs, which are also effective, may be advocated by some authors. My goal, as well as theirs, is simply to preserve the life of the victim.

Continual revision and updating of essential material is evident in this fifth edition. Changes have occurred in the design of the emergency drug and equipment kit in Chapter 3 (Preparation), as well as Cerebrovascular Accident (Chapter 19), Drug-Related Emergencies (Chapter 22), Chest Pain (Chapter 26), and Cardiopulmonary Resuscitation (Chapter 30). The American Heart Association will meet in Dallas, Texas, in 1999 to review its guidelines for basic (BLS) and advanced cardiac life (ACLS) support. Changes in technique are likely to be forthcoming when the AHA publishes its new recommendations under the title *ECC* [Emergency Cardiac Care] *2000*.

As a demonstration of the continuing change in the management of specific emergencies, let us look at the bare bones emergency kit that has been recommended by this author over the years. In the first edition of this text, the basic [module one] emergency drug kit contained 13 recommended drugs (eight injectable, five noninjectable). This number fell continually in succeeding editions to six (four injectable, two noninjectable) in editions 2 (1982) and 3 (1987), and to four (two injectable and two noninjectable) in edition 4 (1993). This latest edition presents a basic emergency drug kit with the addition of three drugs, including that "good old wonder drug," aspirin.

The basic format of the text—based upon clinical signs and symptoms rather than on a systems-oriented approach—remains quite well received and is continued in this fifth edition. Increased emphasis is placed upon the management scheme for all medical emergencies: **P** . . . position, **A** . . . airway, **B** . . . breathing, **C** . . . circulation, and **D** . . . definitive care. Management of medical emergencies need not, and should not, be complicated. Emphasizing this concept throughout the textbook should make it somewhat easier for the entire office staff to grasp the importance of certain basic steps in life saving [**P, A, B, C, D**].

As with the previous editions of this text, I have been quite fortunate to have been associated with a number of persons who helped to make the task of revision somewhat more tolerable and, to whatever degree possible, enjoyable. As I have discovered with each previous edition, it is impossible to mention everyone involved in the production of this book. However, I must mention several persons without whose help and guidance this volume would not have been completed: Norman Goldberg and Martin Fong, my photographers, and Dr. Rhonda J. Everett, Robert Gire, J. Perry Ormiston, Dr. Howard Boller, Anna Caresson, and Stephanie Ayuas, all of whom participated as photographic models and tolerated all sorts of injustices in the name of science and education.

I would like to thank all the people whom I have worked with at Mosby over these years. One person, Ms. Melba Steube, who recently retired from Mosby, deserves special thanks from me. Over the years, Melba was the person responsible for prodding a reluctant and, truth be known, lazy author to get the lead out. Melba Steube will be greatly missed.

Reader input concerning the previous editions of this text and their suggestions of new items for inclusion in future editions have proved to be of inestimable value. I greatly appreciate, and indeed wish to solicit, comments from my readers.

**Stanley F. Malamed, DDS**

# Contents

# MEDICAL EMERGENCIES
## in the
## DENTAL OFFICE

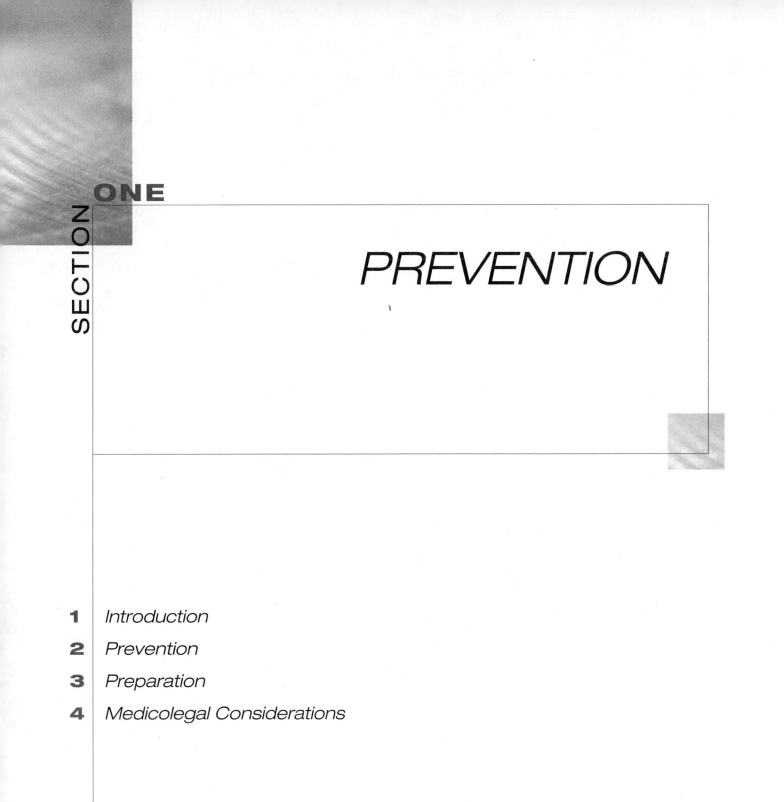

SECTION **ONE**

*PREVENTION*

# Introduction

LIFE-THREATENING emergencies can and do occur in the practice of dentistry. They can happen to anyone—a patient, doctor, member of the office staff, or person who is merely accompanying a patient. Although the occurrence of life-threatening emergencies in dental offices is infrequent, a number of factors exist today that can increase the likelihood of such incidents. These include (1) the increasing number of older persons seeking dental care, (2) the therapeutic advances in the medical profession, (3) the growing trend toward longer dental appointments, and (4) the increasing use and administration of drugs in dentistry.

Fortunately, other factors exist to minimize the development of life-threatening situations. These include a pretreatment physical evaluation of each patient, which consists of a medical history questionnaire, dialogue history, and physical examination, and possible modifications in dental care to minimize medical risks. For example, McCarthy[1] has estimated that through the effective implementation of stress-reduction procedures, all but about 10% of life-threatening situations in the dental office can be prevented. He said, "10% of all nonaccidental deaths are classified as sudden, unexpected deaths . . . unpreventable."

## Morbidity

In spite of the most meticulous protocols designed to prevent the development of life-threatening situations, emergencies still occur. Consider, for example, newspaper articles describing the sudden and unexpected deaths of young, well-conditioned athletes.[2,3] Such emergencies can happen in any environment. The occurrence of such a tragedy inside a dental office is not a surprising event given the stress many patients associate with dental care. This text studies emergency situations that develop in dental practice. However, dental practitioners first must understand that no medical emergency is entirely unique to dentistry. For instance, even local anesthetic overdose is seen outside dentistry in cocaine abuse.

Table 1-1 presents the combined findings of two surveys, one completed by Fast, Martin, and Ellis[4] in 1985 and the other by Malamed[5] in 1992. A total of 4309 survey respondents from all 50 U.S. states and 7 Canadian provinces reported 30,608 emergencies over 10 years. Of those, 96.6% answered positively to the following question: "In the past ten years, has a medical emergency occurred in your dental office?" (Doctors used their own definitions of emergency situations.)

The overwhelming majority of these situations (15,407) involved syncope (fainting), usually a benign occurrence. (Beware the word *benign* in any description of an emergency. When improperly managed, any emergency can turn into a catastrophe.) On the other hand, a significant number of reported emergencies were related to the cardiovascular (3381), central nervous (1663), and respiratory (2718) systems, all of which are potentially life threatening.

Table 1-2 presents a summary of those life-threatening situations that occurred at the School of Dentistry clinics at the University of Southern California from 1973 through mid-1998. Although most situations arose while the patient was undergoing treatment, others developed while the patient was not in the dental chair. Some patients experienced episodes of orthostatic (postural) hypotension in the restroom, several suffered convulsive seizures in the waiting room, and one suffered a seizure just outside the clinic entrance. In one instance, an adult accompanying a patient developed an allergic skin reaction after ingesting aspirin to treat a headache.[4] In two other instances a dental student viewing pictures of acute maxillofacial injuries in a lecture hall and a dentist treating a patient suffered episodes of vasodepressor syncope. Such examples merely stress the need for dental practitioners to be prepared in case of emergencies.

Although any medical emergency can develop in the dental office, some are seen more frequently than others. Most such situations are entirely stress induced (for example, pain, fear, and anxiety) or involve preexisting conditions that are exacerbated when patients are placed in stressful environments. Stress-induced situations include vasodepressor syncope and hyperventilation, whereas preexisting medical conditions that can be exacerbated by stress include

table **1-1**   *Emergencies in private-practice dentistry*

| EMERGENCY SITUATION | NUMBER REPORTED |
| --- | --- |
| Syncope | 15,407 |
| Mild allergic reaction | 2,583 |
| Angina pectoris | 2,552 |
| Postural hypotension | 2,475 |
| Seizures | 1,595 |
| Asthmatic attack (bronchospasm) | 1,392 |
| Hyperventilation | 1,326 |
| "Epinephrine reaction" | 913 |
| Insulin shock (hypoglycemia) | 890 |
| Cardiac arrest | 331 |
| Anaphylactic reaction | 304 |
| Myocardial infarction | 289 |
| Local anesthetic overdose | 204 |
| Acute pulmonary edema (heart failure) | 141 |
| Diabetic coma | 109 |
| Cerebrovascular accident | 68 |
| Adrenal insufficiency | 25 |
| Thyroid storm | 4 |
| TOTAL | 30,608 |

Data from Fast TB, Martin MD, Ellis TM: Emergency preparedness: a survey of dental practitioners, *J Am Dent Assoc* 112:499-501, 1986; and Malamed SF: Managing medical emergencies, *J Am Dent Assoc* 124:4-53, 1993.

table **1-2**   *Emergencies at the University of Southern California School of Dentistry (1973-June 1998)*

| EMERGENCY SITUATION | NUMBER REPORTED |
| --- | --- |
| **Type** | |
| Convulsive seizures | 45 |
| Vasodepressor syncope | 41 |
| Hyperventilation | 39 |
| Hypoglycemia | 24 |
| Postural hypotension | 18 |
| Mild allergic reaction | 15 |
| Angina pectoris | 14 |
| Acute asthmatic attacks | 11 |
| Acute myocardial infarction | 1 |
| **Victim** | |
| Patient (during treatment) | 129 |
| Patient (before or after treatment) | 45 |
| Dental personnel | 24 |
| Other persons in dental office | 10 |

most acute cardiovascular emergencies, broncho-spasm (asthma), and seizures. The effective management of pain and anxiety in the dental office is therefore essential in the prevention and minimization of potentially catastrophic situations.

Drug-related adverse reactions comprise another category of life-threatening situations that occur more often than dentists expect. The most frequent are associated with local anesthetics, the drugs most commonly used in dentistry. Psychogenic reactions, drug overdose, and drug allergy are just a few of the problems associated with the administration of local anesthetics. The overwhelming majority of such cases are stress related (psychogenic); however, other reactions (overdose, allergy) represent responses to the drugs themselves. Most adverse drug responses are preventable. Therefore thorough knowledge of drug pharmacology and proper drug administration are critical in the prevention of drug-related complications.

Matsuura[4] evaluated medical emergency situations in dental offices in Japan (Tables 1-3 and 1-4). Only 1.5% of the emergency situations occurred in the waiting room. The greatest percentage of medical emergencies, 54.9%, took place during the administration of local anesthesia, which is the most stressful procedure performed in the dental office. About 22% of these emergencies developed during dental treatment and 15% in the dental office after the completion of treatment. Most such emergencies were orthostatic (postural) hypotension or vasodepressor syncope.

The type of dental care being administered at the time of each emergency is illuminating. More than 65% of cases developed during two types of dental care—tooth extraction (38.9%) and pulp extirpation (26.9%). The emergencies most likely occurred because the patient experienced sudden, unexpected pain. In one instance a local anesthetic was administered to a patient complaining of a sensitive tooth, most likely a mandibular molar, and pain control was achieved. After treatment began, the patient experienced an unexpected spasm of intense pain as either the drill neared the pulp chamber or the tooth being extracted was moved. The pain triggered the release of endogenous catecholamines, which in turn added to the creation of an emergency. Thus the importance of clinically adequate pain control in safe dental care cannot be overstated.

## table **1-3** Occurrence of systemic complications

| TIME OF COMPLICATION | % |
| --- | --- |
| Immediately before treatment | 1.5 |
| During or after local anesthesia | 54.9 |
| During treatment | 22.0 |
| After treatment | 15.2 |
| After leaving dental office | 5.5 |

Data from Matsuura H: Analysis of systemic complications and deaths during treatment in Japan, *Anesth Prog* 36:219-228, 1990.

## table **1-4** Treatment performed at time of complication

| TREATMENT | % |
| --- | --- |
| Tooth extraction | 38.9 |
| Pulp extirpation | 26.9 |
| Unknown | 12.3 |
| Other treatment | 9.0 |
| Preparation | 7.3 |
| Filling | 2.3 |
| Incision | 1.7 |
| Apicoectomy | 0.7 |
| Removal of fillings | 0.7 |
| Alveolar plastics | 0.3 |

Data from Matsuura H: Analysis of systemic complications and deaths during dental treatment in Japan, *Anesth Prog* 36:219-228, 1990.

# Death

Most emergency situations that occur in dental practice potentially can threaten the patient's life. However, only on rare occasions does a patient actually die in a dental office (Figure 1-1). Although accurate statistics on dental morbidity and mortality are difficult to obtain, various investigators and organizations, including the Southern California Society of Oral Surgeons[5,6] and the American Dental Association,[7] have undertaken surveys of dental practices.

In a 1962 American Dental Association survey of nearly 4000 dentists, 45 deaths in dental offices were reported.[7] In addition, 7 such deaths occurred in the waiting room before the patients had been treated. In a survey of Texas dentists, Bell[8] reported 8 deaths in dental offices, 6 of which occurred in the offices of general practitioners and 2 in oral surgery practices; 1 death occurred in a waiting room before treatment. Only 2 deaths were associated with the administration of general anesthetics.

More recently, Lytle[6] reported 8 deaths associated with the administration of general anesthesia in a 20-year period (1 death in every 673,000 general anesthetic administrations), Robinson[9] reported 8 deaths related to the use of anesthetics, and Adelman[10] documented 3 deaths resulting from aspiration of dental

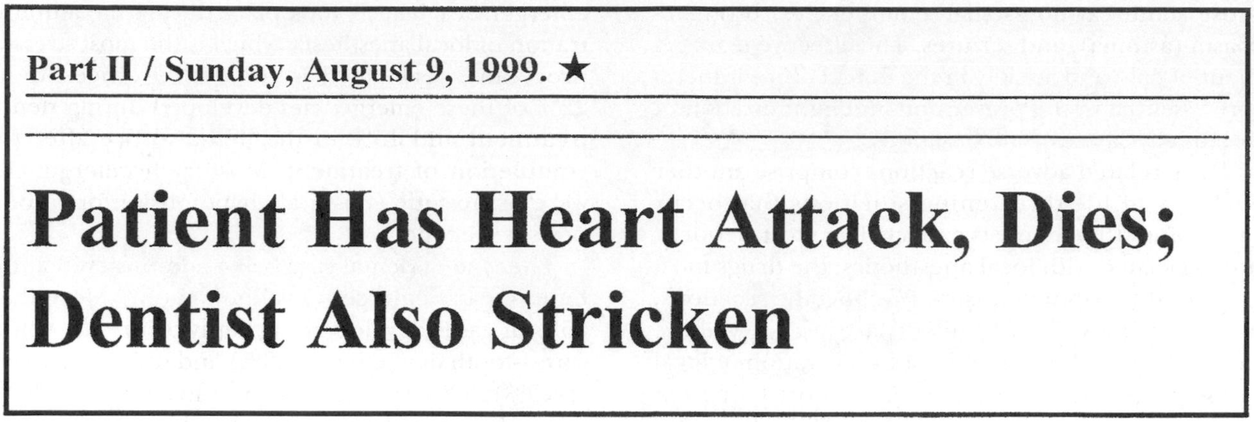

Part II / Sunday, August 9, 1999. ★

# Patient Has Heart Attack, Dies; Dentist Also Stricken

**Figure 1-1**  A dentist and a patient both are stricken with heart attacks.

appliances. In fact, any of the emergencies mentioned in the previous section potentially could double or triple these numbers. Failure to properly recognize and treat clinical signs and symptoms can turn a relatively innocuous situation into an office tragedy.

Adequate pretreatment physical evaluation, combined with proper use of the many techniques of pain and anxiety control, can help prevent many emergencies and deaths. I firmly believe that all dental practitioners must pursue prevention vigorously. Chapter 2 of this text is devoted to this goal, as are other excellent textbooks.[11,12]

Unfortunately, the most stringent precautions cannot prevent the occurrence of deaths. Each year in the United States, 10% of all nonaccidental deaths occur suddenly and unexpectedly in relatively young persons believed to be in good health. The usual cause of death is a lethal cardiac dysrhythmia, most often ventricular fibrillation. Preventive measures cannot entirely eliminate this event, so dental practitioners must be prepared. All members of the dental team must recognize and manage such emergencies. Lytle's survey[5] of the Southern California Society of Oral and Maxillofacial Surgeons (SCSOMS) documented two dental patients who suffered cardiac arrest and successfully were resuscitated. In both cases the dental office had easy access to the proper resuscitative equipment, and the office team acted promptly and effectively.

However, not all such deaths occur within the confines of the dental office. The stress associated with dental treatment can trigger events that may result in a patient's death days after the appointment. In the SCSOMS survey,[5] 10 such incidents were reported. Of particular interest are 3 deaths caused by myocardial infarction and 1 caused by cerebrovascular accident.

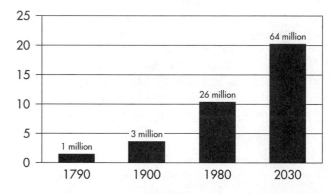

**Figure 1-2**  The most rapidly growing segment of the U.S. population is the group 65 and older because of the large number of aging post–World War II baby boomers.

Another death reportedly was related to an allergic reaction to propoxyphene hydrochloride, which the dentist prescribed for postoperative pain relief.

McCarthy[1] estimates that one or two treatment-related deaths will occur throughout the career of the typical dental practitioner. He further predicts that the number of office-related deaths will increase to 5 if dental patients are observed for 7 days after treatment.

## Risk Factors

### INCREASED NUMBER OF OLDER PATIENTS

The life expectancy of persons born in the United States has increased steadily during this century. In 1900 the life expectancy for a white male was 40 years and for a white female, 49 years. In 1996 these figures were 73.8 for white males and 79.6 for white females

| table **1-5** | Life expectancy in the United States | | | | |

| YEAR | TOTAL | WHITE MALE | WHITE FEMALE | AFRICAN-AMERICAN MALE | AFRICAN-AMERICAN FEMALE |
|---|---|---|---|---|---|
| 1996 | 76.1 | 73.8 | 79.6 | 66.1 | 74.2 |
| 1981 | 74.2 | 71.1 | 78.5 | 64.4 | 73 |
| 1975 | 72.5 | 68.7 | 76.5 | N/A | N/A |
| 1970 | 70.8 | 67.1 | 74.6 | 60 | 68.3 |
| 1960 | 69.7 | 66.6 | 73.1 | N/A | N/A |
| 1950 | 68.2 | 66.6 | 71.1 | N/A | N/A |
| 1940 | 62.9 | 60.8 | 65.2 | N/A | N/A |
| 1930 | 59.7 | 58.1 | 61.6 | N/A | N/A |
| 1920 | 54.1 | 53.6 | 54.6 | N/A | N/A |
| 1910 | 47.3 | 46.3 | 48.2 | N/A | N/A |
| 1900 | N/A | 40 | 49 | N/A | N/A |

Data from Division of Vital Statistics, National Center for Health Statistics, 1985; and 1996 statistics from *Monthly Vital Statistics Report* 46:1(supp)2-11, 1997.

(Table 1-5). Aging post-World War II baby boomers have turned the most rapidly growing segment of the U.S. population into those 65 and older (Figure 1-2), and these increasing numbers of older Americans are seeking dental care.

Although many older patients appear to be in good health, the dental practitioner must always be on the lookout for significant subclinical disease. All major organ systems (cardiovascular, hepatic, renal, pulmonary, endocrine, and central nervous) must be monitored in older patients, but the cardiovascular system is of particular significance. Cardiovascular function and efficiency decrease as part of the normal aging process. In some instances, decreased efficiency may manifest itself as heart failure or angina pectoris, but overt signs are not always apparent. When subjected to stress (pain, fear, anxiety), the cardiovascular system may not be able to meet the body's demands for increased oxygen and nutrients, a lack of which can lead to the development of acute cardiovascular complications such as life-threatening dysrhythmias and anginal pain.

Cardiovascular disease is the leading cause of death in persons over 65 years in the United States today (Box 1-1). Situations that might have proved innocuous to a person at a younger age may well prove to be harmful 20 years later. This relative inability of older persons to tolerate undue stress was demonstrated in a survey of the effects of age in fatally injured automobile drivers. Baker and Spitz[13] found the proportion of drivers aged 60 years or older to be five times as high among those killed as among drivers who survived multivehicle crashes.

Many drivers 60 years and over died after crashes that did not prove fatal to younger drivers. The cor-

| box **1-1** | *Top five causes of death by age group in 1995* |

**1-4 years**
1. Accidents and adverse effects
2. Congenital anomalies
3. Malignant neoplasms
4. Homicide and legal intervention
5. Diseases of the heart

**5-14 years**
1. Accidents and adverse effects
2. Malignant neoplasms
3. Homicide and legal intervention
4. Congenital anomalies
5. Suicide

**15-24 years**
1. Accidents and adverse effects
2. Homicide and legal intervention
3. Suicide
4. Malignant neoplasms
5. Diseases of the heart

**25-44 years**
1. HIV infection
2. Accidents and adverse effects
3. Malignant neoplasms
4. Diseases of the heart
5. Suicide

**45-64 years**
1. Malignant neoplasms
2. Diseases of the heart
3. Accidents and adverse effects
4. Cerebrovascular diseases
5. Chronic obstructive pulmonary disease

**65 years and older**
1. Diseases of the heart
2. Malignant neoplasms
3. Cerebrovascular diseases
4. Chronic obstructive pulmonary disease
5. Pneumonia and influenza

Modified from Anderson RN, Kochanek KD, Murphy SL: Report of final mortality statistics, 1995, *Monthly Vital Statistics Report*, vol 45, no 11, suppl 2, table 7, 1997, Hyattsville, Md, National Center for Health Statistics, pp 22-23.

box **1-2** | *Changes in geriatric patients*

**Central Nervous System**
Decreased number of brain cells
Cerebral arteriosclerosis
    CVA
    Decreased memory
    Emotional changes
Parkinsonism

**Cardiovascular system**
Coronary artery disease
    Angina pectoris
    Myocardial infarction
    Dysrhythmias
    Decreased contractility
High blood pressure
    Renovascular disease
    Cerebrovascular disease
    Cardiac disease

**Respiratory System**
Senile emphysema
Arthritic changes in thorax
Pulmonary problems related to pollutants
Interstitial fibrosis

**Genitourinary system**
Decreased renal blood flow
Decreased number of functioning glomeruli
Decreased tubular reabsorption
Benign prostatic hypertrophy

**Endocrine system**
Decreased response to stress
Type II-adult-onset diabetes mellitus

Modified from Lichtiger M, Moya F: *Curr Rev Nurse Anesth* 1(1):1, 1978.
*CVA*, Cerebrovascular accident.

table **1-6** | *Pulmonary changes in patients 65 years and older*

| FUNCTION | PERCENTAGE COMPARED WITH CAPACITY AT AGE 30 |
|---|---|
| Total lung capacity | 100 |
| Vital capacity | 58 |
| $O_2$ uptake during exercise | 50 |
| Maximum breathing capacity | 55 |

Data from Lichtiger M, Moya F: *Curr Rev Nurse Anesth* 1(1):1, 1978.

box **1-3** | *Factors increasing risk during dental treatment*

Increased number of older patients
Medical advances
    Drug therapy
    Surgical techniques
Longer appointments
Increased drug use
    Local anesthetics
    Sedatives
    Analgesics
    Antibiotics

relation of age and length of survival suggests that whereas younger drivers recover from injuries, many older drivers succumb to complications. The aging process involves both physiologic and pathologic changes that may alter the patient's ability to successfully adapt to stress.

Box 1-2 lists changes older patients frequently encounter. Decrease in tissue elasticity is a major physiologic change that has a significant effect on all the body's organs. For example, in a 75-year-old individual, cerebral blood flow is 80% of what it was at age 30, cardiac output has declined to 65%, and renal blood flow has decreased to 45%. The latter potentially can affect the actions of certain drugs, primarily those that rely principally on urinary excretion to remove the drug and its metabolites from the body.

Penicillin, tetracycline, and digoxin, for example, exhibit greatly increased beta half-lives in older patients.

Decreased tissue elasticity also affects the lungs. Pulmonary compliance decreases with age and can progress to senile emphysema. Chronic exposure to smoke, dust, and pollutants can decrease respiratory function in older patients, producing disorders such as asthma and chronic bronchitis. Pulmonary function in the older patient is considerably diminished compared with that of the younger patient (Table 1-6).

However, within the last two decades, dental practitioners have begun treating more patients over 60 years who retain most of their natural dentition. These patients require the full range of dental care—periodontics, endodontics, crowns, bridges, restorative work, implants, and oral surgery. Because of their ages and the possibility of preexisting physical disabilities, these patients are much less able to handle the stress normally involved in planned treatment. This reduced tolerance for stress should indicate to the dental practitioner that older patients are greater medical risks during dental treatment, even in the absence of a clinically evident disease (Box 1-3). In addition, the dental practitioner must take every step to minimize this risk (see Stress Reduction Protocols[9] in Chapter 2).

## MEDICAL ADVANCES

With age, the incidence of disease rises. Diabetic patients and patients with cardiovascular diseases (heart failure, arteriosclerosis) face significantly longer life expectancies today than they did 20 or 30 years ago. Many patients who were confined to their homes or wheelchairs, unable to work and unlikely to seek dental care, today live fairly normal lives because of advances in drug therapy and surgical technique. Radiation and chemotherapy enable many cancer victims to live longer. Surgical procedures such as the coronary artery bypass and graft operation and heart valve replacement have become commonplace, permitting previously incapacitated patients to pursue active lifestyles. Single- and multiple-organ transplants have higher success rates and are performed with greater frequency than in past years. Newer and more effective drug therapies are available for the management of chronic disorders such as high blood pressure, diabetes, and human immunodeficiency virus.

These medical advances are truly significant. They also mean that dental practitioners must manage the oral-health needs of potentially at-risk patients, many of whom suffer from chronic disorders that are merely being kept under control or managed, not cured. McCarthy[1] has termed these persons "the walking wounded, accidents looking for a place to happen."

## LONGER APPOINTMENTS

In recent years many doctors have increased the lengths of their typical dental appointments. Although appointments of less than 60 minutes are still commonplace, many doctors now schedule 1- to 3-hour treatment sessions. Dental care can be stressful for the patient, doctor, and staff members, and longer appointments naturally create more stress. Medically compromised patients are more likely to react adversely under these conditions than are healthy individuals, but even healthy patients can suffer stress, which can create unforeseen complications. Stress reduction has become an important concept in the prevention of medical emergencies.

## INCREASED DRUG USE

Drugs play an integral part in dentistry. Drugs for the prevention of pain, the reduction of anxiety, and the treatment of infection are an important part of every doctor's armamentarium. However, all drugs have multiple effects; no drug is absolutely risk free. Knowledge of the pharmacologic actions of a drug and of proper technique will greatly decrease the occurrence of drug-related emergencies.

In addition, many dental practitioners must work with patients who ingest drugs not prescribed by a doctor. Halpern[14] found that 18% of his patients were taking some form of medication. This incidence rose with age; 41% of patients over 60 years were taking one or more medications regularly. Dental practitioners must take special care to anticipate and recognize complications related to either the pharmacologic actions of a drug or the complex interactions between commonly used dental drugs and other medications. For example, orthostatic hypotension is associated with many drugs used in the management of high blood pressure.

Other examples include the potentially lethal interactions between the monoamine-oxidase inhibitors and opioids (for example, meperidine and fentanyl) or between epinephrine and noncardiospecific β-adrenergic blockers. This text aims in part to increase the dental practitioner's awareness of possible high-risk patients so that appropriate modifications can be incorporated into the planned treatment. A second aim is to increase prompt recognition and effective management of such situations, which will continue to occur in spite of the most stringent prevention efforts.

Goldberger[15] wrote, "When you prepare for an emergency, the emergency ceases to exist." The ultimate aim in the management of any emergency is the preservation of life. This primary goal is the thread that holds together each section in this text.

# Classification of Life-Threatening Situations

Several methods are available for the classification of medical emergencies. The traditional approach has been the systems-oriented classification, which lists major organ systems and discusses life-threatening situations associated with those systems (Box 1-4).

Although a systems approach often is considered suitable for educational purposes, from a clinical perspective it is lacking. A second classification method divides emergency situations into two broad categories—cardiovascular and noncardiovascular emergencies, which both can be broken down further into stress-related and non–stress-related emergencies. This system offers a very general breakdown of life-threatening emergencies that is particularly useful to doctors.* Combining the systems provides two divisions from which to work—cardiovascular

---

*The term *doctor* is applied generically throughout the rest of this text. The term describes the individual charged with the direction and management of emergency situations, often the dentist for the purposes of this text.

box **1-4**   *Systems-oriented classification*

| | |
|---|---|
| Infectious diseases | Obstetrics and gynecology |
|   Immune system | Nervous system |
|     Allergies |   Unconsciousness |
|     Angioneurotic edema |     Vasodepressor syncope |
|     Contact dermatitis |     Orthostatic hypotension |
|     Anaphylaxis |     Convulsive disorders |
|   Skin and appendages |     Epilepsy |
|   Eyes |   Drug-overdose reactions |
|   Ears, nose, and throat |   Cerebrovascular accident |
|   Respiratory tract |   Endocrine disorders |
|     Asthma |     Diabetes mellitus |
|     Hyperventilation |     Hyperglycemia |
|   Cardiovascular system |     Hypoglycemia |
|     Arteriosclerotic heart disease |   Thyroid gland |
|     Angina pectoris |     Hyperthyroidism |
|     Myocardial infarction |     Hypothyroidism |
|     Heart failure |   Adrenal gland |
|   Blood |     Acute adrenal |
|   Gastrointestinal tract and liver |       insufficiency |

box **1-5**   *Cardiac-oriented classification*

**Noncardiovascular emergencies (stress related)**

Vasodepressor syncope
Hyperventilation
Seizure
Acute adrenal insufficiency
Thyroid storm
Asthma (bronchospasm)

**Noncardiovascular emergencies (non-stress related)**

Orthostatic hypotension
Overdose reaction
Hypoglycemic reactions
Hyperglycemia
Allergy

**Cardiovascular emergencies (stress related)**

Angina pectoris
Acute myocardial infarction
Acute heart failure
Cerebral ischemia and infarction

**Cardiovascular emergencies (non-stress related)**

Acute myocardial infarction

versus noncardiovascular and stress-related versus non–stress-related emergencies (Box 1-5).

This classification can assist the doctor in the preparation of a workable treatment protocol for the prevention of such a situation. The risk of developing a stress-related emergency may be reduced through the incorporation in dental care of several stress-reducing modifications. Such factors include the use of psychosedative techniques, effective pain control, and limitations on the length of dental treatments. A complete description of these factors is found in Chapter 2.

Although the cardiac system is effective in emergency prevention, doctors need a method that can help them recognize and manage such situations. Therefore they must abandon classifications based on organ systems. In most real-life clinical situations, doctors often are unaware of patients' underlying pathologic conditions. The doctor must recognize and initiate management of potentially life-threatening situations using only the most obvious clinical signs and symptoms as guides. For this reason a classification of emergency situations based on clinical signs and symptoms has proved useful since the first publication of this book in 1978.

Of necessity, the doctor bases the initial management of most emergency situations on these clinical clues until a more definitive diagnosis can be obtained. Commonly seen signs and symptoms include alterations of consciousness (unconsciousness, impaired consciousness), respiratory distress, seizures, drug-related emergencies, and chest pain. In each situation a successful outcome depends on the doctor's adherence to a defined treatment protocol. Once such steps have been employed successfully, additional (secondary) steps can steer the doctor toward a more definitive diagnosis, which can help correct the problem.

This text is set up through use of defined protocols and steps of management. Each major section is devoted to a common symptom complex. Each section contains a list of the more common manifestations of that symptom complex. Basic management procedures for the problem are discussed and followed by a detailed review of that category's more common emergencies. Each section closes with a differential diagnosis (Box 1-6).

These classifications are designed to place each life-threatening situation in the category that most closely represents the usual clinical manifestation of the problem. Several situations also could be included in classifications other than the ones in which they have been placed. For example, acute myocardial infarction and cerebrovascular accident are possible causes of unconsciousness, but full discussions

| box **1-6** | *Common medical emergencies in the dental office* |

Unconsciousness
    Vasodepressor syncope
    Orthostatic hypotension
    Acute adrenal insufficiency
Respiratory distress
Airway obstruction
Hyperventilation
Asthma (bronchospasm)
Heart failure and acute pulmonary edema
Altered consciousness
    Diabetes mellitus: hyperglycemia and hypoglycemia
    Thyroid gland dysfunction (hyperthyroidism and hypothyroidism)
    Cerebrovascular accident
Seizures
Drug-related emergencies
    Drug-overdose reactions
    Allergy
Chest pain
    Angina pectoris
    Acute myocardial infarction
Cardiac arrest and cardiopulmonary resuscitation

of these emergencies are found in their more commonly encountered clinical manifestations—chest pain for myocardial infarction and altered consciousness for cerebrovascular accident.

# Outline of SPECIFIC Emergency Situations

In the discussion of each emergency situation various factors will be presented. Included are the following headings and the aim of each:

1. General considerations: An introductory section presents general information about the situation. Definitions and synonyms are included when relevant.
2. Predisposing factors: Discussions focus on the incidence and cause of the disorder and those factors that can predispose a patient to experience a life-threatening situation.
3. Prevention: This section builds on previous sections to prevent acute exacerbation of the disorder. The medical history questionnaire, vital signs, and dialogue history are used to determine a risk category for each patient based on the system developed by the American Society of Anesthesiologists. Suggestions for specific dental treatment modifications complete the discussion.

4. Clinical manifestations: This section focuses on the clinically evident signs and symptoms that help doctors recognize the disorder.
5. Pathophysiology: Discussion centers on the pathologic process underlying clinical signs and symptoms. A fuller understanding of the problem's cause can better enable the doctor to manage the situation.
6. Management: The step-by-step management of clinical signs and symptoms is this section's aim.
7. Differential diagnosis: Each section then closes with a chapter devoted to helping the doctor identify the probable cause of that patient's emergency.

## REFERENCES

1. McCarthy EM: Sudden, unexpected death in the dental office, *J Am Dent Assoc* 83:1091, 1971.
2. Drooz A: Gathers collapses, then dies, *Los Angeles Times,* March 5, 1990, C-1.
3. Schoolgirl dies during basketball drill. *New York Times,* November 20, 1988.
4. Matsuura H: Analysis of systemic complications and deaths during dental treatment in Japan, *Anesth Prog* 36:219-228, 1990.
5. Lytle JJ: Anesthesia morbidity and mortality survey of the Southern California Society of Oral Surgeons, *J Oral Surg* 32:739, 1974.
6. Lytle JJ, Stamper EP: The 1988 anesthesia survey of the Southern California Society of Oral and Maxillofacial Surgeons, *Oral Surg* 47(8):834-842, 1989.
7. Moen BD, Ogawa GY: *The 1962 survey of dental practice,* Chicago, 1963, American Dental Association.
8. Bell WH: Emergencies in and out of the dental office: a pilot study of the State of Texas, *J Am Dent Assoc* 74:778, 1967.
9. Robinson EM: Death in the dental chair, *J Forensic Sci* 34(2):377-380, 1989.
10. Adelman GC: Asphyxial deaths as a result of aspiration of dental appliances: a report of three deaths, *J Forensic Sci* 23(2):389-395, 1985.
11. Little JW and Falace DA: *Dental management of the medically compromised patient,* ed 5, St Louis, 1997, Mosby.
12. McCarthy FM: *Essentials of safe dentistry for the medically compromised patient,* Philadelphia, 1989, WB Saunders.
13. Baker SP, Spitz WU: Age effects and autopsy evidence of disease in fatally injured drivers, *JAMA* 214:1079, 1970.
14. Halpern IL: Patient's medical status: a factor in dental treatment, *Oral Surg* 39:216, 1975.
15. Goldberger E: Treatment of cardiac emergencies, ed 5, St Louis, 1990, Mosby.

# 2

# *Prevention*

**A**CCORDING to McCarthy,[1] a complete system of physical evaluation for all prospective dental patients can prevent approximately 90% of life-threatening situations. The remaining 10% (so-called sudden, unexpected deaths) occur in spite of all preventive efforts. Goldberger[2] stated, "When you prepare for an emergency, the emergency ceases to exist." This statement is accurate in that preparation for an emergency diminishes the danger or possibility of morbidity and death. Prior knowledge of a patient's physical condition enables the doctor to incorporate modifications into the planned dental treatment. In other words, "To be forewarned is to be forearmed."

This chapter* provides a detailed discussion of the most important components of physical evaluation, which can lead to a significant reduction in the occurrence of acute medical emergencies when used properly. (This chapter will be referred to frequently throughout the rest of the text.)

## Evaluation Goals

This section describes a comprehensive but easily employed physical evaluation. The steps described enable the doctor to assess accurately potential risk before

---

*Portions of this chapter have appeared in a slightly different form in Malamed SF: *Sedation: a guide to patient management,* ed 3, St Louis, 1995, Mosby.

beginning treatment.* Box 2-1 and the following list the goals each doctor should pursue:

1. Determine the patient's ability to physically tolerate the stress involved in the planned treatment.
2. Determine the patient's ability to psychologically tolerate the stress involved in the planned treatment.
3. Determine whether treatment modifications are required to enable the patient to better tolerate the stress involved in the planned treatment.
4. Determine whether the use of psychosedation is warranted:

    Determine which sedation technique is most appropriate.

    Determine whether contraindications exist to any drugs to be used in the planned treatment.

The first two goals involve the patient's ability to tolerate the stress involved in dental treatment. That stress may be either physiologic or psychologic. Many if not most patients with preexisting medical conditions are less able to tolerate the usual levels of stress associated with dental treatment. These patients are more likely to undergo acute exacerbations of their preexisting conditions when exposed to such stress. Examples of such preexisting conditions include angina pectoris, epilepsy, asthma, and sickle cell disease. Although most patients are able to tolerate dental treatment, the doctor must determine before treatment begins (1) the potential problem, (2) the level of severity of the problem, and (3) the potential effect on the planned dental treatment.

Excessive stress also may be detrimental to a person who is not medically compromised. Fear, anxiety, and pain—especially sudden, unexpected pain—can lead to acute changes in the body's homeostasis. Many dental patients experience fear-related (psy-chogenic) emergencies, including hyperventilation and vasodepressor syncope (fainting).

The third goal in physical evaluation is to determine whether the planned treatment requires modification to better enable the patient to tolerate the stress. In some instances a healthy patient physically can handle the treatment but is unable psychologically to tolerate it.

The medically compromised patient also benefits from treatment modifications aimed at the minimization of stress. Doctors always must remember that medically compromised patients often fear dental treatment, which can increase the risk of a medical emergency when combined with their reduced tolerance for stress. Stress-reduction protocols, which are discussed later in this chapter, aid the doctor in the minimization of treatment-related stress. When the patient requires some assistance to cope with dental treatment, the doctor may consider psychosedation. Determining the need for these techniques, selecting the most appropriate technique, and choosing the most appropriate drug(s) for the patient are part of the final goal of the physical evaluation.

## Physical Evaluation

The term *physical evaluation* describes the steps involved in the fulfillment of the aforementioned goals. Physical evaluation in dentistry consists of the medical history questionnaire, physical examination, and dialogue history. Armed with this information, the doctor can better (1) determine the physical and psychologic status of the patient, which enables the doctor to assign that patient a risk factor classification; (2) seek medical consultation; and (3) institute appropriate treatment modifications.

### MEDICAL HISTORY QUESTIONNAIRE

The use of a written, patient-completed medical history questionnaire is a moral and legal necessity in the practice of medicine and dentistry. In addition, a medical history questionnaire provides the doctor with valuable information about the physical and psychologic condition of the patient.

Many questionnaire forms are available. However, most are simply modifications of two basic types—the American Dental Association (ADA) short form medical history and the ADA long form medical history. The short form, usually one page, provides basic information about a patient's medical history and ideally is suited for a doctor who has considerable clinical experience in physical evaluation. To use the short

---

*I am often asked, "What is this risk?" The risk in dental care is that an adverse situation may develop during treatment.

---

box **2-1**    *Goals of physical evaluation*

1. Determine the patient's ability to **physically** tolerate the stress involved in the planned treatment.
2. Determine the patient's ability to **psychologically** tolerate the stress involved in the planned treatment.
3. Determine whether **treatment modifications** are required to enable the patient to better tolerate the stress involved in the planned treatment.
4. Determine whether the use of **psychosedation** is warranted.
    a. Determine which sedation technique is most appropriate.
    b. Determine whether contraindications exist to any of the drugs to be used in the planned treatment.

form effectively, the doctor must have a firm grasp of the appropriate dialogue history required to aid in the determination of risk. The doctor also must be experienced in the use and interpretation of physical evaluation techniques. Unfortunately, most doctors employ a short form or a modification primarily as a patient convenience. The long form, usually two or more pages, provides a detailed summary of the patient's past and present physical condition. It is used most often in teaching capacities, for which it is ideal.

Because of the increasing use of computers in today's world, numerous computer-generated history questionnaires are now available. A positive response to a question about a medical condition or problem prompts the computer to formulate additional questions designed to help the doctor determine the degree of risk associated with the condition.

Any medical history questionnaire also can prove to be entirely worthless. The ultimate value of the questionnaire rests in the ability of the doctor to interpret the significance of the answers and elicit additional information through physical examination and dialogue history. The adult and pediatric medical history questionnaires used at the University of Southern California (USC) School of Dentistry perhaps have combined the best of both the short and the long forms[3] (Figures 2-1 and 2-2). Although both the long and short form medical history questionnaires are valuable in the determination of a patient's physical condition during treatment, a criticism of most available health history questionnaires is their lack of questions relating to the patient's attitudes toward dentistry. It is recommended therefore that one or more questions be included that relate to this all-important subject: Do you feel very nervous about having dentistry treatment? Have you ever had a bad experience in the dental office?

Following is a list of each question on the USC medical history questionnaire, with a discussion of the significance of each:

## Medical History Questionnaire

**1. Are you having pain or discomfort at this time?**

*Comment:* The primary thrust of this question is related to dentistry. Its purpose is to determine what prompted the patient to seek dental care. If pain or discomfort is present, the doctor may need to treat the patient immediately, whereas in a more normal situation, treatment can be delayed until future visits.

**2. Do you feel very nervous about having dental treatment?**

**3. Have you ever had a bad experience in a dental office?**

*Comment:* I have found that many adults are reluctant to admit to the doctor, hygienist, or assistant their fears about treatment for fear of being labeled a "baby." This is especially true of young men in their late teens or early twenties; they attempt to "take it like a man" or "grin and bear it" rather than admit their fears. All too often, such macho behavior results in an episode of vasodepressor syncope. Whereas many such patients do not offer verbal admissions of fear, I have found that these same patients may volunteer the information in writing. (Additional ways a doctor can determine a patient's anxiety are discussed later in this chapter.)

**4. Have you been hospitalized during the past 2 years?**

*Comment:* Knowing why a patient was hospitalized can enable the doctor to evaluate the patient's ability to tolerate the stress involved in the planned dental treatment.

**5. Have you been under the care of a medical doctor during the past 2 years?**

*Comment:* As with question 4, knowledge of any problems for which the patient required medical intervention can increase significantly the doctor's ability to evaluate the patient's condition before treatment.

**6. Have you taken any medicine or drugs during the past 2 years?**

*Comment:* Because many patients make a distinction between the terms *drug* and *medication,* questionnaires must use both to determine what drugs (pharmaceutically active substances) a patient has taken. Unfortunately, in today's world the term *drug* often connotes the illicit use of medications (for example, opioids). In the minds of many patients, people "do" drugs but "take" medications for the management of medical conditions.

Doctors must be aware of the medications and drugs their patients take to control and treat medical disorders. Frequently, patients take medications without knowing the condition the medications are designed to treat; some patients do not even know the names of medications they are taking. Thus doctors must have available one or more means of identifying these medications and of determining their indications, side effects, and potential drug interactions. Many excellent sources are available, including the *Physicians' Desk Reference* (PDR)[4] and others.[5,6] The *ADA Guide to Dental Therapeutics* is an invaluable reference to the drugs that are commonly employed in dentistry and to the medications most often prescribed by physicians. Potential complications and drug interactions are stressed.

Knowledge of the drugs and medications their patients are taking permits doctors to identify medical disorders, possible side effects—some of which may be of significance in dental treatment (for example, postural hypotension)—and possible interactions between those medications and the drugs administered during dental treatment (Table 2-1).

**7. Are you allergic to (that is, experience itching, rashes, or swelling of the hands, feet, or eyes) or made sick by penicillin, aspirin, codeine, or any drugs or medications?**

*Comment:* Question 7 seeks to determine whether the patient has had any adverse reactions to drugs. Such reactions

## MEDICAL HISTORY

*CIRCLE*

1. Are you having pain or discomfort at this time? .............................. YES    NO
2. Do you feel very nervous about having dental treatment? ....................... YES    NO
3. Have you ever had a bad experience in a dental office? ....................... YES    NO
4. Have you been hospitalized during the past 2 years? ........................... YES    NO
5. Have you been under the care of a medical doctor during the past 2 years? ......... YES    NO
6. Have you taken any medicine or drugs during the past 2 years? ................... YES    NO
7. Are you allergic to (that is, experience itching, rashes, swelling of the hands, feet, or eyes) or made sick by penicillin, aspirin, codeine, or any drugs or medications? ..... YES    NO
8. Have you ever had any excessive bleeding requiring special treatment? ............. YES    NO
9. Circle any of the following that you have had or have at present:

| | | | | |
|---|---|---|---|---|
| Heart Failure | Heart Surgery | Hay Fever | Glaucoma | Venereal Disease |
| Heart Disease or Attack | Artificial Joint | Sinus Trouble | Pain in Jaw Joints | (Syphilis, Gonorrhea) |
| Angina Pectoris | Anemia | Allergies or Hives | AIDS | Cold Sores |
| High Blood Pressure | Stroke | Diabetes | Hepatitis A (infectious) | Genital Herpes |
| Heart Murmur | Kidney Trouble | Thyroid Disease | Hepatitis B (serum) | Epilepsy or Seizures |
| Rheumatic Fever | Ulcers | X-ray or Cobalt Treatment | Liver Disease | Fainting or Dizzy Spells |
| Congenital Heart Lesions | Emphysema | Chemotherapy (Cancer, Leukemia) | Yellow Jaundice | Nervousness |
| Scarlet Fever | Cough | Arthritis | Blood Transfusion | Psychiatric Treatment |
| Artificial Heart Valve | Tuberculosis (TB) | Rheumatism | Drug Addiction | Sickle Cell Disease |
| Heart Pacemaker | Asthma | Cortisone Medicine | Hemophilia | Bruise Easily |

10. When you walk up stairs or take a walk, do you ever have to stop because of pain in your chest, shortness of breath, or extreme fatigue? .......................... YES    NO
11. Do your ankles swell during the day? .............................. YES    NO
12. Do you use more than two pillows to sleep? ................................ YES    NO
13. Have you lost or gained more than 10 pounds in the past year? ................. YES    NO
14. Do you ever awaken short of breath? ................................ YES    NO
15. Are you on a special diet? .................................... YES    NO
16. Has your medical doctor ever said you have a cancer or tumor? ................. YES    NO
17. Do you have any disease, condition, or problem not listed here? ................. YES    NO
18. WOMEN:    Are you pregnant now? ............................... YES    NO
             Are you practicing birth control? ............................ YES    NO
             Do you anticipate becoming pregnant? ........................... YES    NO

*To the best of my knowledge, all the preceding answers are true and correct. If I ever have any change in my health, or if my medicines change, I will inform the doctor of dentistry at the next appointment without fail.*

_____       _____       _____
*Date*                    *Faculty Signature*        *Signature of Patient, Parent or Guardian*

## MEDICAL HISTORY / PHYSICAL EVALUATION UPDATE

*Date*     *Addition*     *Student/Faculty Signatures*

_____   _____   _____   _____

_____   _____   _____   _____

_____   _____   _____   _____

**Figure 2-1**  Medical history questionnaire. Room for periodic updates is provided on the University of Southern California questionnaire. (From Malamed SF: *Sedation: a guide to patient management*, ed 3, St Louis, 1995, Mosby.)

Child's Name: _____  Date of Birth: _____  Age _____  Date: _____

Address: _____  Telephone: ( )

Physician's name (Medical Doctor): _____  Telephone: ( )

*Please circle the appropriate answer*

1. Does your child have a health problem? .......... YES  NO
2. Was your child a patient in a hospital? ........... YES  NO
3. Date of last physical exam: _____
4. Is your child now under medical care? ........... YES  NO
5. Is your child taking medication now? ........... YES  NO
   If so, for what? _____
6. Has your child ever had a serious illness or operation?  YES  NO
7. If so, explain: _____
8. Does your child have (or ever had) any of the following diseases?
   a. Rheumatic fever or rheumatic heart disease ... YES  NO
   b. Congenital heart disease .................. YES  NO
   c. Cardiovascular disease (heart trouble, heart attack, coronary insufficiency, coronary occlusion, high blood pressure, arteriosclerosis, stroke) ....... YES  NO
   d. Allergy?  Food □,  Medicine □,  Other □ .. YES  NO
   e. Asthma □  Hay Fever □ ................. YES  NO
   f. Hives or a skin rash ..................... YES  NO
   g. Fainting spells or seizures ............... YES  NO
   h. Hepatitis, jaundice or liver disease .......... YES  NO
   i. Diabetes .............................. YES  NO
   j. Inflammatory rheumatism (painful or swollen joints) ................ YES  NO
   k. Arthritis .............................. YES  NO
   l. Stomach ulcers ........................ YES  NO
   m. Kidney trouble ........................ YES  NO
   n. Tuberculosis (TB) ..................... YES  NO
   o. Persistent cough or cough up blood .......... YES  NO
   p. Veneral disease ........................ YES  NO
   q. Epilepsy .............................. YES  NO
   r. Sickle Cell disease ...................... YES  NO
   s. Thyroid disease ........................ YES  NO
   t. AIDS ................................. YES  NO
   u. Emphysema ........................... YES  NO
   v. Psychiatric treatment .................... YES  NO
   w. Cleft lip/palate ........................ YES  NO
   x. Cerebral palsy ......................... YES  NO
   y. Mental retardation ..................... YES  NO
   z. Hearing disability ...................... YES  NO
   aa. Developmental disability .................. YES  NO
       If yes, explain: _____
   bb. Was your child premature? ................ YES  NO
       If yes, how many weeks _____
   cc. Other: _____
9. Does your child have to urinate (pass water) more than six times a day? ........................ YES  NO
10. Is your child thirsty much of the time? ............ YES  NO
11. Has your child had abnormal bleeding associated with previous surgery, extractions or accidents? .... YES  NO
12. Does he/she bruise easily? ..................... YES  NO

13. Has he/she ever required a blood transfusion? ..... YES  NO
14. Does he/she have any blood disorders such as anemia, etc? ................................. YES  NO
15. Has he/she ever had surgery, x-ray or chemotherapy for a tumor, growth, or other condition? .......... YES  NO
16. Does your child have a disability that prevents treatment in a dental office? .................. YES  NO
17. Is he/she taking any of the following?
    a. Antibiotics or sulfa drugs ................. YES  NO
    b. Anticoagulants (blood thinners) .............. YES  NO
    c. Medicine for high blood pressure ............. YES  NO
    d. Cortisone or steroids ..................... YES  NO
    e. Tranquilizers .......................... YES  NO
    f. Aspirin ............................... YES  NO
    g. Dilantin or other anticonvulsant .............. YES  NO
    h. Insulin, tolbutamide, Orinase, or similar drug ... YES  NO
    i. Any other? _____
18. Is he/she allergic to, or has he/she ever reacted adversely to, any of the following?
    a. Local anesthetics ....................... YES  NO
    b. Penicillin or other antibiotics ................ YES  NO
    c. Sulfa drugs ........................... YES  NO
    d. Barbituates, sedatives, or sleeping pills ......... YES  NO
    e. Aspirin ............................... YES  NO
    f. Any other? _____
19. Has he/she any serious trouble associated with any previous dental treatment? ..................... YES  NO
    If so, please explain: _____
20. Has your child been in any situation which could expose him/her to x-rays or other ionizing radiators? ...... YES  NO
21. Last date of dental examination: _____
22. Has he/she ever had orthodontic treatment (worn braces)? ............................. YES  NO
23. Has he/she ever been treated for any gum diseases (gingivitis, periodontitis, trenchmouth, pyorrhea)? ........... YES  NO
24. Does his/her gums bleed when brushing teeth? .... YES  NO
25. Does he/she grind or clench teeth? .............. YES  NO
26. Has he/she often had toothaches? ................ YES  NO
27. Has he/she had frequent sores in his/her mouth? .. YES  NO
28. Has he/she had any injuries to his/her mouth or jaws?  YES  NO
    If yes, explain: _____
29. Does he/she have any sores or swellings of his/her mouth or jaws? ............................. YES  NO
30. Have you been satisfied with your child's previous dental care? ................................ YES  NO

ADOLESCENT WOMEN:
31. Are you pregnant now, or think you may be? ....... YES  NO
32. Do you anticipate becoming pregnant? ........... YES  NO
33. Are you taking the Pill? ....................... YES  NO

To the best of my knowledge, all of the preceding answers are true and correct. If my child ever has a change in his/her health or his/her medicines change, I will inform the doctor at the next appointment without fail.

Parent's Signature: _____  Date _____

MEDICAL HISTORY / PHYSICAL EXAMINATION REVIEW

| Date | Addition | Student/Faculty Signatures | |
|------|----------|----------------------------|---|
| ____ | _____ | _____ | _____ |
| ____ | _____ | _____ | _____ |
| ____ | _____ | _____ | _____ |

**Figure 2-2**  University of Southern California pediatric medical history questionnaire.

table **2-1**  *Dental drug interactions*

| DENTAL DRUG | INTERACTING AGENTS | RESULTING EFFECT |
| --- | --- | --- |
| Anesthetics, general | Antidepressants | Hypotension |
| | Antihypertensives | Hypotension |
| Antihistamines | Alcohol | CNS depression |
| | Phenothiaxine (Compazine, Thorazine) | Increased sedation |
| Anticholinergics (atropine) | Antihistamines | Increased anticholinergic effect |
| | Levodopa | Increased anticholinergic effect |
| | Phenothiazine (Compazine, Thorazine) | Increased anticholinergic effect |
| | Antidepressants, tricyclic (Vivactil, Surmontil, Tofranil) | |
| Barbiturates | Alcohol | Enhanced sedation, increased |
| | Anticoagulants, oral | Decreased anticoagulant effect |
| | Antidepressants, tricyclic (Vivactil, Surmontil, Tofranil) | Decreased antidepressant effect |
| | β-Adrenergic blockers (Lopressor, Inderal) | Decreased β-blocker effect |
| | Corticosteroids | Decreased steroid effect |
| | Digitoxin (digitalis) | Decreased digitoxin effect |
| | Doxycycline | Decreased doxycycline effect |
| | Griseofulvin (Fulvicin, Grisactin, Grifulvin, Grivate) | Decreased griseofulvin effect |
| | Phenothiazine | Decreased phenothiazine effect |
| | Quinidine | Decreased quinidine effect |
| | Rifampin | Decreased barbiturate effect |
| Benzodiazepines | Alcohol | Enhanced sedation |
| | Barbiturates | Enhanced sedation increased respiratory depression |
| Carbamazepine | Anticoagulants, oral | Decreased anticoagulant effect |
| | Doxycycline | Decreased doxycycline effect |
| | Propoxyphene | Increased carbamazepine effect |
| Cephalosporin antibiotics | Aminoglycoside antibiotics | Increased nephrotoxicity |
| | Ethacrynic acid | Increased nephrotoxicity |
| | Furosemide | Increased nephrotoxicity |
| Clindamycin | Curariform drugs | Neuromuscular blockade |
| | Lomotil | Increased diarrhea, colitis |
| Corticosteroids | Barbiturates | Decreased corticosteroid effect |
| | Ephedrine | Decreased dexamethasone effect |
| | Phenytoin | Decreased corticosteroid effect |
| | Rifampin | Decreased corticosteroid effect |
| Erythromycin | Lincomycin | Decreased antimicrobial effect |
| Fluoride | Aluminum hydroxide | Decreased fluoride absorption |

Modified from Council on Dental Therapeutics: *J Am Dent Assoc* 107:885, 1983.
*CNS,* Central nervous system; *MAO,* monoamine oxidase.

are not uncommon; those most frequently reported usually are labeled allergic reactions. However, in spite of the great frequency with which allergy is reported, true documented and reproducible allergic drug reactions are relatively rare. The doctor must evaluate thoroughly all adverse reactions to drugs, especially when the doctor plans to administer or prescribe closely related medications for the patient during dental treatment (see Chapters 16 through 20).

**8. Have you ever had any excessive bleeding requiring special treatment?**

*Comment:* Bleeding disorders such as hemophilia can lead to modification of certain forms of dental therapy (for example,

surgery and local anesthetic administration) and must therefore be made known to the doctor before treatment is begun.

**9. Circle any of the following ailments that you have had or have at present.**

*Comment:* Following is a list of some of the more common ailments afflicting the U.S. adult population:

**Heart failure**

*Comment:* The degree of heart failure must be assessed through dialogue history. When a patient experiences a more serious condition, such as congestive heart failure (CHF) or dyspnea (labored breathing) at rest, that patient requires strict treatment

**table 2-1** | *Dental drug interactions—cont'd*

| DENTAL DRUG | INTERACTING AGENTS | RESULTING EFFECT |
|---|---|---|
| Lincomycin | Curariform drugs | Neuromuscular blockade |
| | Kaolin, pectin | Decreased lincomycin effect |
| | Diphenoxylate-atropine and similar products (Lomotil, Latropine) | Increased diarrhea, colitis |
| Meperidine | Barbiturates | Increased CNS depression |
| | Curariform drugs | Increased respiratory depression |
| Furoxone matulate | MAO inhibitors (Marplan, Nardil, Parnate) | Hypertension |
| Phenothiazine | Alcohol | Increased sedation (promethazine) |
| | Guanethidine | Decreased phenothiazine effect |
| | Levodopa | Decreased levodopa effect |
| | Lithium | Decreased phenothiazine effect |
| Propoxyphene | Alcohol | Increased respiratory depression |
| | Carbamazepine | Increased carbamazepine effect |
| | Curariform drugs | Increased respiratory depression |
| Salicylates (aspirin) | Acetazolamide | Increased salicylate CNS toxicity |
| | Antacids | Decreased salicylate levels |
| | Anticoagulants, oral | Increased bleeding risk |
| | Dipyridamole | Increased effect on platelet function |
| | Hypoglycemics | Increased hypoglycemia |
| | Methotrexate | Increased methotrexate toxicity |
| | Probenecid | Decreased uricosuric effect |
| Sympathomimetic amines (epinephrine, phenylephrine, nordefrin) | Antidepressants, tricyclic (Vivactil, Surmontil, Tofranil) | Hypertension, hypertensive crisis |
| | Antihypertensive drugs | Decreased hypertensive effect |
| | β-Adrenergic blockers (Lopressor, Inderal) | Hypertension with epinephrine |
| | Halogenated anesthetics | Cardiac dysrhythmias |
| | Digitalis drugs | Tendency for cardiac dysrhythmias |
| | Indomethacin | Severe hypertension |
| | MAO inhibitors (Marplan, Nardil, Parnate) | Hypertensive crisis |
| Tetracycline | Antacids | Decreased tetracycline effect |
| | Barbiturates | Decreased doxycycline effect |
| | Bismuth subsalicylate | Decreased tetracycline effect |
| | Carbamazepine | Decreased doxycycline effect |
| | Iron, oral | Decreased tetracycline effect |
| | Methoxyflurane | Increased nephrotoxicity |
| | Milk and dairy products | Decreased tetracycline effect |
| | Phenytoin | Decreased doxycycline effect |
| | Zinc sulfate | Decreased tetracycline effect |

modifications. In this situation the doctor must judge whether the patient needs supplemental oxygen ($O_2$) during treatment. Whereas most CHF patients are classified according to the American Society of Anesthesiologists' (ASA) Physical Status Classification System as ASA II (mild CHF without disability) or ASA III (disability developing with exertion or stress) risks, dyspnea while the patient is at rest creates ASA IV risk. (The ASA physical evaluation system is discussed in detail later in this chapter.)

### Heart disease or attack

*Comment:* *Heart attack* is the lay term for a myocardial infarction (MI). The doctor must know the time that has elapsed since the patient suffered the MI, the severity of the MI, and the degree of residual damage that the patient suffered to decide whether to modify treatment. Dental treatment should be postponed 6 months after an MI. Most post–myocardial infarction patients are considered ASA III risks; however, a patient who suffered an MI less than 6 months before treatment should be considered an ASA IV risk. Where little or no residual damage to the myocardium is present, the patient is an ASA II risk.

### Angina pectoris

*Comment:* A history of angina (defined in part as chest pain brought on by exertion and alleviated by rest) usually

table **2-2** *Prophylactic regimens for dental, oral, respiratory, and esophageal procedures*

| SITUATION | AGENT | REGIMEN* |
|---|---|---|
| Standard general prophylaxis | Amoxicillin | Adults, 2 g; children, 50 mg/kg orally 1 hour before procedure |
| Inability to take oral medications | Ampicillin | Adults, 2 g IM or IV; children, 50 mg/kg IM or IV 30 minutes before procedure |
| Allergy to penicillin | Clindamycin or | Adults, 600 mg; children, 20 mk/kg orally 1 hour before procedure |
| | Cephalexin† or cefadroxil† or | Adults, 2 g; children, 50 mg/kg orally 1 hour before procedure |
| | Azithromycin or clarithromycin | Adults, 500 mg; children, 15 mg/kg orally 1 hour before procedure |
| Allergy to penicillin and inability to take oral medications | Clindamycin or | Adults, 600 mg; children, 20 mg/kg IV 30 minutes before procedure |
| | Cefazolin† | Adults, 1 g; children, 25 mg/kg IM or IV 30 minutes before procedure |

Modified from Dajani AS and others: Prevention of bacterial endocarditis: recommendations by the American Heart Association, *J Am Dent Assoc* 128(8):1142-1151, 1997; and American Dental Association, American Academy of Orthopaedic Surgeons: Advisory statement: antibiotic prophylaxis for dental patients with total joint replacements, *J Am Dent Assoc* 128(7):1004-1008, 1997.
*IM*, Intramuscular; *IV*, intravenous.
*Total doses for children should not exceed those for adults.
†Cehpalosporins should not be prescribed for individuals with immediate-type hypersensitivity reactions (for example, urticaria, angioedema, or anaphylaxis) to penicillins.

indicates the presence of a significant degree of coronary artery atherosclerosis. The risk factor for the typical patient with stable angina is ASA III. Stress reduction is strongly recommended in these patients. Patients with unstable or recent-onset angina represent ASA IV risks.

### High blood pressure

*Comment:* Elevated blood pressure measurements are common in the dental environment primarily because of the added stress many patients associate with dental treatment. Whenever a patient reports a history of high blood pressure, the doctor must determine the names of the patient's medications, the potential side effects of those medications, and the possible interactions with other medications. (Guidelines for clinical evaluation of risk [ASA categories] based on adult blood pressure determinations are discussed later in the chapter.)

### Heart murmur

*Comment:* Heart murmurs are common, and not all murmurs are clinically significant. The doctor should determine whether a murmur is functional (nonpathologic, or ASA II) or whether clinical signs and symptoms of either valvular stenosis or regurgitation are present (ASA III or IV) and whether antibiotic prophylaxis is warranted. A major clinical symptom of a significant (organic) murmur is undue fatigue. Table 2-2 provides guidelines for antibiotic prophylaxis. These were revised in June 1997.[7,8] Box 2-2 categorizes cardiac problems as to their requirements for antibiotic prophylaxis, and Box 2-3 addresses prophylaxis and dental procedures specifically.

### Rheumatic fever

*Comment:* A history of rheumatic fever should prompt the doctor to perform an in-depth dialogue history for rheumatic heart disease. If rheumatic heart disease is present, antibiotic prophylaxis can minimize the risk of the patient developing subacute bacterial endocarditis. Depending on the severity of the disease and the presence of a disability, rheumatic heart disease can confer an ASA II, III, or IV risk. Additional therapy modifications may be advisable.

### Congenital heart lesions

*Comment:* The doctor must perform an in-depth dialogue history to determine the nature of the lesion and the degree of disability it produces. Patients can represent ASA II, III, or IV risks. The doctor may recommend medical consultation, especially for the pediatric patient, to judge the lesion's severity. Most dental treatments require prophylactic antibiotics.

### Scarlet fever

*Comment:* Produced by group A β-hemolytic streptococci, scarlet fever rarely results in cardiovascular sequelae such as valvular damage. However, where such damage is present, antibiotic prophylaxis is required. An adult patient with a history of childhood scarlet fever who does not have negative permanent sequelae may be considered an ASA I risk (if all other history factors are negative).

### Prosthetic heart valve

*Comment:* Patients with prosthetic (artificial) heart valves are no longer uncommon. The doctor's primary concern is the

box **2-2** *Cardiac conditions associated with endocarditis*

**Endocarditis prophylaxis recommended**

*High-risk category*

Prosthetic cardiac valves, including bioprosthetic and homograft valves

Previous bacterial endocarditis

Complex cyanotic congenital heart disease (for example, single-ventricle states, transposition of great arteries, tetralogy of Fallot)

Surgically constructed systemic pulmonary shunts or conduits

*Moderate-risk category*

Most other congenital cardiac malformations (other than those listed in this box)

Acquired valvular dysfunction (for example, rheumatic heart disease)

Hypertrophic cardiomyopathy

Mitral valve prolapse with valvar regurgitation or thickened leaflets*

**Endocarditis prophylaxis not recommended**

*Negligible-risk category*

*(no greater risk than general population)*

Isolated secundum atrial septal defect

Surgical repair of atrial septal defect, ventricular septal defect, or patent ductus arteriosus (with no residual effects beyond 6 months)

Previous coronary artery bypass graft surgery

Mitral valve prolapse without valvar regurgitation*

Physiologic, functional, or innocent heart murmurs*

Previous Kawasaki disease without valvar dysfunction

Previous rheumatic fever without valvar dysfunction

Cardiac pacemakers (intravascular and epicardial) and implanted defibrillators

Modified from Dajani AS and others: Prevention of bacterial endocarditis: recommendations by the American Heart Association, *J Am Dent Assoc* 128(8):1142-1151, 1997; and American Dental Association, American Academy of Orthopaedic Surgeons: Advisory statement: antibiotic prophylaxis for dental patients with total joint replacements, *J Am Dent Assoc* 128(7):1004-1008, 1997.

box **2-3** *Dental procedures and endocarditis prophylaxis*

**Endocarditis prophylaxis recommended***

Dental extractions

Periodontal procedures, including surgery, scaling and root planing, probing, and recall maintenance

Dental implant placement and reimplantation of avulsed teeth

Endodontic (root canal) instrumentation or surgery beyond the apex

Subgingival placement of antibiotic fibers or strips

Initial placement of orthodontic bands but not brackets

Intraligamentary local anesthetic injections

Prophylactic cleaning of teeth or implants where bleeding is anticipated

**Endocarditis prophylaxis not recommended**

Restorative dentistry† (operative and prosthodontic) with or without retraction cord‡

Local anesthetic injections (nonintraligamentary)

Intracanal endodontic treatment and post placement and buildup

Placement of rubber dams

Postoperative suture removal

Placement of removable prosthodontic or orthodontic appliances

Taking of oral impressions

Fluoride treatments

Taking of oral radiographs

Orthodontic appliance adjustment

Shedding of primary teeth

Modified from Dajani AS and others: Prevention of bacterial endocarditis: recommendations by the American Heart Association, *J Am Dent Assoc* 128(8):1142-1151, 1997; and American Dental Association, American Academy of Orthopaedic Surgeons: Advisory statement: antibiotic prophylaxis for dental patients with total joint replacements, *J Am Dent Assoc* 128(7):1004-1008, 1997.

*Prophylaxis is recommended for patients with high- and moderate-risk cardiac conditions.

†Restorative dentistry includes restoration of decayed teeth (filling of cavities) and replacement of missing teeth.

‡Clinical judgment may indicate antibiotic use in selected circumstances that may create significant bleeding.

determination of the appropriate antibiotic regimen. Prophylactic guidelines[8] list these requirements; however, the doctor should be advised to consult with the patient's physician (for example, the cardiologist or cardiothoracic surgeon) before treatment. Prosthetic heart valve patients usually represent ASA II or III risks.

**Heart pacemaker**

*Comment:* Pacemakers are implanted beneath the skin of the upper chest or the abdomen, and pacing wires extend into the myocardium. The most frequent indication for the use of a pacemaker is the presence of a clinically significant dysrhythmia. Fixed-rate pacemakers provide hearts with regular, con-

tinuous rates regardless of the heart's inherent rhythm, whereas the more common demand pacemakers activate only when the rhythm of the heart falls into an abnormal range. Although there is little indication for the administration of antibiotics in these patients, medical consultation is suggested prior to the start of treatment in order to obtain the specific recommendations of the patient's physician. The patient with a pacemaker usually is an ASA II or III risk during dental treatment.

**Implanted defibrillator**

*Comment:* In recent years patients who represent a significant risk of sudden unexpected death (e.g., cardiac arrest) due to electrical instability of the myocardium (e.g., ventricular fibrillation) have had implantable defibrillators placed below the skin of their abdomen. Medical consultation is recommended strongly for these patients.

### Heart Surgery

*Comment:* Heart surgery can include any procedure—from the implantation of a pacemaker to a valve replacement to a coronary artery bypass surgery or a heart transplant. When a patient provides a positive response to a question about such surgery, the doctor must perform a vigorous dialogue history to determine what implications the procedure may have on dental treatment. The degree of risk in these patients varies from an ASA II to V.

### Prosthetic joint replacement

*Comment:* Approximately 450,000 total joint arthroplasties are performed annually in the United States. An expert panel of dentists, orthopedic surgeons, and infectious disease specialists convened by the ADA and the American Academy of Orthopaedic Surgeons performed a thorough review of the available data to determine the need for antibiotic prophylaxis to prevent hematogenous prosthetic joint infections in dental patients who have undergone total joint arthroplasties. The panel concluded that antibiotic prophylaxis is not recommended for dental patients with pins, plates, and screws or those who have undergone total joint replacements. However, doctors should consider premedication in a small number of patients who may be at increased risks for the development of hematogenous total joint infection (Box 2-4).[9]

### Anemia

*Comment:* Anemia is a relatively common adult ailment, especially among young adult women (iron-deficiency anemia). The doctor must determine the type of anemia present. The ability of the blood to carry $O_2$ or give up $O_2$ molecules to other cells is decreased in anemic patients. This decrease may be significant during procedures in which hypoxia is likely to develop.

Although hypoxia should never occur during dental treatment, the use of deeper levels of intramuscular (IM) or intravenous (IV) sedation without supplemental $O_2$ administration is more likely to produce hypoxia, which can be an even more dangerous situation in anemic patients. ASA risk factors vary from II to IV depending on the severity of the $O_2$ deficit. Sickle cell anemia can occur in some black patients, in which case the doctor must differentiate between sickle cell disease and sickle cell trait. In addition, congenital or idiopathic methemoglobinemia is a relative contraindication to the administration of the amide local anesthetic prilocaine.[10]

### Stroke

*Comment:* The doctor must pay close attention to stroke, cerebrovascular accident (CVA), or brain attack (a term that is increasingly used in the lay press), because a patient who has suffered a CVA is at a greater risk of suffering another CVA or

---

box **2-4**    *Patients at risk for developing hematogenous total joint infection*

**Immunocompromised or immunosuppressed patients**

Patients with inflammatory arthropathies: rheumatoid arthritis, systemic lupus erythematosus
Patients with disease-, drug-, or radiation-induced immunosuppression

**Other patients**

Patients with insulin-dependent (type 1) diabetes
Patients who have had joint placement within past 2 years
Patients who have had previous prosthetic joint infections
Malnourished patients
Hemophiliacs

Data from American Dental Association, American Academy of Orthopaedic Surgeons: Advisory statement: antibiotic prophylaxis for dental patients with total joint replacements, *J Am Dent Assoc* 128(7):1004-1008, 1997.

---

a seizure during hypoxia. If the doctor uses sedation at all, only light levels such as those provided through inhalation sedation or IV conscious sedation are recommended. The doctor should be especially sensitive to transient cerebral ischemia, a precursor to CVA; this condition represents an ASA III risk. The post-CVA patient is an ASA IV risk within 6 months of the CVA, becoming an ASA III risk 6 or more months after the incident (if recovery is uneventful). In rare cases the post-CVA patient can be an ASA II risk.

### Kidney dysfunction

*Comment:* The doctor should evaluate the nature of the renal disorder. Treatment modifications including antibiotic prophylaxis may be appropriate for several chronic forms of renal disease. Functionally anephric patients are categorized as ASA IV risks, whereas patients with most other forms of renal dysfunction represent either ASA II or III risks. Box 2-5 shows a sample dental referral letter for a patient on long-term hemodialysis treatment because of chronic kidney disease.

### Ulcers

*Comment:* The presence of stomach or intestinal ulcers may be indicative of acute or chronic anxiety and the possible use of medications such as tranquilizers, H1-inhibitors, and antacids. Knowledge of which drugs are being taken is important before additional drugs are administered in the dental office. Recently the U.S. Food and Drug Administration made several H1-inhibitors over-the-counter drugs. Because many patients do not consider such drugs "real" medications, the doctor must specifically question the patient about them. The presence of ulcers does not itself represent an increased risk during treatment. In the absence of additional medical problems, the patient may represent an ASA I or II risk.

| box 2-5 | *Dental referral letter* |

Dear Doctor:

The patient who bears this note is undergoing long-term chronic hemodialysis treatment because of chronic kidney disease. In providing dental care to this patient, please observe the following precautions:

1. Dental treatment is most safely done 1 day after the last dialysis treatment or at least 8 hours thereafter. Residual heparin may make hemostasis difficult. (Some patients are on long-term anticoagulant therapy.)
2. We are concerned about bacteremic seeding of the arteriovenous shunt devices and heart valves. We recommend prophylactic antibiotics before and after dental treatment. Antibiotic selection and dosage can be tricky in renal failure. We recommend 3 g of amoxicillin 1 hour before the procedure and 1.5 g 6 hours later. For patients with penicillin allergies, 1 g of erythromycin 1 hour before the procedure and 500 mg 6 hours later is recommended.

Sincerely,

Courtesy Kaiser Permanente Medical Center, Los Angeles, Calif.

### Emphysema

*Comment:* Emphysema is a form of chronic obstructive pulmonary disease (COPD), also called *chronic obstructive lung disease* (COLD). The emphysematous patient has a decreased respiratory reserve from which to draw if the body's cells require additional $O_2$, which they often do during stress. Supplemental $O_2$ therapy during dental treatment is recommended in severe cases of emphysema; however, the severely emphysematous patient should not receive more than 3 L of $O_2$ per minute.[11] This restriction helps ensure the doctor does not eliminate the patient's hypoxic drive, which is the emphysematous patient's primary stimulus for breathing. The emphysematous patient is an ASA II, III, or IV risk depending on the degree of the disability.

### Cough

*Comment:* A chronic cough can indicate active tuberculosis or other chronic respiratory disorders such as chronic bronchitis. Cough associated with an upper respiratory infection confers an ASA II classification on the patient, whereas chronic bronchitis in a patient who has smoked more than one pack of cigarettes daily for many years may indicate chronic lung disease and confer on the patient an ASA III risk. The doctor must weigh carefully the risks before administering central nervous system (CNS) depressants—especially those such as opioids and barbiturates, which depress the respiratory system more than others—in patients who exhibit signs of diminished respiratory reserve (ASA III and IV).

### Tuberculosis

*Comment:* The doctor first must determine whether the disease is active or arrested. (Arrested tuberculosis is an ASA II risk.) Medical consultation and treatment modification are recommended when such information is not easily determined. Inhalation sedation with nitrous oxide and $O_2$ is not recommended for patients with active tuberculosis (ASA III or IV) because of the likelihood that the rubber goods (reservoir bag and conducting tubing) may become contaminated and the difficulty in their sterilization. However, for doctors who treat many patients with tuberculosis and other infectious diseases, disposable rubber goods for inhalation sedation units are recommended.

### Asthma

*Comment:* Asthma (bronchospasm) is marked by a partial obstruction of the lower airway. The doctor must determine the nature of the asthma (intrinsic [allergic] versus extrinsic [nonallergic]), frequency of the episodes, causative factors, method of management for acute episodes, and drugs the patient is taking to minimize the risk that an acute episode may develop. Stress is a common factor in acute asthmatic episodes. The well-controlled asthmatic represents an ASA II risk, whereas the well-controlled but stress-induced asthmatic is an ASA III risk. Patients whose acute episodes are uncontrolled or difficult to terminate (requiring hospitalization) are ASA III or IV risks.

### Hay fever

*Comment:* Hay fever indicates that the patient is allergic to a foreign protein (for example, pollen, animal dander, dust, or dirt) and represents an ASA II risk. If possible, elective dental care should be postponed, if possible, during acute exacerbation of the hay fever.

### Sinus trouble

*Comment:* Sinus problems can indicate the presence of an allergy (ASA II), which should be pursued in the dialogue history, or upper-respiratory tract infection (ASA II) such as a common cold. The patient may experience some respiratory distress when placed in a supine position; distress may also be present if rubber dam is used. Specific treatment modifications—postponing treatment until the patient is able to breathe more comfortably, limiting the degree of recline in the dental chair, and foregoing use of rubber dam—are advisable.

### Allergies or hives

*Comment:* The doctor must evaluate the patient's allergies thoroughly before administering dental treatment or drugs. The importance of this question and its full evaluation cannot be overstated. The doctor must complete a vigorous dialogue history before dental treatment, especially when a presumed or documented history of drug allergy is present. The presence of allergies alone represents ASA II risks. No emergency situation is as frightening to health professionals as the acute, systemic allergic reaction, known as *anaphylaxis.* Prevention of this life-threatening situation is ever more gratifying than treatment once it develops.

### Diabetes

*Comment:* A patient who responds positively to this question requires further inquiry to determine the type, severity, and degree of control of the diabetic condition. A patient with type I (insulin-dependent diabetes mellitus, or IDDM) or type II (non–insulin-dependent diabetes mellitus, or NIDDM) diabetes mellitus is not usually a great risk during the administration of dental care or drugs. The NIDDM patient is usually an ASA II risk; the well-controlled IDDM patient, an ASA III risk; and the poorly controlled IDDM patient, an ASA III or IV risk.

The greatest concerns during dental treatment relate to the possible effects of dental care on subsequent eating and development of hypoglycemia (low blood sugar). Patients leaving a dental office with residual soft tissue anesthesia, especially in the mandible, usually defer eating until sensation returns, a period of possibly many hours. Diabetic patients may have to modify their insulin doses if they do not maintain normal eating habits.

### Thyroid disease

*Comment:* The clinical presence of thyroid dysfunction—either hyperthyroidism or hypothyroidism—should prompt the doctor to use caution in the administration of certain drug groups (for example, epinephrine to hyperthyroid patients and CNS depressants to hypothyroid patients). In most instances, however, the patient already has seen a physician and undergone treatment for their thyroid disorder by the time they seek dental treatment. In this case the patient is in a euthyroid state (normal blood levels of thyroid hormone) because of surgical intervention, irradiation, or drug therapy. The euthyroid state represents an ASA II risk, whereas clinical signs and symptoms of hyperthyroidism or hypothyroidism represent ASA III or, in rare instances, ASA IV risks.

### Radiation therapy
### Chemotherapy (cancer, leukemia)

*Comment:* The presence or prior existence of cancer of the head or neck may require specific modification of dental therapy. Irradiated tissues have decreased resistance to infection, diminished vascularity, and reduced healing capacity. However, no specific contraindication exists to the administration of medication for pain or anxiety control in these patients. Many patients with cancer also may be receiving long-term therapy with CNS depressants such as antianxiety drugs, hypnotics, and opioids. Consultation with the patient's oncologist is recommended before dental treatment. A past or current history of cancer does not necessarily increase the ASA risk status. However, patients who are cachectic or hospitalized and are in poor physical condition may represent ASA IV or V risks.

### Arthritis
### Rheumatism
### Cortisone Medicine

*Comment:* A history of arthritis may be associated with chronic use of salicylates (aspirin) or other nonsteroidal anti-inflammatory drugs (NSAIDs), some of which may alter blood clotting. (Indeed, low-dose aspirin has demonstrated its effectiveness in minimizing the risk of another myocardial infarction in patients recovering from myocardial infarctions.[12]) Arthritic patients who are receiving long-term corticosteroid therapy may suffer an increased risk of acute adrenal insufficiency, especially when the patient recently has stopped taking the steroid. Such patients may require reinstitution of steroid therapy or a modification (increase) in the corticosteroid doses during dental treatment so that they will be able to respond more appropriately to any additional stress associated with the treatment.

Because of possible difficulties in positioning the patient comfortably, modifications may be necessary to accommodate the patient's physical disability. Most patients receiving corticosteroids are categorized as ASA II or III risks depending on the reason for the medication and the degree of disability present. Patients with significantly disabling arthritis are ASA III risks.

### Glaucoma

*Comment:* For patients with glaucoma, the need to administer a drug that diminishes salivary gland secretions will need to be addressed. Anticholinergics, such as the drugs atropine, scopolamine, and glycopyrrolate, are contraindicated in patients with glaucoma because these drugs produce an increase in intraocular pressure. Patients with glaucoma are usually ASA II risks.

### Pain in the jaw joints

*Comment:* Cases of chronic temporomandibular joint pain are becoming increasingly common. Before the patient undergoes treatment, possible causes of the pain should be evaluated. For example, bruxism can indicate that the patient is under unusual stress, a condition that can be managed via oral antianxiety drugs or other psychotropics. The doctor should determine the names of the drugs the patient is taking, their potential side effects, and any drug interactions. TMJ pain itself does not increase a patient's ASA risk.

### Acquired immunodeficiency syndrome

*Comment:* Patients who have tested positive for human immunodeficiency virus (HIV) are representative of every area of the population. The usual barrier techniques should be employed to minimize the risk of cross infection to both the patient and staff members. Patients who are HIV positive are considered ASA II, III, IV, or V risks depending on the progress of the infection.

**Hepatitis A (infectious)**
**Hepatitis B (serum)**
**Hepatitis C**
**Liver disease**
**Yellow jaundice**
**Blood transfusion**
**Drug addiction**

*Comment:* These diseases or problems either are transmissible (AIDS and hepatitis A and B) or can indicate hepatic dysfunction. A history of blood transfusion or past or present history of drug addiction should alert the doctor to a probable increase in the risk of hepatic dysfunction or AIDS. (Hepatic dysfunction is especially important in the parenteral drug abuse patient.) Hepatitis C is responsible for more than 90% of cases of posttransfusion hepatitis, but only 4% of cases are attributable to blood transfusions; up to 50% of cases are related to IV drug use. Incubation of hepatitis C averages 6 to 7 weeks. The clinical illness is mild, usually asymptomatic, and characterized by a high rate (>50%) of chronic hepatitis.[13]

### Hemophilia

*Comment:* The doctor must thoroughly evaluate hemophilia and other bleeding disorders before beginning any procedure, especially those in which bleeding may occur. The doctor is advised to avoid (whenever possible) the administration of regional nerve blocks in which the risk of positive blood aspiration is great. Techniques include the inferior alveolar nerve block and posterior superior alveolar nerve block. In most instances, alternative techniques for pain control should be considered. Hemophiliacs are categorized as ASA II, III, or IV risks.

**Venereal disease (syphilis, gonorrhea)**
**Cold sores**
**Genital herpes**

*Comment:* When treating such patients, dentists and staff members risk infection. When oral lesions are present, dental care should be postponed if possible. Standard barrier techniques, protective gloves, eyeglasses, and masks provide operators with a degree of (but not total) protection. Such patients usually represent ASA II and III risks but may be IV or V risks in extreme situations.

### Epilepsy or seizures

*Comment:* Seizures are common dental emergencies. Even well-controlled epileptics may suffer seizures in stressful environments such as the dental office. The doctor must determine the type, frequency of occurrence, and drug(s) used to control the seizure before beginning dental treatment. Doctors often must modify the treatment (for example, use stress-reduction techniques) for patients with known seizure disorders. Epileptics whose conditions are under control are ASA II risks; patients who retain less control represent ASA III or IV risks.

### Fainting or dizzy spells

*Comment:* A positive response may indicate a patient's chronic postural (orthostatic) hypotension, symptomatic hypotension or anemia, or transient ischemic attack (TIA), a form of prestroke. In addition, patients with certain types of seizure disorders, such as the "drop attack," may report fainting or dizzy spells. The doctor may be advised to perform further evaluation, including a consultation with the patient's primary-care physician. A transient ischemic attack represents an ASA III risk, whereas chronic postural hypotension is normally a II or III risk.

**Nervousness**
**Psychiatric treatment**

*Comment:* The doctor should be aware of any nervousness (in general or specifically related to dentistry) or history of psychiatric care before treating the patient. Such patients may be receiving a number of medications to manage their disorders, drugs that may interact with those the doctor uses to control pain and anxiety (see Table 2-1). Medical consultation should be considered in many such cases. Extremely fearful patients are ASA II risks, whereas patients receiving psychiatric care and drugs represent II or III risks.

### Sickle cell disease

*Comment:* Sickle cell disease is seen in black patients exclusively. Periods of unusual stress or $O_2$ deficiency (hypoxia) can precipitate a sickle cell crisis. The administration of supplemental $O_2$ during treatment is strongly recommended for those with sickle cell disease. Patients with sickle cell trait represent ASA II risks, whereas those with sickle cell disease are II or III risks.

### Bruise easily

*Comment:* A positive response to this question may indicate the presence of a bleeding disorder, which should be evaluated before the start of dental care. Results of the evaluation should determine the ASA risk factor.

Questions 10 through 14 may alert the doctor to one of the conditions in question 9 of which the patient is unaware. Unfortunately, many persons cannot accurately gauge their current health and do not receive regular physical examinations. In addition, many diseases begin insidiously, producing a gradual onset of clinical signs and symptoms over a period of months or years. Patients who are diagnosed as diabetic are almost always amazed to hear that they probably had been diabetic for many years prior to their diagnosis. When told of the presenting signs and symptoms, many state that they have had them for years. Because some patients are unaware that they may suffer from one or more of the disorders listed in question 9, a series of questions was designed to list commonly observed signs and symptoms associated with many medical disorders. A positive response to any of questions 10 through 14 should trigger a detailed dialogue history to determine the dental implications.

**10. When you walk up stairs or take a walk, do you ever have to stop because of pain in your chest, shortness of breath, or extreme fatigue?**

*Comment:* Although the patient may have responded negatively in question 9 to the presence of angina, heart failure, or pulmonary emphysema, clinical signs and symptoms of heart or lung disease may be evident. However, a positive response to this question does not always indicate that the patient suffers such a disease. To more accurately determine the patient's status before the start of dental care, further evaluation is suggested.

**11. Do your ankles swell during the day?**

*Comment:* Swollen ankles (pitting edema or dependent edema) indicate possible CHF. However, varicose veins, pregnancy, and renal dysfunction are other causes of ankle edema. In addition, healthy persons who stand on their feet for long periods (for example, mail carriers and dental staff members) also may exhibit edematous ankles.

**12. Do you use more than two pillows to sleep?**

*Comment:* Persons with severe CHF exhibit orthopnea, the inability to breathe comfortably when lying down. These patients usually require additional (e.g., 4) pillows under their back, which in effect sits them up in bed so that they are able to breathe more comfortably during sleep. This condition, referred to as "four-pillow orthopnea," increases the patient's risk during dental treatment and requires modification. The doctor may place a note in the patient's chart instructing staff members not to position the patient at more than a 45-degree recline (or the appropriate degree for the patient) to increase that patient's comfort during treatment. The use of rubber dam may be contraindicated in patients who demonstrate difficulty breathing at rest as it may significantly impair their breathing.

**13. Have you lost or gained more than 10 pounds in the past year?**

*Comment:* The question refers primarily to an unexpected gain or loss of weight, not intentional dieting. Unexpected weight changes may indicate heart failure, hypothyroidism (increased weight), hyperthyroidism, widespread carcinoma, uncontrolled diabetes mellitus (weight loss), or a number of other disorders.

**14. Do you ever awaken from sleep short of breath?**

*Comment:* Paroxysmal nocturnal dyspnea (PND), the sudden onset of shortness of breath while sleeping, usually indicates severe left ventricular failure or severe pulmonary disease. Patients who exhibit PND require treatment modifications, including changes in position. ASA classifications range from III to V. There are other more benign reasons for this symptom to develop, such as the occurrence of nightmares.

**15. Are you on a special diet?**

*Comment:* The doctor should be alerted to any dietary alterations resulting from certain medical disorders (diabetes, high blood pressure, heart failure, elevated cholesterol) or the patient's attempt to lose weight. Severe dieting, such as fasting or fad dieting, can upset the body's biochemical homeostasis and increase the patient's risk for development of medical problems.

In recent years many people have sought to lose weight using a combination of two drugs—phentermine and fenfluramine (Fen-Phen).[14] Although the combination did produce the desired weight loss, several severe, potentially lethal complications arose. Primary pulmonary hypertension, a potentially fatal disorder, reportedly occurs about 30 times more frequently in patients receiving anorectic agents for more than 3 months, compared with those not taking the drugs.

These popular anorectics are associated closely with the development of valvular heart disease. The risks of primary pulmonary hypertension and valvular heart disease and the occurrence of convulsions, coma, and death with overdose appear equally likely with dexfenfluramine and fenfluramine. In late 1997 the Food and Drug Administration withdrew this drug combination from the American market. However, doctors should be alerted to the possibility of valvular heart disease in patients who received these drugs for prolonged periods. Medical consultation should be considered if the patient's cardiac status is in doubt.[15]

**16. Has your medical doctor ever said you have a cancer or tumor?**

*Comment:* This question refers to the comments made previously concerning radiation treatment and chemotherapy (see the question 9 comment).

**17. Do you have any disease, condition, or problem not listed here?**

*Comment:* The patient is encouraged to comment on specific matters not previously discussed. Examples of several possibly significant disorders include acute intermittent porphyria, atypical plasma cholinesterase, and malignant hyperthermia.

**18. Women: Are you pregnant now?**

Are you practicing birth control?

Do you anticipate becoming pregnant?

*Comment:* Pregnancy represents a relative contraindication to extensive elective dental care, particularly during the first trimester. Consultation with the patient's physician usually is recommended. Although the use of local anesthetics is permitted during pregnancy, the doctor should evaluate the risk versus the benefits to be gained from the use of most sedative drugs. Of the available sedation techniques, inhalation sedation with nitrous oxide and $O_2$ is recommended. Use of oral, IM, or IV routes is not contraindicated but should be reserved for those patients for whom other techniques are unavailable.

**To the best of my knowledge, all the preceding answers are true and correct. If I ever have any change in my health, I will inform the doctor of dentistry at the next appointment without fail.**

*Comment:* This final statement is important from a medicolegal standpoint because although instances of purposeful lying on health histories are rare, they do occur. This statement must be accompanied by the date on which the history was completed and the signatures of the patient (or the parent or guardian if the patient is a minor or is not legally competent) and the doctor who reviews the history. This in effect becomes a contract obliging the patient, parent, or guardian to report any changes in the patient's health or medications. Brady and Martinoff[16] demonstrated that a patient's analysis of personal health frequently is overly optimistic and that pertinent health matters sometimes are not immediately reported.

The questionnaire must be updated regularly, approximately every 6 months or after any prolonged lapse in treatment. In most instances the entire medical history questionnaire need not be redone. The doctor need only ask the following questions:

1. **Have you experienced any change in your general health since the last dental visit?**
2. **Are you now under the care of a medical doctor? If so, what is the condition being treated?**
3. **Are you currently taking any drugs or medications?**

If any of these questions elicits a positive response, a detailed dialogue history should follow. For example, a patient may answer that no change has occurred in general health but may want to notify the doctor of a minor change in condition, such as the end of a pregnancy or the recent diagnosis of NIDDM or asthma.

In either situation a written record of having updated the history should be entered into the patient's progress notes or on the health history form. When the patient's health status has changed significantly since the last history was completed, the entire history should be redone (for example, if a patient recently has been diagnosed with cardiovascular disease and must manage it with many medications).

In reality, most persons do not undergo significant changes in their health with any regularity. Thus one health history questionnaire may remain current for many years, and the ability to demonstrate that a patient's medical history was updated regularly becomes all the more important.

The questionnaire should be completed in ink. The doctor makes a correction or deletion by drawing a single line through the original entry without obliterating it. The doctor then adds and initials the change and records the date. The doctor also should enter a written notation on the chart when the patient reveals significant information during the dialogue history. As an example, when a patient answers positively to the question about a heart attack, the doctor's notation may read "1986" (the year the myocardial infarction occurred).

## PHYSICAL EXAMINATION

Although the medical history questionnaire is extremely important in the overall assessment of a patient's physical and psychological status, it does have some limitations. For the health history to be valuable, patients must (1) be aware of their own states of health and any medical conditions and (2) be willing to share this information with the dentist.

Most patients do not knowingly deceive the dentist by omitting important information from their medical history questionnaires, but such cases have been recorded. For example, a patient who sought treatment for an acutely inflamed tooth decided to withhold from the doctor the fact that he had suffered a myocardial infarction 2 months earlier because he knew that to inform the doctor of this would mean that the doctor probably would not perform the treatment that the patient desired.[17] The more likely cause of unintentional misinformation is that the patient is unaware that a problem exists. Many "healthy" persons do not visit their physicians for regular checkups. In fact, recent information suggests that annual medical visits be discontinued in healthy patients under 40 years because the annual physical examination has not proven as valuable an aid in preventive medicine as researchers once believed.[18]

Most patients simply do not visit their physicians on a regular basis, doing so only when they feel ill. Therefore both the patient and the doctor may be unaware of a medical disorder. Simply because a patient feels good does not mean that patient is necessarily healthy. Many disorders can be present in subclinical states for months or years without exhibiting any overt signs or symptoms. When such signs and symptoms, like shortness of breath or undue fatigue, do occur, patients often mistake them for more benign problems.

The first few questions on most history forms establish the length of time since the patient's last physical examination. Thus the doctor can gauge the value of answers to questions dealing with specific diseases in question 9. Because of these problems, patient-completed medical history questionnaires are not always reliable, the doctor must seek additional sources for information concerning the patient's physical status. A physical examination provides much of this information. Physical examination in dentistry consists of the following steps:

- Monitoring of vital signs
- Visual inspection of the patient
- Function tests as indicated
- Auscultation, monitoring (via electrocardiogram), and laboratory tests of the heart and lungs as indicated

Minimal physical evaluation of prospective patients should consist of measurement of the vital signs and visual inspection of the patient. The primary value of this examination is that it provides the doctor with important firsthand information about the patient's physical status, whereas the questionnaire provides historical, anecdotal information.

Physical examination should be completed at an initial visit before the doctor begins dental treatment. Vital signs obtained at this preliminary appointment, known as *baseline* vital signs, serve two functions. First, they help determine a patient's ability to tolerate the stress involved in the planned treatment. Second, baseline vital signs are used as a standard during the management of emergency situations in comparison with readings obtained during the emergency.

## VITAL SIGNS

The six vital signs are as follows:
1. Blood pressure
2. Heart rate (pulse) and rhythm
3. Respiratory rate
4. Temperature
5. Height
6. Weight

Baseline vital signs should be obtained before dental treatment begins. Although the screaming 3-year-old and the difficult-to-manage disabled adult may present difficulties, the doctor should make every effort to record vital signs for each patient.

Blood pressure and heart rate and rhythm always should be recorded when possible. Respiratory rate also should be evaluated whenever possible but usually must be done surreptitiously. Temperature recording may be part of the routine evaluation but more often is recorded in situations in which it is deemed necessary (for example, when infection is present or the patient appears feverish). Height and weight measurements may be obtained in most instances by asking the patient but should be measured when the response appears inconsistent with visual appearance. Weight is of considerable importance when parenteral (IM) sedation is to be used.

The following information provides techniques for the recording and interpretation of vital signs.

**Blood pressure**    The following technique is recommended for the accurate determination of blood pressure.[19] A stethoscope (Figure 2-3) and sphygmomanometer, or blood pressure cuff, (Figures 2-4 and 2-5) are necessary. The most accurate and reliable of these devices is the mercury gravity manometer (see Figure 2-5). The aneroid manometer (see Figure 2-4), probably the most frequently employed, is calibrated to show results in millimeters of mercury (mmHg, or torr) and is also quite accurate if well maintained. Rough handling of the aneroid manometer can lead to erroneous readings. The aneroid manometer should be recalibrated at least annually, checked against a mercury manometer.

In recent years many automatic blood pressure monitoring devices have become available primarily for home monitoring. The earliest such device lacked accuracy, sensitivity, and reliability; however, many newer devices now possess all three qualities. Their costs range from well under $100 (Figure 2-6) to several thousands of dollars (Figure 2-7). (All values are in U.S. dollars.)

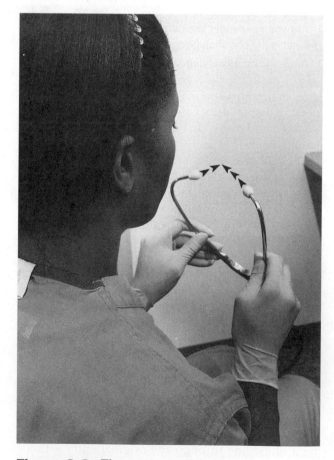

**Figure 2-3**  The earpieces of the stethoscope are inserted in an anterior direction.

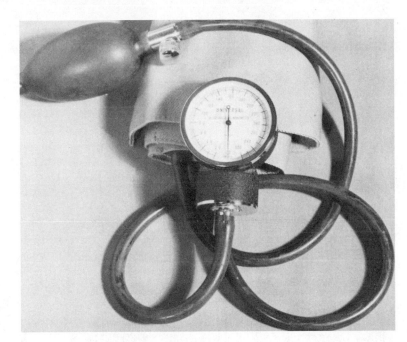

**Figure 2-4**  Aneroid manometer.

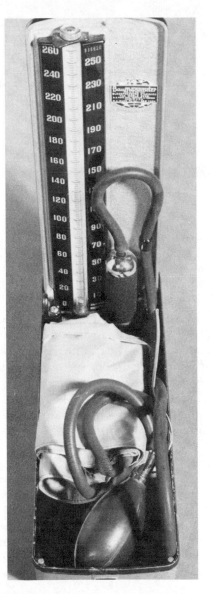

**Figure 2-5**  Mercury gravity manometer.

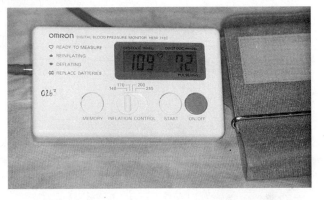

**Figure 2-6**  Automatic blood pressure device.

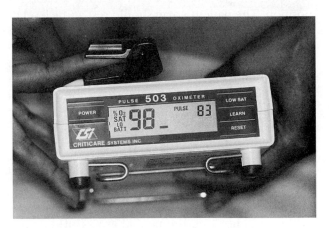

**Figure 2-7**  Vital signs monitor.

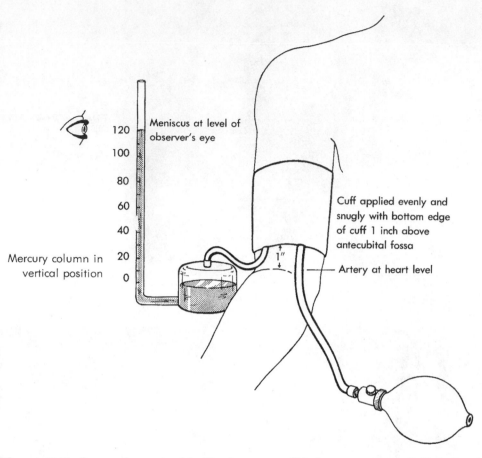

120 — Meniscus at level of observer's eye
100
80
60
40
Mercury column in    20
vertical position      0

Cuff applied evenly and snugly with bottom edge of cuff 1 inch above antecubital fossa
1"
Artery at heart level

**Figure 2-8**    Proper placement of the blood pressure cuff (sphygmomanometer). (From Burch GE, DePasquale NP: *Primer of clinical measurement of blood pressure*, St Louis, 1962, Mosby.)

For the routine preoperative recording of blood pressure, the patient should be seated in an upright position. The patient's arm should rest at the level of the heart, relaxed, slightly flexed, and supported on a firm surface. The patient should be permitted to rest at least 5 minutes before the blood pressure is recorded. This permits the patient to relax so that the blood pressure recorded is closer to the patient's usual baseline reading. During this time the doctor may perform other noninvasive procedures, such as a review of the medical history questionnaire.

Before it is placed on the arm, the blood pressure cuff should be deflated. The cuff should be wrapped evenly and firmly around the arm, with the center of the inflatable portion over the brachial artery and the rubber tubing along the medial aspect of the arm. The lower margin of the cuff should be placed approximately 1 inch (2 to 3 cm) above the antecubital fossa. A cuff is too tight if two fingers cannot fit under the lower edge of the cuff. A tight cuff decreases venous return from the arm, which results in erroneous measurements (elevated diastolic pressure). A cuff is too loose (a more frequent problem) if it can be pulled off the arm with a gentle tug. A slight resistance should be present when a cuff is properly applied (Figure 2-8).

The radial pulse in the wrist is palpated while the pressure in the cuff is increased rapidly to a point approximately 30 mmHg above the point at which the radial pulse disappears. The cuff then should be deflated slowly at 2 to 3 mmHg per second until the radial pulse reappears. This is called *palpatory systolic pressure.* Pressure in the cuff then should be released.

Determination of blood pressure by the more accurate auscultatory method requires palpation of the brachial artery, which is located on the medial aspect of the antecubital fossa (Figure 2-9). The earpieces of the stethoscope should be placed facing forward (see Figure 2-3), firmly in the recorder's ears. The diaphragm of the stethoscope must be placed firmly on the medial aspect of the antecubital fossa, over the brachial artery. To reduce noise, the stethoscope should not touch the blood pressure cuff or rubber tubing. The blood pressure cuff should be inflated

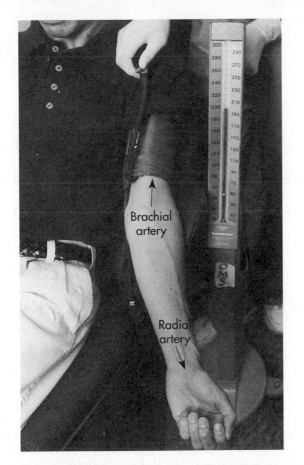

**Figure 2-9**  Location of the brachial and radial arteries. The brachial artery is located on the medial half of the antecubital fossa, whereas the radial artery is on the lateral volar aspect of the wrist.

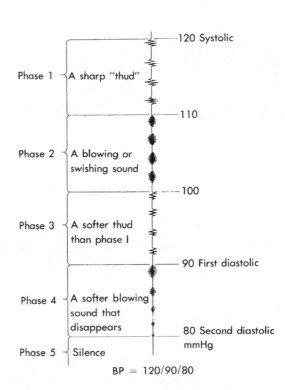

**Figure 2-10**  Korotkoff sounds. Systolic blood pressure is recorded during the first phase, and diastolic blood pressure is recorded at the point in which sound disappears (fifth phase). (From Burch GE, DePasquale NP: *Primer of clinical measurement of blood pressure*, St Louis, 1962, Mosby).

rapidly to a level 30 mmHg above the previously determined palpatory systolic pressure. Pressure in the cuff should be released gradually (2 to 3 mmHg per second) until the first sound is heard through the stethoscope. A light tapping sound is heard as the pressure decreases. This first sound is the systolic blood pressure.

As the cuff deflates further, the sound undergoes changes in quality and intensity (Figure 2-10). As the cuff pressure approaches the diastolic pressure, sounds become dull and muffled and then cease. The diastolic blood pressure can be determined best when the sounds cease completely. In some instances, however, the sounds do not stop completely. Thus the point at which the sounds become muffled serves as the diastolic pressure. The cuff should be deflated slowly to a point 10 mmHg beyond the point of disappearance and then totally deflated.

If additional recordings are necessary, at least 15 seconds should elapse before the cuff is reinflated. This period permits blood trapped in the arm to flow

elsewhere, providing a more accurate reading. Blood pressure is recorded on the patient's chart or sedation and anesthesia record as a fraction—130/90 R (right) or L (left) depending on the arm used to obtain the reading.

Awareness of the errors involved in proper blood pressure recording decreases the likelihood of unnecessary medical consultation, which can burden the patient financially and cause the patient to lose faith in the doctor. Some relatively common errors associated with the recording of blood pressure include the following:

- Loose application of the blood pressure cuff provides false elevated readings, which are probably the most common errors.
- Use of the wrong cuff size can result in erroneous readings. A normal adult blood pressure cuff placed on an obese patient's arm produces falsely elevated readings. This same cuff applied to the arm of a child or a thin adult produces falsely decreased readings. Sphygmomanometers are available in

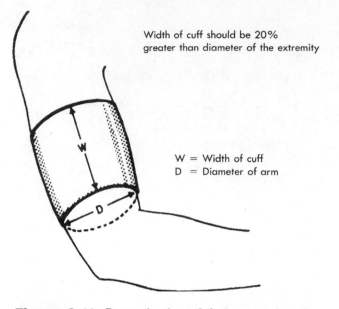

**Figure 2-11** Determination of the proper size of a blood pressure cuff. (From Burch GE, DePasquale NP: *Primer of clinical measurement of blood pressure,* St Louis, 1962, Mosby.)

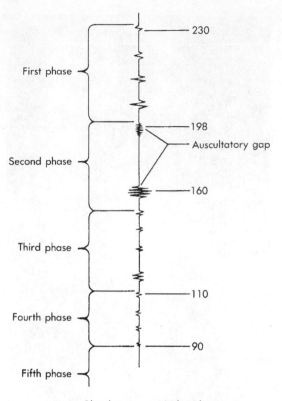

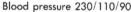

Blood pressure 230/110/90

**Figure 2-12** Korotkoff sounds, illustrating an auscultatory gap. Sound is heard at 230 mmHg, disappears at 198 mmHg, and reappears at 160 mmHg. All sound is lost (fifth phase) at 90 mmHg. (From Burch GE, DePasquale NP: *Primer of clinical measurement of blood pressure,* St Louis, 1962, Mosby.)

many sizes. The width of the compression cuff should be approximately 20% greater than the diameter of the extremity on which the blood pressure is being recorded (Figure 2-11). Doctors may want to keep handy a pediatric cuff and a thigh cuff in addition to the adult cuff.

- An *auscultatory gap* may occur. This gap represents a loss of sound between systolic and diastolic pressures, with the sound reappearing at a lower level (Figure 2-12). For example, systolic sounds are noted at 230 mmHg; however, the sound then disappears at 198 mmHg, reappearing at approximately 160 mmHg. All sound is lost at 90 mmHg. If the person taking the blood pressure has not palpated (estimated) the systolic blood pressure before auscultation, the cuff may be inflated to some arbitrary pressure, such as 165 mmHg. At this pressure, no sound is heard because the value lies within the auscultatory gap.

  Sounds first are noticed at 160 mmHg and disappear at 90 mmHg, levels well within treatment limits for adults (Table 2-3). In reality, however, this patient's blood pressure is 230/90, a significantly elevated pressure that represents a greater risk to the patient during dental care. Although the auscultatory gap occurs infrequently, the possibility of error can be eliminated through use of the palpatory

technique. A pulse is palpable in the gap even when the sound disappears. Although the auscultatory gap has no pathologic significance, it is found most often in patients with high blood pressure.

- The patient may be anxious. Anxiety can cause transient elevations in blood pressure, primarily systolic pressure. Such an elevation is even more likely in the patient who is scheduled to undergo sedation to manage their dental fears. Thus baseline vital signs should be taken during a visit before the start of dental treatment, perhaps at the initial office visit when vital sign measurements should be close to normal.

- Blood pressure is based on the Korotkoff sounds produced by the passage of blood through obstructed, partially obstructed, or unobstructed arteries (see Figure 2-10). Watching a mercury column or needle on an aneroid manometer for pulsations leads to the recording of falsely elevated

table **2-3**   *Guidelines for blood pressure in adults*

| BLOOD PRESSURE (mmHg OR TORR) | ASA CLASSIFICATION | DENTAL THERAPY CONSIDERATIONS |
|---|---|---|
| <140 and <90 | I | 1. Observe routine dental management.<br>2. Recheck in 6 months. |
| 140 to 159 and/or 90 to 94 | II | 1. Recheck blood pressure before dental treatment for three consecutive appointments; if all measurements exceed these guidelines, medical consultation is recommended.<br>2. Observe routine dental management.<br>3. Implement stress reduction protocol as indicated. |
| 160 to 199 and/or 95 to 114 | III | 1. Recheck blood pressure in 5 minutes.<br>2. If still elevated, perform medical consultation before beginning dental therapy.<br>3. Observe routine dental therapy.<br>4. Implement stress reduction protocol. |
| >200 and/or >115 | IV | 1. Recheck blood pressure in 5 minutes.<br>2. Perform immediate medical consultation if pressure is still elevated.<br>3. Do not perform dental therapy, routine or emergency,* until elevated blood pressure is corrected.<br>4. Perform emergency dental therapy with drugs (analgesics, antibiotics).<br>5. Refer to hospital if immediate dental therapy indicated. |

*When the blood pressure of the patient is slightly above the cutoff for category IV and when anxiety is present, the use of inhalation sedation may diminish the blood pressure (via the elimination of stress) below the 200/115 level. The patient should be advised that if the nitrous oxide and oxygen succeeds in decreasing the blood pressure below this level, the planned treatment can proceed. However, if the blood pressure remains elevated, the planned procedure must be postponed until the elevated blood pressure has been lowered to a more acceptable range.

systolic pressures. These pulsations are observed approximately 10 to 15 mmHg before the initial Korotkoff sounds are heard.

• Use of the right or left arm produces differences in recorded blood pressure. A difference of 5 to 10 mmHg exists between the arms, with the left arm producing slightly higher measurements.

*Guidelines for clinical evaluation.* The USC physical evaluation system is based on the ASA Physical Status Classification System, which classifies patients into five risk categories based on their medical histories and physical evaluations (see page 41). Table 2-3 presents blood pressure recordings by ASA classifications.

Adult patients in the ASA I range (<140/<90 mmHg) should have their blood pressures recorded every 6 months unless specific dental procedures require more frequent monitoring. Parenteral or inhalation routes of drug administration demand more frequent recording of vital signs. Ideally the administration of local anesthesia also should be preceded by a monitoring of blood pressure. Patients whose blood pressures place them into the ASA, II, III, or IV categories for blood pressure should be monitored more frequently. Patients with known high blood pressure

should have their blood pressure monitored at each visit to determine whether it is adequately controlled.

According to the recommendations, routine blood pressure monitoring in all patients minimizes the occurrence of acute complications associated with high blood pressure (for example, CVA and chest pain). When parenteral or inhalation sedation techniques or general anesthesia are employed, a greater need exists for baseline and preoperative vital sign recording. A comparison of postoperative and baseline vital signs helps the doctor determine a patient's recovery from the effects of CNS depressants and readiness for discharge.

Yet another reason the routine monitoring of blood pressure should be emphasized relates to emergency management. After assessment and management in each emergency are completed, certain specific steps may be necessary for definitive treatment. Primary among these is the monitoring of vital signs, particularly blood pressure. Blood pressure recorded during an emergency situation is an important indicator of the cardiovascular system's status. However, unless a baseline (nonemergency) blood pressure was recorded previously, the measurement obtained during the emergency is of less significance. A recording during an emergency of 80/50 mmHg is less ominous if the preoperative reading was 110/70 than if it was 190/110. In all situations the absence of blood pressure is an indication for cardiopulmonary resuscitation.

Normal blood pressure values in younger patients are lower than those in adults. Table 2-4 presents normal ranges of blood pressure measurements for infants and children.

**Heart rate and rhythm**  Heart rate (pulse) and rhythm can be measured through the use of any readily accessible artery. Most commonly employed for routine (nonemergency) measurement are the brachial artery, located on the medial aspect of the antecubital fossa, and the radial artery, located on the radial and volar aspects of the wrist. Other arteries, such as the carotid and femoral, also can be used but rarely are in routine situations because they are not as accessible. In emergency situations the carotid artery should be palpated in lieu of others because it delivers oxygenated blood to the brain. Prompt and accurate location of this artery is essential in emergency situations. (Locating the carotid artery [in the neck] is reviewed in Chapter 5.)

When palpating for a pulse, the doctor should press the fleshy portions of the index and middle fingers onto the patient's skin gently enough to feel the pulsation but not so firmly that the pressure occludes the artery. The thumb should not be used to monitor a pulse because it contains its own artery that pulsates. Situations have arisen in which the measured heart rate has been the doctor's, not the victim's. Furthermore, in the infant the precordium is no longer recommended as the site to determine the presence of an effective heartbeat.[20] The brachial artery in the upper arm is the preferred site (Figure 2-13).

*Guidelines for clinical evaluation.*  The following three factors should be evaluated when heart rate and rhythm are monitored:

1. Heart rate (recorded as beats per minute)
2. Heart rhythm (regular or irregular)
3. Pulse quality (thready, strong, bounding, or weak)

The heart rate should be evaluated for a minimum of 30 seconds, ideally for 1 minute. The normal resting heart rate for an adult ranges from 60 to 110 beats per minute. This rate is frequently lower in well-conditioned athletes and elevated in apprehensive patients. However, clinically significant pathologic processes also can produce slow (<60 = bradycardia) or rapid heart rates (>110 = tachycardia). Any adult heart rate under 60 or above 110 beats per minute should receive further evaluation. When no obvious cause for the deviation in rate is discernible (for ex-

ample, endurance sports or anxiety), medical consultation should be considered.

The normal pulse maintains a relatively regular rhythm, known as a *normal sinus rhythm* or NSR (Figure 2-14). Occasional premature ventricular contractions (PVCs) are so common that they are not necessarily considered abnormal (Figure 2-15). Smoking, fatigue, stress, various medications (such as epinephrine), and alcohol all can produce PVCs. However, when PVCs

| table **2-4** | *Normal blood pressure measurements** | |
|---|---|---|
| **AGE (YR)** | **MEAN SYSTOLIC ±2 SD** | **MEAN DIASTOLIC ±2 SD** |
| Newborn | 80 ± 16 | 46 ± 16 |
| 6 mo-1 yr | 89 ± 29 | 60 ± 10† |
| 1 | 96 ± 30 | 66 ± 25† |
| 2 | 99 ± 25 | 64 ± 25† |
| 3 | 100 ± 25 | 67 ± 23† |
| 4 | 99 ± 20 | 65 ± 20† |
| 5-6 | 94 ± 14 | 55 ± 9 |
| 6-7 | 100 ± 15 | 56 ± 8 |
| 7-8 | 102 ± 15 | 56 ± 8 |
| 8-9 | 105 ± 16 | 57 ± 9 |
| 9-10 | 107 ± 16 | 57 ± 9 |
| 10-11 | 111 ± 17 | 58 ± 10 |
| 11-12 | 113 ± 18 | 59 ± 10 |
| 12-13 | 115 ± 19 | 59 ± 10 |
| 13-14 | 118 ± 19 | 60 ± 10 |

From Nadas AS, Fyler DC: *Pediatric cardiology,* ed 3, Philadelphia, 1972, WB Saunders.
*SD,* Standard deviation.
*Modified from data in the literature; figures have been rounded off to the nearest decimal place.
†In this study the point of muffling was taken as the diastolic pressure.

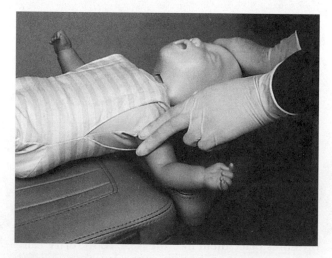

**Figure 2-13**  The best way to determine an infant's pulse is through location of the brachial artery, located on the medical side of the upper arm.

are present at a rate of five or more per minute in a patient with other risk factors for coronary artery disease, medical consultation should be considered. When palpating the pulse, PVCs are detected clinically as breaks in a generally regular heart rate in which a longer than normal pause (skipped beat) is noted and followed by the resumption of normal rhythm.

In reality a PVC is a contraction of the ventricles before enough blood is present in their chambers to produce a pulse wave in a peripheral artery. Unusually frequent PVCs (more than five per minute in a patient with other cardiovascular disease risk factors) indicate myocardial irritability and may presage severe dysrhythmias* such as ventricular fibrillation (Figure 2-16).

*The terms *dysrhythmia* and *arrhythmia* are used interchangeably to describe irregularities in the heart's rhythm. In fact, the term *dysrhythmia* is the more correct because the prefix *dys* means "abnormal"; thus a *dysrhythmia* is an abnormal rhythm. The prefix *a* means the "absence of"; thus *arrhythmia* describes the absence of a rhythm, or asystole (a flat line on an electrocardiogram).

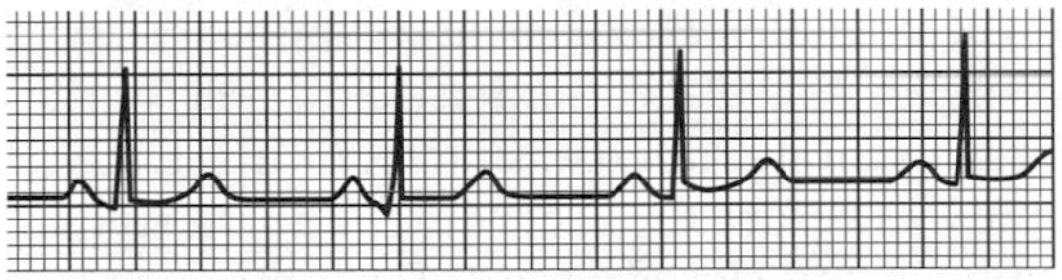

**Figure 2-14** Normal sinus rhythm. (From Berne RM, Levy MN: *Physiology,* ed 4, St Louis, 1998, Mosby.)

Indeed, patients with high numbers of PVCs are considered prime candidates for implanted defibrillators.

A second important disturbance in pulse is termed *pulsus alternans*. This disturbance is not truly a dysrhythmia but a regular heart rate characterized by a pulse in which strong and weak beats alternate. The alternating contractile force of a diseased left ventricle produces the disturbance. Pulsus alternans is observed frequently in left ventricular failure, severe arterial high blood pressure, and coronary artery disease. Medical consultation is indicated.

Accurate diagnosis of a cardiac dysrhythmia via palpation of an artery alone is difficult if not impossible. However, consultation with the patient's physician and possible testing (for example, electrocardiography) helps in determining the nature of the dysrhythmia and its significance to the planned dental treatment.

The quality of the pulse commonly is described as bounding, thready, strong, or weak. These adjectives relate to the "feel" of the pulse and are used to describe different conditions. For example, a patient with severe arterial high blood pressure may exhibit a strong, bounding pulse, whereas the pulse of a patient with hypotension and signs of shock may be described as weak and thready. Table 2-5 demonstrates the normal pulse rates for children, which are more rapid than those in adults.

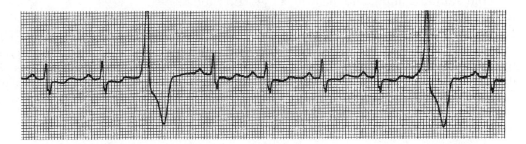

**Figure 2-15** The third and eighth complexes show unifocal premature ventricular contractions. (From Zalis EG, Conover MH: *Understanding electrocardiography: physiological and interpretive concepts,* St Louis, 1972, Mosby.)

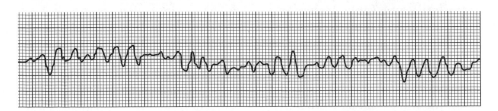

**Figure 2-16** Ventricular fibrillation. (From Berne RM, Levy MN: *Physiology,* ed 4, St Louis, 1998, Mosby.)

| table **2-5** | Average pulse rates for children |
|---|---|

| AGE (YR) | LOWER LIMITS OF NORMAL | AVERAGE | UPPER LIMITS OF NORMAL |
|---|---|---|---|
| Newborn | 70 | 120 | 170 |
| 1-11 mo | 80 | 120 | 160 |
| 2 | 80 | 110 | 130 |
| 4 | 80 | 100 | 120 |
| 6 | 75 | 100 | 115 |
| 8 | 70 | 90 | 110 |
| 10 | 70 | 90 | 110 |

From Behrman RE, Vaughn VC, III: *Nelson textbook of pediatrics,* ed 12, Philadelphia, 1983, WB Saunders.

| table **2-6** | Respiratory rates by age |
|---|---|

| AGE (YR) | RATE/MINUTE |
|---|---|
| Neonate | 40 |
| 1 wk | 30 |
| 1 | 24 |
| 3 | 22 |
| 5 | 20 |
| 8 | 18 |
| 12 | 16 |
| 21 | 12 |

**Respiratory rate**    Determination of the respiratory rate must be made surreptitiously. Patients aware that their breathing is being observed usually do not breathe normally. Therefore respiration should be monitored immediately after the heart rate is ascertained. The doctor's fingers should be left on the patient's radial or brachial pulse after the pulse rate has been determined, and the doctor counts respirations by observing the rise and fall of the chest for a minimum of 30 seconds, ideally for 1 minute.

*Guidelines for clinical evaluation.* The normal respiratory rate for an adult is 16 to 18 breaths per minute. Bradypnea (slow breathing rate) may be produced by opioid administration, and tachypnea (rapid breathing rate) is seen with fever and alkalosis. The most commonly observed change in breathing in dental practice is hyperventilation, an abnormal increase in the rate and depth of respiration that is almost always a manifestation of anxiety. Hyperventilation also is seen in patients with diabetic acidosis. Extreme psychologic stress is the most common reason for hyperventilation in dental settings.

Any significant variation in respiratory rate or depth should be evaluated fully before the doctor begins dental treatment. The absence of spontaneous ventilation is always abnormal and is an indication for artificial ventilation. Table 2-6 presents the normal range of respiratory rates for different age groups.

Blood pressure, heart rate and rhythm, and respiratory rate all provide information about the patient's cardiorespiratory system. These measurements should be recorded as part of the routine physical evaluation of all prospective patients. Recording of the remaining vital signs—temperature, height, and weight—is desirable but optional. However, in cases in which parenteral medications are to be administered, especially in lighter-weight, younger patients, recording of a patient's weight is of considerable importance.

**Temperature**    Temperature should be monitored orally if possible. The thermometer, sterilized and shaken down, is placed under the tongue of the patient, who should not eat, smoke, or drink anything 10 minutes before the recording. The thermometer remains in the closed mouth for 2 minutes before removal. Disposable thermometers (Figure 2-17), digital thermometers (Figure 2-18), and forehead thermometers (Figure 2-19) also are gaining acceptance today.

*Guidelines for clinical evaluation.* The normal oral temperature of 98.2° F (37° C) is merely an average. The true normal range encompasses 97° to 99.6° F (36.1° to 37.5° C). Temperatures vary slightly, from 0.5° to 2.0° F, throughout the day; the lowest temperatures are in the early morning and highest in the late afternoon. Fever represents an increase in temperature beyond 99.6° F (37.5° C). Temperatures above 101° F (38.3° C) usually indicate the presence of an active pathologic process.

The cause of the fever must be determined before treatment begins. If the fever is related to a dental infection, immediate treatment and antibiotic and antipyretic therapy are indicated. If the patient's temperature is 104° F (40° C) or higher, medical consultation is suggested. With elevated temperature, elective dental care is contraindicated and treatment is limited to drug administration (antibiotics and antipyretics) because the patient is less able than usual to tolerate stress.

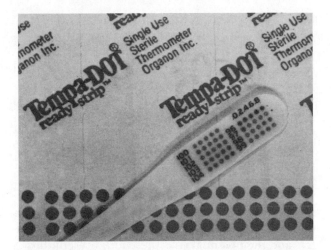

**Figure 2-17** Disposable thermometer. (From Malamed SF: *Sedation: a guide to patient management,* St Louis, ed 3, 1995, Mosby.)

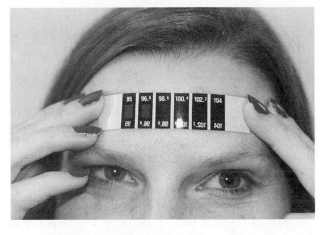

**Figure 2-19** Forehead thermometer.

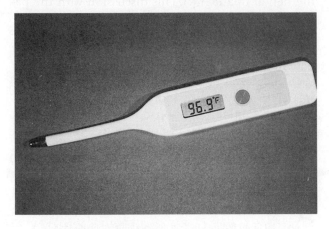

**Figure 2-18** Digital thermometer.

**Height and weight** Patients should be asked their height and weight, two variable measurements. Numerous insurance companies have developed charts of normal height and weight ranges available for doctors' offices.

*Guidelines for clinical evaluation.* Patients at either end of the normal distribution curve for height and weight should be screened carefully. Gross obesity or extreme underweight may indicate of an active pathologic process. Patients with various endocrine disorders such as Cushing's syndrome may be obese; those with pulmonary tuberculosis, malignancy, the latter stages of AIDS, and hyperthyroidism may be extremely underweight. In all instances of gross obesity or extreme underweight, medical consultation before treatment is recommended. Excessively

tall persons are referred to as *giants,* whereas persons who are decidedly shorter than normal are called *dwarfs.* In both instances, endocrine gland dysfunction may be present. Medical consultation relative to the planned dental treatment is usually unnecessary.

## VISUAL INSPECTION

Visual observation can provide the doctor with valuable information about the patient's medical status and level of apprehension about dental treatment. Observation of the patient's posture, body movements, speech, and skin may help the doctor in the diagnosis of disorders that previously may have gone undetected.

Patients with CHF and other chronic pulmonary disorders often must sit more upright in the dental chair than other patients because of the presence of severe orthopnea (for example, three- or four-pillow orthopnea). The arthritic patient with a rigid neck may need to rotate the entire trunk when turning toward the doctor or viewing an object from the side. Recognition of these factors better enables the doctor to determine necessary treatment modifications.

In addition, involuntary body movements occurring in conscious patients may indicate significant disorders. Tremor is noted in disorders such as fatigue, multiple sclerosis, parkinsonism, hyperthyroidism, and hysteria and nervous tension (the latter being prominent in dental settings).

The character of a patient's speech also may be significant. A CVA can cause muscle paralysis and lead to speech difficulties. Epileptic patients on long-term anticonvulsant therapy may exhibit sluggish speech patterns. Anxiety about the impending dental treatment also can be detected in speech. Rapid responses to questions or nervous voice quivers can indicate increased anxiety and the possible need for sedation during dental treatment.

Other possible disorders can be detected from the presence of specific, nondental odors on the patient's breath. Patients with diabetic acidosis and ketosis often have the sweet, fruity odor of acetone on the breath, whereas patients with uremia often emit the smell of ammonia. The most probable detectable breath odor is alcohol, which should alert the doctor to the possibility of heightened anxiety or drug abuse.

The feel and color of the patient's skin are other important sources of information. The doctor can learn a great deal by greeting patients with a welcoming handshake. The skin of a very apprehensive person is cold and wet, that of a patient with a hyperthyroid condition is warm and wet, and that of a patient with diabetic acidosis is warm and dry. The color of a patient's skin also is significant. Pallor (a loss of color) can indicate anemia or heightened anxiety (that is, presyncope). Cyanosis can indicate the presence of heart failure, chronic pulmonary disease, methemoglobinemia or polycythemia and is most noticeable in the nail beds and mucous membranes (lips). Flushed skin may suggest apprehension, hyperthyroidism, or elevated temperature, whereas jaundice may indicate past or present hepatic disease. However, each such observation also has a benign explanation that should be considered.

Additional factors revealed through the visual examination include (1) the presence of prominent jugular veins in a patient seated upright, an indication of possible right ventricular failure (or of an overly tight collar); (2) clubbing of the fingers, which can indicate chronic cardiopulmonary disease; (3) swelling of the ankles, which is seen in cases of right ventricular failure, varicose veins, renal disease, and occasionally in near-term pregnancy; and (4) exophthalmos, which can indicate hyperthyroidism. (Each such finding is discussed more completely in the prevention section within specific chapters.)

For a more complete discussion of the art of observation and its importance in medical diagnosis, the reader should consult additional sources.[21,22]

## ADDITIONAL EVALUATION PROCEDURES

After the completion of the written medical history questionnaire, recording of vital signs, and physical examination, a more in-depth evaluation of specific medical disorders should be performed. This examination can include auscultation of the heart and lungs, testing of blood glucose levels, retinal examination, function tests for cardiorespiratory status (for example, the breath-holding test), electrocardiographic examination, and blood chemistries. At present, many such tests are used in dental offices but only irregularly. Explanation and evaluation of many of these tests are beyond the scope of this text, but specific tests (for example, blood-glucose testing and cardiopulmonary function) are referred to in later chapters for the management of specific situations.

**Dialogue history**    The doctor now must determine the significance of any disorders the patient suffers and the potential risks these may present during the planned dental treatment. (By risk, this text describes that of the patient's medical problem becoming acutely exacerbated during or immediately after the dental treatment.) This discussion with the patient is termed the *dialogue history,* in which the doctor must use all available knowledge of the pathologic process to assess the degree to which the patient is at risk. (Dialogue history is emphasized in each chapter in the discussion on the prevention of specific emergency situations.)

For example, in response to a positive reply in question 9 to the presence of diabetes, the following questions may be included in the dialogue history:

### At what age did you develop diabetes?

*Comment:* This question is designed to help determine whether the disease manifested itself while the patient was a juvenile or an adult. Juvenile-onset diabetes is usually type I, or insulin-dependent diabetes mellitus (IDDM), whereas adult-onset diabetes more likely represents type II, or non–insulin-dependent diabetes mellitus (NIDDM).

### How do you control your diabetes?

*Comment:* The question should provide enough information to determine whether the diabetes is IDDM or NIDDM. Patients with IDDM are more likely to develop acute complications associated with diabetes, primarily hypoglycemia.

### How often do you monitor your blood sugar, and what are the recordings? (monitoring the degree of control the patient maintains over the disease)

### Have you been hospitalized for your diabetic condition? Why?

*Comment:* A history of hospitalization for low blood sugar (hypoglycemia) may alert the doctor to seek outside assistance more immediately if a problem develops with this patient during treatment. In addition, hospitalization because of chronic complications of diabetes should alert the doctor to seek signs and symptoms of arteriosclerosis.

The following dialogue history may be initiated if a patient records a positive answer for question 9 under angina pectoris:

**What precipitates your angina?**
**How frequently do you suffer anginal episodes?**
**How long do your anginal episodes last?**
**Describe a typical anginal episode.**
**How does nitroglycerin affect the anginal episode?**
**Has there been any change in the frequency, intensity, or radiation of pain of your angina in the past several weeks?**

(These questions and some possible responses will be discussed more completely in Chapter 27.)

# Anxiety Recognition

Thus far the primary aim in the evaluation of a prospective patient has been to determine the patient's physical ability to handle the stress involved in the planned dental treatment. Few questions have been directed at the patient's psychologic outlook toward dentistry in general and the treatment in particular. The traditional (long-form) medical history questionnaire asks questions such as: "Do you have fainting spells or seizures?" and "Have you had any serious trouble associated with any previous dental treatment?" Most short-form medical histories ignore questions about anxiety.

Heightened anxiety and fear of dentistry can lead to the acute exacerbation of medical problems such as angina, seizures, and asthma and stress-related problems such as hyperventilation and vasodepressor syncope. One goal in patient evaluation is to determine whether the patient is psychologically able to tolerate the stress associated with the planned dental treatment. Three methods are available to allow the doctor to recognize the presence of anxiety. The first is the medical history questionnaire; second, the anxiety questionnaire; and third, the art of observation.

## PSYCHOLOGIC EXAMINATION

### Medical history questionnaire

This chapter previously discussed the inclusion of one or more questions relating to a patient's attitudes toward dentistry in the medical history questionnaire. Professionals at the USC School of Dentistry have found that patients who will not verbally admit their fears to the doctor often indicate on the questionnaire that they are apprehensive. An affirmative response to either question 2 or question 3 should alert the doctor to begin a more in-depth dialogue history with the patient to determine the cause of the fear.

**Anxiety questionnaire**    An additional aid in the recognition of anxiety is the anxiety questionnaire (Box 2-6) devised by Corah.[23] Used since 1973 at the USC School of Dentistry, this questionnaire has been a reliable aid in the recognition of anxiety. Answers to individual questions are scored 1 through 5 (with "a" being assigned a score of 1 and "e" being assigned a 5). The maximum score possible is 20. Scores of 8 or above indicate higher-than-normal levels of anxiety that should be addressed by the doctor before treatment begins.

box **2-6**    *Anxiety questionnaire*

1. If you had to go to the dentist tomorrow, how would you feel about it?
   a. I would look forward to it as a reasonably enjoyable experience.
   b. I would not care one way or the other.
   c. I would be very uneasy about it.
   d. I would be afraid that it would be unpleasant and painful.
   e. I would be very frightened of what the dentist might do.
2. When you are waiting in the dentist's office for your turn in the chair, how do you feel?
   a. Relaxed
   b. A little uneasy
   c. Tense
   d. Anxious
   e. So anxious that I almost break out in a sweat or almost feel physically sick
3. When you are in the dentist's chair waiting for him or her to get the drill ready and begin working on your teeth, how do you feel?
   a. Relaxed
   b. A little uneasy
   c. Tense
   d. Anxious
   e. So anxious that I almost break out in a sweat or almost feel physically sick
4. You are in the dentist's chair to have your teeth cleaned. While you are waiting and the dentist is getting out the instruments with which to scrape your teeth around the gums, how do you feel?
   a. Relaxed
   b. A little uneasy
   c. Tense
   d. Anxious
   e. So anxious that I almost break out in a sweat or almost feel physically sick
5. In general, do you feel uncomfortable or nervous about receiving dental treatment?
   a. Yes
   b. No

From Corah NL: Development of a dental anxiety scale, *J Dent Res* 48:596, 1969.

**Observation**    In the absence of such questions or an affirmative response to such questions, careful observation of the patient can enable the doctor and staff members to recognize unusually anxious patients. Some patients may admit to the doctor and staff that they are quite apprehensive; however, the vast majority of apprehensive adult patients do everything possible to conceal this anxiety. These patients usually feel that their fear of dentistry is irrational and probably childish. They do not wish to tell the doctor of their fears because they are afraid of being labeled a "baby." Because of this pervasive attitude, dental staff members must be trained to seek out and recognize clinical signs and symptoms of heightened patient anxiety. Whereas a number of levels exist into which anxiety may be subdivided, for the purposes of this discussion two are presented—severe (neurotic) and moderate.

Patients with severe anxiety usually do not attempt to hide this fact from the doctor. In fact, these patients often do anything within their power to avoid undergoing dental treatment. It is estimated that between 6% and 14% (14 million to 34 million) of Americans actively avoid dental visits completely because of fear and that another 20% to 30% dislike them enough to make only occasional visits.[24] Such patients constitute the severe anxiety group. When in the dental office, they may be recognized by the following signs:

- Increased blood pressure and heart rate
- Trembling
- Excessive sweating
- Dilated pupils

Severely anxious patients most commonly appear in the dental office when they have severe toothaches or infections. The patients normally say that they have had the problem for quite some time and have attempted every available means of home remedy (for example, toothache drops). The reason for finally visiting the dental office is that the patient has not been able to sleep for a few nights because of intense pain that no home remedy can alleviate. Such patients are driven to the dental office by extreme discomfort and usually expect to have the tooth removed.

These patients represent management problems. Although they wish to have their problems treated, their underlying fears of dentistry often make them unable to tolerate the procedure when it is time for treatment to begin. In addition, the doctor often is faced with the unpleasant prospect of having to either extract an acutely inflamed tooth or extirpate the pulp of an acutely sensitive tooth, two situations in which achieving clinically adequate pain control in any patient may be difficult.

Because of these factors, severely anxious patients frequently are candidates for the use of either IV sedation or general anesthesia. Oral, IM, or inhalation sedation, when used as suggested, have little likelihood of success, primarily because of their limited effectiveness or the constraints that are properly placed on their use. Children with severe anxiety are frequently candidates for either IM or IV (deep) sedation or for general anesthesia.

Therefore assuming that adult patients may attempt to hide their fears, the doctor and staff members should observe clues before and during the patient's treatment. Front-office personnel, such as the receptionist, may overhear patients in the waiting room talking amongst themselves. Patients also may ask important questions of the receptionist, such as, "Is the doctor gentle?" or "Does the doctor use gas?" The receptionist should be trained to inform the doctor immediately whenever a patient makes a statement that may indicate an increased level of concern about upcoming treatment. All chairside personnel also should be on the lookout for signs of increased anxiety. Shaking the patient's hand as a greeting may help these staff members perceive signs of anxiety, such as cold, sweaty palms in an office that is not particularly cool.

Discussing a patient's prior dental experiences also may indicate the level of anxiety. A patient with a history of emergency treatment only (for example, extractions or incision and drainage) who cancels or does not appear for subsequent appointments may be a high-anxiety patient. The same may be true for the patient with a history of multiple canceled appointments. The doctor should discuss this history with the patient to determine the reasons behind this pattern of treatment (or nontreatment).

Once the patient is seated in the dental chair, the doctor and staff members should watch and listen carefully. Apprehensive patients remain alert and on guard at all times. They sit at the edge of the chair, and their eyes roam around the room, taking in everything. They are afraid of surprises, and their posture appears unnaturally stiff, with tense arms and legs. They may nervously fiddle with a handkerchief or tissue, occasionally unaware of such actions, and exhibit the white-knuckle syndrome, in which the knuckles turn white from severe clenching. The patient may exclaim, "Gee, it's hot in here!" to explain diaphoresis (sweating) of the palms or forehead.

The moderately apprehensive patient often is overly willing to aid the dentist. Actions are carried

---

box **2-7**   *Clinical signs of moderate anxiety*

**Reception area**

Questions to receptionist regarding injections or use of sedation
Nervous conversations with other patients in waiting room
History of emergency dental care only
History of canceled appointments for nonemergency treatment
Cold, sweaty palms

**In dental chair**

Unnaturally stiff posture
Nervous play with tissue or handkerchief
White-knuckle syndrome
Perspiration on forehead and hands
Overwillingness to cooperate with doctor
Quick answers

---

out quickly, usually without thought. These patients answer the doctor's questions quickly, usually too quickly. Box 2-7 summarizes the clinical signs of moderate anxiety.

Once the dentist recognizes anxiety, whether through the questionnaire or observation, the patient must be confronted. A straightforward approach is surprisingly successful. The dentist may say, "Mr. Smith, I see from your medical history that you have had several unpleasant experiences in a dental office. Would you kindly describe these to me?" After noticing anxiety, the dentist might say, "Mrs. Smith, you appear to be somewhat nervous today. Is something bothering you?" I have been astonished at how rapidly patients drop all pretense at being calm once they realize that the doctor is aware of their fears. They usually say, "Doctor, I didn't think you could tell." Once the fears are in the open, the dentist should try to determine their exact source (for example, injections or drills). Once the source of a patient's fears is known, steps can be implemented to minimize their occurrence.

A moderately anxious patient usually is treatable. In most cases, conscious sedation effectively can manage such patients. Conscious sedation may be performed with a drug (pharmacosedation) or non-drug technique (iatrosedation). General anesthesia is needed only rarely in the effective management of the moderately fearful patient.

## DETERMINATION OF MEDICAL RISK

After completing the physical examination and thorough dental exam and deciding on a tentative treatment plan, the doctor must gather all the information and answer the following questions:

- Is this patient capable, both physiologically and psychologically, of tolerating in relative safety the stress involved in the proposed dental treatment plan?
- Is the patient at a greater risk (of morbidity or mortality) than normal during the planned dental care?
- If the patient does represent an increased risk, what treatment modifications if any should be employed to minimize this risk during the planned dental treatment?
- Is the risk too great for the patient to be managed safely in the dental office?

The USC School of Dentistry has developed a physical evaluation system that attempts to assist the doctor in categorizing patient risk during dental treatment. This evaluation system is designed to place each patient into an appropriate risk category so that dental care can be provided in greater comfort and safety. The system is based on the ASA Physical Status Classification System.

### ASA physical status classification system

In 1962 the American Society of Anesthesiologists adopted what is referred to now as the ASA Physical Status Classification System.[25] The classification represents a method by which the doctor can estimate the medical risk to a patient who is scheduled to receive anesthesia for a surgical procedure. The system was designed primarily for patients who were to receive a general anesthetic, but since its introduction the classification system has been used for all surgical patients regardless of anesthetic technique (for example, general anesthesia, regional anesthesia, or conscious sedation). The system has remained essentially unchanged and in continuous use since its introduction and has proven a valuable method in the determination of surgical and anesthetic risk before dental procedures.[26] The classification system is as follows:

ASA I: A normal, healthy patient without systemic disease
ASA II: A patient with mild systemic disease
ASA III: A patient with severe systemic disease that limits activity but is not incapacitating
ASA IV: A patient with an incapacitating systemic disease that is a constant threat to life
ASA V: A moribund patient not expected to survive 24 hours with or without an operation

ASA E: Emergency operation of any variety, with E preceding the number to indicate the patient's physical status (for example, ASA E-III)

When this system was adopted for use in a typical outpatient dental setting, the ASA V classification was eliminated. An effort has been made to correlate the remaining four classifications with possible modifications for dental treatment. Figure 2-20 illustrates the USC physical evaluation record on which a summary of the patient's physical and psychologic status is presented. Each classification is reviewed, and clinical examples of each are listed.

*ASA I.* ASA I patients are considered normal and healthy. Review of their medical history, physical evaluation, and other evaluation parameters indicate no abnormalities. The heart, lungs, liver, kidneys, and CNS appear to be in good health. Physiologically, ASA I patients should be able to tolerate the stress involved in a dental treatment plan without added risk of serious complications. Psychologically, such patients also should have little or no difficulty handling the treatment. ASA I patients are able to walk up one flight of stairs or two level city blocks without distress.* Healthy patients with little or no anxiety are classified as ASA I. An ASA I classification is a "green light" for treatment, and treatment modification usually is not required for these patients.

*ASA II.* The ASA II patient has a mild systemic disease or is a healthy (ASA I) patient who demonstrates extreme anxiety and fear toward dental treatment. These patients generally are less stress tolerant than ASA I patients; however, they still represent minimal

---

*Shortness of breath, undue fatigue, and chest pain all are signs of distress.

risks during dental treatment. Routine treatment is permitted as long as some thought is given to the possible modifications or considerations that the patient's condition may warrant. Examples of such modifications include the use of prophylactic antibiotics or sedative techniques, limits on the duration of treatment, and possible medical consultation.

ASA II patients can walk up one flight of stairs or two level city blocks before distress causes them to stop. An ASA II classification should be a "yellow light," warning to the doctor to proceed with caution. Elective dental care is warranted with minimal increase in risk to the patient during therapy. Treatment modifications should also be considered.

Examples of ASA II patients include the following:
- Well-controlled NIDDM
- Well-controlled epilepsy
- Well-controlled asthma
- Well-controlled hyperthyroid or hypothyroid disorders in which patients are under a physician's care and presently have normal thyroid function (considered euthyroid)
- ASA I patients with upper respiratory infections
- Healthy, pregnant women
- Otherwise healthy patients with allergies, especially to drugs
- Otherwise healthy patients with extreme dental fears
- Healthy patients over 60 years of age
- Adults with blood pressures between 140 and 159 mmHg systolic and/or 90 to 94 mmHg diastolic

Generally, the ASA II patient can perform normal activities without experiencing distress (for example, undue fatigue, dyspnea, or precordial pain).

*ASA III.* ASA III patients have severe systemic disease that limits activity but is not incapacitating. At rest, ASA III patients do not exhibit signs and symp-

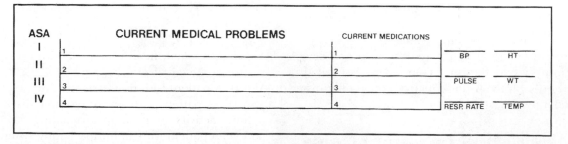

**Figure 2-20**    The physical evaluation section on the health history form provides room for a summary of medical problems, vital signs, and classification according to the American Society of Anesthesiologists' Physical Status Classification System. (From Malamed SF: *Sedation: a guide to patient management,* St Louis, ed 3, 1995, Mosby.)

toms of distress; however, distress is exhibited when the patient experiences either physiologic or psychologic stress. For example, an anginal patient may be normal in the waiting room but develop chest pain when seated in the dental chair. ASA III patients are able to walk up one flight of stairs or two level city blocks, but distress en route forces them to stop. Like ASA II patients, these are "yellow light" patients (proceed with caution). Elective dental care is not contraindicated, but the patient's risk during treatment is increased. Serious consideration should be given to the possible implementation of treatment modifications.

Examples of ASA III patients include the following:
- Stable angina pectoris
- Status postmyocardial infarction more than 6 months before treatment with no residual signs or symptoms
- Status post-CVA more than 6 months before treatment with no residual signs and symptoms
- Well-controlled IDDM
- CHF with orthopnea and ankle edema
- COPD: emphysema or chronic bronchitis
- Exercise-induced asthma
- Less well-controlled epilepsy
- Hyperthyroid or hypothyroid disorders when patients are symptomatic
- Adults with blood pressures between 160 to 199 mmHg systolic and/or 95 to 114 mmHg diastolic

ASA III patients usually can perform normal activities without experiencing distress (for example, undue fatigue, dyspnea, or precordial pain) but may need rest during an activity should they become distressed.

*ASA IV.* ASA IV patients have an incapacitating systemic disease that is a constant threat to their lives. These patients have severe medical problems that are of greater significance to their health than the planned dental treatment. Whenever possible, elective dental care should be postponed until the patient's medical condition has improved at least to an ASA III classification.

ASA IV patients are unable to walk up one flight of stairs or two level city blocks. Distress is present even at rest. These patients present in the dental office exhibiting clinical signs and symptoms of disease. An ASA IV classification is a "red light," warning that the risk involved in treatment of the patient is too great to permit elective care. The management of dental emergencies, such as infection and pain, should be treated as conservatively as possible in the dental office until the patient's condition improves.

Whenever possible, treatment should be noninvasive, consisting of the prescription of medications such as analgesics for pain and antibiotics for infection. In situations in which immediate intervention is necessary (for example, incision and drainage, extraction, pulpal extirpation), the patient should receive such care within the confines of an acute care facility (i.e., hospital). Although hospitalized patients are still at risk, their chances of survival may be increased in the event an acute medical emergency arises.

Examples of ASA IV patients include the following:
- Unstable angina pectoris (preinfarction angina)
- Myocardial infarction within the past 6 months
- CVA within the past 6 months
- Adult blood pressure greater than 200 mmHg or 115 mmHg
- Severe CHF or COPD (requiring $O_2$ supplementation or confinement in a wheelchair)
- Uncontrolled epilepsy (with a history of hospitalization)
- Uncontrolled IDDM (with a history of hospitalization)

*ASA V.* ASA V patients are moribund and are not expected to survive more than 24 hours with or without the planned surgery. ASA V patients almost always are hospitalized, terminally ill patients. They may be referred to as DNAR (do not attempt resuscitation) or "no code" patients. Resuscitation efforts are not instituted if the patient suffers respiratory or cardiac arrest. Elective dental treatment definitely is contraindicated; however, emergency care in the realm of palliative treatment (that is, pain relief) may be necessary. An ASA V classification is a "red light" for dental care.

Examples of ASA V patients include the following:
- End-stage renal disease
- End-stage hepatic disease
- End-stage cancer
- End-stage infectious disease
- End-stage cardiovascular disease
- End-stage respiratory disease

The ASA classification system is not only helpful in the determination of treatment risk but is also easy to employ. Classification is especially easy when a patient has but one isolated medical problem, such as the previous examples provided with each category. However, many patients suffer multiple ailments, in which case determination of the appropriate ASA classification may be more difficult. In such situations the doctor must weigh the significance of each disease and choose an appropriate category.

The ASA physical status classification system is not meant to be inflexible; rather, it should function as a relative value system based on a doctor's clinical judgment and assessment of the relevant clinical data available. When the doctor is unable to determine the clinical significance of one or more disease entities, consultation with the patient's physician or other medical or dental colleague is recommended. In all cases, however, the treating doctor ultimately must decide to either treat or postpone treatment. The ultimate responsibility for the health and safety of a patient rests solely in the hands of the treating doctor.

ASA I, II, and III patients are candidates for both elective and emergency dental treatment. The degree of risk represented by these patients increases with each successive category, as do the indications for treatment modification.

## MEDICAL CONSULTATION

A number of steps are involved in a typical medical consultation (Box 2-8). A dentist should not seek a medical consultation until the patient's dental and physical evaluations are completed. The dentist should be prepared to discuss fully with the patient's physician the proposed dental treatment plan and any anticipated problems. One of the most important considerations in medical consultation is the determination of the patient's ability to tolerate in relative safety the stress involved in the proposed dental treatment. The advice of the patient's regular physician should be carefully considered. Whenever doubt remains after a consultation, a second opinion, perhaps from a specialist in the specific area of concern, should be sought.

After a satisfactory consultation, the dentist next must consider the implementation of steps to minimize the perceived risk to the patient. The dentist holds the final responsibility for the dental treatment plan and its risks. Risk cannot be shared with the patient's physician. In most cases, medical consultation alters the dental plan minimally or not at all. Specific treatment modifications represent potentially important steps the dentist may undertake to decrease the patient's risk. (Specific modifications are discussed in the following section.)

## STRESS-REDUCTION PROTOCOL

At this point in the pretreatment evaluation, all relevant history and physical evaluation data have been reviewed, and a physical status classification has been assigned. Most patients are classified as ASA I or II

| box 2-8 | *Medical consultation* |

- Obtain the patient's dental and medical histories.
- Complete the physical examination, including both oral and general examination.
- Provide a tentative treatment plan based on the patient's oral needs.
- Make a general systemic assessment (choose a physical status category).
- Consult the patient's physician, when appropriate, via telephone:
  - Physician's receptionist
    - Introduce yourself and give the patient's name.
    - Ask to speak with the physician.
  - Physician:
    - Introduce yourself.
    - Give the patient's name and the reason for the visit to you.
    - Relate briefly your summary of the patient's general condition.
    - Ask for additional information about the patient.
    - Present your treatment plan briefly, including medications to be used and the degree of stress anticipated.
    - Discuss any problems.
  - After consultation:
    Write a complete report of the conversation for records and obtain a written report from the physician if possible.

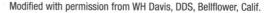
Modified with permission from WH Davis, DDS, Bellflower, Calif.

risks, a few as ASA III, and only a very small percentage as ASA IV. The percentages in each category change as the ages of the patients increase. In a study of the health histories and ASA classifications of more than 4000 dental patients in the Netherlands, percentages of ASA I and II patients decreased and percentages of ASA III and IV patients increased as the ages of the participants increased. Patients completed risk-related, patient-administered questionnaires. Classifications determined (all patients) for ASA I were 63.3%; for ASA II, 25.7%; for ASA III, 8.9%; and for ASA IV, 2.1%.[27]

Most dental procedures can prove stressful to patients. Stress may be of either a physiologic (pain or strenuous exercise) or psychologic nature (anxiety or fear). In either case, however, one of the body's responses to stress involves an increase in the release of catecholamines (epinephrine and norepinephrine) from the adrenal medulla and other tissue storage sites into the cardiovascular system, resulting in an increase in the body's cardiovascular workload (increased heart rate, strength of myocardial contraction, and myocardial $O_2$ requirement).

Although ASA I patients may be able to tolerate such changes in cardiovascular activity, ASA II, III, and IV patients increasingly are less able to withstand them safely. For example, patients with angina may respond to increased stress with episodes of chest pain, and various dysrhythmias may develop. Patients with CHF may develop acute pulmonary edema. Even patients with noncardiovascular disorders can respond adversely when faced with increased levels of stress. For example, patients with asthma may develop acute episodes of breathing difficulty (bronchospasm), and epileptic patients may suffer seizures.

Unusual degrees of stress in ASA I patients may be responsible for several psychogenically-induced emergency situations such as hyperventilation or vasodepressor syncope. Interviews with apprehensive dental patients have demonstrated that many patients begin to worry a day or two before their dental appointment. Such patients may have trouble sleeping the night before an appointment and arrive feeling fatigued and even less able to tolerate stress. The risk presented by these patients during dental treatment is increased even further.

The stress reduction protocol[28] listed in Box 2-9 includes two series of procedures that, when used either individually or collectively, minimize patient stress during treatment, which decreases the degree to which the patient is at risk. This protocol is based on the belief that the prevention or reduction of stress should begin before the appointment, continue throughout treatment, and follow through into the postoperative period, if necessary.

### Recognition of medical risk and anxiety

Recognition of risks and anxieties represents the starting point for the management of stress. Medical risk assessment is determined accurately through strict adherence to the measures previously described in this chapter, which include the medical history questionnaire, physical examination, and dialogue history. The recognition of anxiety is often a more difficult task. As previously discussed, visual observation and verbal communication with the patient can provide the doctor with important clues to the presence of dental anxiety.

### Medical consultation

Medical consultation with a patient's primary-care physician should be considered in those situations in which the doctor is uncertain about the degree to which the patient is at risk. Medical consultation is neither required nor recommended for all patients with medical problems. However, a consultation should be sought when the treating doctor is uncertain about the nature of the patient's disorder or the possible interactions between the

---

box **2-9**    *Stress-reduction protocols*

#### Normal, healthy, anxious patient (ASA I)

- Recognize the patient's level of anxiety.
- Premedicate the evening before the dental appointment, as needed.
- Premedicate immediately before the dental appointment, as needed.
- Schedule the appointment in the morning.
- Minimize the patient's waiting time.
- Consider psychosedation during therapy.
- Administer adequate pain control during therapy.
- Length of appointment variable.
- Follow up with postoperative pain and anxiety control.
- Telephone the highly anxious or fearful patient later the same day that treatment was delivered.

#### Medical risk patient (ASA II, III, IV)

- Recognize the patient's degree of medical risk.
- Complete medical consultation before dental therapy, as needed.
- Schedule the patient's appointment in the morning.
- Monitor and record preoperative and postoperative vital signs.
- Consider psychosedation during therapy.
- Administer adequate pain control during therapy.
- Length of appointment variable; do not exceed the patient's limits of tolerance.
- Follow up with postoperative pain and anxiety control.
- Telephone the higher medical risk patient later on the same day that treatment was delivered.
- Arrange the appointment for the highly anxious or fearful, moderate-to-high-risk patient during the first few days of the week (Monday through Wednesday in most countries; Saturday through Monday in Arabic countries) when the office is open for emergency care and the treating doctor is available.

---

disorder and the planned dental treatment. The doctor always must remember that a consultation is merely a request for additional information to aid in the determination of the degree of risk present and the therapy modification required. The final responsibility for the care and safety of a patient rests with the treating doctor.

**Premedication**    Many apprehensive patients state that their fear of dental treatment is so great that they are unable to get a good night's sleep the night before scheduled treatment. These patients are fatigued the day of the appointment and even less able to tolerate additional stress during treatment. If such a patient is also medically compromised, the risk of an acute exacerbation of the patient's medical problem increases. In an ASA I patient, such additional stress may provoke a psychogenically induced response. Clinical manifestations of increased fatigue include a lowered pain reaction threshold. Such a patient is more likely to interpret what is usually perceived as a nonpainful stimulus as painful than the well-rested patient.

Therefore the doctor should seek to determine whether a patient's heightened anxiety interferes with sleep. Oral sedation is one method a doctor can use to help the patient achieve restful sleep. The doctor may prescribe an antianxiety or sedative-hypnotic drug, such as triazolam or flurazepam, to be taken 1 hour before sleep. The appropriate use of oral antianxiety or sedative-hypnotic agents is an excellent method to help diminish preoperative stress. Other drugs, such as diazepam, oxazepam, hydroxyzine, promethazine, and chloral hydrate, have proved effective in adults and children. The use of barbiturates, such as secobarbital, pentobarbital, and hexobarbital, is not recommended.*

As the scheduled appointment time approaches and the patient's anxiety level heightens, the administration of such a drug approximately 1 hour before the scheduled treatment decreases the patient's anxiety level to such a degree that the thought of dental treatment is no longer frightening. (Oral medications should be administered about 1 hour before the scheduled start of treatment to permit development of the agent's therapeutic blood level.) Patients may take oral medications at home or in the dental office. However, when the doctor prescribes a CNS depressant for administration by the patient at home, the doctor must advise the patient against driving a car or operating other potentially hazardous machinery and document this advice in the chart.

**Appointment scheduling**    Apprehensive or medically compromised patients (including children) are able to tolerate stress best when they are well rested. Therefore the most appropriate time to schedule appointments with these patients is usually in the morning. When the apprehensive patient has an appointment in the afternoon, the patient must contend with the ominous specter of dental appointment, which casts a pall over the day and gives the patient time to worry. The patient becomes more anxious, which increases the likelihood that adverse psychogenic reactions may develop. A morning appointment permits this patient to "get it over with" and continue to perform daily activities without the burden of anxiety.

The medically compromised patient faces a similar situation. As fatigue sets in during the day, the patient is less able to manage increased stress. Before an afternoon appointment a medically compromised patient may have spent many hours at work and in traffic, rendering that patient less able to tolerate the stress of treatment. An earlier appointment provides both the patient and the doctor some degree of flexibility in management.

The doctor also should try to schedule treatment for the moderately to highly anxious medical risk patient early in the week so that if postoperative complications arise, the patient can contact and be seen promptly by the treating doctor. In addition, the doctor routinely should contact such patients later on the same day of dental treatment to check on their condition. Patients greatly appreciate such personal contact, which also helps minimize or prevent posttreatment complications.

**Minimized waiting time**    The apprehensive patient should not have to wait in the dental office for a long time before treatment begins. Anticipation of a procedure often can induce more fear that the actual procedure itself.[29] Sitting and waiting allows the patient to perceive dental office smells, hear dental office sounds, and fantasize about the "terrible things" that are going to happen. Cases of serious morbidity and death have occurred in dental office waiting rooms before treatment.[30] Minimal waiting time is of even greater significance for the apprehensive, medically compromised patient.

**Vital signs (preoperative and postoperative)**    Before beginning treatment on a medically compromised patient, the doctor routinely should measure and record the patient's vital signs. (A trained member of the auxiliary staff also can record vital signs.) Signs recorded should include blood pressure, heart rate and rhythm, and respiratory rate. Comparison of these signs to the patient's baseline values recorded at an earlier visit can indicate the patient's physical status at any given appointment. Although vital sign recordings are particularly relevant in patients with cardiovascular disease, they should be taken and recorded on all medically compromised (all ASA III and appropriate ASA II) patients. Postoperative vital signs also should be measured and recorded in these same patients regularly.

**Psychosedation during therapy**    If additional stress reduction is necessary during dental treatment, any sedation or general anesthesia tech-

---

*Doses of these and other drugs can be found in Malamed SF: *Sedation: a guide to patient management*, ed 3, St Louis, 1995, Mosby.

nique may be used. Nondrug techniques include ia-trosedation and hypnosis, whereas more commonly used pharmacosedation procedures include oral, in-halation, IM, and IV sedation. The primary goal of all these techniques is the same—to decrease or elimi-nate stress in a conscious patient. When appropriate techniques are used properly, this goal is usually achieved without any added risk to the patient. (The use of these techniques in various medical problems is discussed in later chapters.)

### Adequate pain control during therapy

Achieving adequate pain control is essential in effec-tive stress reduction, especially in the medically com-promised patient. For example, patients with clinically significant heart or blood vessel disease may be affected adversely by endogenously released catecholamines; such patients almost always warrant a vasoconstrictor in their local anesthetics. However, the doctor must always use and administer these drugs judiciously. Without adequate control of pain, sedation and stress reduction are impossible to achieve.

### Duration of dental treatment

The length of the treatment period is significant to both med-ically compromised and apprehensive patients. Unless the patient's condition warrants short visits, the doctor should consider the patient's wishes and decide on an appropriate length.

In many cases the apprehensive patient (ASA I or II) may prefer to have as few dental appointments as pos-sible regardless of length; this patient may prefer to manage the dental treatment with 3-hour or longer appointments. However, attempting to satisfy the pa-tient's desire for a longer appointment is inadvisable when the doctor believes that a shorter appointment is warranted. For example, cases of serious morbidity and death have occurred when doctors complied with parents' wishes to complete treatment of their children in one long appointment instead of multi-ple shorter visits.[31]

Unlike the anxious ASA I patient, the medically compromised patient should not undergo long ap-pointments. For many persons, being seated in a den-tal chair for 1 hour is quite stressful. Even a "good" ASA I patient may have some difficulty tolerating 2- or 3-hour dental procedures. Permitting a higher-risk patient to undergo such extended treatment unnec-essarily increases the patient's risk. Dental appoint-ments in the medically compromised patient there-fore should be shorter, never exceeding the limit of the patient's tolerance. Signs that this limit has been reached include evidence of fatigue, restlessness, sweating, and discomfort. The most prudent way to manage the patient at this time is to terminate the procedure as expeditiously as possible and resched-ule treatment for a later date.

### Postoperative control of pain and anxi-ety

Of equal importance to preoperative and intra-operative pain and anxiety control is the management of pain and anxiety after treatment.[32] Posttreatment management is especially relevant for the patient who has undergone a potentially traumatic procedure such as endodontics, periodontal or oral surgery, extensive oral reconstruction, or restorative procedures. The doctor must consider possible complications that might arise during the 24 hours immediately after den-tal care, discuss these with the patient, and take steps to assist the patient in their management. These steps may include any or all of the following:

- Be available by telephone 24 hours a day.
- Monitor pain control and prescribe analgesic med-ication as needed.
- Prescribe antibiotics if a possibility of infection exists.
- Prescribe antianxiety drugs if the patient requires them.
- Prescribe muscle relaxants after prolonged ther-apy or multiple injections into one area (such as inferior alveolar nerve block).

Availability of the doctor by telephone 24 hours a day has become the standard of care in dentistry. With answering services, telephone answering machines, and pagers readily available, the patient expects to be able to contact the doctor whenever necessary.

Several studies have demonstrated that patients consider unexpected pain more uncomfortable than expected pain.[33] If pain is a possibility after a proce-dure, the doctor should forewarn the patient and prescribe an analgesic drug. If the patient experi-ences posttreatment pain and was not warned, the patient immediately may think something has gone wrong. If the doctor discusses the possibility of post-treatment discomfort and the pain never material-izes, the patient remains relaxed and confident in the doctor's abilities.

In addition to the general modifications designed to reduce the patient's stress level, the doctor may consider therapy modifications for medically com-promised patients. Both the general and specific modifications for a given patient should be entered on the patient's permanent record (see Figure 2-20). Examples of specific therapy modifications include the following:

- The doctor may administer humidified $O_2$ intra-operatively through the nasal cannula at a flow of 3 to 4 L per minute (Figure 2-21). This procedure

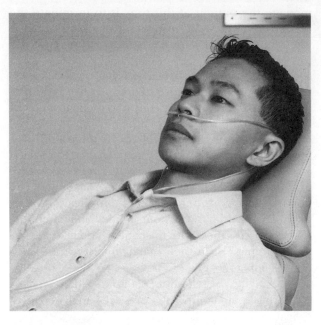

**Figure 2-21** As a therapy modification for medically compromised patients, the doctor may administer supplemental oxygen through a nasal cannula and humidifier.

may be necessary for patients with CHF or COPD who are judged ASA III risks.

- The doctor may modify the patient's positioning during treatment; some patients may be unable to tolerate the recommended supine or semisupine position and may require placement in a more upright position. Patients with significant degrees of orthopnea (three or four pillows) may be unable to breathe comfortably in a supine position.

- The doctor may opt not to use a rubber dam when treating patients with latex allergy or certain cardiovascular or respiratory disorders. If a rubber dam cannot be used, the doctor should warn the patient about the danger of swallowing or aspirating a foreign body (for example, a dental instrument) and make a note on the patient's chart.

Stress-reduction protocols and specific treatment modifications have improved patient management before, during, and after treatment. These protocols have made it possible to manage the dental health needs of a broad spectrum of both anxious and medically compromised patients with minimal complications.

## REFERENCES

1. McCarthy EM: Sudden, unexpected death in the dental office, *J Am Dent Assoc* 83:1091, 1971.

2. Goldberger E: *Treatment of cardiac emergencies,* ed 5, St Louis, 1990, Mosby.

3. McCarthy FM: A new, patient-administered medical history developed for dentistry, *J Am Dent Assoc* 111:595, 1985.

4. *Physicians' Desk Reference,* ed 52, Oradell, NJ, 1998, Medical Economics.

5. Skidmore-Roth L: *Mosby's 1999 nursing drug reference,* St Louis, 1999, Mosby.

6. American Dental Association: *ADA guide to dental therapeutics,* Chicago, 1998, The Association.

7. Dajani AS and others: Prevention of bacterial endocarditis: recommendations by the American Heart Association, *JAMA* 277(22):1794-1801, 1997.

8. Dajani AS and others: Prevention of bacterial endocarditis: recommendations by the American Heart Association, *J Am Dent Assoc* 128(8):1142-1151, 1997.

9. American Dental Association, American Academy of Orthopaedic Surgeons: Advisory statement: antibiotic prophylaxis for dental patients with total joint replacements, *J Am Dent Assoc* 128(7):1004-8, 1997.

10. Wilburn-Goo D, Lloyd LM: When patients become cyantonic: acquired methemoglobinemia, *J Am Dent Assoc* 130(6):826-831, 1999.

11. McCarthy FM: *Essentials of safe treatment for the medically compromised patient,* Philadelphia, 1989, WB Saunders.

12. Ridker PM and others: Clinical characteristics of nonfatal myocardial infarction among individuals on prophylactic low-dose aspirin therapy, *Circulation* 84(2):708-711, 1991.

13. Akahane Y and others: Hepatitis C virus infection in spouses of patients with type C chronic liver disease, *Ann Intern Med* 120(9):748-752, 1994.

14. Vivero LE, Anderson PO, Clark RF: A close look at fenfluramine and dexfenfluramine, *J Emerg Med* 16(2):197-205, 1998.

15. Dentists should exercise caution with fen-phen users, *N Y State Dent J* 63(10):20, 1997.

16. Brady WF, Martinoff JT: Validity of health history data collected from dental patients and patient perception of health status, *J Am Dent Assoc* 101:642, 1980.

17. Prior AJ, Drake-Lee AB: Auditing the reliability of recall of patients of minor surgical procedures, *Clin Otolaryngol* 16(4):373-375, 1991.

18. Dorman JM: The annual physical comes of age, *J Amer Coll Health* 38(5):205-206, 1990 (editorial).

19. American Heart Association: *Recommendations for human blood pressure determination by sphygmomanometry,* Dallas, 1967, The Association.

20. Cavallaro D, Melker R: Comparison of two techniques for determining cardiac activity in infants, *Crit Care Med* 11:189, 1983.

21. Bates B: *A visual guide to physical examination,* ed 3, Philadelphia, 1995, JB Lippincott.

22. Seidel HM and others: *Mosby's guide to physical examination,* ed 4, St Louis, 1999, Mosby.

23. Corah NL, Gale EN, Illig SJ: Assessment of a dental anxiety scale, *J Am Dent Assoc* 97:816, 1981.

24. Milgrom P and others: *Treating fearful dental patients,* Reston, Va, 1985, Reston Publishing.

25. American Society of Anesthesiologists: New classification of physical status, *Anesthesiology* 24:1, 1963.

26. Haynes SR, Lawler PG: An assessment of the consistency of ASA physical status classification allocation, *Anaesthesia* 50(3):195-199, 1995.

27. de Jong KJ, Oosting J, Abraham-Inpijn L: Medical risk classification of dental patients in the Netherlands, *J Public Health Dent* 53(4):219-222, 1993.

28. McCarthy FM: Stress reduction and therapy modifications, *J Calif Dent Assoc* 9:41, 1981.

29. Gale EN: Fears of the dental situation, *J Dent Res* 51:964, 1972.

30. Bell WH: Emergencies in and out of the dental office: a pilot study in the state of Texas, *J Am Dent Assoc* 74:778, 1967.

31. deJulien LE: Causes of severe morbidity/mortality cases, *J Cal Dent Assoc* 11:45, 1983.

32. Goodsen JM, Moore PA: Life-threatening reactions after pedodontic sedation: an assessment of opioid, local anesthetic, and antiemetic drug interaction, *J Am Dent Assoc* 107:239, 1983.

33. Corah N: Development of a dental anxiety scale, *J Res Dent* 48:596, 1969.

# 3

# *Preparation*

**D**ESPITE every effort to prevent them, life-threatening emergencies do occur in dental offices. Prevention, as successful as it may be, is not always enough. The entire dental office staff must be prepared fully to assist in the recognition and management of any potential emergency situation. If every staff member is not prepared, those few serious emergencies every doctor encounters may result in tragedy.

## General Information

Guidelines have been established to help doctors and staff members adequately prepare for the rapid and effective management of life-threatening situations. Most such guidelines have been developed by state boards of dental examiners in connection with the certification of doctors who wish to use parenteral sedation techniques, such as intramuscular (IM) or intravenous (IV) sedation or general anesthesia, in their offices.[1] Specialty groups, such as the American Association of Oral & Maxillofacial Surgeons,[2] the Academy of Pediatric Dentistry,[3] and the American Association of Periodontists have developed similar guidelines. The American Association of Dental Schools has developed curricular guidelines for the teaching of anesthesia and pain control that include recommendations for emergency preparation.[4]

Those primarily affected by these guidelines are doctors who have received advanced education and

51

training degrees in various techniques of drug administration. The guidelines provide lists of required personnel, equipment, and emergency drugs for the safe and effective management of emergency situations and suggest protocols for such management.

Unfortunately, no such guidelines exist for the overwhelming majority of doctors who have not received such advanced training in drug administration or who do not belong to these specialty societies. In addition, the level of training in emergency medicine that most health professionals receive varies considerably. Only a few doctors are experts in emergency medicine, whereas the vast majority possess no more than basic knowledge of emergency care.

Regardless of the doctor's level of training in emergency medicine, staff members should be equally prepared to manage these situations. The doctor always is expected to initiate emergency management and be capable of sustaining a patient's life through application of the steps of basic life support (BLS): (**P** [positioning], **A** [airway], **B** [breathing], and **C** [circulation]). **D** (definitive treatment), including the administration of drugs, is based on the training level of the treating doctor.

Some doctors will find themselves in special situations that require significantly more training than the basic level described in this text. In some parts of the world, including sections of the United States and Canada, sparsely populated areas still exist in which medical care—whether routine or emergency—is not readily available. In my numerous travels, I have met many dentists, assistants, and hygienists from rural areas of Montana, North Dakota, eastern Nevada, Arizona, New Mexico, Alaska, and throughout Canada who themselves handle all the health care needs in large geographic areas.

Many of these practitioners state that they are their area's primary source for emergency medical care because the nearest ambulance service is more than 1 hour away. Many of them are trained in advanced cardiac life support (ACLS) and certified in advanced trauma life support; others possess varying degrees of training as emergency medical technicians and paramedics. Morrow[5] suggests appropriate levels of emergency training for these doctors and recommends that they have immediate access to emergency kits based upon the distance between the dental office and nearest emergency medical facility.

## OFFICE PERSONNEL

Because the doctor cannot be with the patient from the time they walk through the door to the time they leave the office, all office staff members must be prepared to manage problems and emergencies that may arise in the doctor's absence. Preparation of dental staff members and of the office for medical emergencies should include the following minimal requirements:

1. Staff training should include BLS instruction for all members of the dental office staff, recognition and management of specific emergency situations, and emergency "fire drills."
2. Office preparation should include the posting of emergency assistance numbers and the stocking of emergency drugs and equipment.

**Training**  Without a doubt the most important step in the preparation for medical emergencies in the dental office is the training of all office personnel, including nonchairside employees (for example, receptionists and laboratory technicians), in the recognition and management of emergency situations. This training should include an annual refresher course in emergency medicine that includes all possible conditions, such as seizures, chest pain, and respiratory difficulty, rather than a review of BLS only. Continuing education courses are presented at most major dental meetings and through most local dental societies. Lists of scheduled courses are available from the American Dental Association.

**Basic life support**  The aforementioned training must include an understanding of and an ability to perform basic life support (cardiopulmonary resuscitation [CPR]). An understanding of CPR includes knowledge of **P-A-B-C.** All office personnel should be required to obtain certification at the level of a BLS health care provider (American Heart Association) or a professional rescuer (American Red Cross) at least once a year. BLS training should be included in every dental staff member's job description.

The ability of all office personnel to administer BLS is the most important step in the preparation for emergency management. All initial emergency management includes proper BLS administration. (Specific BLS techniques are discussed in detail in Chapters 5 and 30.) Many if not most emergency situations in the dental office are readily manageable through the use of these steps alone. Drug therapy is always relegated to a secondary role.

**Advanced cardiac life support**  Interesting and sobering statistics from the American Heart Association and other sources[6,7] have shown that the application of BLS alone does not provide the patient of an out-of-hospital cardiac arrest a great chance of survival. Survival rates are only 16% when BLS is initiated promptly and efficiently but the implementation of ACLS is delayed for more than 16 minutes. Although 16% may seem a dismal rate of survival, it contrasts dramatically with a 0% survival rate when BLS is not performed. On the other hand, survival rates for out-of-hospital cardiac arrest patients reached 43% in Seattle when rapid implementation of BLS was combined with more readily available (less than 8 minutes) ACLS.[7]

Some medical and dental professionals have used these data to argue against the requirement that dentists and physicians be CPR-certified before they can be licensed. This argument is faulty for two reasons:

1. CPR (BLS) is not used solely in situations of cardiac arrest.* In fact, most health professionals working outside the hospital may never need to use all three steps of BLS as they must with cardiac arrest. However, all health professionals, especially dentists, are required many times in the course of their professional lives to maintain an airway (**A**) and, on fewer occasions, to maintain the patient's breathing (**A + B**) in managing medical emergencies other than cardiac arrest.

2. A second reason why basic life support certification should be a requirement for dental licensure is that dentists are one of the few groups of health professionals permitted to learn and administer ACLS. Though the author does not advocate requiring ACLS for all dentists or for all physicians (though there are some groups for whom such training should be required, as described shortly), it is a plain and simple fact that ACLS will not be effective in the absence of BLS. Those dentists who practice in remote areas of the country where emergency medical assistance is less readily available seriously should consider certification in ACLS.

ACLS training involves the following areas:

1. Adjuncts for airway control and ventilation (including intubation)
2. Patient monitoring and dysrhythmia recognition
3. Defibrillation and synchronized cardioversion
4. Cardiovascular pharmacology
5. Acid-base balance maintenance
6. Venipuncture
7. Resuscitation of infants, including newborns

Although not all dentists need to know how to use these techniques, the steps are invaluable in emergency

situations. ACLS programs are provided by hospitals under the sponsorship of the American Heart Association. Such training is especially valuable to those who use parenteral sedation or general anesthesia in their offices. Local American Heart Association affiliates and in-house training programs at local hospitals or medical centers can provide additional ACLS information.

**Team management**    When office personnel are trained in the recognition and management of emergency situations, each person is able to maintain the life of a patient alone or as a member of a trained emergency team. Although management of most emergencies is possible with a single rescuer (often the doctor), the combined efforts of several trained individuals are usually more efficient. Because most dental offices have more than one staff member present during working hours (when most emergencies occur), a team approach is possible. The emergency team should consist of a minimum of two to three members, each with a predefined role in emergency management. The doctor usually leads the team and directs the actions of the other team members.

Team member 1, usually the doctor, is the person who is with the victim when the emergency is noticed or first reaches the victim. This member's primary task is to initiate BLS (**P-A-B-C**) as indicated by physical assessment of the victim. This individual also activates the office emergency system and calls for help to alert other office personnel to the need for assistance (similar to a "code blue" in a hospital). This member should remain with the victim throughout the emergency unless another team member steps in to relieve member 1. If the initial person at the scene is not the doctor, the doctor assumes the role of team member 1 on arrival.

*Duties of team member 1*
Provide BLS as indicated
Stay with the victim
Alert office staff members

Team member 2 should gather the emergency kit and portable oxygen ($O_2$) system and bring them to the emergency site.

*Duties of team member 2*
Bring emergency kit and $O_2$ to emergency site
Check $O_2$ daily
Check emergency kit weekly

Team member 3 acts as a circulating nurse or assistant. For example, a chairside assistant working alongside the doctor may serve in this capacity if the patient undergoing treatment is the victim of an

---

*I prefer to call this technique *basic life support* (BLS) instead of *cardiopulmonary resuscitation* (CPR). The term *CPR* conjures up images of a patient suffering cardiac arrest on whom chest compressions are being performed. In reality, airway and breathing doubtless are the components most often used in BLS. A movement is under way to change the name *CPR* to *CPCR* (*cardiopulmonarycerebral resuscitation*), a term that more fully describes the primary goal of BLS—the maintenance of normal brain function.

emergency. In another situation, member 3 may be the next person to come to the aid of member 1. Primary functions of member 3 include assisting member 1 with BLS as required, monitoring the victim's vital signs (blood pressure, heart rate and rhythm, respiration), and providing assistance as needed. For example, member 3 may prepare emergency drugs for administration, occasionally administer drugs, position the victim, loosen a collar or belt, activate emergency medical services (EMS) number, or perform all such duties.

Member 3 also may keep a written chronological record of all events, including vital signs, drug administration, and patient response to treatment. In a large medical office building, member 3 may be sent to the building's main entrance to meet the emergency medical technicians and lead them to the victim.

*Duties of team member 3*
Assist with BLS
Monitor vital signs
Prepare emergency drugs for administration
Activate EMS system
Assist as needed
Maintain records
Meet rescue team at building entrance

All office personnel must be able to function in emergency situations. In addition, all team members should be able to perform the duties of every other team member. Thus practice becomes vitally important.

**Emergency practice drills**    If life-threatening situations occurred with any regularity in dentistry, emergency practice sessions would be unnecessary; team members would receive their training under actual emergency conditions. Fortunately, life-threatening situations occur only infrequently. Therefore members of the dental office emergency team quickly become "rusty" because they are not given enough opportunities to practice. Annual refresher courses therefore are invaluable in the maintenance of a functional emergency team.

However, the ability of each team to perform well in the office setting is even more important. Periodic in-office emergency drills help to maintain efficient emergency teams in the absence of true emergency situations. All members of the team should respond exactly as they must under true emergency conditions. Some doctors purchase mannequins and hold frequent mandatory practice sessions at which staff members can practice CPR skills. In addition, instructional videotapes can provide visual examples of proper emergency management in the dental office,

including demonstrations in drug preparation and administration.[8-10]

For instance, the doctor prepares to administer a local anesthetic to a patient. As the syringe is inserted in the patient's mouth, the patient loses consciousness. The doctor (member 1) calls the other team members, using a code word or communication device such as a light or buzzer. Member 2, an assistant working in the back room, locates the portable $O_2$ cylinder and emergency drug kit and brings them to the emergency site while member 3, the chairside assistant, assists the doctor and victim. Member 1 initiates BLS, positioning the patient and ensuring a patent airway.

Member 3 monitors the victim's vital signs, beginning with the heart rate (carotid, brachial, or radial pulse). Under the doctor's supervision, member 2 prepares the $O_2$ for possible use and locates the aromatic ammonia vaporoles. If possible, member 3 will record, in chronological fashion, the vital signs and management of this situation. If the victim does not regain consciousness in a reasonable short period of time, member 2 or 3 activates the EMS system, meets the emergency personnel, and escorts them to the emergency site. If emergency drug administration is warranted, the doctor should, if possible, administer the drugs. However, if this is not possible, the doctor should assign another team member to administer the drugs under careful supervision.

In later chapters this text provides dental staff members with the proper guidelines for the prevention, recognition, and management of emergency situations.

However, emergency teams are effective only if team members practice on a regular basis.

**Office preparation: emergency medical assistance**    Emergency team members must be aware of whom to call when help is needed and when to call them.

*Whom to call.*  Although most office emergencies may be managed efficiently by the office emergency team, some may require additional assistance. The doctor must consider this matter before the situation actually develops. Certain emergency telephone numbers should be available and conspicuously displayed near all office telephones. The doctor may want to include the telephone numbers of local EMS personnel (9-1-1 in the United States and 9-9-9 in Great Britain), a dental or medical professional in close proximity to the office who has been well-trained in emergency management, an emergency ambulance service, and a nearby hospital emergency room.

Most U.S. communities and an increasing number of countries worldwide have instituted universal emergency numbers to expedite activation of fire, police, and EMS personnel. Though varying degrees of sophistication exist, this number usually connects the caller to an emergency operator who screens the call and activates the appropriate response (fire, police, medical). When emergency medical care is required in the dental office, the community EMS is the preferred source for immediate assistance. However, because not all areas have the 9-1-1 system, additional emergency telephone numbers should be posted, if needed.

The team member who calls the EMS operator must try to remain calm and clearly provide the operator with all requested information. The operator may request the nature of the emergency in general terms (for example, whether the patient is conscious or unconscious or has chest pain or seizures) and the location of the office.* The address of the dental office should be posted by every telephone. If the office is located in a large professional building, a team member should wait near the building's main entrance to hold an elevator for emergency personnel and escort them to the emergency site.

The doctor also can enlist the help of a well-trained dental or medical professional in preparation for an emergency. This arrangement should be finalized before help is actually needed, and the doctor should check to ensure this professional is available during the doctor's office hours. I have found that the best-trained individuals in this field are emergency medicine physicians, anesthesiologists (both medical and dental), surgeons (medical), and oral and maxillofacial surgeons (dental).

Unfortunately, the first two groups of physicians are hospital-based and not readily available for assistance outside the hospital. However, most medical and dental surgeons and dental anesthesiologists maintain private practices in the community and may be available. Prior arrangement with these individuals can help prevent misunderstandings and increase their usefulness in emergency situations.

Many emergency ambulance services require that their personnel be trained as emergency medical technicians. These individuals can assist the doctor in the absence of additional help. The level of assistance available in this case will vary, ranging from basic life support to advanced cardiac life support.

The location of the hospital close to the dental office should be determined. This facility should have a 24-hour emergency department staffed with fully trained emergency personnel. All office staff members should determine the nearest fully equipped hospital emergency room to their place of residence. The American Heart Association periodically evaluates hospital emergency departments and awards symbols that are prominently displayed outside emergency departments that successfully meet their requirements (Figure 3-1). Evaluations are made for adult and pediatric emergency departments.

*Whom to call*
EMS (9-1-1)
Nearby medical or dental doctor well trained in
    emergency medicine
Ambulance service
Nearby hospital with American Heart Association-
    approved emergency room

One point worth stressing in an emergency situation is that the telephone number for EMS in most U.S. areas is 9-1-1 (nine-one-one) and not 911 (nine-eleven). In moments of panic, callers may become confused and be unable to locate the 11 (eleven) on the telephone keypad. In a number of recorded inci-

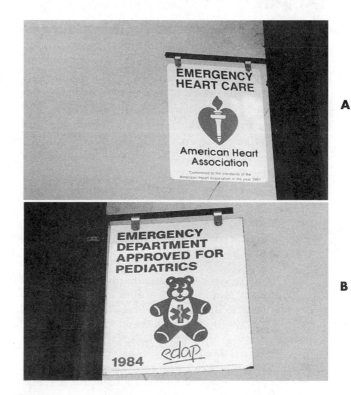

**Figure 3-1** **A,** Emergency heart care seal from American Heart Association. **B,** Pediatric emergency care seal.

*More advanced EMS systems automatically provide the address of the caller if the caller remains on the line for a minimum of 15 seconds. However, address errors have occurred, especially when the address has been changed but the telephone number has not. The caller should confirm the address when placing the call.

dents, this problem has led to a delayed arrival (or nonarrival) of EMS personnel, and the death of the victim.

*When to call.* The designated team member should call for EMS assistance as soon as the individual responsible for the patient's health and safety (usually the doctor) deems it necessary. Never hesitate to seek assistance if any doubt remains as to the nature of the situation or its management. The earlier the assistance is sought, the better.

## EMERGENCY DRUGS AND EQUIPMENT

Emergency drugs and equipment must be available in every dental office. In a survey of 2704 dentists in the United States and Canada, 84% had emergency drugs and equipment available.[11] Although most emergency situations do not demand the administration of drugs, on occasion it may save lives. For example, in acute systemic allergy (anaphylaxis), the administration of epinephrine is essential to the patient's survival. In most instances, however, drug administration is secondary in overall management to BLS.

## COMMERCIAL VERSUS HOMEMADE EMERGENCY DRUG KITS

A number of emergency kits are produced commercially for sale to dental and medical professionals. Although some of these kits are well equipped, others contain drugs and equipment of dubious value in a typical medical or dental office. These kits usually are produced by the manufacturer in conjunction with experts in emergency medicine. The drugs and equipment these kits provide all too often reflect the expertise of the experts, not the level of training of the doctors for whom they are designed.

The Council on Dental Therapeutics of the American Dental Association issued a report on emergency drug kits in 1973.[12] An updated report was published in 1998.[13] The following statement, equally true today, is an excerpt from the 1973 report:

> None of these kits is compatible with the needs of all practitioners, and their promotion is sometimes misleading. All dentists must be prepared to diagnose and treat expeditiously life-threatening emergencies that may arise in their practices. The best way to accomplish this objective is by taking continuing education courses on the subject of emergencies to remain informed on current practices recommended for handling emergencies in the office. A false sense of security may be engendered by the purchase of a kit if the practitioner presumes

that it will fulfill all the needs of an emergency situation. The most important factors in effective treatment of emergencies are the knowledge, judgment, and preparedness of the dentist . . . Since emergency kits should be individualized to meet the special needs and capabilities of each clinician, no stereotyped kit can be approved by the Council on Dental Therapeutics. Practitioners are encouraged to assemble their own individual kit that will be safe and effective in their hands or to purchase a kit that contains drugs that they are fully trained to administer.

Figures 3-2 through 3-5 illustrate a variety of commercially prepared and self-made emergency drug kits.

The best emergency drug kit is one the doctor designs personally to meet that doctor's special requirements and capabilities. In my experience, commercially prepared emergency kits are quickly placed in cabinets, where they remain until an emergency arises. The doctor and staff members spend little if any time familiarizing themselves with the contents of the kit or the indications for the use of its drugs. Worse yet, the doctor may try to use the drugs inside without being familiar with them or with the nature of the patient's problem. The emergency kit quickly becomes a security blanket that provides little security. By preparing an individualized kit, the doctor will become familiar with all the drugs and equipment inside. This inti-

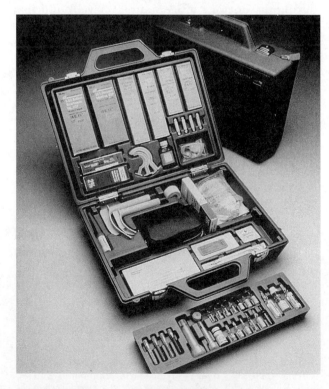

**Figure 3-2** Banyan STAT KIT 600. (Courtesy Banyan International Corporation, Abilene, Texas 79601.)

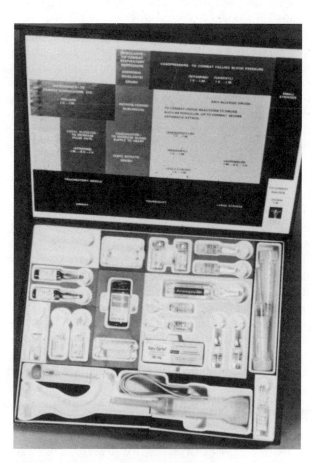

**Figure 3-3** Healthfirst Emergency Kit (Courtesy Healthfirst Corporation, Edmonds, Wash).

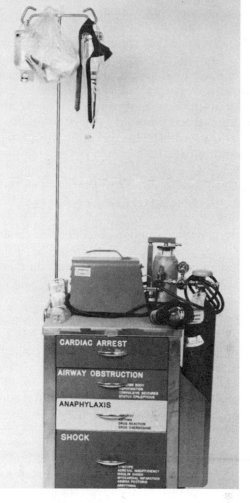

**Figure 3-4** Self-made emergency kit for office with personnel who are well trained in emergency medicine.

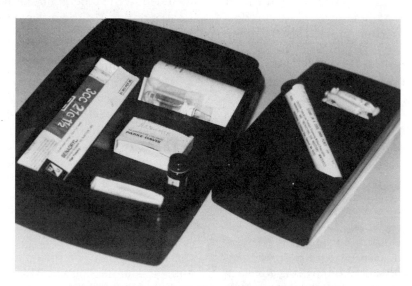

**Figure 3-5** Basic, self-made drug emergency kit.

mate knowledge benefits both the doctor and the patient in an emergency situation.

Each doctor should select items for the emergency kit based on that doctor's training in emergency medicine, the importance of the drug in the successful outcome of the situation, and in some cases, regulations for mandatory drugs and equipment. The latter requirement usually is found in specialty practices such as anesthesiology or parenteral sedation,[1] oral and maxillofacial surgery,[2] pedodontics,[3] and periodontology.

## Emergency Drug Kits

The dental office emergency kit need not and indeed should not be complicated. It should be as simple as possible to use. Pallasch's statement[14] that "complexity in a time of adversity breeds chaos" is all too true. The doctor should remember three things in preparing and using emergency drug kits:

1. Drug administration is not necessary for the immediate management of medical emergencies.
2. Primary management of all emergency situations involves BLS.
3. When in doubt, never medicate.

The emergency kit described in the following sections is a simple, organized collection of drugs and equipment that has been highly effective in the management of life-threatening situations that occur in dental offices. However, the proper management of a patient in most emergency situations does not require drug administration. First and foremost in the management of emergency situations are the steps of BLS (**P-A-B-C**). Only after these steps have been implemented does the doctor consider administering drugs. Even in acute anaphylaxis, in which the patient experiences immediate respiratory distress, circulatory collapse, or both, BLS remains the immediate response, followed almost as rapidly by the administration of epinephrine. Management of all emergency situations follows the **P-A-B-C-D** protocol (**D** . . . definitive management: drugs and EMS).

### ITEMS IN AN EMERGENCY KIT

The following guidelines will aid in the development of a useful and effective dental office emergency kit. Therapeutic categories for inclusion in the kit are listed, suggestions are offered for specific drugs within each group, and selection criteria for each drug mentioned explained.

Doctors should consider including items from each therapeutic category in the emergency kit; however, doctors should select only those drugs with which they are familiar and able to use. Suggested drugs are listed with alternatives in many instances. The doctor must evaluate carefully every item that goes into the emergency drug kit. If the doctor has any doubts about the categories or specific agents, consultation with a physician (preferably a specialist in emergency medicine) or hospital pharmacist is recommended but above all determine their reasons for suggesting a certain drug or drug category over others.

All drugs come with drug-package inserts. Doctors should save this information sheet from each drug included in their kit, read it, and take note of important information about the drug, including its indications, usual doses (pediatric, adult, and geriatric), adverse reactions, and expiration dates. Many doctors transfer this information to an index card for quick reference. The emergency drugs and equipment described in the following sections are presented in four levels, or modules. The design of each of the following modules is based on the doctor's level of training and experience in emergency medicine:

- Module one: basic emergency kit (critical drugs and equipment)
- Module two: noncritical drugs and equipment
- Module three: ACLS
- Module four: antidotal drugs

Two categories of drugs are described for each module—injectable and noninjectable drugs, as well as emergency equipment. Doctors always must remember that the categories of drugs and equipment included in the emergency kit must conform to the level of training of the office personnel who will use it. Emergency kits should be simple but effective. The "KISS" principle (keep it simple, stupid) is an appropriate guideline.

A complete discussion of when and how each item should be used can be found in the sections on management of specific emergencies. The drugs and equipment in the emergency kit are intended for use in patients of any age (pediatric, adult, or geriatric). Doctors must be aware of the distinction in therapeutic doses between patients of different ages; pediatric (and in many cases, geriatric) doses are smaller than adult doses. Specific drug doses are not emphasized in this chapter but are presented in individual discussions of emergency management.

Most injectable emergency drugs are prepared in a 1-ml glass ampule or vial. The number of milligrams of drug present in 1 ml of solution varies from drug

table **3-1** *Injectable drug doses*

| | AGE RANGE (YR) | ml OF SOLUTION | EPINEPHRINE (1:1000) (ml) |
|---|---|---|---|
| Adult | >7 | 1.0 | 0.3 |
| Child | 1-7 | 0.5 | 0.15 |
| Infant | <1 | 0.25 | 0.075 |

to drug. For example, diazepam is 5 mg/ml, whereas diphenhydramine is 50 mg/ml and ephedrine is 10 mg/ml. The 1-ml form of the drug is known as its *therapeutic dose,* or *unit dose.* Thus 1 ml of solution is the usual dose of the drug administered to an adult patient in an emergency situation. For pediatric patients (1 year through 7 years) the therapeutic dose of an injectable drug is 0.5 ml, or one-half the adult dose; for infants under 1 year, the therapeutic dose is 0.25 ml, or one-quarter the adult dose (Table 3-1).

However, epinephrine is a major exception to this basic rule of doses. Although the 1-ml form of 1:1000 epinephrine solution is considered the adult therapeutic dose, a smaller dose—0.3 ml—is recommended, with subsequent doses based on the patient's response. Pediatric and infant epinephrine doses are reduced accordingly (0.15 ml and 0.075 ml of a 1:1000 epinephrine solution).

Noninjectable drugs usually are prepared so that one tablet or spray is the adult therapeutic dose. Many noninjectable drugs also are prepared in pediatric forms to simplify administration. Because both adults and children are seen in most dental offices, the doctor should consider including both forms in the emergency drug kit.

Other items of emergency equipment should be available in both adult and pediatric forms. These include face masks and oropharyngeal and nasopharyngeal airways (if included). Indeed the pediatric dentist must provide a wider range of equipment in both pediatric (for the patient) and adult (for the doctor or staff patient) sizes than the doctor who treats only adults.

## ADMINISTRATION OF INJECTABLE DRUGS

For a drug to exert a therapeutic effect a minimum therapeutic blood level must be achieved in the target organ (for example, the brain [anticonvulsants] or heart [antidysrhythmics]) or target system (skin). In other words, enough of the drug must enter the bloodstream and be transported to the part of the body where it is needed. Therefore the ideal route for emergency drug administration is IV; onset of action is approximately 20 seconds, and the drug effect the most reliable of all routes of administration.

Unfortunately, unless the doctor has established an IV line in the patient before the emergency occurs, many doctors may find its insertion difficult if not impossible during the emergency. Unless a doctor is adept at venipuncture, an alternative route of administration should be employed. Emergency drugs may be administered via the IM route into various sites, most often the anterolateral aspect of the thigh (vastus lateralis), the middeltoid region of the upper arm, and the upper outer quadrant of the gluteal region. IM administered drugs have an onset of action of about 10 minutes with normal tissue perfusion. This is somewhat slower with decreased blood pressure (hypotension). Of these three traditional IM injection sites, the middeltoid provides the most rapid uptake of most drugs (because of its greater tissue perfusion) and is therefore the site of choice. The vastus lateralis is a close second because of its accessibility and anatomic safety. In the younger pediatric patient the vastus lateralis is the preferred IM injection site. Emergency drugs should not be administered in the gluteal region because it lacks vascularity compared with the previous sites. A number of anatomic considerations, especially with pediatric patients, also accompany drug administration in the gluteal region.

One additional site provides an even more effective and rapid uptake than the middeltoid region—the tongue. Emergency drugs can be injected either into the body of the tongue (intralingual injection) or sublingually for a more rapid uptake and onset of clinical action. The drug may be administered into the body of the tongue or floor of the mouth, either intraorally (Figure 3-6, *A*) or extraorally (Figure 3-6, *B*). Onset of action is approximately 5 to 10 minutes in the presence of effective circulation, but slower in patients with hypotension.

The steps of BLS must continue as needed while the emergency team awaits the onset of the drug's action. However, in the absence of effective circulation, neither IV nor IM drugs are effective. In this situation (as in all emergency situations), drugs are secondary to BLS.

In situations where IV access is impossible but a patient has been successfully intubated, the administration of certain drugs (epinephrine, lidocaine, atropine, naxolone, and flumazenil) into the endotracheal tube provides a rapid onset of action as the drug is absorbed from the well-perfused pulmonary vascular bed (Box 3-1).

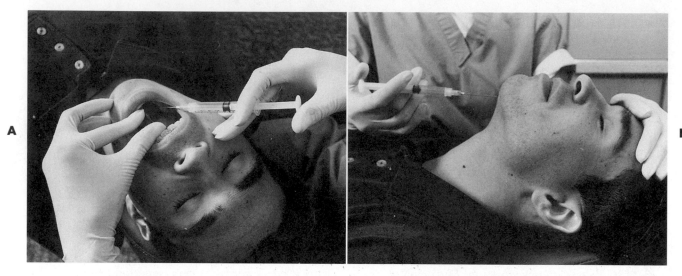

**Figure 3-6** **A,** Intralingual injection—intraoral approach. **B,** Intralingual injection—extra-oral approach.

*Drug administration classified by rate of onset*

1. Endotracheal (when available): epinephrine, lidocaine, atropine, naloxone, and flumazenil only
2. Intravenous
3. Sublingual or intralingual
4. Intramuscular
   a. Vastus lateralis
   b. Middeltoid
   c. Gluteal region

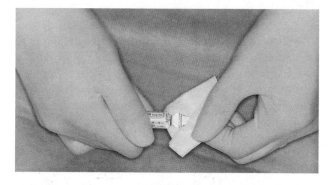

**Figure 3-7** Ampule, held between fingers, cracks at pre-scored neck.

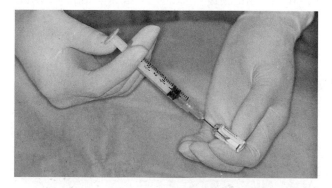

**Figure 3-8** Syringe is loaded with medication.

**Parenteral drug administration** Virtually all injectable emergency drugs can be purchased in preloaded syringes. I strongly believe that these drugs should not be available in preloaded form in the typical dental office because they become too easy to administer. In almost all emergencies, there is no urgent need to administer any drug to the victim other than O₂.

However, I do recommend keeping preloaded syringes of epinephrine because this drug must be administered promptly when an acute allergic reaction develops. With only epinephrine available preloaded, doctors and staff members are less likely to be confused about which drug to administer in an emergency. ACLS drugs normally are available in preloaded form but should be kept separate from other emergency drugs. The time it takes to prepare drugs in syringes for administration can be better used to perform BLS **(P-A-B-C).**

To prepare an injectable emergency drug for either IM or IV administration, the rescuer breaks the unit-dose ampule by covering the prescored neck with a gauze pad (Figure 3-7) and loading the drug into the syringe (Figure 3-8). The individual who administers the drug always must check its printed label to determine the drug's name and dose, especially when ad-

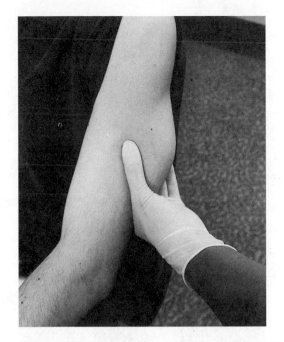

**Figure 3-9** Intramuscular injection—muscle pulled away from bone.

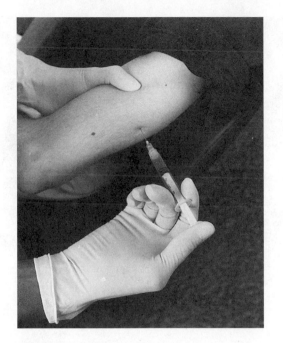

**Figure 3-10** Intramuscular injection—syringe held like dart, needle advanced 1 inch into tissue.

ministering epinephrine, naloxone, and meperidine, which are available in more than one dosage form. Furthermore, when the situation is not urgent, the doctor or staff member should label the loaded syringe with the drug's name and concentration (in milligram/milliliter).

**IM administration**  The following steps outline the technique for the administration of drugs via IM routes:

1. Cleanse the area of needle insertion.
2. Grab the muscle and pull it away from the bone (Figure 3-9).
3. Holding the syringe like a dart, quickly insert the needle into the muscle mass approximately 1 inch (one-half the length of the needle [Figures 3-10 and 3-11]).
4. Aspirate to ensure nonvascular penetration.
5. Quickly administer the drug.
6. Remove the syringe, placing a piece of dry gauze and applying pressure to the injection site for a minimum of 1 to 2 minutes.
7. Rub the area to increase vascularity and rate of drug absorption.

(IM drug administration and venipuncture are reviewed in depth in selected texts.[15])

**IV administration**  The following steps outline the technique of venipuncture.

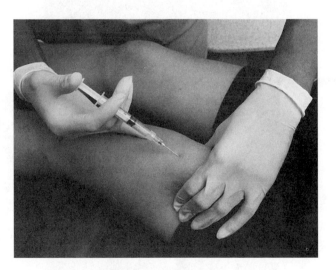

**Figure 3-11**  IM injection in vastus lateralis.

1. Place a tourniquet above the antecubital fossa (Figure 3-12).
2. Have the patient open and close the fist to help distend veins (Figure 3-13). When the patient cannot open and close the fist (as with the unconscious or uncooperative patient), the arm should be placed below the level of the patient's heart to help distend the veins (Figure 3-14).

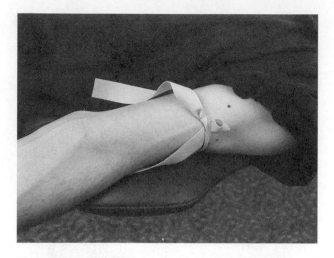

**Figure 3-12**  Intravenous tourniquet placed above antecubital fossa.

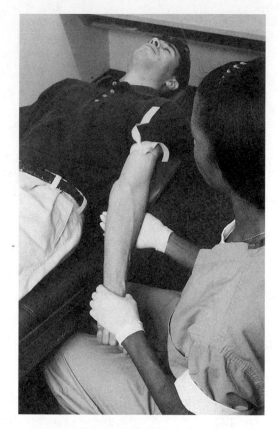

**Figure 3-14**  Veins may be distended by keeping arm below level of heart.

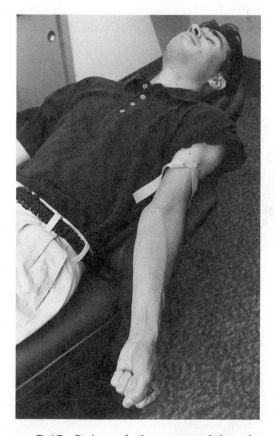

**Figure 3-13**  Patient asked to open and then close fist for help distending veins.

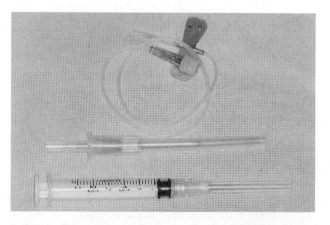

**Figure 3-15**  Scalp vein needle, indwelling catheter, and syringe (*top* to *bottom*).

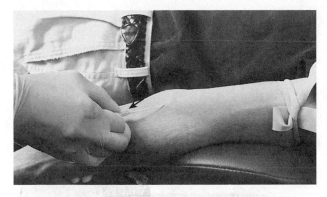

**Figure 3-16**   Needle held at 30° angle for penetration of skin.

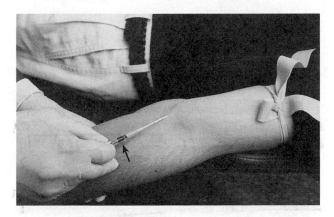

**Figure 3-17**   Return of blood into needle is sign of successful venipuncture.

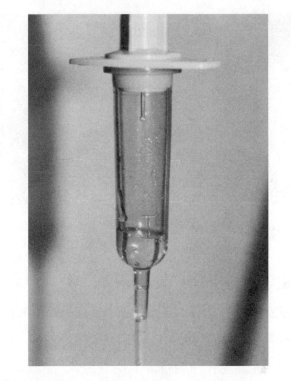

**Figure 3-18**   Infusion set for continuous intravenous infusion.

3. Cleanse and dry the area in which the vein is to be punctured.
4. Angle an indwelling catheter, scalp vein needle, or syringe (Figure 3-15), with the bevel of the needle facing up, at about a 30-degree angle to the vein to be entered (Figure 3-16).
5. Advance the needle into the vein until a return of blood is noted (Figure 3-17).

NOTE: The return of blood into the needle is the only consistent sign of a successful venipuncture.

6. Remove the tourniquet and either start the IV infusion (Figure 3-18) or administer the desired drug (Figure 3-19).
7. Secure the needle with tape to maintain venous access (Figure 3-20).

In dental offices in which the doctor is well versed in emergency drugs and their administration and has a well-trained emergency team, preloaded

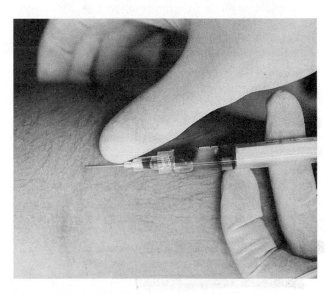

**Figure 3-19**   Needle/syringe in vein. Drug injected directed into vein.

and labeled syringes of emergency drugs are more appropriate. This situation most likely is found when the doctor has been trained in the techniques of general anesthesia or, in certain instances, IV conscious sedation.

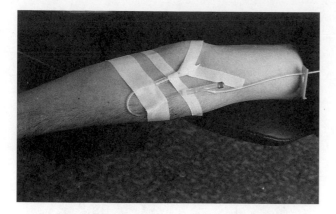

**Figure 3-20** Continuous infusion secured by tape.

# Module One: Critical (Essential) Emergency Drugs and Equipment

What should be included in the minimum, (absolutely basic) emergency kit for a dental or medical office? As always, BLS training is the most significant asset and the first technique to be used in all emergency management. However, a number of injectable and noninjectable drugs and items of equipment should also be considered absolutely essential for inclusion in the dental office emergency kit (Table 3-2).

## CRITICAL INJECTABLE DRUGS

The following two categories of injectable drugs are considered critical in any emergency kit:
1. Epinephrine
2. Histamine blockers

Both drugs are used in the management of an acute allergic reaction, one of the most feared of all emergency situations faced by the health professional.

### Primary injectable: drug for acute allergic reaction (anaphylaxis)

*Drug of choice:* Epinephrine
*Drug class:* Catecholamine
*Alternative drug:* None
*Proprietary:* Ana-Guard, Epipen, Epipen Jr.

Epinephrine (Adrenalin) is the most important emergency drug in medicine. Epinephrine is the drug of choice in the management of the acute (life-threatening) allergic reaction. Epinephrine is valuable in the management of both the respiratory and cardiovascular manifestations of acute allergic reactions. Desirable properties of epinephrine include: (1)

a rapid onset of action; (2) potent action as a bronchial smooth muscle dilator (beta2 properties); (3) histamine-blocking properties; (4) vasopressor actions; and (5) its actions on the heart, which include an increase in heart rate (21%), increased systolic blood pressure (5%), decreased diastolic blood pressure (14%), increased cardiac output (51%), and increased coronary blood flow. Undesirable actions include epinephrine's tendency to predispose the heart to dysrhythmias and its relatively short duration of action.

*Therapeutic indications:* A 1:1000 concentration of epinephrine should be used to treat cases of acute allergic reaction (anaphylaxis, see Chapter 24) and acute asthmatic attack (bronchospasm, see noninjectable drugs and Chapter 13). A 1:10,000 concentration is recommended in the management of cardiac arrest (ACLS, see Chapter 30).

*Side effects, contraindications, and precautions:* Tachydysrhythmias, both supraventricular and ventricular, may develop. Epinephrine should be administered with caution to pregnant women because it decreases placental blood flow and can induce premature labor. When it is used, all vital signs should be monitored frequently. In the setting of the dental office, epinephrine will usually be considered for administration in situations felt to be acutely life-threatening, such as anaphylaxis and (possibly) cardiac arrest. In such situations the advantages of epinephrine administration clearly outweigh any risks. No contraindications exist to epinephrine administration under these conditions.

*Availability:* Epinephrine for parenteral administration is supplied in either a 1:1000 concentration (1g [1000 mg]/l), in which each milliliter contains 1 mg of the agent, or as a 1:10,000 concentration. The 1:1000 concentration is meant for IM and subcutaneous administration only, whereas the 1:10,000 concentration is designed for IV administration. Because the dosage of this drug is critical, it is advisable to have parenteral epinephrine available in preloaded syringe form rather than in a multidose vial. In addition, preloaded syringes permit the drug to be administered quickly, a requirement in the treatment of the acute allergic reaction. It is recommended therefore that epinephrine be available in preloaded syringes and 1-ml ampules.

Because of its short duration of action and because the dose administered is 0.3 mg, multiple administrations are usually necessary during the management of the acute phase of anaphylaxis. Unit-dose (1-ml) ampules are preferred over multidose vials because the unit-dose form prevents the doctor

| table **3-2** | Module one—critical (essential) emergency drugs and equipment |

| | **PRIMARY DRUG** | | | **RECOMMENDED FOR KIT** | |
|---|---|---|---|---|---|
| **CATEGORY** | **GENERIC** | **PROPRIETARY** | **ALTERNATIVE** | **QUANTITY** | **AVAILABILITY** |
| **Injectables** | | | | | |
| Antiallergy | Epinephrine | Adrenalin | None | One preloaded syringe and 3 - 4 × 1-ml ampules | 1:1000 (1 mg/ml) |
| Histamine blocker | Chlorpheniramine | ChlorTrimeton | Diphenhydramine | 3 - 4 × 1-ml ampules | 10 mg/ml |
| **Noninjectables** | | | | | |
| Oxygen | Oxygen | | None | Minimum of 1 E cylinder | |
| Vasodilator | Nitroglycerin | Nitrolingual spray | Nitrostat SL tablets | One metered spray bottle | 0.4 mg/dose |
| Bronchodilator | Albuterol | Proventil, Ventolin | Metaproterenol | One metered dose inhaler | |
| Antihypoglycemic | Sugar | | | Orange juice, nondiet soft drink | |
| Antiplatelet | Aspirin | Many | None | 3 or 4 chewable (162 mg) tablets | 162, 325 mg |

| **EQUIPMENT** | **DESCRIPTION** | **QUANTITY** |
|---|---|---|
| **Emergency equipment** | | |
| Oxygen delivery system | Positive-pressure and demand valve, or bag-valve-mask device and clear full-face masks of various sizes | Minimum of one oxygen delivery system with positive-pressure mask<br>One portable bag-valve-mask device<br>Minimum of 1 child, one small-adult, and one large-adult full-face masks |
| | Pocket mask | One pocket mask per employee |
| Syringes for drug administration | Disposable syringes | 2 - 4 × 2-ml syringes with attached needles for parenteral drug administration |
| Suction and suction tips | High-volume suction system | Office suction system |
| | Large-diameter, round-ended suction tips or tonsillar suction | Minimum of two |
| Tourniquets | Rubber or Velcro tourniquet, rubber tubing, or sphygmomanometer | Three tourniquets and one sphygmomanometer |
| Magill intubation forceps | Blunt-ended scissors with right-angle bend | One pediatric-size forceps |

or other staff member from inadvertently overadministering epinephrine. An overdose of epinephrine can produce significant complications.[16,17]

*Dose:* Although the 1-ml ampule of 1:1000 epinephrine is considered the adult therapeutic dose, epinephrine is administered via the IM or subcutaneous route in a dose of 0.3 to 0.5 ml of solution with additional doses administered as needed. This break with tradition (1 ml as the adult therapeutic dose of an emergency drug) stems from the fact that although 1 mg of epinephrine is the usual therapeutic dose for anaphylaxis, this dose may be excessive for some patients. For instance, the person with significant cardiovascular disease (for example, American Society of Anesthesiologists [ASA] IV, status post–myocardial infarction or high blood pressure, or post–cerebrovascular accident)

who suffers an anaphylactic reaction to an insect bite and receives 1 ml of a 1:1000 epinephrine solution probably will not die from the allergic response. However, the possibility that the epinephrine's action on the patient's cardiovascular system can lead to serious adverse consequences is increased.

Unfortunately, in what may be a near-panic situation (anaphylaxis) the doctor may administer to the victim an overly large dose of epinephrine. Preloaded syringes are available that make it impossible to administer in excess of the predetermined dose (Figure 3-21).[18,19] The syringe's plunger and guide channel are rectangular. However, at the 0.3-ml mark the rectangle shifts 90 degrees, which makes the administration of more than 0.3 ml (0.3 mg) at a time impossible. The plunger must be rotated to administer an additional dose. Such a syringe is highly recommended

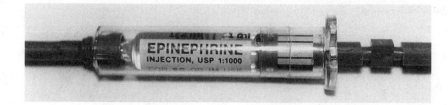

**Figure 3-21**    2-dose epinephrine syringe administers 0.3 mg per dose.

for inclusion in all emergency drug kits. Pediatric forms of these syringes that deliver a dose of 0.15 mg also are available.

*Suggested for emergency kit:* Each kit should have one preloaded syringe (1 ml of 1:1000 [1 mg epinephrine]) and three or four ampules of 1:1000 epinephrine to treat anaphylaxis either via an IM or subcutaneous route.

## Primary injectable: drug for allergic reaction

*Drug of choice:* Chlorpheniramine
*Proprietary:* ChlorTrimeton
*Drug class:* Histamine blocker (antihistamine)
*Alternative drug:* Diphenhydramine

Antihistamines now are categorized as *histamine blockers,* a term that better describes their mode of clinical action. Histamine blockers are valuable in the management of the more common delayed allergic response and in the definitive management of the acute allergic reaction (administered after epinephrine has resolved the life-threatening phase of the reaction). Histamine blockers are competitive antagonists of histamine; they do not prevent the release of histamine from cells in response to injury, drugs, or antigens but do prevent histamine's access to its receptor site in the cell, blocking the response of the effector cell to histamine. Therefore histamine blockers are more potent in preventing the actions of histamine than in reversing these actions once they occur. An interesting action of many histamine blockers is that they are also potent local anesthetics, especially diphenhydramine and tripelennamine.[20,21]

The choice of a specific histamine blocker for the emergency kit was made after considering that most patients seeking dental care are ambulatory and desire to leave the dental office unescorted (probably to drive a car). However, cortical depression (sedation), a potential side effect of many histamine blockers, should prevent the patient from being discharged from the dental office unescorted.

Diphenhydramine HCl (Benadryl) causes sedation in nearly 50% of individuals. On the other hand, chlorpheniramine (ChlorTrimeton), produces less sedation (10%) than diphenhydramine with an equivalent histamine-blocking action.

*Therapeutic indications:* Histamine blockers are recommended in management of delayed-onset allergic reactions, the definitive management of acute allergic reactions, and as local anesthetics when the patient has a history of alleged allergy to local anesthesia (see Chapter 24).

*Side effects, contraindications, and precautions:* Side effects of histamine blockers include central nervous system depression, decreased blood pressure, and thickening of bronchial secretions resulting from the drug's drying action. Because of this drying effect, histamine blockers are contraindicated in the management of acute asthmatic episodes.

*Availability:* Chlorpheniramine is available in 10 mg/ml in 1- and 2-ml ampules and in 1-ml preloaded syringes. Diphenhydramine is available in 10 mg/ml in 10- and 30-ml multidose vials, 50 mg/ml in 1-ml ampules and 10-ml multidose vials, and 1-ml preloaded syringes.

*Suggested for emergency kit:* The emergency kit should contain three or four 1-ml ampules of either chlorpheniramine (10 mg/ml) or diphenhydramine (50 mg/ml). Syringes preloaded with histamine-blockers are not recommended because there is never any urgency associated with their administration.

## CRITICAL NONINJECTABLE DRUGS

The following five noninjectable drugs also are considered critical:
1. Oxygen
2. Vasodilator
3. Bronchodilator
4. Antihypoglycemic
5. Aspirin

## Primary noninjectable: Oxygen (O₂)

*Drug of choice:* Oxygen
*Drug class:* None
*Alternative drug:* None
*Proprietary:* None

Unquestionably the most useful drug in the entire emergency kit is $O_2$, which is supplied in a variety of sizes of compressed gas cylinders. Recommended is the E cylinder, which is quite portable. In emergency situations an E cylinder provides $O_2$ for approximately 30 minutes (when the patient is apneic). Larger cylinders (H cylinders) provide significantly more $O_2$ but are less portable; smaller cylinders (A through D cylinders) contain too little $O_2$ to be clinically effective for more than an extremely short duration. $O_2$ produced through a chemical reaction in small canisters is not adequate for an emergency kit. A portable E cylinder of $O_2$ also should be available in offices in which centrally located nitrous oxide and $O_2$ is available. Because emergencies do occur in areas of the dental office other than in the dental chair, the $O_2$ delivery system must be portable.

*Therapeutic indications:* $O_2$ administration is indicated in any emergency situation in which respiratory distress is evident. Indeed $O_2$ should never be withheld from a patient during a medical emergency.*

*Side effects, contraindications, and precautions:* None with the emergency use of $O_2$, although $O_2$ administration is not indicated in the treatment of hyperventilation.

*Availability:* Compressed gas cylinders come in a variety of sizes. Portability of the emergency $O_2$ cylinder is desirable.

*Suggested for emergency kit:* One E cylinder is the minimum requirement for an emergency kit.

## Primary noninjectable: vasodilator

*Drug of choice:* Nitroglycerin
*Proprietary:* Nitrolingual spray, Nitrostat tablets
*Drug class:* Vasodilator
*Alternative drug:* Amyl nitrite

Vasodilators are used in the immediate management of chest pain as may occur with angina pectoris or acute myocardial infarction. Two varieties of vasodilators are available: nitroglycerin as a tablet and a spray, and an inhalant, amyl nitrite. A patient with a history of angina pectoris usually carries a supply of nitroglycerin.

Tablets remain the most popular form of the drug, but most patients prefer the translingual spray once they have used it. During dental care the patient's nitroglycerin source should be readily accessible. Placed sublingually or sprayed onto the lingual soft tissues, nitroglycerin acts in 1 to 2 minutes. The patient's own drug should be used if at all possible, but if it is unavailable or is ineffective, the emergency kit should contain the 0.4-mg formulation.

The shelf life of nitroglycerin tablets, once exposed to air, is short (about 12 weeks) when the container is not adequately sealed or the tablets are stored in a pill box. In such cases the active nitroglycerin vaporizes, leaving behind nothing but inert filler. This is not problem for an anginal patient who uses only one bottle with 25 tablets. The typical patient with stable angina uses a bottle within 4 to 6 weeks. Most anginal patients, however, have several opened bottles of nitroglycerin available—in their pockets, cars, offices, and homes. The doctor should not use the patient's drug if doubt exists as to when the bottle was opened. Nitroglycerin deterioration is more likely to occur with a dental office's supply of nitroglycerin, which is used (hopefully) only rarely.

Nitroglycerin tablets placed sublingually usually produce a bitter taste and impart a sting. When the bitter taste is absent, the doctor should suspect the drug has become ineffective. A translingual nitroglycerin spray introduced in the United States in 1986 has a significantly longer shelf life than sublingual tablets even after being used once or repeated times and is highly recommended for inclusion in the emergency drug kit.

Amyl nitrite, another vasodilator, is available in inhalant form. It is supplied in a yellow vaporole or a gray cardboard vaporole with yellow printing in doses of 0.3 ml, which when crushed between the fingers and held under the victim's nose produces profound vasodilation in about 10 seconds. The duration of action of amyl nitrite is shorter than nitroglycerin, but its shelf life is considerably longer. Side effects occur with all vasodilators (see following section) but are more significant with amyl nitrite.

*Therapeutic indications:* With chest pain, vasodilators are used as an aid in differential diagnosis, and in the definitive management of angina pectoris (see Chapter 27), the early management of acute myocardial infarction (see Chapter 28), and the management of acute hypertensive episodes.

---

*Although $O_2$ administration is not necessary in the treatment of hyperventilating patients, its administration does not produce a significant adverse reaction.

*Side effects, contraindications, and precautions:* Side effects of nitroglycerin include a transient, pulsating headache, facial flushing, and a degree of hypotension, especially if the patient is in an upright position. Because of its mild hypotensive actions, nitroglycerin is contraindicated in patients who are hypotensive but may be used with some degree of effectiveness in the management of acute hypertensive episodes. Because nitroglycerin as a tablet is an unstable drug (has a short shelf life once opened), it usually must be replaced within 12 weeks after its initial use.

Side effects of amyl nitrite are similar to but more intense than those of nitroglycerin. These include facial flushing, pounding pulse, dizziness, intense headache, and hypotension. Amyl nitrite should not be administered to patients seated in upright positions because significant postural changes develop.

The recent introduction of sildenafil (Viagra) to treat male erectile dysfunction has created another drug-drug interaction. Men who have been receiving nitroglycerin for the treatment of ischemic heart disease have died after ingesting sildenafil, a vasodilating drug.[22]

*Availability:* Nitroglycerin is available in three forms—0.15-, 0.3-, 0.4-, 0.6-mg doses of sublingual tablets, 0.4 and 0.8 mg/dose translingual spray, and 0.3-ml doses of amyl nitrate yellow vaporoles (Figure 3-22).

*Suggested for emergency kit:* Kits should contain one bottle of metered translingual nitroglycerin spray (0.4 mg).

## Primary noninjectable: bronchodilator

*Drug of choice:* Albuterol
*Proprietary:* Proventil, Ventolin
*Drug class:* Bronchodilator
*Alternative drug:* Metaproterenol

Asthmatic patients and patients with allergic reactions manifested primarily by respiratory difficulty require the use of bronchodilators. Although epinephrine remains the drug of choice in the management of bronchospasm, its wide-ranging effects on systems other than the respiratory tract have resulted in the introduction of newer, more specific drugs known as $\beta_2$-*adrenergic agonists*. These drugs, of which albuterol is an example, have specific bronchial smooth muscle–relaxing properties ($\beta_2$) with little or no stimulatory action on the cardiovascular and gastrointestinal systems ($\beta_1$).

In the dental environment, where the doctor may be unaware of the patient's true cardiovascular status, $\beta_2$ agonists appear more attractive for management of acute asthmatic episodes than do drugs with both $\beta_1$- and $\beta_2$-agonist properties such as epinephrine and isoproterenol. As with anginal patients, most asthmatic patients carry their medication (in this case, a bronchodilator) with them at all times. In virtually all situations the bronchodilator is an inhaler that dispenses a calibrated dose, which the patient inhales. Inhalation allows the drug to reach the bronchial mucosa, where it acts directly on bronchial smooth muscle (Figure 3-23).

Before dental treatment begins, asthmatic patients who are at greater risk of bronchospasm (for example, dental phobics) should be asked to make their bronchodilators available. Bronchodilators must be administered precisely as directed. One or two inhalations every 4 to 6 hours is the recommended

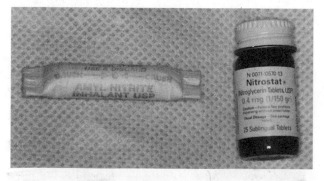

**Figure 3-22**   Vasodilators.

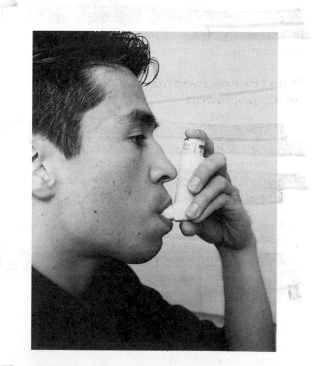

**Figure 3-23**   Bronchodilator self-administered by asthmatic patient.

dosage for albuterol. Nebulized epinephrine (for example, Primatene Mist) should be administered one or two inhalations per hour. In situations in which nebulized agents fail to terminate the attack, other bronchodilators (for example, epinephrine, aminophylline, isoproterenol) must be administered parenterally (via an IM or subcutaneous route).

*Therapeutic indications:* Bronchodilators are used to treat bronchospasm (acute asthmatic episodes) (see Chapter 13) and allergic reactions with bronchospasm (see Chapter 24).

*Side effects, contraindications, and precautions:* Albuterol, like other $\beta_2$ agonists, can have clinically significant cardiac effects in some patients. This response is less likely to develop with albuterol than with other bronchodilators, thus its selection for the emergency kit. Metaproterenol, epinephrine, and isoproterenol mistometers are more likely to produce cardiovascular side effects, including tachycardia and ventricular dysrhythmias. Administration of these latter drugs is contraindicated in patients with preexisting tachydysrhythmias from prior use of the drug (see Chapter 13).

*Availability:* Albuterol inhalers (Ventolin, Proventil), metaproterenol inhalers (Alupent), epinephrine mistometers (Medihaler-Epi; Primatene Mist), and isoproterenol mistometers (Medihaler-Iso).

*Suggested for emergency kit:* One metered albuterol inhaler.

## Primary noninjectable: antihypoglycemic

*Drug of choice:* Orange juice
*Drug class:* Antihypoglycemic
*Alternative drug:* Soft drink (nondiet)
*Proprietary:* None

Antihypoglycemics are useful in the management of hypoglycemic reactions in patients with diabetes mellitus or nondiabetic patients with hypoglycemia (low blood sugar). The diabetic patient usually carries a sugar source such as a candy bar. The dental office also should have such items available for use in the conscious hypoglycemic patient.

For management of the unconscious hypoglycemic patient, refer to the discussion of secondary injectable drugs in this chapter. In certain well-defined and well-controlled situations, thick nonviscous forms of carbohydrate may be used to manage the unconscious hypoglycemic when no injectable source is available and where emergency medical assistance is not readily obtainable. This technique, *transmucosal application of sugar*, is described in Chapter 17.

*Therapeutic indications:* Hypoglycemic states secondary to diabetes mellitus or fasting hypoglycemia in the conscious patient (Chapter 17); emergency management of unconscious hypoglycemic states in the absence of both parenteral medications and rapid access to emergency medical assistance (Chapter 17).

*Side effects, contraindications, and precautions:* Liquid or viscous oral carbohydrates should not be administered to a patient who does not have an active gag reflex or is unable to drink without assistance. Parenteral administration of antihypoglycemics is recommended in these situations. There are no side effects when oral carbohydrates are administered as directed.

Small tubes of decorative icing are useful in certain specific situations in the management of unconscious hypoglycemic patients. These tubes contain a thickened paste of concentrated sugar that can be applied in a thin ribbon to the buccal mucosa in both the maxilla and the mandible (Figure 3-24). Because it is thick, this paste does not run and thus potential airway obstruction is not a danger. Onset of action is slow, at least 20 or 30 minutes before blood sugar levels become elevated. This delay limits the recommendation for its use to situations in which emergency assistance is not immediately available. BLS must be continued while the patient remains unconscious.

*Availability:* Antihypoglycemics come in a variety of forms, including Glucola, Gluco-Stat, Insta-Glucose, nondiet cola beverages, fruit juices, granulated sugar, and tubes of decorative icing.

*Suggested for emergency kit:* Any of the previously mentioned sources can be included in the emergency kit.

## Primary noninjectable: antiplatelet

*Drug of choice:* Aspirin
*Drug class:* Antiplatelet
*Alternative drug:* None

Aspirin has become a recommended antithrombotic drug in the prehospital phase of suspected myocardial infarction. Considered to be the standard antiplatelet agent, aspirin represents the most cost-effective treatment available for patients with

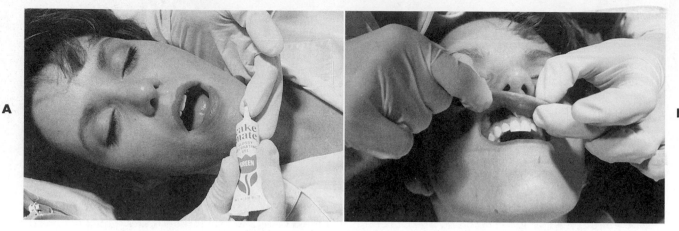

**Figure 3-24**  **A,** Decorative icing applied transmucosally. **B,** Transmucosal sugar applied in thin layer on buccal mucosa.

acute ischemic coronary syndromes. Aspirin irreversibly acetylates platelet cyclooxygenase, removing all cyclooxygenase activity for the life span of the platelet (8 to 10 days).[23] Aspirin stops production of proaggregatory thromboxane $A_2$ and is also an indirect antithrombotic agent. Aspirin also has important nonplatelet effects because it likewise inactivates cyclooxygenase in the vascular endothelium and thereby diminishes formation of antiaggregatory prostacyclin.[23]

The ISIS-2 trial provides the strongest evidence that aspirin independently reduces the mortality of patients with AMI without additional thrombolytic therapy (overall 23% reduction) and is synergistic when used in combination with thrombolytic therapy (42% reduction in mortality).[24] Administration of aspirin is recommended for all patients with suspected AMI or unstable angina.[23] Standard doses range from 160 to 324 mg given orally. Minimal side effects are noted, particularly with the 160-mg dose.

*Therapeutic indications:* Aspirin is recommended in management of patients with suspected myocardial infarction or unstable angina.

*Side effects, contraindications, and precautions:* Definite contraindications to aspirin therapy include ongoing major or life-threatening hemorrhage; a significant predisposition to such hemorrhage, such as a recent bleeding peptic ulcer; or a history of aspirin allergy.

*Availability:* Aspirin is available in 65-, 81-, 162-, and 325-mg tablets, under many brand names.

*Suggested for emergency kit:* The emergency kit should include 3 or 4 "baby" chewable aspirin (162 mg).

## CRITICAL EMERGENCY EQUIPMENT

Critical items of emergency equipment include the following:
1. $O_2$ delivery system
2. Syringes
3. Suction and suction tips
4. Tourniquets
5. Magill intubation forceps

Merely having various items of emergency equipment available does not of itself better equip a dental office or better prepare the staff member for the management of emergency situations. Personnel who are expected to use this equipment must be well trained in its proper use. Unfortunately, many emergency equipment items commonly found in dental and medical offices can be useless and even hazardous if they are used improperly or in the wrong situation. Training in the proper use of equipment, such as the laryngoscope and the oropharyngeal airway, can be achieved best through the care of patients under general anesthesia, a situation not readily available to most dental personnel.

Many items listed in this section are therefore recommended for use only by properly trained individuals. All emergency equipment items classified as secondary and unfortunately several classified as primary (for example, the $O_2$ delivery system) require special training. Although all doctors should be trained in the use of $O_2$ delivery systems, courses in which these techniques are taught are particularly difficult to locate. (Readers interested in such hands-on programs should contact their local dental society, dental school, hospital, or American Heart Association affiliate.)

Therefore dental personnel must use only those pieces of emergency equipment with which they are

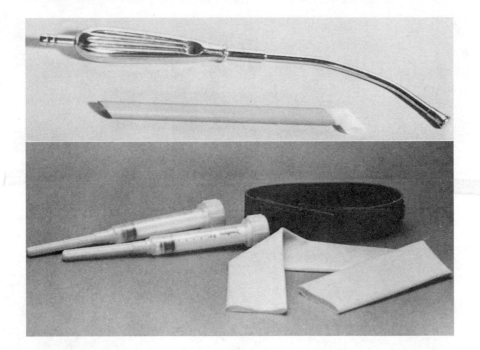

**Figure 3-25**   Primary emergency equipment: tourniquet, syringes, suction, and suction tips.

intimately familiar and have been trained to use properly. The usefulness of the items described here varies with the training of the office personnel. All dental personnel should become proficient in the use of the primary items of equipment.

**O₂ delivery system**   Table 3-3 compares several methods of ventilation.

*Positive pressure:* An $O_2$ delivery system adaptable to the E cylinder allows for the delivery of $O_2$ under positive pressure to the patient. Examples of this device include the positive-pressure/demand valve (Figure 3-25) and the reservoir bag on many inhalation sedation units. The devices should be fitted with a clear face mask, allowing for the efficient delivery of 100% $O_2$ while permitting the rescuer to inspect visually the victim's mouth for the presence of foreign matter (for example, vomitus, blood, saliva, water). Face masks should be available in child, small-adult, and large-adult sizes.

*Bag-valve-mask device:* A portable, self-inflating bag-valve-mask device (Ambu-bag, PMR; Figure 3-26) is a self-contained unit that may be easily transported to any site within a dental office. This is an important feature since not all emergencies will develop within the dental operatory and it may be necessary to resuscitate a person in other areas, such as the waiting room or restroom. A source of positive-pressure oxygen or ambient air or enriched $O_2$ (>21%, <100%)

| table **3-3** | *Comparison of ventilation method* |
|---|---|
| **TECHNIQUE** | **% OXYGEN** |
| Mouth-to-mouth | 16 |
| Mouth-to-mask | 16 |
| Bag-valve-mask | 21 |
| Bag-valve-mask + oxygen | >21-<100 |
| Postitive pressure mask | 100 |

attached to an oxygen delivery tube must also be available in these areas. With either device the rescuer must be able to maintain both an airtight seal and a patent airway with one hand while using the other hand to activate the device and ventilate the victim (Figure 3-27).

*Pocket mask:* The pocket mask is a clear full-face mask, identical in shape and application to the positive-pressure and bag-valve-mask devices (Figure 3-28). Unlike these devices, however, the rescuer must apply exhaled air ventilation (16% $O_2$) into the inlet on top of the mask to ventilate the victim. Exhalation occurs passively through a one-way valve located on the side of the mask. In this way, the rescuer does not rebreathe the victim's exhaled air. The pocket mask also is available with a supplemental $O_2$ port, permitting attachment of the mask to an $O_2$ tube, and deliver enriched $O_2$ ventilation.

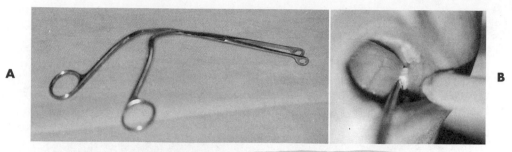

**Figure 3-26** **A,** Magill intubation forceps. **B,** Magill intubation forceps enable small objects to be readily removed from oral cavity.

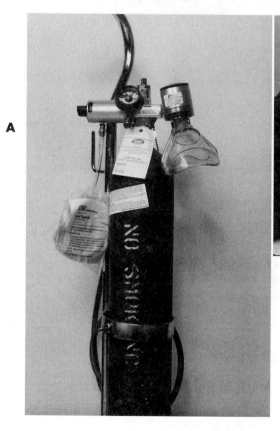

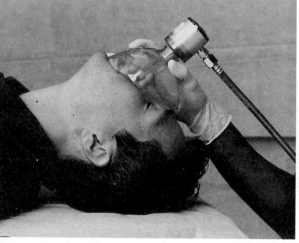

**Figure 3-27**  Positive-pressure O₂ system.

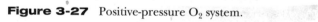

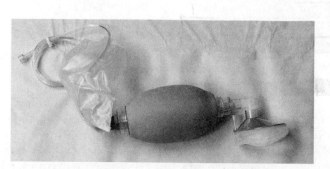

**Figure 3-28**  Self-inflating bag-valve-mask. Permits delivery of atmospheric air (21% oxygen) or oxygen-enriched air. Clear face mask is preferred to opaque.

Small enough to fit easily into a pocket or purse, the pocket mask enables the rescuer to provide mouth-to-mask ventilation to a nonbreathing victim in place of mouth-to-mouth ventilation. The pocket mask also helps individuals overcome the so-called "yuck" factor, which refers to the fact that a significant percentage of victims requiring artificial ventilation regurgitate, presenting with a pharynx and oral cavity filled with vomitus ("yuck").

The rescuer also can use the pocket mask to ventilate a pediatric patient by simply inverting the mask, holding the narrow nose-side of the mask in the cleft of the chin and the wider chin-side on the bridge of the child's nose (Figure 3-29). Because of increased concern in the health professions about the transmission of hepatitis and HIV virus as a result of direct physical contact with bodily fluids, the pocket mask (or any mask for that matter) is an ideal choice to provide the rescuer positive psychologic support. In addition, the low cost of the mask (under $20) is another reason why all dental office personnel should have their own pocket mask.

*Suggested for emergency kit:* One portable O₂ cylinder (E cylinder) with a positive-pressure mask, one portable self-inflating bag-valve-mask device, and one pocket mask for each staff member. Several sizes—child, small-adult, and large-adult—of clear full-face masks also should be available; specialty practices should stock additional mask sizes.

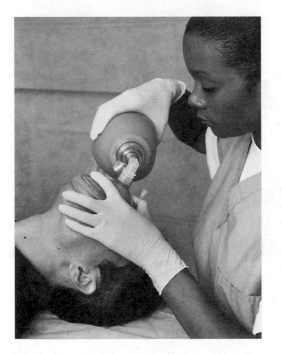

**Figure 3-29**  Hand positions with bag-valve-mask device.

NOTE: Advanced training is required for the safe and effective use of masks used for ventilation.

### Syringes

Plastic disposable syringes equipped with an 18- or 21-gauge needle are used in parenteral drug administration. Although many sizes are available, the 2-ml syringe is adequate for the delivery of emergency drugs (Figure 3-30).

*Suggested for emergency kit:* Two to four 2-ml disposable syringes with 18- or 21-gauge needles.

### Suction and aspirating apparatus

A strong suction system and a variety of large-diameter suction tips are essential items of emergency equipment. The disposable saliva ejector, commonly found in dental offices, is entirely inadequate in situations in which any other than the tiniest object must be evacuated from a patient's mouth. Aspirator tips should be rounded to ensure that there is little risk of bleeding should it become necessary to suction the hypopharynx. Plastic evacuators and tonsil suction tips are quite adequate for this purpose (see Figure 3-30).

*Suggested for emergency kit:* A minimum of two plastic evacuators or tonsil suction tips should be available in the emergency kit.

### Tourniquets

A tourniquet will be required if IV drugs are to be administered. In addition, three tourniquets are needed to perform a bloodless phlebotomy in the management of acute pulmonary edema (see Chapter 14). A sphygmomanometer (blood pressure cuff) can be used as a tourniquet, as may a simple piece of latex tubing (see Figure 3-30).

*Suggested for emergency kit:* Three tourniquets and a sphygmomanometer should be included in each kit.

### Magill intubation forceps

The Magill intubation forceps is designed to aid in the placement of an endotracheal tube during nasal intubation. The Magill intubation forceps is a blunt-ended scissors with a right-angle bend (Figure 3-31). This design permits the forceps to grasp objects deep in the hypopharynx such as the endotracheal tube.

The use of gloves is now the standard of care in dentistry, and a number of recently published reports have described dental items, such as crowns and endodontic files, being dislodged and lying in the posterior region

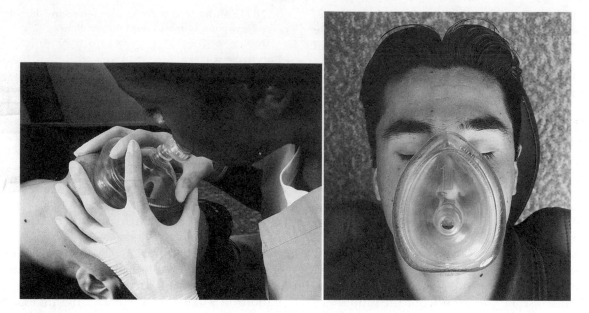

**Figure 3-30**  Pocket mask.

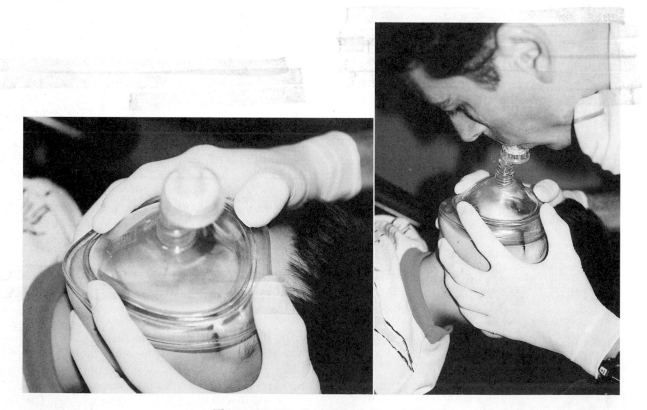

**Figure 3-31**  Pocket mask for a child.

of the patient's oral cavity. There is usually nothing readily available on an instrument tray that can adequately and easily be used to retrieve such objects. The Magill intubation forceps is designed to perform this function and is highly recommended for inclusion in every emergency kit.

*Suggested for emergency kit:* One pediatric-size Magill intubation forceps.

# Module Two: Secondary (Noncritical) Emergency Drugs and Equipment

Drugs and equipment included in this level, though important and valuable in the management of emergency situations, are not considered critical elements of the office emergency kit (Table 3-4). Only doctors who have been trained in the use of these drugs

should consider including them in the office kit. Doctors who administer parenteral sedation may be required by their state or specialty organization to maintain many of these drugs in their emergency kits.

## SECONDARY INJECTABLE DRUGS

Seven drug categories are included in this level:
1. Anticonvulsants
2. Analgesics
3. Vasopressors
4. Antihypoglycemics
5. Corticosteroids
6. Antihypertensives
7. Anticholinergics

### Secondary injectable: anticonvulsant
*Drug of choice:* Midazolam
*Proprietary:* Versed
*Drug class:* Benzodiazepine
*Alternative drug:* Diazepam

table **3-4**   *Module two—secondary (noncritical) drugs and equipment*

| CATEGORY | PRIMARY DRUG | | | RECOMMENDED FOR KIT | |
|---|---|---|---|---|---|
| | GENERIC | PROPRIETARY | ALTERNATIVE | QUANTITY | AVAILABILITY |
| **Injectables** | | | | | |
| Anticonvulsant | Midazolam | Versed | Diazepam | 1 × 5-ml vial | 5 mg/ml |
| Analgesic | Morphine sulfate | — | Meperidine | 2 × 2-ml ampules | 10 mg/ml |
| Vasopressor | Methoxamine | Vasoxyl | Phenylephrine | 2 or 3 × 1-ml ampules | 10 mg/ml |
| Antihypoglycemic | 50% dextrose solution | — | Glucagon | 1 × 50-ml vial (IV) | |
| Corticosteroid | Hydrocortisone sodium succinate | Solu-Cortef | — | 1 × 2-ml vial | 50 mg/ml |
| Antihypertensive | Esmolol | Brevibloc | Propranolol | 2 × 100 mg/ml vial | 100 mg/ml |
| Anticholinergic | Atropine | — | — | 2 or 3 × 1-ml ampules | 0.5 mg/ml |
| | | | | or 2 × 10-ml syringes | 1.0 mg/10 ml |
| **Noninjectables** | | | | | |
| Respiratory stimulant | Aromatic ammonia | — | — | 1-2 boxes | 0.3 ml/vaporole |
| Antihypertensive | Nifedipine | Procardia | — | 1 bottle | 10-mg capsules |

| EQUIPMENT | DESCRIPTION | QUANTITY |
|---|---|---|
| **Emergency equipment** | | |
| Cricothyrotomy equipment* | Scalpel or cricothyrotomy device | 1 scalpel with disposable blade or cricothyrotomy device |
| Artificial airways* | Plastic or rubber oropharyngeal and nasopharyngeal airways | Assorted adult and pediatric airways |
| Equipment for endotracheal intubation* | Laryngoscope and blades (curved or straight) | Minimum of one and spare batteries |
| | Endotracheal tubes | Assorted adult and pediatric sizes |

*IV,* Intravenous; *HCl,* hydrochloride.
*Use of these devices requires significant advanced training to ensure their safe and effective use.

Seizure disorders may occur in the dental office under several circumstances, including epileptic seizures, overdose reactions to local anesthetics, obstructed airway in an unconscious patient, and febrile convulsions. Only rarely will an anticonvulsant be required to terminate seizure activity. An anticonvulsant should be considered for inclusion in the emergency kit so that is readily available. The choice of an anticonvulsant has become somewhat simpler since the introduction of the benzodiazepines.

Until about 30 years ago, barbiturates were the drugs of choice in the management of acute seizure disorders. With its introduction in 1960, diazepam became the preferred anticonvulsant. Because seizure disorders are characterized by stimulation of the central nervous, respiratory, and cardiovascular systems followed by a period of depression of these same systems, drugs that depress these systems at therapeutic doses are more likely to produce postseizure complications.

When barbiturates are administered to terminate seizure activity, the patient's postseizure depression is accentuated and prolonged because of the pharmacologic actions of the barbiturate. When the seizure activity is significant, the ensuing postictal period of depression usually is profound, leading to compromised respiration and a period of hypotension. When barbiturates are used to terminate seizures, the ensuing depression will likely be intensified, leading to respiratory arrest and a profound cardiovascular depression or collapse. If the doctor is not adept at recognizing and managing this situation, the patient can face more risks after the seizure than during it.

Unlike barbiturates, benzodiazepines usually terminate seizure activity without significant depression of the respiratory and cardiovascular systems. For many years, diazepam was the anticonvulsant drug of choice because of its ability to terminate seizures without producing profound postictal depression. Its lack of water solubility, however, limited its use to IV administration.* It was highly unlikely that a physician or dentist who was not technically proficient in venipuncture would be able to start an IV line on a patient during a generalized tonicoclonic seizure. Where this was possible, diazepam was the preferred drug.

With the introduction of midazolam, a water-soluble benzodiazepine that is effective as an anticonvulsant both IV and IM became available. Although IV administration still is preferred, the IM route is now available.

---

*The recent introduction of water-soluble diazepam (Dizac) has made IM administration of the drug and its clinical effects more predictable.

IM midazolam provides clinical action within 10 to 15 minutes. (Time of onset is dependent upon blood pressure and tissue perfusion).[25]

*Therapeutic indications:* Midazolam is used to treat prolonged seizures (see discussion of status epilepticus in Chapter 21), local anesthetic-induced seizures (see Chapter 23), hyperventilation (see discussion of sedation in Chapter 12), and thyroid storm (see discussion of sedation in Chapter 18).

*Side effects, contraindications, and precautions:* The major clinical side effect noted with benzodiazepines when used as anticonvulsants is respiratory depression or arrest. However, with careful titration during administration, this effect is less likely to occur. Compared with barbiturates, benzodiazepine-induced respiratory depression is considerably more mild.

*Availability:* Midazolam (Versed [USA], Hypnovel and Dormicum [Europe, Great Britain]) is available in 5 mg/ml in 1-, 2-, 5-, and 10-ml vials and in 2-ml preloaded syringes and in 1 mg/ml in 2-, 5-, and 10-ml vials. Diazepam (Valium) is available in 5 mg/ml in 2-ml ampules and 10-ml vials and in 2-ml preloaded syringes.

*Suggested for emergency kit:* One 5-ml vial of midazolam (5 mg/ml).

## Secondary injectable: analgesic
*Drug of choice:* Morphine sulfate
*Proprietary:* None
*Drug class:* Opioid agonist
*Alternative drug:* Meperidine

Analgesics are used in emergency situations in which acute pain or anxiety is present. In most instances the pain or anxiety increases the workload of the heart (which increases the myocardial $O_2$ requirement) which may prove detrimental to the patient's well-being. Two such circumstances include acute myocardial infarction and congestive heart failure. The analgesic drugs of choice include the opioid agonists morphine sulfate and meperidine (Demerol).

*Therapeutic indications:* Intense, prolonged pain or anxiety; acute myocardial infarction (see Chapter 28); and congestive heart failure (see Chapter 14).

*Side effects, contraindications, and precautions:* Opioid agonists are potent central nervous and respiratory system depressants. Vigilant monitoring of vital signs is mandatory whenever these drugs are used. Use of opioid agonists is contraindicated in victims of injury and multiple trauma; the drugs should be used with care in any person with compromised respiratory function. (Naloxone can be administered to reverse the respiratory depressant actions of opioid agonists and other opioid-agonist properties and of analgesia [see Module Four—antidotal drugs]). Opioid analgesics should be administered IV to victims suspected of having acute myocardial infarction. This group of drugs should not be included in the emergency drug kit unless the doctor and staff members are trained in IV drug administration.

*Availability:* Morphine sulfate is available in 8, 10, and 15 mg/ml (in 2-ml ampules and 20 ml vials), and meperidine comes in 50 and 100 mg/ml (in 1-ml ampules and 20- and 30-ml vials).

*Suggested for emergency kit:* Emergency kits may contain 10 mg/ml morphine sulfate (two 2-ml ampules) or 50 mg/ml meperidine (2 ml ampules).

NOTE: In recent years, emergency medical services in many countries have employed mixtures of nitrous oxide ($N_2O$) and $O_2$ in place of opioid analgesics in the management of pain associated with acute myocardial infarction. Concentrations of $N_2O$ have varied between 35% and 50%. At these levels a mixture of 35% to 50% $N_2O$ and 50% to 65% $O_2$ decreases pain, sedates the patient, and provides that patient 2½ to 3 times ambient levels of $O_2$ (see Chapter 28). When available, $N_2O$-$O_2$ may be used in place of opioid analgesics. This is especially important where direct IV access is unobtainable. In its absence, however, an opioid analgesic should be considered for inclusion in the emergency kit.

Opioid agonists are schedule II drugs, which means that they must be maintained in a secure location in the dental office. A schedule II classification precludes their physical presence in the emergency drug kit, which should be readily accessible at all times.

## Secondary injectable: vasopressor

*Drug of choice:* Methoxamine
*Proprietary:* Vasoxyl
*Drug class:* Vasopressor
*Alternative drug:* Phenylephrine

Although one potent vasopressor—epinephrine—already is included in the emergency kit, most emergencies in the dental office in which a vasopressor is needed will not require epinephrine. Epinephrine is used primarily in the management of acute allergic reactions and rarely is indicated in the management of clinically mild to moderate hypotension. Epinephrine elicits an extreme antihypotensive response. In addition to an increase in blood pressure, this drug increases the heart's workload through its effect on heart rate and

strength of cardiac contractions; it also increases the irritability of the myocardium thereby sensitizing it to dysrhythmias.

In most clinical situations listed below (see Therapeutic Indications), the victim's systolic blood pressure has fallen to about 60 to 80 mmHg and has not returned to its baseline level in an appropriate time period. A drug should be available which will elevate the systolic blood pressure approximately 30 to 40 mmHg for a sustained period, allowing the body to return to a more normal functional state. Furthermore, in most instances the cardiovascular status of the patient is unknown unless electrocardiographic monitoring is being employed. For this reason, it is desirable to have available a vasopressor that produces a moderate increase in blood pressure without an undue increase in the myocardium's workload.

Methoxamine (Vasoxyl) and phenylephrine (Neo-Synephrine) both produce moderate blood pressure elevations through peripheral vasoconstriction (α-receptor agonists). Methoxamine produces sustained action but has little effect on the myocardium or central nervous system; its vasopressor action is associated with a marked increase in peripheral resistance and without an increase in cardiac output. A compensatory bradycardia accompanies the rise in blood pressure produced by methoxamine. The onset of the pressor action is almost immediate after IV administration and can persist for up to 60 minutes. After intramuscular injection, the pressor response develops within 15 minutes and persists for 90 minutes. Phenylephrine acts similarly; a 5-mg IM dose causes the systolic blood pressure to elevate 30 mmHg and diastolic blood pressure to elevate 20 mmHg, and the response lasts for 50 minutes. As with methoxamine, a pronounced and persistent bradycardia is noted (average decline in heart rate from 70 to 44 beats per minute).

*Therapeutic indications:* Vasopressors are used to manage hypotension, in which the status of the patient's heart is unknown and the intent is to raise the blood pressure without undue cardiac stimulation. Possible uses include the following:
- Syncopal reactions (see Section II)
- Drug overdose reactions (see Chapter 23)
- Postseizure states (see Chapter 21)
- Acute adrenal insufficiency (see Chapter 8)
- Allergy (see Chapter 24)

*Side effects, contraindications, and precautions:* Parenteral administration of most vasopressors is contraindicated in patients with high blood pressure or ventricular tachycardia. The drugs must be used with extreme caution in patients with hyperthyroidism, bradycardia, partial heart block, myocardial disease, or severe atherosclerosis.

*Availability:* Methoxamine (Vasoxyl) is available in 10 mg/ml and 20 mg/ml (1-ml ampules and 10-ml vials), and phenylephrine (Neo-Synephrine) is available in 10 mg/ml (1-ml ampules).

*Suggested for emergency kit:* Methoxamine, 10 mg/ml (two to three 1-ml ampules or phenylephrine, 10 mg/ml (two to three 1-ml ampules).

NOTE: Vasopressors are used only infrequently for the management of hypotensive states. Other nonpharmacologic means are available for the elevation of blood pressure, such as the positioning of the patient in the supine position with the feet elevated or the administration of IV fluids (D5&W, lactated Ringers). A number of anesthesiologists have told me that the only vasopressor they administer is epinephrine—and then only when no blood pressure is present.

### Secondary injectable: antihypoglycemic
*Drug of choice:* Dextrose, 50% solution
*Proprietary:* None
*Drug class:* Antihypoglycemic
*Alternative drug:* Glucagon

In the management of low blood sugar (hypoglycemia), the mode of therapy depends largely on the patient's level of consciousness. Oral carbohydrate administration is preferred, but when a patient is unconscious or severely obtunded, 50 ml of a 50% dextrose solution should be administered IV. When the IV route is not available, glucagon may be administered via the IM route.

Glucagon, normally produced in the pancreas, elevates the blood glucose level by mobilizing hepatic glycogen and converting it to glucose. Glucagon is effective only when hepatic glycogen is available; it is ineffective in the treatment of starvation or chronic hypoglycemic states. As soon as the patient begins to respond (that is, regains consciousness and is able to swallow) oral carbohydrates should be administered.

*Therapeutic indications:* Antihypoglycemics are used in the treatment of hypoglycemia (see Chapter 17) and as a diagnostic aid in unconsciousness or seizures of unknown origin (see Chapter 9).

*Side effects, contraindications, and precautions:* 50% dextrose solution, which must be administered IV, may produce tissue necrosis if extravascular infiltration occurs. There are no specific contraindications to the use of 50% dextrose. Administration of a bo-

lus of 50% dextrose to an already hyperglycemic patient does not significantly elevate blood sugar levels. Glucagon administered either via IV or IM routes is contraindicated in patients in starvation states or with chronic hypoglycemia.

*Availability:* 50% dextrose is available in 50-ml glass ampules, whereas glucagon is available in 1 mg (1 unit) of dry powder with 1 ml of diluent and in 10 mg of dry powder with 10 ml of diluent.

*Suggested for emergency kit:* 50% dextrose (1 vial), if IV route is available or 1 mg/ml (two or three 1-ml vials) of glucagon for IV or IM administration.

### Secondary injectable: corticosteroid
*Drug of choice:* Hydrocortisone sodium succinate
*Proprietary:* Solu-Cortef
*Drug class:* Adrenal glucocorticosteroid
*Alternative drug:* None

Corticosteroids are used to manage acute allergic reactions—but only after the rescuer has brought the acute, life-threatening phase under control through the use of BLS, epinephrine, and histamine blockers. Corticosteroids are valuable primarily in the prevention of recurrent anaphylactic episodes. Corticosteroids also are used to manage acute adrenal insufficiency.

The onset of action for corticosteroids is slow, even when the drugs are administered IV.[26] Because maximum effectiveness may not occur for up to 60 minutes after IV administration, many doctors and researchers question the effectiveness of these drugs in the management of allergic reactions in patients with normally functioning adrenal glands. The antiallergic effects of corticosteroids are likely simple manifestations of the nonspecific antiinflammatory action of the adrenal glucocorticoids (hydrocortisone and cortisone). The use of dexamethasone (Decadron) and methylprednisolone sodium succinate (Solu-Medrol) are contraindicated in patients with acute adrenal insufficiency. Therefore hydrocortisone sodium succinate is the corticosteroid of choice for the dental emergency kit. Corticosteroids are considered second-line drugs primarily because of their slow onset of action.

*Therapeutic indications:* Corticosteroids are used in the definitive management of acute allergy (see Chapter 24) and in the treatment of acute adrenal insufficiency (see Chapter 8).

*Side effects, contraindications, and precautions:* There are no contraindications to the administration of corticosteroids in the management of life-threatening medical emergencies. When the drug is administered for nonemergency treatment (for example, the prevention of edema during surgery or for pruritus), many factors must be considered, such as the presence of a preexisting infection, peptic ulcer, or hyperglycemia. (A pharmacology text or *Physicians' Desk Reference* can provide more detailed information.)

*Availability:* Hydrocortisone sodium succinate (Solu-Cortef) is available in 50 mg/ml (2-ml vials).

*Suggested for emergency kit:* Hydrocortisone sodium succinate (one 2-ml vial).

## Secondary injectable: antihypertensive
*Drug of choice:* Esmolol
*Proprietary:* Brevibloc
*Drug class:* β-Adrenergic blocker
*Alternative drug:* Propranolol

The need to administer drugs to manage a hypertensive crisis (excessively elevated blood pressure) is extremely uncommon. First, the incidence of extreme acute blood pressure elevation is rare; second, there are many ways other than the parenteral administration of antihypertensive drugs to decrease a patient's blood pressure. Indeed, in interviews with hundreds of dentists who regularly administer parenteral sedation and general anesthesia, I have not found a single one who has needed to administer a drug to decrease excessively elevated blood pressure. Oral drugs, such as nifedipine and nitroglycerin, may be administered in most situations to decrease blood pressure slightly. The inclusion of an antihypertensive drug in the emergency kit is in response to state requirements for general anesthesia permits (and in a few states for parenteral sedation).

Not long ago, drugs such as diazoxide (Hyperstat) were used to manage acute hypertensive episodes or for controlled hypotensive anesthesia. These drugs decrease blood pressure by relaxing vascular smooth muscle in peripheral arterioles. Cardiac output is increased as blood pressure is reduced, and both coronary artery and renal blood flows are maintained. The urgency of the use of these drugs in the management of dental office emergencies is no longer recommended because other, more controllable agents are available.

For example, esmolol (Brevibloc) is a beta$_1$-selective (cardioselective) adrenergic receptor blocking agent with a very short duration of action (elimination half-life [IV] is approximately 9 minutes). Esmolol is indicated for use as an antidysrhythmic agent in patients with paroxysmol supraventricular tachycardia (PSVT) and for the management of intraoperative and postoperative tachycardia and hypertension. When used in

management of PSVT esmolol produced significant drops in blood pressure in between 20% and 50% of patients. Hypotension was significant (<90 mmHg systoic or <50mmHg diastolic) in 12% of these patients. Owing to the short duration of esmolol (~30 minutes via IV) this hypotensive effect is short-lived. β-adrenergic and nonselective β-adrenergic receptor-blocking actions. After IV administration, the α- to β-blockade ratio is 1:7. Labetalol produces a dose-related decrease in blood pressure without reflex tachycardia or a significant reduction in heart rate (presumably through its mixture of both α- and β-blockade). Because of its α blockade, decreases in blood pressure are greater when the patient is standing than when the patient is in a supine position, in which signs of postural hypotension may develop. When administered to patients (who are in supine positions) for the management of severe hypertension, an initial IV dose of 0.25 mg/kg (17.5 mg for a 70-kg patient), the drug decreases blood pressure by an average of 11/7 mmHg.

*Therapeutic indications:* Acute hypertensive episodes

*Side effects, contraindications, and precautions:* Esmolol is contraindicated in patients with sinus bradycardia, heart block greater than first degree, cardiogenic shock or overt heart failure. Potentially significant hypotension can develop with any dose of esmolol, but is more likely to be seen with doses beyond 200 ucg/kg/min. Patients receiving esmolol should be closely monitored. In patients with CHF esmolol in higher doses may precipitate more severe cardiac failure. In both situations, hypotension and cardiac failure, discontinuation of esmolol leads to reversal of clinical signs and symptoms within 30 minutes. Extravascular injection of the 20 mg/ml concentration of esmolol may lead to serious localized reactions and skin necrosis. This is less common with the 10 mg/ml solution.

*Availability:* Esmolol is available as 2.5 g in a 10-ml ampule which is diluted to a 10-mg/ml concentration prior to infusion, and as a 100-mg/ml solution which is also diluted to 10-mg/ml prior to administration.

*Suggested for emergency kit:* Two ampules 100 mg/ml with diluent.

## Secondary injectable: parasympathetic blocking agent
*Drug of choice:* Atropine
*Drug class:* Anticholinergic
*Alternative drug:* None
*Proprietary:* None

Atropine, a parasympathetic blocking agent, is recommended for the management of symptomatic bradycardia (adult heart rate of <60 beats per minute). By enhancing discharge from the sinoatrial node, atropine can provoke tachycardia (adult heart rate >110 beats per minute). Atropine is beneficial in situations in which the patient's heart has an overload of parasympathetic activity (more than vagus nerve stimulation). Extremely fearful patients are likely to develop this response. When stimulated, the vagus nerve decreases sinoatrial node activity, which slows the heart rate. When the heart rate becomes overly slow, cerebral blood flow is decreased and clinical signs and symptoms of cerebral ischemia develop. By blocking this vagal effect, atropine acts to maintain adequate cardiac output and cerebral circulation.

Atropine also is considered an essential component of ACLS, in which it is used to manage hemodynamically significant bradydysrhythmias (significant heart block and asystole).

*Therapeutic indications:* Atropine is used to treat bradycardia and hemodynamically significant bradydysrhythmias (see Chapter 30).

*Side effects, contraindications, and precautions:* Large doses of atropine (>2 mg) may produce clinical signs of overdose, including hot, dry skin; headache; blurred nearsightedness; dry mouth and throat; disorientation; and hallucinations. Administration of atropine is contraindicated in patients with glaucoma or prostatic hypertrophy. However, in life-threatening situations the benefits of atropine administration usually outweigh the possible risks. Atropine can increase the degree of partial urinary obstruction associated with prostatism; the drug also is contraindicated in older patients with narrow-angle glaucoma.

*Availability:* Atropine is available in 0.5 mg/ml in 1-ml vials and as 1 mg/ml in 10-ml preloaded syringes.

*Suggested for emergency kit:* Two or three ampules of 0.5 mg/ml (for IM administration) or two 10-ml syringes with 1 mg per syringe (for IV administration).

## SECONDARY NONINJECTABLE DRUGS

Two noninjectable drugs are considered at this level:
1. Respiratory stimulants
2. Antihypertensives

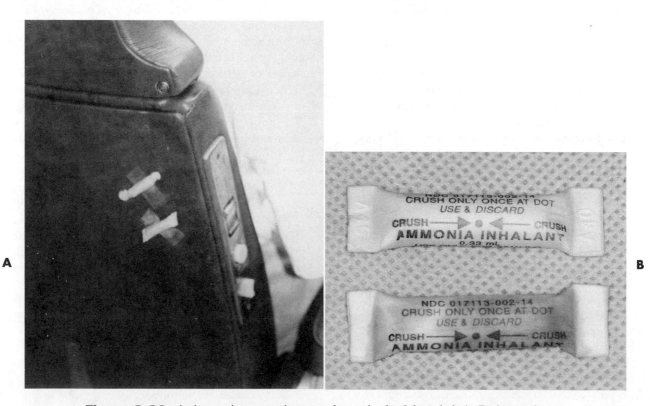

**Figure 3-32** **A,** Aromatic ammonia vaporoles on back of dental chair. **B,** Aromatic ammonia vaporole darkens *(bottom)* when used.

## Secondary noninjectable: respiratory stimulant

*Drug of choice:* Aromatic ammonia
*Proprietary:* None
*Drug class:* Respiratory stimulant
*Alternative drug:* None

Aromatic ammonia is the agent of choice for inclusion in the emergency kit as a respiratory stimulant. It is available in a silver-gray vaporole, which is crushed and placed under the breathing victim's nose until respiratory stimulation is effected. Aromatic ammonia has a noxious odor and irritates the mucous membrane of the upper respiratory tract, stimulating the respiratory and vasomotor centers of the medulla. This action in turn increases respiration and blood pressure. Movement of the arms and legs often occurs in response to ammonia inhalation; these movements further increase blood flow and raise blood pressure, especially in the patient who has been positioned properly.

*Therapeutic indications:* Aromatic ammonia is used to treat respiratory depression not induced by opioid analgesics; vasodepressor syncope (see Chapter 6).

*Side effects, contraindications, and precautions:* Ammonia should be used with caution in persons with chronic obstructive pulmonary disease or asthma; its irritating effects on the mucous membranes of the upper respiratory tract may precipitate bronchospasm.

*Availability:* Silver-gray vaporoles containing 0.3 ml of aromatic ammonia.

*Suggested for emergency kit:* One to two boxes of vaporoles.

NOTE: After $O_2$, aromatic ammonia is the most commonly used drug in the emergency kit. I keep one or two vaporoles close to every dental unit (for example, taped behind the back of the headrest) so that when the drug is needed, time is not wasted searching for it (Figure 3-32). The vaporoles should be located so that the doctor or staff member can reach them without having to leave the patient. In addition, several vaporoles should be kept in the emergency kit for use in other areas of the dental office.

## Secondary noninjectable: antihypertensive

*Drug of choice:* Nifedipine
*Proprietary:* Procardia
*Drug class:* Calcium channel blocker
*Alternative drug:* Nitroglycerin

Two drugs that help manage acute elevations in blood pressure—esmolol for parenteral administration and nitroglycerin for sublingual or translingual administration have previously been discussed. The need for yet another antihypertensive drug is minimal, especially in view of the fact that the need for antihypertensive drug administration in dental office situations is extremely slight.

Nifedipine primarily is used to manage angina, especially vasospastic or Prinzmetal's variant angina. As is seen with nitroglycerin, a modest and usually well-tolerated hypotension commonly is observed as a side effect of nifedipine administration. The occasional patient also may experience excessive and less well-tolerated hypotension, especially if the patient is standing or seated upright.

Many doctors and researchers lately have questioned the use of nifedipine in the treatment of hypertensive events. Grossman and others[27] stated: "Given the seriousness of the reported adverse events, the use of nifedipine capsules for hypertensive emergencies and pseudoemergencies should be abandoned. Adverse events cited include: cerebrovascular ischemia, stroke, numerous instances of severe hypotension, acute myocardial infarction, conduction disturbances, fetal distress, and death."

*Therapeutic indications:* Hypertension; acute anginal pain (see Chapter 27).

*Side effects, contraindications, and precautions:* Excessive hypotension may be noted, especially when nifedipine is administered to patients already receiving β-blockers and are undergoing anesthesia with high doses of fentanyl.

*Availability:* Nifedipine comes in 10-mg or 20-mg capsules.

*Suggested for emergency kit:* One bottle of 10-mg capsules.

## SECONDARY EMERGENCY EQUIPMENT

Items described in this section are adjunctive to the basic techniques of airway management presented in the primary equipment section of this chapter and in Chapter 5. These items are recommended only for persons who have received the advanced training required to use them safely and effectively.[28] They are not meant to serve as substitutes for the basic techniques of airway management.

Secondary emergency equipment items include the following:
1. Scalpel or cricothyrotomy needle
2. Artificial airways
3. Laryngoscope and endotracheal tubes

### Scalpel or cricothyrotomy device

When all other noninvasive procedures have failed to secure a patent airway, a cricothyrotomy may have to be performed. The emergency kit should contain an instrument that can be used to create an opening into the trachea below the obstruction. A scalpel or specially designed cricothyrotomy device is recommended (Figure 3-33) (see Chapter 11).

*Suggested for emergency kit:* One scalpel with a disposable blade and one cricothyrotomy device should be included in the emergency kit.

NOTE: Advanced training is required for safe and effective use of these devices.

### Artificial airways

Plastic or rubber oropharyngeal or nasopharyngeal airways are used to assist in the maintenance of a patent airway in the unconscious patient (Figure 3-34). These devices, which lift the base of the tongue off the posterior pharyngeal wall, are recommended by the American Heart Association only when manual methods in the maintenance of an airway have proved ineffective.[28] Patients who are not deeply unconscious can tolerate the nasopharyngeal airway better, whereas the oropharyngeal airway will induce gagging, regurgitation, or vomiting in patients who are not deeply unconscious. Therefore I suggest inclusion of the nasopharyngeal airway, in a variety of sizes (for example, child, small adult, normal adult), for the office emergency kit.

*Suggested for emergency kit:* At a minimum, the kit should contain one set each of adult and pediatric nasopharyngeal airways.

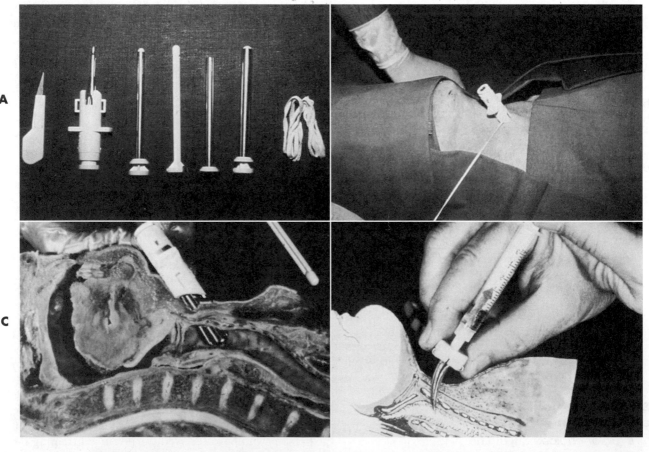

**Figure 3-33**  **A,** *(left to right),* stylet; needle and housing unit; airway; obturator; airways (2); tie. **B,** Airways secured in position. **C,** Anatomic view of positioned airway. **D,** Pediatric cricothyrotomy needle.

NOTE: Advanced training is required for safe and effective use of these devices.

## Advanced airway devices

Many devices are available to aid in the maintenance of a patent airway in the unconscious or semiconscious patient. Among these are the *esophageal obturator airway* (EOA), laryngeal mask airway (LMA), laryngoscope and endotracheal tube. As with the other devices listed in this section, advanced training in the use of each item is absolutely essential.

The *EOA* is a 37-inch, large-bore tube designed to be inserted into and to occlude the esophagus, permitting air to be forced into the victim's trachea and lungs and not the stomach.[29] Although usually easily inserted, even by untrained rescuers, problems can develop that minimize the usefulness of this device. These include possible insertion of the tube into the trachea, thereby entirely obstructing the airway, and the high probability that the victim will vomit when the *EOA* is removed. Because of these potential problems, the American Heart Association lists the following considerations when EOAs are used[30]:

1. Should be used only by trained individuals
2. Should not be used in victims younger than 16 years
3. Should not be used in conscious victims or those who are breathing spontaneously
4. Should not be left in place for more than 2 hours
5. Should not be used forcefully during insertion
6. Suction should be immediately available during insertion and removal

NOTE: The EOA is not recommended for inclusion in the emergency kit unless the doctor and staff members have received training in its proper insertion and removal.

The *laryngeal mask airway* is used widely in Europe for airway control during anesthesia. The airway is a tube (similar to an endotracheal tube) and a small mask with an inflatable circumferential cuff intended for placement in the victim's posterior pharynx that seals the base of the tongue and laryngeal opening. This device has a very high success rate and low complication rate, both of which are achievable with considerable training.[31] The laryngeal mask airway is used in situations in which endotracheal intubation is difficult and increasingly has become the sole means of airway management in many anesthetic procedures.[32]

*Endotracheal intubation* using a laryngoscope to visualize the trachea and an endotracheal tube (Figure 3-35) is a technique of airway maintenance that must be restricted to persons extremely well-trained in its use. Realistically, this limits its usefulness to anesthesiologists, anesthetists, trained paramedical personnel, and those dentists and physicians who have received extensive general anesthesia training.

A number of advantages make endotracheal intubation the preferred technique of airway management. These include the isolation of the airway, which prevents aspiration; the facilitation of ventilation and oxygenation; and providing an avenue for the administration of emergency drugs (for example, epinephrine, lidocaine, atropine, naloxone).[30] The most common mistakes in intubation include accidentally intubating the esophagus and taking more than 30 seconds to intubate. In addition, improper intubation technique often results in fracture of the maxillary anterior teeth.

When used by properly trained individuals, tracheal intubation is a preferred technique of airway management in the unconscious patient.

*Suggested for emergency kit:* A minimum of one laryngoscope and a set of spare batteries and

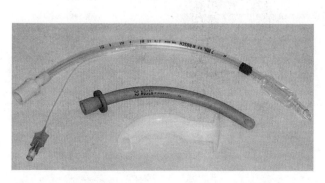

**Figure 3-34** Airway devices *(top to bottom):* endotracheal tube, nasopharyngeal airway and oropharyngeal airway.

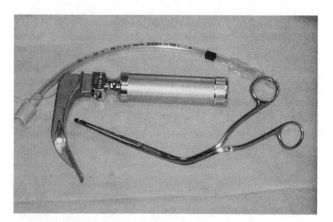

**Figure 3-35** Laryngoscope *(left)*, Magill intubation forceps *(right)*, and endotracheal tube *(bottom)*.

assorted adult- and pediatric-size endotracheal tubes may be included in the emergency kits of doctors trained in their use.

# Module Three: ACLS

A third category of injectable drugs that should be included in the emergency kit are those classified as essential in the performance of ACLS (Table 3-5). These drugs should be considered for inclusion only by doctors who have been certified in ACLS.

## ACLS ESSENTIAL DRUGS

In recent years a number of ACLS drugs previously considered essential have been deemphasized. These include sodium bicarbonate, calcium chloride, bretylium tosylate, and isoproterenol. Essential ACLS drugs include the following:

1. Epinephrine
2. $O_2$
3. Lidocaine
4. Atropine
5. Dopamine
6. Morphine sulfate
7. Verapamil

### ACLS essential: cardiac arrest

*Drug of choice:* Epinephrine
*Proprietary:* Adrenalin
*Drug class:* Endogenous catecholamine
*Alternative drug:* None

Three items form the essentials of ACLS—epinephrine, $O_2$, and defibrillation. Epinephrine (Adrenalin) previously has been discussed as an essential injectable drug in the management of anaphylaxis. Epinephrine is available as a 1-mg dose in preloaded syringes containing either 1 ml (1:1000 concentration) or 10 ml (1:10,000) of solution. The 1:10,000 concentration is for administration IV or endotracheally, whereas the 1:1000 solution is designed for subcutaneous, sublingual, or IM administration.

Epinephrine's importance in cardiac arrest lies in the fact that no other drug can maintain coronary artery blood flow while CPR is in progress, which is essential for preserving a chance of survival in cardiac arrest. Epinephrine also preserves blood flow to the brain. In the absence of drug therapy, cerebral blood flow during CPR is minimal; most blood enters into the common carotid artery and flows into the external carotid branch, not into the internal carotid artery.[33] After the administration of a drug such as epinephrine, with α-adrenergic properties, cerebral blood flow is increased significantly.[34]

*Therapeutic indications:* Cardiac arrest (including ventricular fibrillation, pulseless ventricular tachycardia, asystole, and pulseless electrical activity) (see Chapter 30).

*Side effects, contraindications, and precautions:* In the situations requiring the administration of epinephrine, no contraindications to its use exist. However, doctors should be aware that when large doses are administered to patients not receiving CPR, hypertension frequently results. In addition, epinephrine may induce or exacerbate ventricular ectopy, especially in patients who are receiving digitalis.[35]

*Availability:* Epinephrine is available in 1:10,000 concentration in preloaded 10-ml syringes.

table **3-5**    *Module three—advanced cardiac life support—essential drugs*

| CATEGORY | PRIMARY DRUG | | ALTERNATIVE | RECOMMENDED FOR KIT | |
|---|---|---|---|---|---|
| | GENERIC | PROPRIETARY | | QUANTITY | AVAILABILITY |
| **Injectables** | | | | | |
| Cardiac arrest | Epinephrine | Adrenalin | — | 2 or 3 × 10-ml preloaded syringes | 1:10,000 concentration |
| Oxygen | Oxygen | — | — | 1 E cylinder | |
| Antidysrhythmic | Lidocaine | Xylocaine | Procainamide | 1 preloaded syringe 1 × 5-ml ampule | 100 mg 100 mg |
| Symptomatic bradycardia | Atropine | Atropine | Isoproterenol | 2 × 10-ml syringes | 1.0 mg/10 ml |
| Symptomatic hypotension | Dopamine | Intropin | Dobutamine | 1 or 2 × 5-ml ampules | 80 mg/ml |
| Analgesic | Morphine | Morphine | Meperidine | 2 × 2-ml ampules | 10 mg/ml |
| PSVT* | Verapamil | Isoptin | — | 1 or 2 × 4-ml ampules | 2.5 mg/ml |

*PSVT, Paroxysmal supraventricular tachycardia.

*Suggested for emergency kit:* Two or three preloaded syringes may be included in the kit.

## ACLS essential: O₂

*Drug of choice:* O₂
*Proprietary:* None
*Drug class:* None
*Alternative drug:* None

O₂ already is included in the emergency kit as an essential noninjectable drug. It is essential in cardiac resuscitation and emergency cardiac care. Although exhaled air ventilation provides 16% to 17% O₂ and ambient air ventilation provides 21% O₂, enriched O₂ ventilation, or 100% O₂ ventilation, precludes the possibility of the development of hypoxia if ventilation is adequate.

Absolutely no contraindications exist to the administration of O₂ in emergency situations. Long-term administration of high O₂ concentrations can produce O₂ toxicity, but the duration required for the development of such a situation far exceeds the duration of almost all emergency situations. O₂ must never be withheld or diluted during resuscitation because of the mistaken belief that it is harmful.[30] (See the discussion of O₂ included in Module One in the section on critical noninjectable drugs for a fuller description of the precautions, availability, and recommendations associated with O₂.)

## ACLS essential: antidysrhythmic

*Drug of choice:* Lidocaine
*Proprietary:* Xylocaine
*Drug class:* Local anesthetic, antidysrhythmic
*Alternative drug:* Procainamide

Lidocaine (Xylocaine) is used extensively in the management of cardiac dysrhythmias, especially those of ventricular origin that develop after acute myocardial infarction. Lidocaine is considered the primary antidysrhythmic drug in ACLS. Procainamide also effectively suppresses ventricular ectopy and is recommended for administration when lidocaine has not effectively suppressed life-threatening ventricular dysrhythmias.[36]

*Therapeutic indications:* Lidocaine is administered when premature ventricular contractions (PVCs) occur more than 6 times per minute or with the presence of closely coupled PVCs, multifocal PVCs, or those occurring in bursts of two or more in succession. Lidocaine administration also is indicated in sustained ventricular tachycardia (where a palpable pulse is present) with a pulse and in ventricular fibrillation that is refractory to electrical defibrillation (see Chapter 30).[37]

*Side effects, contraindications, and precautions:* Excessive doses of lidocaine produce myocardial, circulatory, and central nervous system depression. Clinical signs and symptoms of lidocaine overdose include drowsiness, paresthesias, and muscle twitching.[38] More severe overdoses may produce tonic-clonic seizure activity.[39] Decreased hepatic function or hepatic blood flow slows the rate of lidocaine biotransformation, producing prolonged elevated blood levels and a greater risk of lidocaine overdose. Impaired hepatic blood flow frequently is observed in the presence of acute reductions in cardiac output (for example, in myocardial infarction and congestive heart failure.)[40]

*Availability:* Lidocaine is available for IV injection in 5 ml prefilled syringes containing either 50- or 100 mg and in 5 ml ampules of 100 mg.

*Suggested for emergency kit:* One 100-mg preloaded syringe and one 5-ml ampule.

## ACLS essential: symptomatic bradycardia

*Drug of choice:* Atropine
*Proprietary:* Atropine
*Drug class:* Parasympatholytic
*Alternative drug:* Isoproterenol

Atropine is the drug of choice for hemodynamically significant bradydysrhythmias and also is administered during asystole that is refractory to epinephrine administration. A bradydysrhythmia is considered to be hemodynamically unstable when the following conditions are present[30]:

1. Hypotension (defined by ACLS guidelines as systolic blood pressure >90 mmHg)
2. PVCs
3. Altered mental status or symptoms (for example, chest pain or dyspnea)
4. Ischemia
5. Infarction

Isoproterenol is a synthetic sympathomimetic amine with nearly pure β-adrenergic receptor activity. Despite producing a decrease in mean blood pressure, isoproterenol provides increased cardiac output. However, it also markedly increases myocardial O₂ consumption and may therefore induce or exacerbate myocardial ischemia. Although still considered for administration in the management of hemodynamically significant and atropine refractory bradycardia, isoproterenol is no longer the drug of choice. Electronic pacing of the heart has proven more effective than isoproterenol, and does not increase myocardial O₂ requirements. Atropine is one of four drugs that may be administered endotracheally (see Secondary Injectable Drugs).

## ACLS essential: symptomatic hypotension

*Drug of choice:* Dopamine
*Proprietary:* Intropin
*Drug class:* Sympathomimetic amine
*Alternative drug:* Dobutamine

Dopamine (Intropin) is a chemical precursor of norepinephrine. In large doses it stimulates both α- and β-adrenergic receptors. At lower doses it dilates renal, mesenteric, and cerebral arteries.[41] Dopamine also stimulates the release of norepinephrine; it is indicated for administration in hemodynamically significant hypotension in the absence of hypovolemia. When administered, the dose of dopamine should be kept as low as possible to ensure adequate perfusion of vital organs.

Dobutamine is a synthetic sympathomimetic amine that exerts significant inotropic effects by stimulating $\beta_1$- and α-adrenergic receptors in the myocardium.[42] Its β-stimulatory actions greatly outweigh its α-stimulatory actions, usually resulting in a mild vasodilation. In its usual dose, dobutamine is less likely than isoproterenol or dopamine to induce tachycardias. Dopamine is administered IV as an infusion, with the infusion rate altered according to the response of the patient.

*Therapeutic indications:* The primary therapeutic indication for dopamine is to treat hemodynamically significant hypotension in the absence of hypovolemia.

*Side effects, contraindications, and precautions:* Because dopamine produces an increase in heart rate, it may induce or exacerbate supraventricular or ventricular dysrhythmias. In addition, dopamine may alter the imbalance between supply and demand of the myocardium for $O_2$, inducing or exacerbating myocardial ischemia.[43]

Nausea and vomiting frequently are noted with dopamine administration. In patients receiving monoamine oxidase–inhibitors (isocarboxazid, pargyline, tranylcypromine, or phenelzine), dopamine activity may be augmented. These patients should receive no more than one-tenth the usual dose of dopamine.

*Availability:* Dopamine is available as 200 mg, 400 mg, and 800 mg in 5-ml ampules and syringes.

*Suggested for emergency kit:* One or two ampules of 400-mg dopamine (80 mg/ml).

## ACLS essential: analgesia

*Drug of choice:* Morphine
*Proprietary:* Morphine
*Drug class:* Opioid agonist
*Alternative drug:* Meperidine

The management of pain and anxiety during ischemic chest pain is a critical part of overall patient care. Although a number of analgesics are available, morphine is the drug of choice (see discussion on secondary injectable drugs).

## ACLS essential: paroxysmal supraventricular tachycardia

*Drug of choice:* Verapamil
*Proprietary:* Isoptin
*Drug class:* Calcium channel blocker
*Alternative drug:* None

Verapamil (Isoptin) is the second calcium channel blocker discussed in this section. Nifedipine, discussed as a secondary noninjectable drug for the management of hypertensive situations, is another. Verapamil is included in the ACLS category because it is extremely effective in the management of supraventricular tachycardia.[44] Verapamil slows conduction through the atrioventricular node, reducing ventricular response to atrial flutter and fibrillation. Although verapamil may be administered orally, in the context of ACLS it should be administered IV.

*Therapeutic indications:* In emergency cardiac care, verapamil is used primarily to treat paroxysmal supraventricular tachycardia that does not require cardioversion. When verapamil proves ineffective in the management of PSVT, synchronized cardioversion is recommended.

*Side effects, contraindications, and precautions:* A transient decrease in arterial pressure may be noted because of peripheral vasodilation in response to verapamil.[45] Verapamil is not indicated for ventricular tachycardia; it may induce severe hypotension and predispose a patient to ventricular fibrillation.[46]

*Availability:* Verapamil is available for injection in 2.5 mg/ml in 2-ml and 4-ml ampules.

*Suggested for emergency kit:* One or two 4-ml ampules.

For a complete discussion of all aspects of ACLS, the doctor should consult one of the available recommended references.[30,47] In addition, ACLS certification at (minimally) the provider level helps the doctor better understand how properly to use the drugs mentioned in this section.

# Module Four: Antidotal Drugs

Four categories of injectable drugs are used to manage emergency situations that arise in response to the administration of drugs used primarily for sedation via the IM and IV routes or general anesthesia (Table 3-6). These drugs should be maintained in the emergency kit only as warranted by the nature of the dental practice. For example, an opioid antagonist is not essential when opioid agonists are not used in patient management.

## ANTIDOTAL DRUGS

Categories of antidotal drugs include the following:
1. Opioid antagonist
2. Benzodiazepine antagonist
3. Antiemergence delirium drug
4. Vasodilator

### Antidotal drug: opioid antagonist

*Drug of choice:* Naloxone
*Proprietary:* Narcan
*Drug class:* Thebaine derivative
*Alternative drug:* Nalbuphine

The most significant side effect of parenterally administered opioid agonists is their ability to produce respiratory depression by diminishing the responsiveness of the brain's respiratory centers to arterial carbon dioxide. Thus the patient's breathing rate is decreased. Opioid antagonists have been available since 1951 (nalorphine, levallorphan). Although these agents reversed opioid-induced respiratory depression, when administered to patients with non–opioid-induced respiratory depression, both nalorphine and levallorphan were able to produce their own respiratory depression and of enhancing barbiturate-induced respiratory depression.

Naloxone (Narcan) became available in the late 1960s and today remains the only opioid antagonist free of any agonistic properties. Naloxone also reverses other properties of opioids, namely analgesia, and sedation.[48] This action is not entirely innocuous; if opioids are administered for postsurgical analgesia, naloxone administration antagonizes this effect, leaving the patient with unmanaged postsurgical pain. Naloxone may be administered endotracheally in situations in which IV access is not available. Administered IV or endotracheally, improved respiratory function is noted within 2 minutes.

Nalbuphine, an opioid agonist-antagonist, has been used successfully to reverse respiratory depression induced by opioid agonists.[49] Because nalbuphine has its own agonist properties, it provides excellent reversal of opioid-induced respiratory depression, but does not entirely remove postsurgical analgesia or sedation because of its own analgesia-inducing properties.

*Therapeutic indications:* Naloxone is indicated for use in opioid-induced depression, including respiratory depression (see Chapter 23).

*Side effects, contraindications, and precautions:* When administered via IV or endotracheal tube, naloxone's effects last only 30 minutes. A recurrence of respiratory depression may be observed if the opioid previously administered is of longer duration (for example, morphine). IM administration of a second naloxone dose after the IV dose is common. Although this dose is slower in onset, its duration is considerably longer than the IV dose. This regimen minimizes a possible recurrence of respiratory depression.

table **3-6** | *Module four—antidotal drugs*

| CATEGORY | PRIMARY DRUG | | | RECOMMENDED FOR KIT | |
| | GENERIC | PROPRIETARY | ALTERNATIVE | QUANTITY | AVAILABILITY |
| --- | --- | --- | --- | --- | --- |
| **Injectables** | | | | | |
| Opioid antagonist | Naloxone | Narcan | Nalbuphine | 2 × 1-ml ampules | 0.4 mg/ml |
| Benzodiazepine antagonist | Flumazenil | Romazicon | — | 1 × 10-ml multidose vial | 0.1 mg/ml |
| Antiemergence delirium | Physostigmine | Antilirium | — | 2 or 3 × 2-ml ampules | 1 mg/ml |
| Vasodilator | Procaine | Novocain | — | 2 × 2-ml ampules | 10 mg/ml |

It is important to remember that in the presence of opioid-induced respiratory depression, naloxone administration is neither the most important nor the first step in patient management. Airway patency and ventilation are primary considerations. Naloxone must be administered with extreme care to persons with known or suspected physical dependence on opioids. Naloxone's abrupt and complete reversal of opioid agonist effects may precipitate acute withdrawal syndrome.

*Availability:* Naloxone is available for adults in 0.4 mg/ml in 1-ml ampules and 10-ml vials. The drug is available for pediatric administration in 0.02 mg/ml in 2-ml ampules.

*Suggested for emergency kit:* Two 1-ml ampules of 0.4 mg/ml naloxone.

## Antidotal drug: benzodiazepine antagonist

*Drug of choice:* Flumazenil
*Proprietary:* Romazicon
*Drug class:* Benzodiazepine antagonist
*Alternative drug:* None

Although the benzodiazepines have been described as the most nearly ideal agents for anxiety control and sedation, a number of potential adverse reactions are associated with their administration. Emergence delirium, excessive duration of sedation, and possibly (though unlikely in most instances) significant respiratory depression are but a few side effects. The availability of a specific antagonist for benzodiazepines adds another degree of safety to IV (and to a lesser extent IM) sedation.

Flumazenil (Romazicon) has been demonstrated to produce a rapid reversal of sedation and to improve the patient's ability to comprehend and obey commands.[50] The duration of anterograde amnesia associated with midazolam was reduced from 121 minutes without flumazenil to 91 minutes with flumazenil.[50,51] Flumazenil also decreased the recovery time from midazolam sedation, increased alertness, and provided a decreased amnesic effect in the geriatric population (72 ± 9 years). Two patients, however, became anxious following flumazenil administration.[52] The availability of flumazenil is recommended wherever benzodiazepines such as diazepam, midazolam, or lorazepam are administered parenterally.

*Therapeutic indications:* Flumazenil is used to reverse the clinical actions of parenterally administered benzodiazepines (see Chapter 23).

*Side effects, contraindications, and precautions:* Flumazenil has been demonstrated to produce a rebound anxiety state is some patients.[52]

*Availability:* Flumazenil (Romazicon) is available in 0.1 mg/ml in 5-ml and 10-ml multidose vials.

*Suggested for emergency kit:* One 10-ml multidose vial of flumazenil.

## Antidotal drug: antiemergence delirium

*Drug of choice:* Physostigmine
*Proprietary:* Antilirium
*Drug class:* Reversible anticholinesterase
*Alternative drug:* None

Several drugs that are commonly used parenterally to induce sedation can produce what is known as *emergence delirium.* Scopolamine and the benzodiazepines, diazepam and midazolam, are most likely to produce this phenomenon, in which the patient appears to lose contact with reality. The patient also may exhibit increased muscular movement and may seem to speak but make only unintelligible sounds. Physostigmine (Antilirium), a reversible cholinesterase that can cross the blood-brain barrier, has become the drug of choice in the management of emergence delirium. Physostigmine is recommended for inclusion in the emergency drug kit if scopolamine, benzodiazepines, or other drugs that may induce emergence delirium are administered parenterally.

*Therapeutic indications:* Physostigmine is used to reverse emergence delirium (see Chapter 23).

*Side effects, contraindications, and precautions:* Side effects noted with physostigmine administration include increased salivation, possible emesis, and involuntary urination and defecation. The first two actions are most common. If administered too rapidly, physostigmine can produce all these effects plus bradycardia and hypersalivation, which can lead to respiratory difficulty. Atropine, an antagonist and antidote for physostigmine, should always be available whenever physostigmine is administered. Physostigmine should not be administered to patients with asthma, diabetes, cardiovascular disease, or mechanical obstruction of the gastrointestinal or genitourinary tracts.

*Availability:* Physostigmine is available as Antilirium in 1 mg/ml in 2-ml ampules.

*Suggested for emergency kit:* Two or three ampules.

### Antidotal drug: vasodilator
*Drug of choice:* Procaine
*Proprietary:* Novocain
*Drug class:* Local anesthetic
*Alternative drug:* None

A local anesthetic that also possesses significant vasodilating properties is recommended for inclusion in the emergency kit whenever IM or IV drugs are used. Procaine (Novocain) administration is indicated for extravascular injection of an irritating chemical and for accidental intraarterial drug administration. In both instances the problems are localized tissue irritation and compromised circulation in either a localized area (extravascular administration) or a limb (intraarterial administration). Procaine is an excellent vasodilator and anesthetic, both of which make it ideal for administration in the previously mentioned situations.

*Therapeutic indications:* Procaine is used to manage vasospasm and compromised circulation following intraarterial drug injection and to manage pain and vascular compromise following extravascular administration of irritating drugs.

*Side effects, contraindications, and precautions:* Allergy to ester-type local anesthetics is not uncommon. Procaine should not be administered to patients with histories (either documented or alleged) of allergy to "Novocain."

*Availability:* Procaine is available as a 1% (10 mg/ml) solution in 2-ml and 6-ml ampules.

*Suggested for emergency kit:* Two 2-ml ampules.

## Organization of the Emergency Kit

The emergency drug kit need not and indeed should not be complicated. Four levels or modules of drugs and equipment were presented:
1. Module one: basic emergency kit (critical drugs and equipment)
2. Module two: noncritical drugs and equipment
3. Module three: ACLS
4. Module four: antidotal drugs

Doctors should match their educational backgrounds and clinical experiences with these different drugs before including them in the office emergency kit. Only those drugs and items of equipment with which the doctor is thoroughly familiar should be considered for inclusion. Minimally, Module one (critical drugs and equipment) should be available in all offices.

A simple place in which to store emergency drugs and equipment is in a fishing tackle box or plastic box with several compartments. Larger kits may be stored in mobile tool cabinets. Labels should be applied to compartments in which each drug is stored and should list both the drug's generic name (for example, epinephrine) and proprietary name (for example, Adrenalin) to avoid possible confusion during an emergency.

In addition, the office staff should keep written records of the expiration dates of each of the drugs in the emergency kit, and each drug should be replaced prior to that date. Expired drugs and empty $O_2$ cylinders are ineffective in the management of any emergency situation. An office staff member should be assigned to check the emergency drug kit at least once a week and check all emergency equipment daily—especially the $O_2$ cylinders—to ensure that all emergency items are ready for use. Records of all emergency drug and equipment inspections should be entered in a bound (not a loose-leaf) notebook. The emergency kit and equipment must be kept in an area that is readily accessible to all office personnel. The back of a storage closet is not the place for life-saving equipment.

Occasionally, office personnel may run into difficulty purchasing the small quantities of drugs required for the emergency kit. Most drug wholesalers sell these drugs in prepackaged boxes of 12 or 25 units, but in most instances only two or three ampules are required for the office emergency kit. In such cases, office personnel may want to contact a hospital pharmacy, which is more likely to dispense small quantities of the required drugs, or an anesthesia supply house.*

Although this text has recommended each office make its own emergency kit, commercially prepared kits do have one advantage. With these kits, soon-to-be-outdated drugs are automatically replaced (at a cost) by mail. When the doctor does not have ready access to a source of emergency drugs, this service may prove beneficial.

To assess whether your office is prepared to manage life-threatening situations, each emergency team member should ask the following question: "If I were in need of emergency medical care, would I want it to be in my office and managed by my dental team?"

*Contact Southern Anesthesia and Surgical Supply at 1-800-624-5926 or fax 1-800-344-1237 or www.southernanesthesia.com

## REFERENCES

1. American Dental Association House of Delegates: *The use of conscious sedation, deep sedation, and general anesthesia in dentistry,* Chicago, November, 1985, The Association.

2. American Association of Oral and Maxillofacial Surgeons: *Parameters of care for oral and maxillofacial surgery: a guide for practice, monitoring and evaluation,* Rosemont, Ill, 1995, The Association.

3. American Academy of Pediatric Dentistry: Guidelines for the elective use of conscious sedation, deep sedation, and general anesthesia in pediatric patients, *Pediatr Dent* 18(6):30-81, 1996.

4. American Dental Association: *Guidelines for teaching the comprehensive control of pain and anxiety in dental education,* Chicago, 1989, The Association.

5. Morrow GT: Designing a drug kit, *Dent Clin North Am* 26(1):21-33, 1982.

6. Weaver WD and others: Factors influencing survival after out-of-hospital cardiac arrest, *J Am Coll Cardiol* 7:752, 1986.

7. Eisenber MS, Bergner L, Hallstrom A: Cardiac resuscitation in the community: importance of rapid provision and implications for program planning, *JAMA* 241:1905, 1979.

8. Block Drug Company: *Vital response crisis management system,* Jersey City, NJ, 1988, The Company (videotape).

9. Healthfirst Corporation: *Emergency medicine,* Seattle, 1991, The Corporation (videotape).

10. Academy of General Dentistry: *Medical emergencies: video journal of dentistry 3:3,* Chicago, 1994, The Academy (videotape).

11. Malamed SF: Managing medical emergencies, *J Am Dent Assoc* 124:40-53, 1993.

12. American Dental Association Council on Dental Therapeutics: Emergency kits, *J Am Dent Assoc* 87:909, 1973.

13. American Dental Association: *ADA guide to dental therapeutics,* Chicago, 1998, The Association.

14. Pallasch TJ: This emergency kit belongs in your office, *Dent Management,* pp 43-45, August 1976.

15. Malamed SF: *Sedation: a guide to patient management,* ed 3, St Louis, 1995, Mosby.

16. Woodard ML, Brent LD: Acute renal failure, anterior myocardial infarction, and atrial fibrillation complicating epinephrine abuse, *Pharmacotherapy* 18(3):656-658, 1998.

17. Cohen M: Epinephrine: tragic overdose, *Nursing* 26(4):13, 1996.

18. Hollister-Stier Laboratories, Spokane, Washington.

19. Epipen, Epipen Jr: Center Laboratories, Division of EM Pharmaceuticals, Inc, Port Washington, NY.

20. Malamed SF: The use of diphenhydramine HCl as a local anesthetic in dentistry, *Anesth Prog* 20:76, 1973.

21. Pollack CV Jr, Swindle GM: Use of diphenhydramine for local anesthesia in "caine"-sensitive patients, *J Emerg Med* 7(6):611-614, 1989.

22. Israel bans import of sildenafil citrate after six deaths in the US, *BMJ* 316(7145):1625, 1998.

23. Opie LH: Pharmacologic options for treatment of ischemic disease. In Smith TW, editor: *Cardiovascular therapeutics: a companion to Braunwald's heart disease,* Philadelphia, 1996, WB Saunders.

24. ISIS-2 (Second International Study of Infarct Survival) Collaborative Group: Randomized trial of intravenous streptokinase, oral aspirin, both, or neither among 17,187 cases of suspected acute myocardial infarction, ISIS-2, *Lancet* 2(8607):349, 1988.

25. Raines A and others: Comparison of midazolam and diazepam by the IM route for the control of seizures in a mouse model of status epilepticus, *Epilepsia* 31(3):313-317, 1990.

26. Streeten DHP: Corticosteroid therapy. I. Pharmacological properties and principles of corticosteroid use, *JAMA* 232:944, 1975.

27. Grossman E and others: Should a moratorium be placed on sublingual nifedipine capsules given for hypertensive emergencies and pseudoemergencies? *JAMA* 76(16):1328-31, 1996.

28. American Heart Association Emergency Cardiac Care Committee and Subcommittees: Guidelines for cardiopulmonary resuscitation and emergency cardiac care. IX. Ensuring effectiveness of communitywide emergency cardiac care, *JAMA* 268(16): 2289-2295, 1992.

29. Johannigman JA and others: Out-of-hospital ventilation: bag-valve device vs transport ventilator, *Acad Emerg Med* 2(8):719-24, 1995.

30. Cummins RO, editor: *Textbook of advanced cardiac life support,* Dallas, 1997, American Heart Association Subcommittee on Advanced Cardiac Life Support.

31. Pennant JH, White PF: The laryngeal mask airway: its uses in anesthesiology, *Anesthesiology,* 79:144-63, 1993.

32. Verghese C, Brimacombe JR: Survey of laryngeal mask airway usage in 11,910 patients: safety and efficacy for conventional and nonconventional usage, *Anesth Analg* 82(1):129-33, 1996.

33. Paradis NA, Koscove EM: Epinephrine in cardiac arrest: a critical review, *Ann Emerg Med* 19:1288-91, 1990.

34. Koehler RC and others: Beneficial effect of epinephrine infusion on cerebral and myocardial blood flows during CPR, *Ann Emerg Med* 14:744, 1985.

35. Packer M, Gottlieb SJ, Kessler PD: Hormone-electrolyte interactions in the pathogenesis of lethal cardiac arrhythmias in patients with control of arrhythmias, *Am J Med* 80(suppl 4A):23, 1986.

36. Giardina EG, Heissenbuttel RH, Bigger JT Jr: Intermittent intravenous procainamide to treat ventricular arrhythmias, *Ann Intern Med* 78:183, 1973.

37. Olson DW and others: A randomized comparison study of bretylium tosylate and lidocaine in resuscitation of patients from out-of-hospital ventricular fibrillation in a paramedic system, *Ann Emerg Med* 13:807, 1984.

38. Benowitz N and others: Lidocaine disposition kinetics in monkey and man. I. Prediction of a perfusion model, *Clin Pharmacol Ther* 16:87, 1974.

39. Collingsworth KA, Kalman SM, Harrison DC: The clinical pharmacology of lidocaine as an antiarrhythmic drug, *Circulation* 50:1217, 1974.

40. Thomson PD and others: Lidocaine pharmacokinetics in advanced heart failure, liver disease, and renal failure in humans, *Ann Intern Med* 78:499, 1973.

41. Weiner N: Norepinephrine, epinephrine, and the sympathomimetic amines. In Hardman JG, Limbird LE, editors: *Goodman & Gilman's the pharmacological basis of therapeutics,* ed 9, New York, 1996, McGraw-Hill.

42. Leier CV: Acute inotropic support. In Leier CV, editor: *Cardiotonic drugs: a clinical survey,* New York, 1986, Marcel Dekker.

43. Mueller HS, Evans R, Ayers S: Effect of dopamine on hemodynamics and myocardial metabolism in shock following acute myocardial infarction in man, *Circulation* 57:361, 1978.

44. McGoon MD and others: The clinical use of verapamil, *Mayo Clin Proc* 57:495, 1982.

45. Singh BN, Collett JT, Chew CY: New perspectives in the pharmacologic therapy of cardiac arrhythmias, *Prog Cardiovasc Dis* 22:243, 1980.

46. Stewart RB, Bardy GH, Greene HL: Wide complex tachycardia: misdiagnosis and outcome after emergency therapy, *Ann Intern Med* 104:766, 1986.

47. Grauer K, Cavallaro D: *ACLS: certification, preparation, and a comprehensive review,* St Louis, 1993, Mosby.

48. Pallasch TJ, Gill CJ: Naloxone-associated morbidity and mortality, *Oral Surg* 52:602, 1981.

49. Magruder MR, Delaney RD, DiFazio CA: Reversal of narcotic-induced respiratory depression with nalbuphine hydrochloride, *Anesth Rev* 9(4):34, 1982.

50. Rodrigo MR, Rosenquist JB: The effect of Ro 15-1788 (Anexate) in conscious sedation produced with midazolam, *Anaesth Intensive Care* 15:185, 1987.

51. Wolff J and others: Ro 15-1788 for postoperative recovery: a randomized clinical trial in patients undergoing minor surgical procedures under midazolam anaesthesia, *Anaesthesia* 41:1001, 1986.

52. Ricou B and others: Clinical evaluation of a specific benzodiazepine antagonist (Ro 15-1788): studies in elderly patients after regional anaesthesia under benzodiazepine sedation, *Br J Anaesth* 58:1005, 1986.

# 4

# Medicolegal Considerations

**Kenneth S. Robbins**

**R**ECENTLY, much has been written about the legal implications of the practice of dentistry. Each year 7% to 8% of dentists are sued. These percentages represent more than 15,000 lawsuits against dentists every year. The growing tendency of patients to sue is disquieting. Realizing that these suits are only a small fraction of all malpractice claims against dentists further intensifies the problem; most claims are settled by insurance agencies before they even become lawsuits. As the number of dentists and lawyers continues to increase, claims and lawsuits against dentists also increase.

Most patients bring claims and lawsuits against their dentists alleging that the treatment performed produced an undesirable result. Patients frequently complain that parts of their mouths were damaged severely, particularly that nerve damage resulted in temporary or permanent loss of sensation or partial loss of mouth control. Although malpractice complaints in dentistry that arise as a result of medical emergencies comprise only a minority of the total number of lawsuits against dentists, the life-and-death nature of medical emergencies makes these cases among the most serious; the potential injury to the patient and the liability of the dentist both are high.

As Dr. Malamed demonstrates, medical emergencies for which the dentist and staff members should be prepared have substantially more serious implications for both the patient and the dentist than the less severe circumstances that give rise to most lawsuits.

Lawsuits that seek damages because of temporary paresthesia, broken needles, or permanent cosmetic injuries pale in comparison to lawsuits alleging that a patient suffered brain damage or death from improperly administered cardiopulmonary resuscitation (CPR) during cardiac arrest.

Lawsuits resulting from medical emergencies are based on injuries and medical consequences to the patient that often precipitate the highest jury verdicts and the highest defense costs; they are the multimillion-dollar cases. The high potential jury verdict and the high cost of defense increase the probability that the individual practitioner's and the profession's dental malpractice insurance may skyrocket. Another potentially devastating risk to dentists in these cases is that multimillion-dollar verdicts may exceed the amount of insurance coverage available to a practitioner, putting the dentist's assets and income at risk.

Therefore taking time to consider how dentists can avoid being sued and what they can do to win when they are sued is invaluable. One important step requires that the dentist ask patients to fill out medical history questionnaires. Each dentist then should keep the forms and continually update them. In addition to the University of Southern California questionnaire provided in Chapter 2, the American Dental Association's long form is another valuable source (Figure 4-1). These forms are accepted throughout the profession and may become important evidence for the dentist if a patient brings suit.

# Frequently Asked Questions

What is the expected standard of care when a patient or other individual suffers a medical emergency in the dental office? Is this standard lower than the standard of care in a nonemergency? In a genuine medical emergency, does the Good Samaritan statute exempt the dentist from civil liability? (Most states' Good Samaritan statutes help free the doctor from liability if the doctor renders a patient life-saving treatment in good faith without expecting to be compensated for the service.) If an emergency is truly an unforeseen combination of circumstances, how can the dentist be held liable for it?

These are some of the many questions I have been asked as a trial-oriented defense attorney. Ultimately, a judge and no jury—or more frequently a jury—is left to answer the question at hand. Therefore the lawyer always must examine the context within which the judge or jury answers these difficult questions. In the following pages, I provide a brief review of the most crucial aspects of the trial process. The information describes the logical basis required to understand and apply the legal principles involved in such lawsuits and the legal expectations of dentists under such circumstances.

# The Jury System

Unless a dentist has agreed expressly with a patient to use alternatives to the judicial system to resolve a dispute (for example, arbitration or mediation), the existing judicial system in a particular community and state must resolve a malpractice complaint. More particularly, if a patient files suit alleging injury because of negligence during a medical emergency in the dental office, the case ultimately must be resolved at a trial by jury. The defendant may doubt that the jury members can make sense of the enormous volume of evidence presented in a trial and return the proper verdict. They can, however, and they do. The result depends on the evidence, the law, and the quality of trial counsel.

Long ago, well-heeled people resolved important disputes through professionals adept at some form of one-on-one combat (for example, knights at a joust). Whoever hired the victorious combatant won the dispute. In the modern world, those professionals have been replaced by a different kind of combatant. Lawyers now oppose each other with legal, not lethal, results; the consequences, however, are just as important to those who do the hiring. Opposing attorneys try to uncover as many facts as possible to assist a nonpartisan third party—the judge or jury—in deciding who should win and lose. Ideally, if attorneys for both sides excel equally at their craft, a judge or jury can decide the outcome with sufficient evidence on both sides. Sadly, advocates are not usually equal, and greater incentives to win frequently are provided to the patient's attorneys than to the attorneys hired by insurance companies on the dentist's behalf.

Plaintiffs' attorneys usually are hired on a contingency-fee basis, which means that they are entitled to a percentage of the damages (money) they obtain for their clients (generally 25% to 40%, but sometimes as much as 75%). Therefore plaintiffs' attorneys have built-in incentives to win their clients' cases. Defense attorneys, however, do not accept contingency fees as compensation. Virtually all dentists are defended in a lawsuit by an attorney who is paid by the hour—the same fee, win or lose.

The professionalism among defense attorneys should be sufficiently high to negate the presumption that an attorney with a vested interest in a victory per-

**Copies of the Medical History Are Available Through the Order Department
of the American Dental Association**

# MEDICAL HISTORY

Name _____ Sex _____ Date of Birth: _____

Address _____

Telephone _____ Height _____ Weight _____

Date _____ Occupation _____ Marital Status _____

### DIRECTIONS

If the answer is YES to the question, put a circle around "YES."

If the answer is NO to the question, put a circle around "NO."

Answer all questions by circling either YES or NO, and fill in all blank spaces when indicated.

Answers to the following questions are for our records only and will be considered confidential.

1. Are you in good health? . . . . . . . . . . . . . . . . . . . . . . . . . . . . . . . . . . . . . . . . . . . . . . . . . . . YES    NO
   a.  Has there been any change in your general health within the past year? . . . . . . . . . . . . YES    NO

2. My last physical examination was on _____

3. Are you now under the care of a physician? . . . . . . . . . . . . . . . . . . . . . . . . . . . . . . . . . . . . YES    NO
   a.  If so, what is the condition being treated? _____

4. The name and address of my physician is _____

   _____

   _____

5. Have you had any serious illness or operation? . . . . . . . . . . . . . . . . . . . . . . . . . . . . . . . . . YES    NO
   a.  If so, what was the illness or operation? _____

6. Have you been hospitalized or had a serious illness within the past five (5) years? . . . . . . . . YES    NO
   a.  If so, what was the problem? _____

7. Do you have or have you had any of the following diseases or problems?
   a.  Rheumatic fever or rheumatic heart disease . . . . . . . . . . . . . . . . . . . . . . . . . . . . . . . . YES    NO
   b.  Congenital heart lesions . . . . . . . . . . . . . . . . . . . . . . . . . . . . . . . . . . . . . . . . . . . . . . YES    NO
   c.  Cardiovascular disease (heart trouble, heart attack, coronary insufficiency, coronary
       occlusion, high blood pressure, arteriosclerosis, stroke) . . . . . . . . . . . . . . . . . . . . . YES    NO
       1)  Do you have pain in chest upon exertion? . . . . . . . . . . . . . . . . . . . . . . . . . . . . YES    NO
       2)  Are you ever short of breath after mild exercise? . . . . . . . . . . . . . . . . . . . . . . . YES    NO
       3)  Do your ankles swell? . . . . . . . . . . . . . . . . . . . . . . . . . . . . . . . . . . . . . . . . . . . YES    NO
       4)  Do you get short of breath when you lie down, or do you require extra pillows
           when you sleep? . . . . . . . . . . . . . . . . . . . . . . . . . . . . . . . . . . . . . . . . . . . . . . . . YES    NO
   d.  Allergy . . . . . . . . . . . . . . . . . . . . . . . . . . . . . . . . . . . . . . . . . . . . . . . . . . . . . . . . . . . YES    NO
   e.  Asthma or hay fever . . . . . . . . . . . . . . . . . . . . . . . . . . . . . . . . . . . . . . . . . . . . . . . . YES    NO
   f.  Hives or a skin rash . . . . . . . . . . . . . . . . . . . . . . . . . . . . . . . . . . . . . . . . . . . . . . . . . YES    NO
   g.  Fainting spells or seizures . . . . . . . . . . . . . . . . . . . . . . . . . . . . . . . . . . . . . . . . . . . . YES    NO
   h.  Diabetes . . . . . . . . . . . . . . . . . . . . . . . . . . . . . . . . . . . . . . . . . . . . . . . . . . . . . . . . . YES    NO
       1)  Do you have to urinate (pass water) more than six times a day? . . . . . . . . . . . . YES    NO
       2)  Are you thirsty much of the time? . . . . . . . . . . . . . . . . . . . . . . . . . . . . . . . . . . . YES    NO
       3)  Does your mouth frequently become dry? . . . . . . . . . . . . . . . . . . . . . . . . . . . . YES    NO
   i.  Hepatitis, jaundice or liver disease . . . . . . . . . . . . . . . . . . . . . . . . . . . . . . . . . . . . . YES    NO
   j.  Arthritis . . . . . . . . . . . . . . . . . . . . . . . . . . . . . . . . . . . . . . . . . . . . . . . . . . . . . . . . . . YES    NO
   k.  Inflammatory rheumatism (painful, swollen joints) . . . . . . . . . . . . . . . . . . . . . . . . . YES    NO
   l.  Stomach ulcers . . . . . . . . . . . . . . . . . . . . . . . . . . . . . . . . . . . . . . . . . . . . . . . . . . . . YES    NO
   m.  Kidney trouble . . . . . . . . . . . . . . . . . . . . . . . . . . . . . . . . . . . . . . . . . . . . . . . . . . . . YES    NO
   n.  Tuberculosis . . . . . . . . . . . . . . . . . . . . . . . . . . . . . . . . . . . . . . . . . . . . . . . . . . . . . . YES    NO
   o.  Do you have a persistent cough or cough up blood? . . . . . . . . . . . . . . . . . . . . . . . . . YES    NO
   p.  Low blood pressure . . . . . . . . . . . . . . . . . . . . . . . . . . . . . . . . . . . . . . . . . . . . . . . . . YES    NO
   q.  Venereal disease . . . . . . . . . . . . . . . . . . . . . . . . . . . . . . . . . . . . . . . . . . . . . . . . . . . YES    NO
   r.  Other _____

*Continued*

**Figure 4-1**  American Dental Association long-form medical history questionnaire.

8. Have you had abnormal bleeding associated with previous extractions,
   surgery, or trauma? . . . . . . . . . . . . . . . . . . . . . . . . . . . . . . . . . . . . . . . . . . . .   YES    NO
   a.  Do you bruise easily? . . . . . . . . . . . . . . . . . . . . . . . . . . . . . . . . . . . . . . .   YES    NO
   b.  Have you ever required a blood transfusion? . . . . . . . . . . . . . . . . . . . . . .   YES    NO
       If so, explain the circumstances _____
       _____

9. Do you have any blood disorder such as anemia? . . . . . . . . . . . . . . . . . . . . . .   YES    NO

10. Have you had surgery or x-ray treatment for a tumor, growth, or other condition
    of your head or neck? . . . . . . . . . . . . . . . . . . . . . . . . . . . . . . . . . . . . . . . . .   YES    NO

11. Are you taking any drug or medicine? . . . . . . . . . . . . . . . . . . . . . . . . . . . . . .   YES    NO
    If so, what? _____

12. Are you taking any of the following?
    a.  Antibiotics or sulfa drugs . . . . . . . . . . . . . . . . . . . . . . . . . . . . . . . . . . .   YES    NO
    b.  Anticoagulants (blood thinners) . . . . . . . . . . . . . . . . . . . . . . . . . . . . . .   YES    NO
    c.  Medicine for high blood pressure . . . . . . . . . . . . . . . . . . . . . . . . . . . . . .   YES    NO
    d.  Cortisone (steroids) . . . . . . . . . . . . . . . . . . . . . . . . . . . . . . . . . . . . . . .   YES    NO
    e.  Tranquilizers . . . . . . . . . . . . . . . . . . . . . . . . . . . . . . . . . . . . . . . . . . . .   YES    NO
    f.  Aspirin . . . . . . . . . . . . . . . . . . . . . . . . . . . . . . . . . . . . . . . . . . . . . . . . .   YES    NO
    g.  Insulin, tolbutamide (Orinase) or similar drug . . . . . . . . . . . . . . . . . . . .   YES    NO
    h.  Digitalis or drugs for heart trouble . . . . . . . . . . . . . . . . . . . . . . . . . . . .   YES    NO
    i.  Nitroglycerin . . . . . . . . . . . . . . . . . . . . . . . . . . . . . . . . . . . . . . . . . . . .   YES    NO
    j.  Antihistamine . . . . . . . . . . . . . . . . . . . . . . . . . . . . . . . . . . . . . . . . . . .   YES    NO
    k.  Oral contraceptive or other hormonal therapy . . . . . . . . . . . . . . . . . . . .   YES    NO
    l.  Other _____

13. Are you allergic or have you reacted adversely to any of the following?
    a.  Local anesthetics . . . . . . . . . . . . . . . . . . . . . . . . . . . . . . . . . . . . . . . . .   YES    NO
    b.  Penicillin or other antibiotics . . . . . . . . . . . . . . . . . . . . . . . . . . . . . . . .   YES    NO
    c.  Sulfa drugs . . . . . . . . . . . . . . . . . . . . . . . . . . . . . . . . . . . . . . . . . . . . . .   YES    NO
    d.  Barbiturates, sedatives, or sleeping pills . . . . . . . . . . . . . . . . . . . . . . . .   YES    NO
    e.  Aspirin . . . . . . . . . . . . . . . . . . . . . . . . . . . . . . . . . . . . . . . . . . . . . . . . .   YES    NO
    f.  Iodine . . . . . . . . . . . . . . . . . . . . . . . . . . . . . . . . . . . . . . . . . . . . . . . . . .   YES    NO
    g.  Codeine or other narcotics . . . . . . . . . . . . . . . . . . . . . . . . . . . . . . . . . .   YES    NO
    h.  Other _____

14. Have you had any serious trouble associated with any previous dental treatment? . . . . . . . .   YES    NO
    If so, explain _____
    _____

15. Do you have any disease, condition, or problem not listed above that you think
    I should know about? . . . . . . . . . . . . . . . . . . . . . . . . . . . . . . . . . . . . . . . . .   YES    NO
    If so, please explain _____

16. Are you employed in any situation that exposes you regularly to x-rays or other
    ionizing radiation? . . . . . . . . . . . . . . . . . . . . . . . . . . . . . . . . . . . . . . . . . . .   YES    NO

17. Are you wearing contact lenses? . . . . . . . . . . . . . . . . . . . . . . . . . . . . . . . . . .   YES    NO

## WOMEN

18. Are you pregnant? . . . . . . . . . . . . . . . . . . . . . . . . . . . . . . . . . . . . . . . . . . . . .   YES    NO

19. Do you have any problems associated with your menstrual period? . . . . . . . . . . . . . . . .   YES    NO

Chief Dental Complaint:

_____
                Signature of Patient

_____
                Signature of Dentist

**Figure 4-1—cont'd**   American Dental Association long-form medical history
questionnaire.

forms better. The primary difference between the two types of attorneys is that a plaintiff's attorney who chooses cases carefully often generates a substantially higher fee revenue than a defense attorney, who often must maintain highly competitive hourly rates. Thus the insurance company in a meritorious case pays the plaintiff's lawyer a fee that is usually higher than the fee it pays its own defense attorney. This is done to keep that insurance carrier's expenses as low as possible; it is particularly notable in multimillion-dollar cases, in which the patient's attorney receives a substantial percentage of a gigantic award. Again, the professionalism and trial expertise of defense attorneys should remain unaffected by the different fee arrangements, and the quality of services rendered ideally should be as high for defendants as for plaintiffs. The disparity in incentives, however unfortunate, can create disparity in legal services.

A skilled plaintiff's attorney takes cases based on the outcome that attorney estimates the lawsuit is worth. If the facts of the potential lawsuit indicate that a jury may not decide favorably for the patient, the attorney often does not take the case at all or accepts it with the understanding that the potential lawsuit has a reduced settlement value. I believe that when plaintiffs' attorneys take weak cases and settle them for reduced but substantial amounts, dentists, insurance companies, and defense attorneys encourage this practice each time they approve such settlements.

An astute plaintiff's attorney should request a copy of the patient's chart to review and to have examined by another dentist before agreeing to accept the patient's case. A well-documented chart demonstrating satisfactory patient care discourages the plaintiff's attorney from accepting the case from the start. Therefore thorough documentation by the dentist is not only important at trial but also extremely important in determining whether the patient finds an attorney to file the lawsuit at all.

Once a lawsuit is filed with the court, a sheriff serves the dentist with a complaint and a summons, either by mail or by notice in a newspaper. Within a prescribed time after service—usually 30 days or less—the dentist must file an answer or take the risk that the judge may issue a default judgment against the defendant (the dentist). Between the time that the notice is served and the complaint answered, the dentist must hire an attorney. Generally, the dentist's insurance carrier assigns a lawyer to the case. However, dentists should decide long before a potential lawsuit arises who they would wish to represent them.

Depending on the population of the community, an insurance company usually employs one to three attorneys in that community who normally perform all the defense work on behalf of individuals that the company insures. Sometimes the attorney the company selects is not someone that the dentist would have hired. Therefore all dentists should become familiar—before the threat of a lawsuit—with those attorneys in the community who excel in dental malpractice defense. Before purchasing malpractice insurance, the dentist should agree with the insurance carrier on the choice of a lawyer in the event of a lawsuit. The worst time to make a well-reasoned decision—one that could affect the rest of the dentist's life—is after the dentist has been served notice of a lawsuit and has less than a month to obtain representation.

After the dentist's attorney has filed an answer to the complaint, a process known as *discovery* begins. No longer does any excuse exist for attorneys on either side to be ignorant of any important facts. Liberal rules in this area allow the use of many discovery tools. These include written interrogatories, or questions to be answered by each party; depositions, in which witnesses testify under oath during discovery; requests for production of records by either side; and requests that either side admit certain facts. Discovery permits both parties and their attorneys to learn as much as possible about the merits of the strengths and weaknesses of the other side's case.

The dentist should expect to be kept abreast of all important developments in the lawsuit. A feeling of teamwork should develop between the dentist and the defense attorney; each has expertise that the other needs. A clear example of productive teamwork is when the defense attorney plans for the dentist to be present during the deposition of the patient's expert witness. That expert may have more difficulty criticizing a dentist who is sitting across the table. Often, the dentist also should be present during the patient's deposition.

In addition, these depositions provide excellent opportunities for the dentist to evaluate the quality of the defense attorney. Another example of teamwork is when the dentist offers the defense attorney assistance in the understanding of complex dental and medical issues. Such collaboration also provides the dentist an excellent opportunity to evaluate the plaintiff's most incriminating evidence and to decide the best way to proceed.

## Burden of Proof and Res Ipsa Loquitur

With few exceptions, the plaintiff has what is called the *burden of proof* in any case, including a lawsuit against a dentist. This means that for a patient to win the case, a jury must find that the plaintiff proved the following things:

1. That the dentist was at fault
2. That the dentist's fault was the cause of injury to the patient
3. That the injury must be compensated in dollars and cents (damages), which the dentist must pay to the patient and in serious cases to the patient's family

Therefore in almost all cases in which a dentist is sued, the dentist may take comfort in the fact that the burden is not on the defendant (dentist) to disprove any of the issues; rather, the plaintiff must prove the alleged wrongdoing. In practical terms, however, the best defense for the defense attorney is often the offense. The attorney produces evidence that disproves fault by the dentist (that is, proves the dentist did not injure the patient). Like a good boxer, a good defense attorney always is prepared at trial to take the lead—to counter the plaintiff's punch—with appropriate evidence. This decision is made as late as possible in the process.

The reader may note some qualification in my statement that the patient has the burden of proof in all instances. The law has carved out an interesting and logical exception to a plaintiff's responsibility to prove fault. That exception is known as *res ipsa loquitur*, commonly shortened to *res ipsa*. Literally translated, this phrase means "the thing speaks for itself." Expressed simply, this concept applies to lawsuits in which the result itself indicates that the dentist must have committed some wrongdoing; otherwise, the harm would not have occurred.

For instance, if the dentist or oral surgeon performed a surgical procedure that required the use of small sponges and a sponge was left in the patient's gum and discovered later, the plaintiff would not have to prove that the dentist was at fault. In this case, the dentist would have to prove that the sponge that was left behind in the patient's tissue was not the dentist's fault. Few areas of dentistry exist in which the burden of proof is shifted to the dentist because of the doctrine of res ipsa loquitur. Few if any lawsuits arising out of medical emergencies fall into this category.

## The Expert Witness

A crucial part of the plaintiff's burden of proving the three indispensable elements of a case against the dentist is the procurement of expert testimony. Except in cases of res ipsa loquitur, the plaintiff tries to prove the case through the use of expert testimony. The patient's attorney retains an expert witness, who gives testimony that includes opinions on the appropriate standard of care and whether the dentist met that standard in the treatment of the patient.

Cases involving medical emergencies require the testimony of an expert witness because lay members of the jury are not considered competent to judge cases against dentists without expert testimony (except in res ipsa loquitur cases). The testimony of a witness who is qualified by the court as an expert, who states under oath that the dentist failed to meet the standard of care, and who adds that the injury in question was a result of the dentist's breach of this standard of care becomes an indispensable part of the plaintiff's case. Except in cases of res ipsa loquitur, courts in most states dismiss lawsuits against dentists before trial if the plaintiff has not obtained expert testimony against the dentist.

On the other hand, the defendant dentist and the defense attorney also may retain an expert witness to counter the testimony of the plaintiff's expert. Because the plaintiff has the burden of proof, the dentist need not obtain an expert witness to testify at trial. But if a plaintiff has an expert witness, an experienced defense attorney rarely fails to secure an expert witness on behalf of the dentist.

In some cases, however, the dentist need not obtain an expert witness. The appropriate strategies and counterstrategies in the use of expert witnesses at trial alone could fill an entire book. I have defended cases through trial, though rarely, in which the defendant dentists may well be their own best expert witnesses; however, this strategy must be used carefully. Of course, selection of the expert witness is extremely important. It is a rare person who can testify equally effectively at trial in many different professional and geographic areas.

The selection and use of expert witnesses demonstrate the great care, thought, and psychology both sides must exercise in case preparation and trial. A lawsuit tried solely on the basis of the strategy of the attorneys and the credibility of expert witnesses would be much like a football game without officials. From the beginning of the lawsuit to the conclusion of the trial, a judge always is available to provide answers when the lawyers cannot agree and to interject into each case the principles of law by which all cases are governed—standard of care, negligence, proximate cause of the injuries, and guidelines for awarding of damages.

Although the precise wording of these legal concepts may vary somewhat from state to state, their interpretation is sufficiently broad to allow meaningful discussions about their application in virtually all states. Discussion of several of these important concepts provides dentists a better understanding of what the law expects from them in terms of anticipation, prevention, and successful treatment of a medical emergency in the dental office. These concepts are the cornerstones of a successful defense.

## Standard of Care

A jury must find that the dentist acted negligently before the patient can recover damages. The terms *negligence* and *malpractice* are used synonymously in lawsuits against health care providers. In a dental malpractice case, a judge usually tells the jury that negligence is (1) doing something that an ordinarily prudent dentist would not do under the same or similar circumstances or (2) not doing something that a reasonably prudent dentist would do under the same or similar circumstances. The judge instructs the jury that negligence is the failure to practice ordinary care. This standard seems easy enough to determine as it applies to an automobile driver who does not watch the road or a shop owner who leaves a slippery substance on the floor of the shop, but how does a jury apply the principle of negligence to a dentist?

This is the point at which the testimony of the expert witness enters the picture. The judge's instructions guide the jury with regard to the indispensable expert testimony in almost all cases against dentists; the judge instructs the jury that in the case, each side may call an expert witness to define the standard of care and testify how the defendant dentist met or failed to meet that standard. The judge informs the jury that individuals ordinarily may not enter the courtroom and offer opinions. Usually, witnesses may testify to facts only—those things that they saw or heard or those documents or information they have in their possession that may assist the jury in making a decision.

However, the procedure differs in a lawsuit in which a jury must determine whether a dentist is at fault. In that case, expert witnesses—those individuals who possess special training and experience and whom the court has acknowledged to possess the skill or education necessary to offer opinions to the jury— may testify. Then the jury may consider their opinions. The judge informs the jury members that they need not consider any of the opinions given and may weigh the credibility of the expert witnesses by the same criteria they use for all other witnesses.

The crux of the testimony of each expert witness in a dental malpractice lawsuit is whether the dentist was negligent. In most states an expert witness may not testify to a belief that the dentist was negligent.

However, the expert may provide an opinion about whether the dentist fell within or below the acceptable standard of care. In doing so, the expert may not use personal standards but must use what that expert believes is the standards of the community. In recent years the community standard has been expanded to match the national community standard. Therefore in almost all lawsuits in all courts across the country, each defendant dentist is held to a national standard of care, which the expert witnesses must establish in testimony. However, experts frequently do not agree on the definition of the national standard, and this point remains one of contention.

The previous information has been provided to demonstrate the importance of expert witnesses in the plaintiff's case. Without expert testimony on behalf of the plaintiff, who has the burden of proof, no evidence exists regarding the acceptable standard of care, which the jury must use to conclude whether the dentist's treatment lived up to that standard. Many people in many different professions are qualified as experts in the proper response to medical emergencies in the dental office. They include CPR instructors, paramedics, specially trained nurses, medical doctors, and of course dentists. They create an abundance of potential expert witnesses who are qualified to testify either for or against the dentist.

## Forseeability of the Emergency

An underlying principle of our legal system is the concept of foreseeability. If the consequences of an act are foreseeable and result in harm, liability may be imposed. A cardiac arrest or an idiosyncratic reaction to medication or anesthesia in a dental office arguably may not be foreseeable events. However, experience tells us that although medical emergencies are not predictable, the fact that they do occur makes them foreseeable. This logic most probably is the reason that companies with many employees and those with direct contact with the public—such as department stores, hotels, and restaurants—are upgrading and maintaining higher standards in case medical emergencies do arise.

More and more service-oriented employees are learning how to administer procedures like CPR correctly. At the time of publication of the fourth edition of this book, whether an individual could bring a successful lawsuit against department store personnel for failure to respond properly to that person's cardiac arrest remained questionable. However, as the community standard for response to cardiac arrests is upgraded and as expectations rise as to how service-oriented employees should respond to medical emergencies, this possibility may become a reality. Someday a department store employee may be held liable for negligence if that employee does not have the training needed to treat an individual suffering cardiac arrest.

Given such a possibility, little doubt exists that the expectations of the standards of care in the treatment of medical emergencies are higher in medical facilities, including dental offices. From experience in malpractice cases, I have learned that certain circumstances and practices within a dental office are much more likely to precipitate a medical emergency than those within a department store. This higher likelihood of emergency helps explain the higher expectation of care.

What are some of the foreseeable circumstances or factors likely to precipitate a medical emergency in the dental office? Many people experience fear and anxiety at the mere thought of an upcoming dental appointment. By the time these people actually reach the office waiting room, their fears and anxieties can cause measurable metabolic changes. Sometimes, anger and frustration at having to sit in the waiting room a long time add to the metabolic changes and can increase the risk that an emergency may develop. However, a short waiting period is no guarantee; even patients who are seen immediately often experience substantially more stress in a dental office than in most other environments.

A highly stressed patient is not the ideal candidate to receive anesthetics or medications. Furthermore, once treatment begins, the administration of anesthetics or medications increases the risk that a medical emergency may develop in anxious and nonanxious patients alike. Virtually every anesthetic agent and medication is associated with some adverse or idiosyncratic reaction and side effects. The *Physicians' Desk Reference* (PDR) or the drug-package insert accompanying each anesthetic or medication lists reactions that reportedly have been associated with that drug's administration. Additionally almost every anesthetic agent and medication that a dentist uses can and has produced bizarre medical reactions. Dentists also must remember that those reactions published in the drug-package insert and the *PDR* are associated with the use of a particular anesthetic or medication; in fact the drug's use may have absolutely nothing at all to do with the ensuing medical emergency.

However, even if the emergency was not related to the use of a particular drug, the published warning in the *PDR* is a reliable source to which the patient's expert witness may refer in court. The witness may say to the jury, "The adverse reaction to the anesthetic is something the dentist knew about or should have known about; it is listed as a known side effect in the pharmaceutical bible, the *PDR*, which every prescriber and administrator of medication has or should have. The same information is included with every vial and every package of medication that is opened in the dentist's office." The *PDR* excerpt for that medication thus becomes evidence against the dentist to which the jury can later refer during deliberations.

The *PDR* excerpt also can be used as evidence of notice to the dentist—evidence that the dentist used the anesthetic or medication daily on many patients and therefore had a duty to know all its reported side effects and adverse reactions. Consequently, the plaintiff's attorney may argue, the dentist should have anticipated and treated correctly the adverse reaction or side effect the patient experienced. Of course, the defense attorney can counter through that side's expert witnesses, witnesses from pharmaceutical companies or the FDA, or even from the *PDR* that the side effects, adverse reactions, and incidents reportedly associated with use of the medication are based on reports made by health care providers that may never have been investigated and verified. However, the jury may interpret this kind of evidence as a rationalization. The dentist's attorney always must anticipate this reaction and prepare to respond successfully.

The previous information demonstrates that the *PDR*, in presenting information that offers protection to the pharmaceutical companies, also contains invaluable information every dentist should know and use in practice. If a dentist stays current with the *PDR*, that dentist also can prevent having the patient use this resource against the dentist in a lawsuit. Plaintiffs' attorneys experienced in dental malpractice know that every dental office should contain a *PDR* or in its absence a drug-package insert for each type of anesthesia or medication the office stocks. If a dentist fails to consult the *PDR*, the plaintiff's attorney may attempt to prove that an emergency occurred because the dentist failed to keep up with the latest literature on drugs used in the office.

Therefore all dentists should know thoroughly the drugs they use. An excellent way to do this is to consult the *PDR* and its updates throughout the year. This information will allow the dentist to identify patients for whom special precautions may have to be taken. Notes should be made in those patients' charts if the dentist deems that reevaluation of medications or further evaluation of medical history is necessary. Such follow-up notations can become important courtroom evidence on the dentist's behalf; they also can provide convincing proof that the dentist practices excellent dentistry.

# Handling of the Emergency

In the preface to this book, Dr. Malamed stated that with proper patient management, virtually all medical emergencies can be prevented. Frankly, I believe that within a legal and perhaps medical context this is a rather severe standard to which the dentist is expected to adhere. Rather, I believe that all medical emergencies are foreseeable and that dentists and staff members therefore should be properly trained and equipped to confront the medical emergency as well as reasonably can be anticipated.

However, all dentists should be aware of ways in which they can help avoid the unforeseen emergency. A dentist can increase the chances a patient may suffer a medical emergency by practicing poor bedside (actually chairside) manner, including keeping a patient waiting overly long. In addition, the dentist and staff members can fail to identify genuine anxiety and stress, fail to allay it, or perhaps fail to postpone treatment until a patient's anxiety has been allayed. As far as adverse and idiosyncratic reactions to medications are concerned, preventive measures do exist that dentists can and probably should take based on the current national standards of dental practice.

## HISTORY

As discussed in Chapter 2 and stressed throughout this text, all dentists must obtain a full and complete medical history before treating a patient. Even if the patient is in severe pain and suffering what the dentist considers a dental emergency, a thorough medical history should be obtained from the patient or a person familiar with the patient, such as a spouse or parent. Few if any dental emergencies do not allow the dentist at least a few minutes to ask questions vital to that patient's well-being.

Knowledge of such problems as liver disorders, food and drug allergies, and heart problems is indispensable in the proper care and treatment of a patient. Failure to gather such information can be the most damaging evidence of all. If a thorough medical history would have contraindicated a certain anesthetic or medication and the dentist's administration of that drug results in a serious medical emergency, the patient or the patient's family could convince a jury successfully that the dentist was negligent. Chapter 2 presents several excellent examples of medical history questionnaires.

For the protection of both the dentist and the patient, the dentist should require that each patient complete the questionnaire before initial treatment. Because the medical history in some categories of patients, particularly the young and the elderly, may change markedly from year to year, dentists should require that patients update their medical-history forms annually. If a dentist has not treated a patient for several months, either the dentist or an office staff member should ask whether the patient's medical condition has undergone any changes or whether a physician has treated the patient for anything other than common, garden-variety illnesses; this practice should rule out any major problems before treatment.

In addition, the dentist should note on the chart that the patient was asked such questions since the last visit and should record carefully the patient's responses. For example, a patient suffers a serious adverse reaction in a dental office as a result of medication the dentist administered during treatment; that patient files a lawsuit that goes to trial. A jury is not likely to believe the testimony of a dentist or staff member who claims to recall that the patient stated nothing of any medical consequence had happened since the last dental visit—unless that statement is in writing.

To discredit the verbal statement, a skilled plaintiff's attorney simply must establish the fact that in the months and years since the plaintiff's visit, the dentist has seen several thousand patients and cannot possible recall one patient's statement. In effect the jury is asked to view the dentist's memory with great suspicion. However, if a significant medical event did occur and the patient did not inform the dentist, a written negative response to such a question can support the dentist's credibility years later; this information is difficult evidence for the patient and the plaintiff's attorney to discredit at the trial.

If a patient's medical history requires clarification, the dentist should contact the patient's primary-care physician and make a notation in that patient's chart about the content of the consultation. Patients' charts should include the names and phone numbers of their primary-care physician for this purpose. The dentist should indicate in a phone call to the physician that the dentist is taking notes on the information discussed and should suggest the physician do the same. These notations may prove extremely important at a trial.

## INFORMED CONSENT

In the past two decades, a national standard for informed consent has developed. Different courts in different states may vary in how informed consent should be obtained, but in essence informed consent requires that a dentist explain to a patient the following information in sufficient detail so that the patient understands:

1. Reasons for care and treatment
2. Diagnosis
3. Prognosis
4. Alternatives
5. Nature of care and treatment
6. Risks involved (inherent risks included)
7. Expectations of success
8. Possible results if the patient does not undergo care and treatment or does not follow instructions

As with other topics previously discussed, informed consent alone could fill several chapters of a book. However, informed consent has an interesting twist in the context of medical emergencies. Arguably, the more thorough a dentist is in explaining the risks involved in a procedure and in documenting discussion of those risks with the patient, the stronger the evidence may be against that dentist if a medical emergency does arise during treatment. For instance, an oral surgeon warns a patient that cardiac arrest is a known reaction to a certain anesthetic; that patient subsequently experiences cardiac arrest under the anesthetic in question. The oral surgeon thus may have difficulty explaining to a jury that the reaction was an unforeseeable emergency and therefore impossible for which to prepare. Consequently, the more thorough a dentist is in warning patients about possible risks, the more prepared that dentist should be to prevent or treat those risks.

To the extent that a plaintiff's attorney can demonstrate or prove that medical emergencies occur with a higher frequency in a dentist's office than in many other situations, dentists are expected to be more prepared to prevent or treat such emergencies. Throughout this text, Dr. Malamed discusses the kinds of emergencies dentists should anticipate and how they should treat patients who suffer them; that information need not be repeated here. However, I do want to emphasize that proper response to a medical emergency often requires effective and efficient teamwork. Such teamwork is particularly vital in a situation in which CPR must be administered.

Therefore each dental office should be staffed with appropriately trained personnel who know their assigned tasks in case a medical emergency does develop. For example, who will telephone for an ambulance? Where will the emergency response equipment, including oxygen, be kept, and whose responsibility will it be to bring that equipment to the patient? In many circumstances, CPR cannot be administered effectively by only one person, so dentists who do not ensure that someone other than

themselves knows the CPR techniques may not be protected in court. Because CPR administration is a foreseeable circumstance with which most dentists will be confronted at some time, all office members should be familiar with proper CPR technique and maintain current CPR certification. In addition, dentists should hold occasional CPR office drills and maintain records of such drills that include which staff members participated. These records effectively can refute a plaintiff's contention that a patient died during cardiac arrest because office members lacked CPR training. Whereas CPR is not always effective in saving patients' lives, the dentist should not leave to chance the possibility of being held liable for a patient's death simply because that dentist failed to document employee CPR training and practice drills.

As soon as possible after an emergency, the dentist should note in the chart what happened to the patient—from the initiation of treatment to the conclusion of the emergency or until paramedics or physicians assumed care of the patient. If the emergency is handled correctly, these notes are invaluable in the dentist's trial defense. Because the dentist is responsible for job-related negligence of associates and employees, the dentist must ensure that each member of the dental team is well trained so that an employee's act or omission does not create liability for that dentist. Although a dentist may respond superbly to a medical emergency, problems may arise if staff members are negligent because they lack proper training.

Often, paramedics may handle medical emergencies more expertly than dentists; they may not want the dentist to accompany them to the hospital. The dentist should offer assistance as needed before the paramedics depart for the hospital. Whatever the paramedics decide, both the dentist's offer to continue assistance en route to the hospital and the paramedics' response to that offer should be documented.

## A Lower Standard for Emergencies?

The law does not require that the dentist or any other health care practitioner respond to an emergency in the same way that individual would respond to a nonemergency. In other words the standard of care the law expects of a dentist in an emergency is lower than the standard expected in a nonemergency. However, it is the jury that decides whether a dentist was negligent in an emergency on the basis of the answer to one question—Did the dentist and staff members respond as an ordinarily prudent dentist or staff member would have responded in the same or similar circumstances?

The dentist and staff members are held to the standard of the ordinarily prudent practitioner to the extent that the medical emergency can be shown to have been foreseeable and to the extent that evidence demonstrates that the dentist and staff members should have been prepared. Although the standard of care in emergencies is not as high as that in nonemergencies, emergency situations do have their own standards of conduct. If the dentist and staff members meet these standards, they are not held liable; if they fail to meet them, they may be held liable for a patient who suffered injury or even death.

In addition, all dentists should remember that medical emergencies resulting from dental treatment may occur after the patient has left the office. If a patient begins to experience an adverse reaction to a medication at home and calls, or asks someone to call, the dental office, the dentist and staff must be prepared to treat a potential emergency. The dentist and emergency team members should discuss a preplanned response to such a situation so that they can provide the patient or family member with proper and immediate instructions. A dentist's failure to respond to such a circumstance may itself precipitate a lawsuit. If a patient cannot get the attention of the dentist at the time of the phone call, that patient may later respond with an attention-getting lawsuit.

# Good Samaritan Considerations

Good Samaritan statutes, which differ somewhat from state to state, provide the dentist with some degree of protection from frivolous patient lawsuits. Most such statutes state that health care providers should not be held liable for death or injury (except in situations of gross negligence) in cases in which they render emergency, life-and-death treatment in good faith to individuals who are not their patients (that is, individuals for whose treatment they do not expect to be compensated).

However, a patient who suffers a medical emergency in a dental office usually does not fall under the protection of the state's Good Samaritan statute. Because the victim of the emergency is the dentist's patient, the dentist has an obligation to treat that patient. However, if a nonpatient of the dentist, such as the patient's family member, happens to be in the waiting room and requires an emergency response, the Good Samaritan defense may apply.

# Proactive Measures

Each dentist should establish a relationship with an experienced malpractice defense lawyer in case a lawsuit arises. Dentists also should keep in touch with that lawyer and seek legal advice just as a patient seeks periodic checkups for preventive care. A prudent dentist also should urge the community dental association or society to invite lawyers who specialize in dental malpractice cases to meetings; such lawyers can familiarize area dentists with the requirements for informed consent requirements and other specifics of state law.

In addition, dentists should stay abreast of the statutes and cases that affect dentistry so that they can tailor their practices to meet the requirements of the law. Prudent dentists learn how other dentists equip and prepare their offices and staff members for medical emergencies and ensure that their levels of preparedness are comparable to or exceed the standard in dentistry. This standard of care is not perfection—particularly when the dentist or staff member is responding to a medical emergency.

Although today's health care professionals are defending themselves against more lawsuits than ever, lawsuits can be prevented. Furthermore, if lawsuits do occur, they can be defended successfully. The prevention or successful defense of lawsuits depends on how each dentist and dental team meet the challenges of increased litigation. By preventing lawsuits or providing information leading to a successful defense, dentists not only protect themselves but also maintain the presumption that they care about their patients and take prudent precautions to protect them. If a dentist follows the suggestions provided in this chapter, practices within the standard of reasonableness, maintains continuing dental education, and documents office procedures and patient charts, the law supports that dentist.

One last word: courage. If dentists have competent, experienced counsel and a strong defense, they should have the courage to go through with a trial, if necessary. Settling claims or lawsuits outside court if the dentist should and can win in court only encourages additional lawsuits. By going through with a trial and winning the suit, dentists not only vindicate themselves and their staff members but also discourage similar lawsuits and become better dentists.

# *UNCONSCIOUSNESS*

# 5

## Unconsciousness

### General Considerations

*N* the recent past the loss of consciousness was not an uncommon occurrence in the practice of dentistry. In surveys of dental practices by Fast[1] and Malamed,[2] vasodepressor syncope (common faint) was the medical emergency most often reported, accounting for more than 50% of all emergency situations. Although any number of other causes can produce a loss of consciousness (Schultz[3] presents 33 potential causes in a differential diagnosis of syncope [Box 5-1]), the initial steps in the management of unconsciousness, regardless of cause, remain the same; these steps are directed primarily toward certain basic, life-sustaining procedures—**P** (position), **A** (airway), **B** (breathing), and **C** (circulation).

In most instances the loss of consciousness is transient, and administration of the aforementioned basic yet crucial procedures is all that proper management will be required. However, other causes of unconsciousness do require significant additional attention once these steps have been taken (**D** [definitive care]).

This section discusses several of the more common emergency situations that may result in the loss of

*Throughout this and subsequent chapters, emergency procedures are explained under the assumption that the doctor performs the life-saving duties. However, staff members may assume some or all of those duties if the doctor is unavailable.

box **5-1**   *Differential diagnosis of syncope*

Neurogenic causes
    Breath holding
    Carotid sinus disease
    Vasovagal syncope
    Vasodepressor syncope
    Orthostatic hypotension
    Glossopharyngeal neuralgia
    Seizure disorders
Vascular causes
    Cerebrovascular disease
        Tussive (cough) syncope
        Cerebrovascular accident
    Pulmonary embolism
    Aortic arch syndromes
Endocrinopathies
    Hypoglycemia
    Addisonian crisis
    Pheochromocytoma
    Hypothyroidism
Exposure to toxins and drugs
Psychogenic problems
Cardiogenic causes
    Valvular heart disease
    Dysrhythmia
    Myocardial infarction
    Certain congenital heart anomalies
    Hypertrophic cardiomyopathy
    Pacemaker syndrome
Disorders of oxygenation
    Anemia
    High altitude exposure
    Barotrauma
    Decompression sickness

Modified from Raven P, editor: *Emergency medicine: concepts and clinical practice,* ed 4, St Louis, 1998, Mosby.

box **5-2**   *Terms associated with unconsciousness*

**anoxia**  Absence or lack of oxygen

**coma**  From the Greek term *koma,* meaning deep sleep; most often used to designate a state of unconsciousness from which the patient cannot be roused even by powerful stimulation (Huff[4] defining coma as "that altered state that exists in a patient manifesting inappropriate responses to environmental stimuli who maintains eye closure throughout the stimuli").

**consciousness**  From the Latin term *conscius,* meaning aware; implies that an individual is capable of responding appropriately to questions or commands and that protective reflexes, including the ability of the individual to independently maintain a patent airway, are intact[5]

**faint**  Sudden, transient loss of consciousness

**hypoxia**  Low oxygen content

**syncope**  From the Greek term *synkope;* a sudden, transient loss of consciousness without prodromal symptoms that is followed within seconds to minutes (<30 minutes) by resumption of consciousness, usually with the premorbid status intact[6]

**unconsciousness**  A lack of response to sensory stimulation[7]

## Predisposing Factors

Table 5-1 outlines possible causes for a patient's loss of consciousness in the dental office and includes their frequency of occurrence. A glance at this list will indicate to the reader that many causes exist for the loss of consciousness. Although many causes do exist, a closer examination reveals that three factors, when present, increase the likelihood that a patient may experience an alteration or loss of consciousness. These factors include (1) stress, (2) impaired physical status, and (3) the administration or ingestion of drugs.

In dental settings, stress is the primary cause in most cases of unconsciousness. Vasodepressor syncope, the most common cause of unconsciousness in dentistry, is commonly a manifestation of unusually high levels of stress. Syncope occurring during venipuncture or the intraoral injection of a local anesthetic is a typical example of vasodepressor syncope.[8,9]

Impaired physical status (ASA III or IV) is a second factor that increases the likelihood of syncope. Many of the causes listed in Table 5-1 are not usually associated with the onset of syncope but may progress to unconsciousness if the underlying problem is not recognized promptly or if the patient is debilitated.

consciousness. Box 5-2 lists terms and definitions that are associated with unconsciousness and are found in the following chapters.

The terms *syncope* and *faint* commonly are used interchangeably to describe the transient loss of consciousness caused by reversible disturbances in cerebral function. Throughout this text the term *syncope* will be used to describe this occurrence. However, readers must remember that syncope is only a symptom and that although syncopal episodes may occur in healthy individuals, they may also be indicative of serious medical disorders. Any loss of consciousness, however brief, represents a potentially life-threatening situation requiring prompt recognition and effective management.

| table **5-1** | *Possible causes of unconsciousness in the dental office* |

| CAUSE | FREQUENCY | DISCUSSION |
|---|---|---|
| Vasodepressor syncope | Most common | Unconsciousness (Section Two) |
| Drug administration or ingestion | Common | Drug-related emergencies (Section Six) |
| Orthostatic hypotension | Less common | Unconsciousness (Section Two) |
| Epilepsy | Less common | Seizures (Section Five) |
| Hypoglycemic reaction | Less common | Altered consciousness (Section Four) |
| Acute adrenal insufficiency | Rare | Unconsciousness (Section Two) |
| Acute allergic reaction | Rare | Drug-related emergencies (Section Six) |
| Acute myocardial infarction | Rare | Chest pain (Section Seven) |
| Cerebrovascular accident | Rare | Altered consciousness (Section Four) |
| Hyperglycemic reaction | Rare | Altered consciousness (Section Four) |
| Hyperventilation | Rare | Altered consciousness (Section Four) |

When a patient with impaired physical status is exposed to undue physiologic or psychologic stress, the chances are even greater that this patient may react adversely to the situation. Individuals with underlying cardiovascular disease may respond with sudden death secondary to cardiac dysrhythmias, which are precipitated by the same physiologic stress that can cause vasodepressor syncope in a healthy individual.[10]

A third factor potentially associated with the loss of consciousness is the administration or ingestion of drugs. The three major categories of drugs used in dentistry are analgesics (nonopioids, including nonsteroidal antiinflammatory drugs, opioid analgesics, and local anesthetics), antianxiety agents (sedative-hypnotics and tranquilizers), and antibiotics. Drugs in the first two categories are central nervous system (CNS) depressants and therefore produce alterations in consciousness (for example, sedation) or the loss of consciousness. Some of these drugs, primarily the opioid agonists, predispose the ambulatory dental patient to orthostatic (postural) hypotension (see Chapter 7). Opioids and drugs such as barbiturates and other sedative-hypnotics, if administered in large doses, may induce the loss of consciousness as the patient enters the second or third stage of anesthesia (Guedel's classification[11]).*

Local anesthetics are the most commonly used drugs in dentistry, and because they must be injected, they play a major predisposing role in syncope. Researchers conservatively estimated that dental practitioners in the United States alone inject more than 1 million cartridges of local anesthetics each day, yet morbidity and mortality from these drugs remains incredibly low.[12] However, life-threatening situations can and do develop with the use of local anesthetics. The overwhelming majority of adverse reactions are stress induced (fear and anxiety)[13]; however, reactions that are directly related to the local anesthetics themselves do sometimes occur. These include overdose (toxic) reactions and allergy. (Adverse reactions to local anesthetics and other common dental drugs are discussed more fully in Section Four.)

## Prevention

Loss of consciousness can be prevented in many, if not most, instances by a thorough pretreatment medical and dental evaluation of the prospective patient. Important elements of this evaluation include a determination of the patient's ability to tolerate the stress—both physiologic and psychologic—associated

---

*The stages of anesthesia may be explained best through an explanation of the basic pattern with which general anesthetics and all other CNS depressants act; they progressively depress the CNS. CNS depressants, such as general anesthetics, tranquilizers, sedative-hypnotics, and alcohol, first depress the cerebral cortex, producing a loss of sensory function followed by a loss of motor function. The basal ganglia and cerebellum then become depressed, followed by the spinal cord and medulla. Medullary depression leads to depression of the respiratory and cardiovascular systems, the usual cause of death from drug overdose. Guedel[11] described four stages of anesthesia based on the previous information. Stage 1, analgesia or altered consciousness, corresponds to the action of these drugs on the higher cortical (sensory) centers. The various techniques that encompass psychosedation are included in this stage. Stage 2, delirium excitement, corresponds to the increasing depressant action of these drugs on the higher motor centers. The patient is unconscious during this stage. Stages 1 and 2 comprise the induction phase of general anesthesia. In stage 3, surgical anesthesia, spinal reflexes are depressed, producing skeletal muscle relaxation. Stage 4, medullary paralysis, corresponds to the depression of the respiratory and cardiovascular centers of the medulla, first producing respiratory arrest and then cardiovascular collapse.

with the planned treatment. Use of a medical history questionnaire and physical examination of the patient, followed by a dialogue history may uncover medical or psychologic disabilities that may predispose a patient toward syncope. Detection of these disabilities permits the doctor to modify the planned treatment to better accommodate the patient's physical or psychologic status.

Because many adult patients frequently seek to hide their fears, determination of a patient's anxiety towards dental treatment often is difficult to uncover. Since 1973 the University of Southern California has successfully used a method to help doctors recognize fearful patients. This consists of a short anxiety questionnaire (see Chapter 2) included in the medical history that each patient must complete before treatment begins. The form was modeled after Corah's questionnaire,[14] which presents the patient with a series of questions related to their attitudes toward various components of dental treatment.

Once dental fear and anxiety is confirmed, the dentist can use any of a number of conscious sedation techniques to reduce stress during treatment. These include nondrug procedures, such as iatrosedation and hypnosis; pharmacosedative procedures, including oral, rectal, intranasal, and intramuscular sedation; inhalation sedation with nitrous oxide and oxygen; and intravenous sedation. When used properly, conscious sedation can significantly reduce the medical and psychologic risks associated with dental treatment. However, as previously mentioned, the use of drugs will always be associated with risk factors of which the doctor administering the agents must be aware and be capable of recognizing and managing. According to McCarthy,[15] 90% of potential emergency situations can be prevented through the proper use of preliminary patient evaluation and appropriate use of conscious sedation and pain control.

Another major factor in the prevention of the loss of consciousness was the introduction of sit-down dentistry, in which patients are treated while they lie in a supine or slightly recumbent position. The supine position (ideally with the feet elevated about 10 to 15 degrees) prevents the development of cerebral anoxia, the most common mechanism producing syncope. Increasing use of the supine position during treatment has dramatically decreased the number of episodes of syncope that occur in dental offices.

## Clinical Manifestations

An unconscious patient is incapable of responding to sensory stimulation and has lost protective reflexes (for example, swallowing or coughing) accompanied by a lack of the ability to maintain a patent airway. Primary management of unconsciousness is directed at the reversal of these clinical manifestations.

Clinical signs and symptoms associated with incipient loss of consciousness (presyncope) and the actual state of unconsciousness (syncope) vary somewhat depending on the primary cause of the situation. For this reason the precise clinical manifestations of presyncope and syncope are discussed in greater detail under specific situations (see Chapters 6 through 9).

## Pathophysiology

In his classic test on fainting, Engle[16] classified the mechanisms that produce syncope into four categories (Table 5-2):

1. Reduced cerebral metabolism resulting from inadequate delivery of blood or $O_2$ to the brain
2. Reduced cerebral metabolism resulting from general or local metabolic deficiencies
3. Direct or reflex effects on that part of the CNS that regulates consciousness and equilibrium
4. Psychic mechanisms affecting levels of consciousness with their respective mechanism or mechanisms (categories 1 to 3) of action.

Hypotension is the most common cause of loss of consciousness in humans.

**table 5-2** | *Classification by mechanism of the causes of unconsciousness*

| MECHANISM | CLINICAL EXAMPLE |
|---|---|
| Inadequate delivery of blood or oxygen to the brain | Acute adrenal insufficiency |
| | Hypotension |
| | Orthostatic hypotension |
| | Vasodepressor syncope |
| Systemic or local metabolic deficiencies | Acute allergic reaction |
| | Drug ingestion and administration |
| | Nitrites and nitrates |
| | Diuretics |
| | Sedatives-opioids |
| | Local anesthetics |
| | Hyperglycemia |
| | Hyperventilation |
| | Hypoglycemia |
| Direct or reflex effects on nervous system | Cerebrovascular accident |
| | Convulsive episodes |
| Psychic mechanisms | Emotional disturbances |
| | Hyperventilation |
| | Vasodepressor syncope |

## INADEQUATE CEREBRAL CIRCULATION

The most common mechanism of syncope is a sudden decrease in the delivery of blood to the brain. Vasodepressor syncope (common faint) and orthostatic hypotension are the most frequently encountered clinical examples of this condition. Physiologic disturbances that decrease the blood supply to the brain include the following:

- Dilation of the peripheral arterioles
- Failure of normal peripheral vasoconstrictor activity (orthostatic hypotension)
- A sharp drop in cardiac output (from heart disease, dysrhythmias, or decreased blood volume)
- Constriction of cerebral vessels as carbon dioxide is lost through hyperventilation
- Occlusion or narrowing of the internal carotid or other arteries to the brain
- Life-threatening ventricular dysrhythmias

The first four factors rarely produce unconsciousness when the patient is in the supine position. Management of all six factors is directed at an increase in the supply of well-oxygenated blood to the brain.

## OXYGEN DEPRIVATION

A generalized decrease in skeletal muscle tone equivalent to that noted in Guedel's third stage of anesthesia accompanies a loss of consciousness. The tongue, a mass of skeletal muscle, loses its tone and because of the effect of gravity, falls posteriorly into the hypopharynx, producing either a complete or partial obstruction of the airway (Figure 5-1). In the unconscious patient, hypopharyngeal obstruction by the base of the relaxed tongue always occurs when the head is flexed and almost always when the head is maintained in midposition.[17,18] Resuscitation of the unconscious patient focuses primarily on relief of this obstruction. Until the obstruction is removed, the patient continues to receive hypoxic levels of $O_2$ (partial obstruction) or becomes anoxic (total obstruction), with a decreasing likelihood of successful resuscitation.[19]

The vital importance of airway management and oxygenation in the maintenance of consciousness may be explained as follows: Under normal conditions the brain derives most of its energy from the oxidation of glucose. To maintain this energy source, the brain must receive a continuous supply of glucose and $O_2$. Without $O_2$, some glucose still can be metabolized into lactic acid to provide limited energy, but this source cannot fulfill the brain's requirements for more than a few seconds, rapidly leading to the loss of consciousness.

The human brain, which accounts for only 2% of total body mass, uses approximately 20% of the total $O_2$ and 65% of the total glucose the body consumes.[20] To do this, approximately 20% of the total blood circulation per minute must reach the brain. When the supply of either fuel is diminished, brain function is affected rapidly. The cerebral blood flow of a normal individual situated in the supine position is an estimated 750 ml per minute. Thus at any given time the blood circulating through the brain contains 7 ml of $O_2$, an amount adequate to supply the brain's requirements for less than 10 seconds. Rossen, Kabat, and Anderson[21] performed experiments in which the human brain was deprived of $O_2$ by a sudden and complete arrest of cerebral circulation. Individuals lost consciousness within 6 seconds.

Complete airway obstruction, in which the victim becomes anoxic, leads to permanent brain damage within 4 to 6 minutes and cardiac arrest within 5 to 10 minutes. In a study of dogs asphyxiated for 5 minutes, 50% of survivors sustained gross brain damage; after 10 minutes of asphyxiation, all demonstrated significant brain damage.[19] Some authorities contend that periods of anoxia for as short as 3 minutes may cause permanent brain damage.[22] Partial airway obstruction, in which the victim receives hypoxic levels of $O_2$, can produce similar results, although more slowly and through more complex pathways. In either case the doctor and staff members must be able to initiate the steps of basic life support (BLS) rapidly and effectively.

Adequate ventilation has been termed the *sine qua non* of resuscitation.[23] Once a patient has been secured, and only then, should the doctor proceed to more definitive life suppport measures (chest compression or drug administration).

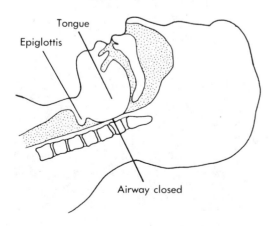

**Figure 5-1**  In an unconscious victim the tongue falls backward against the wall of the pharynx, producing airway obstruction.

## GENERAL OR LOCAL METABOLIC CHANGES

Changes in the quality of blood perfusion to the brain that are caused by chemical or metabolic derangements also may provoke the loss of consciousness or may predispose a patient to its occurrence. The most frequently encountered clinical situations that lead to syncope through this mechanism include hyperventilation, hypoglycemia, the administration or ingestion of drugs, and the acute allergic reaction. In these cases the patient will not regain consciousness until the underlying chemical or metabolic cause is corrected.

## ACTIONS ON THE CENTRAL NERVOUS SYSTEM

Loss of consciousness associated with alterations within the brain itself or through reflex effects on the CNS manifests clinically as convulsions and cerebrovascular accidents.

## PSYCHIC MECHANISMS

Psychic mechanisms, such as emotional disturbances, are the most common causes of transient losses of consciousness in dental settings and include several clinical situations discussed previously. Vasodepressor syncope and hyperventilation are included in this category.

# Management

Immediate management of the unconscious victim is predicated on two objectives:
1. Recognition of unconsciousness
2. Management of the unconscious victim, including the recognition of possible airway obstruction and management

## RECOGNITION OF UNCONSCIOUSNESS

*Step 1: Assessment of consciousness.* The doctor first must determine whether the victim is conscious or unconscious; distinguishing between the two is critical because many of the following steps of BLS should not be performed on a conscious individual. For this reason the following three criteria based on the previously discussed definition of unconsciousness should be used:
1. Lack of response to sensory stimulation
2. Loss of protective reflexes
3. Inability to maintain a patent airway

The first of these criteria is the most useful to the rescuer, who must rapidly assess a victim's level of consciousness. The latter two—loss of protective reflexes and the inability to maintain a patent airway—are also clinical manifestations of unconsciousness but are used less frequently to assess the condition.

The American Heart Association[24] recommends that the rescuer gently shake the victim's shoulder and shout loudly, "Are you all right?" to determine whether the victim lacks a response to sensory stimulation. If the victim does not respond to the shake-and-shout maneuver (Figure 5-2), the rescuer should assume that the victim is unconscious and immediately proceed with the steps of BLS.

Pain is another stimulus that may be used to determine the victim's level of consciousness. Peripheral pain, such as pinching of the suprascapular region, usually evokes a motor response from the patient (for example, deep inhalation, limb movement, forehead furrowing, or spoken words). Absence of such a response to a painful stimulus also indicates unconsciousness (greater CNS depression). If the victim does not respond, the doctor should institute BLS procedures.

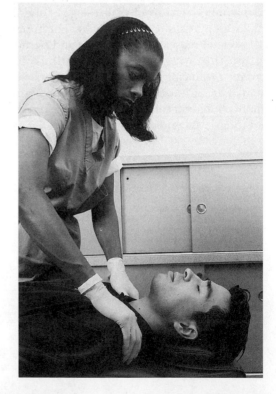

**Figure 5-2**  Unconsciousness is determined by performing the "shake-and-shout" maneuver, gently shaking the shoulders and calling the victim's name.

*Step 2: Terminate dental procedure.*

*Step 3: Summoning of help.* If the victim does not respond to peripheral stimulation, the rescuer should call for assistance immediately by activating the dental office emergency system (see Chapter 3).

## MANAGEMENT OF THE UNCONSCIOUS PATIENT

The loss of consciousness depresses many of the body's vital functions, including its protective reflexes—choking, coughing, sneezing, and swallowing—and the ability of the victim to maintain an open, or patent, airway. The following steps allow the rescuer to maintain these vital functions until the victim either recovers spontaneously or is transported to a hospital equipped with the resources for more definitive management.

*Step 4:* **P**—*position victim.* As soon as unconsciousness is recognized, the victim is placed in the supine (horizontal) position with the brain at the same level as the heart and with the feet elevated slightly (a 10- to 15-degree angle). Rescuers should avoid the head-down (Trendelenburg) position because gravity pushes the abdominal viscera superiorly up into the diaphragm, restricting respiratory movement and diminishing the effectiveness of breathing.[25] A primary objective in the management of unconsciousness is the delivery of oxygenated blood to the brain, and the supine position best enables the heart to accomplish this goal. A slight elevation of the feet to approximately 10 to 15 degrees can further increase the return of blood to the heart. This position is achieved easily in most contoured dental chairs (Figure 5-3). Extra head supports, such as pillows,

should be removed from the headrest of the dental chair when the victim loses consciousness (Figure 5-4).

One situation requiring modification of this basic positioning is the loss of consciousness in a pregnant woman near term. Positioning a woman who is in the latter stages of pregnancy in the supine position may actually lead to a decrease in the return of venous blood to the heart, which decreases the blood supply available for delivery to the brain. The gravid uterus may obstruct or diminish blood flow through the inferior vena cava on the right side of the abdomen, trapping large amounts of blood in the legs. Normal, healthy pregnant women have lost consciousness simply lying on their backs on hard surfaces. If a third-trimester pregnant woman loses consciousness while seated in a dental chair, the doctor or staff member should quickly lower the chair to the supine position, turn the patient onto her right side, and tuck a blanket or pillow under the left side of her back to help her maintain that position.[26] The gravid uterus no longer lies directly over the vena cava, and the return of venous blood from the legs remains unimpeded.

*Step 5:* **A**—*assess and open airway.* In virtually all cases of unconsciousness, some degree of airway obstruction will be present. Therefore after the victim is positioned the next step must be establishment of a patent airway. Opening of the airway and restoration of breathing are the most basic and important steps of

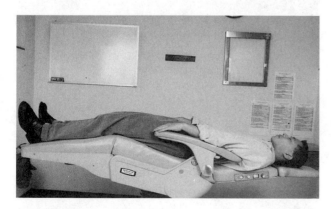

**Figure 5-3** The unconscious victim should be positioned with the thorax and brain at the same level and the feet elevated slightly (about 10 or 15 degrees). The position aids in the return of venous blood to the heart.

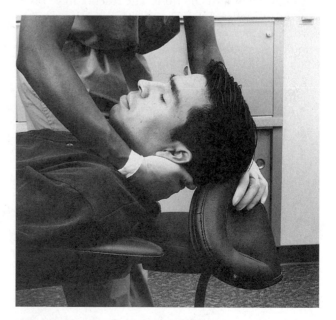

**Figure 5-4** Any extra head supports, such as pillows, should be removed from the headrest of the dental chair when the victim loses consciousness.

BLS. These steps can be performed quickly under most circumstances and without adjunctive equipment or assistance.

*Head-tilt technique.* The head-tilt procedure comprises the initial and most important step in the maintenance of a patent airway. This technique usually is augmented with the chin-lift technique. The formerly used head tilt–neck lift technique was abandoned after research demonstrated that the head tilt–chin lift procedure is more effective.[27]

The rescuer performs the head-tilt procedure by placing a hand on the victim's forehead and applying a firm, backward pressure with the palm (Figure 5-5). In situations in which the victim retains some degree of muscle, head tilt alone may provide a patent airway. When a lesser degree of muscle tone is present, use of the chin-lift or jaw-thrust technique in conjunction with head-tilt may be necessary.

*Jaw-thrust technique (if necessary).* Although head tilt is effective in reestablishing airway patency in most situations, occasionally an airway may remain obstructed. In most instances, additional forward displacement of the mandible performed with the jaw-thrust maneuver adequately removes this obstruction (Figure 5-6). To perform the technique, the rescuer's fingers are placed behind the posterior border of the ramus of the mandible; the rescuer displaces the mandible forward, dislocating it while tilting the head backward. The rescuer's thumbs then retract the lower lip, which allows the victim to breathe through the mouth and nose. The rescuer must be situated behind the top of the supine victim's head to perform the procedure properly, and the rescuer's elbows should rest on the surface on which the victim lies.

Carrying out the jaw-thrust maneuver also provides the rescuer the chance to gauge the victim's degree of unconsciousness. As previously mentioned, peripheral pain is a potent sensory stimulus, and dislocation of the mandible is painful. Thus the victim's response to this procedure tells the rescuer how deeply unconscious that victim is. A movement or an audible response is considered a positive sign because the victim is not deeply unconscious. In addition, the ease with which the rescuer can dislocate the mandible is another gauge of the depth of a victim's unconsciousness. Profound unconsciousness produces a marked loss of muscle tone throughout the body, and dislocation of the mandible becomes easier to perform. This ease is in sharp contrast to the doctor's attempt to dislocate the mandible in a patient who is conscious or only slightly unconscious; in these

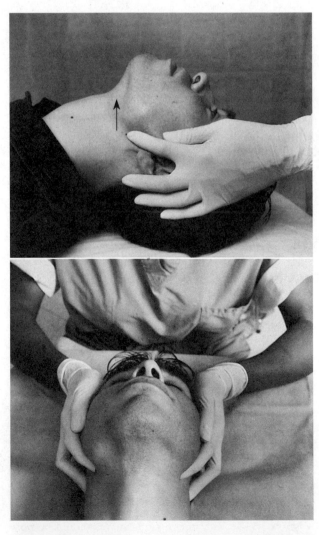

A

B

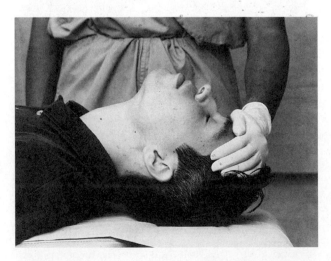

**Figure 5-5**  To perform the head-tilt procedure, the rescuer places one hand on the victim's forehead and applies firm, backward pressure with the palm to achieve the tilt.

**Figure 5-6**  To perform the jaw-thrust technique, the rescuer must grasp the angles of the mandible with both hands and displace the mandible forward. **A,** Side view. **B,** Top view. When possible neck injury is a consideration, the jaw-thrust without head tilt is the preferred technique.

patients the degree of muscle tone that remains makes dislocating the mandible more difficult and the patient's discomfort more intense.

The modified jaw-thrust technique (without head tilt) is the safest initial approach to opening of the airway of a victim with a suspected neck injury (an unlikely occurrence in the dental office) because the rescuer need not extend the victim's neck to complete the procedure. The rescuer must support the neck carefully without tilting it backward or turning it from side to side.

*Head tilt–chin lift technique.* To maintain an airway using the head tilt–chin lift technique (Figure 5-7), the rescuer places the fingers of one hand under the bony symphysis region of the victim's mandible to lift the tip of the mandible up and bring the chin forward. Because the tongue is attached to the mandible, it is pulled forward and off the posterior pharyngeal wall. Lifting the mandible forward also tilts the head backward, aiding in head tilt. The tips of the rescuer's fingers should be placed only on bone, not on the soft tissues of the chin. Compressing these soft tissues increases airway obstruction, pushing the tongue farther upward into the oral cavity. The rescuer should lift the victim's chin, almost bringing the teeth in contact with one another. In addition, the rescuer must try to avoid closing the victim's mouth completely during this procedure.

Research conducted during the past 20 years has provided evidence that the head tilt–chin lift technique of airway management provides the most consistently reliable airway.[27] The previously recommended head

tilt–neck lift technique offered no advantage and put patients with neck injuries in danger (Figure 5-8). For this reason the American Heart Association changed its guidelines for airway management to state that the head tilt–chin lift technique is the preferred method.[24]

All the previously discussed head-tilt maneuvers stretch the tissues between the larynx and mandible, lifting the base of the tongue and epiglottis from the posterior pharyngeal wall (Figure 5-9). These techniques relieve anatomic airway obstruction caused by soft tissues in approximately 80% of unconscious patients.[23] The rescuer must take care to maintain the victim's head in this position at all times until consciousness returns.

It is important to extend the head sufficiently to elevate the tongue and establish a patent airway but to avoid overextension of the head, which increases the risk of possible damage to the victim's vertebrae and spinal cord. One method by which the rescuer can gauge an appropriate tilt is to examine the relationship of the tip of the victim's chin to the earlobes. When the head is not extended, the unconscious victim's airway is obstructed and the tip of the chin lies well below the earlobes (Figure 5-10). When the head is properly extended, this relationship is altered so that the tip of the victim's chin points up into the air in line with the earlobes. This line should

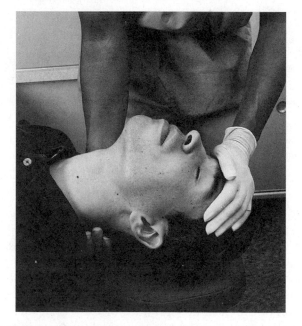

**Figure 5-7** To perform the head tilt–chin lift technique, the rescuer places the fingers of one hand on the bony anterior portion of the victim's mandible and the other hand on the victim's forehead. The head is then rotated backward, the preferred technique for airway maintenance.

**Figure 5-8** To perform the head tilt–neck lift technique, the rescuer places one hand beneath the victim's neck and the other hand on the victim's forehead and rotates the neck backward. Head tilt–neck lift is no longer recommended.

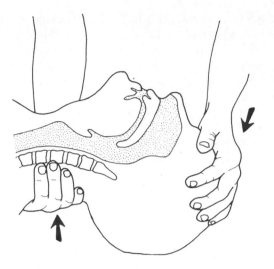

**Figure 5-9**  Head tilt stretches the soft tissues of the neck, lifting the victim's tongue off the pharynx and opening the airway.

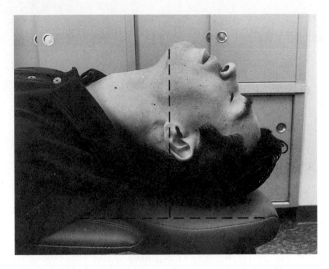

**Figure 5-11**  When the victim's head is extended properly, the tip of the chin points up into the air in line with the earlobes, lifting the mandible and tongue off the pharyngeal wall.

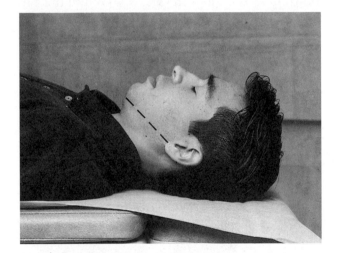

**Figure 5-10**  When the head is not extended, the chin, mandible, and tongue are forced into the airway, producing obstruction.

| table 5-3 | Anatomic differences between adult and infant airways |
| --- | --- |

| DIFFERENCE | SIGNIFICANCE |
| --- | --- |
| Infant head larger than adult head | Do not need to elevate infant head to align axes |
| Infant mouth and nose smaller | Infant requires mouth-to-mouth and nose resuscitation |
| Infant tongue larger relative to oral cavity | Increases potential for obstruction |
| At 1 year, tracheal diameter less than the width of a pencil | Increases potential for obstruction |
| At 2 years the glottic opening only 6.5 mm | Increases potential for obstruction |
| Cricoid cartilage ring narrowest segment of infant airway; glottic closure narrowest in the adult | Precludes use of cuffed endotracheal tubes of patient less than 12 years |
| Infant cricothyroid membrane not palpable | Precludes cricothyrotomy |
| Air passages in infants smaller than in adults | Decreases airway reserve and increases vulnerability to obstruction: finger sweep contraindicated because increased potential for obstruction |

Modified from Kastendieck JG: Airway management. In Rosen P, editor: *Emergency medicine: concepts and clinical practice*, ed 2, St Louis, 1988, Mosby.

be perpendicular to the surface on which the victim is lying (Figure 5-11).

In the unconscious adult it is unlikely that the head will be overextended; the opposite—failure to extend the head far enough—is a more common problem. In the infant or child, however, overextension of the head may produce or exacerbate airway obstruction. Because of anatomic differences in the sizes of the upper airways and tracheas in children and adults, the child's head need not be extended as far in head-tilt as an adult's head (Table 5-3). Extension of the child's head to the same degree as that of an adult may lead to airway obstruction as the narrowest portion of the trachea is compressed. Although the degree of extension previously suggested usually produces a patent airway in a child, it must be modified as the need arises.

table **5-4**    *Determination of airway patency and breathing*

| CLINICAL SIGNS | DIAGNOSIS | MANAGEMENT |
| --- | --- | --- |
| Can feel and hear air at nose and mouth *and* see chest and abdominal movement | Airway patent; patient breathing | Maintain airway |
| Can feel and hear air at nose and mouth *but* see no chest and abdominal movement | Airway patent; patient breathing | Maintain airway |
| Cannot feel or hear air at mouth and nose *and* chest and abdominal movements heaving and erratic | Patient attempting to breathe, but airway obstruction still present | Repeat head tilt; if necessary use jaw thrust technique |
| Cannot feel or hear air at mouth and nose *and* no chest and abdominal movements evident | Respiratory arrest | Proceed to step 6b; begin artificial ventilation |

*Step 6a:* **B**—*Assess airway patency and breathing.* After performing head tilt–chin lift, the rescuer must assess the patency of the airway (Table 5-4). The victim may be breathing spontaneously or inadequately or may not be breathing at all. During this assessment the rescuer must maintain the victim's head in the extended position previously established by head tilt–chin lift. The rescuer should lean over the victim, placing their ear 1 inch from the nose and mouth while looking toward the victim's chest (Figure 5-12).

Using the look-listen-and-feel technique, the rescuer then determines whether the victim is breathing. Seeing the chest or abdomen move indicates that the victim is attempting to breathe but not necessarily effectively exchanging air. Feeling or hearing air at the victim's nose and mouth indicates an adequate exchange of air. In addition, the rescuer may not notice chest or abdominal movement if the victim is fully clothed. However, if the rescuer can feel and hear the victim's breath, visual signs of chest movement are not necessary to determine the adequacy of ventilation.

NOTE: Seeing a victim's chest move does not guarantee that the victim actually is breathing (exchanging air) but simply that the victim is trying to breathe. Hearing and feeling the exchange of air against the rescuer's cheek is a sign that the victim is breathing spontaneously.

If the unconscious victim is exchanging air adequately, the airway is maintained via head tilt–chin lift and the dental team proceeds with additional management, including the administration of $O_2$ and the monitoring of vital signs (blood pressure, heart rate, and respiratory rate). If no air can be felt or heard at the mouth and nose and there is no evidence of chest or abdominal movement, a tentative diagnosis of respiratory arrest is made and artificial ventilation is started immediately (step 6b).

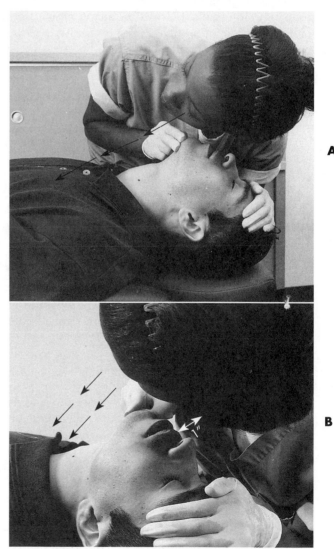

**A**

**B**

**Figure 5-12**  The look-listen-feel technique. While maintaining head tilt, the rescuer assesses airway patency by placing their ear 1 inch from the victim's nose and mouth **(A)** and watching the chest for spontaneous respiratory movements **(B)**.

| table **5-5** | *Causes of partial airway obstruction* | |
|---|---|---|
| **SOUND** | **PROBABLE CAUSE** | **MANAGEMENT** |
| Snoring | Hypopharyngeal obstruction by the tongue | Repeat head tilt; proceed to jaw thrust maneuver, if necessary |
| Gurgling | Foreign matter (blood, water, vomitus) in airway | Suction airway |
| Wheezing | Bronchial obstruction (asthma) | Administer bronchodilator (via inhalation only if conscious; IM or IV if unconscious) |
| Crowing | Laryngospasm (partial) | Suction airway; positive-pressure oxygen |

*IM,* Intramuscular; *IV,* intravenous.

If, in the presence of visible but labored chest or abdominal movements, the rescuer cannot feel or hear airflow at the mouth and nose or detects minimal air exchange along with noisy airflow, airway obstruction, either complete or partial, is present. In this case the rescuer should repeat head tilt–chin lift (see step 5) and recheck the victim for its effectiveness (see step 6a). In the presence of continued airway obstruction, the rescuer must proceed immediately to the next step of airway maintenance.

If the rescuer discovers evidence of foreign matter in the airway after a check for airway patency, the material must be removed before attempting artificial ventilation (if necessary). Various causes of partial or complete airway obstruction are associated with sounds that may prove diagnostic (Table 5-5). Partial airway obstruction produces noise; complete airway obstruction produces silence, an ominous "sound." Foreign matter, primarily liquid, in the hypopharynx produces a gurgling sound similar to that produced when air bubbles through water. Common materials present include saliva, blood, water, or vomitus. Regardless of the nature of the material, the rescuer must remove it from the airway as quickly as possible. A large volume of foreign matter may lead to complete airway obstruction. In addition, particulate material (vomitus) may enter the trachea, creating complete obstruction of the respiratory tract and leading to the victim's asphyxiation and death unless corrected promptly (see Chapters 10 and 11).

The unconscious victim will have previously been placed in the supine position. When the rescuer believes that foreign material is blocking the airway, the victim should be tilted back even further so that their head is lower than the level of their heart (the Trendelenburg position) with the head turned to one side (Figure 5-13). Lowering the victim's head allows the foreign material to pool in the upper portion of the airway, which is more readily accessible to the rescuer. Turning the victim's head to the side allows the foreign material to pool in the most dependent side of the

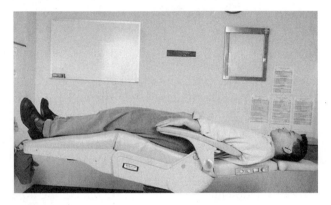

**Figure 5-13** In the Trendelenburg position the victim should be tilted back even further in the dental chair so that the head is below the level of the heart and *(not shown)* turned to one side.

mouth, facilitating its removal and ensuring that the upper side of the mouth is free of material, thus creating a patent airway.

NOTE: Breathing, as discussed in this section, refers to the actual exchange of air through the victim's mouth and nose. The rescuer must distinguish this action from chest movement, which occurs during any attempt at breathing. Chest movement may be present in the absence of adequate air exchange through the victim's mouth and nose.

Immediately after carrying out these two steps, the rescuer should place two fingers in the victim's mouth and remove anything in the oral cavity that can be removed. The sweeping motion of the fingers should begin in the upper portion of the mouth, move posteriorly, and finally move downward and anteriorly (Figure 5-14). A high-volume suction can be used instead of the fingers. Suction tips should be rounded so that the rescuer can place them blindly, if necessary, into the posterior areas of the mouth or into the hypopharynx without fear of inducing bleeding (from the delicate and highly

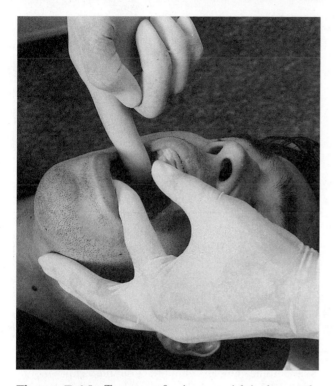

**Figure 5-14**  To remove foreign materials in the mouth, the rescuer must hold the victim's mouth open while using the available fingers to sweep the oral cavity and remove any materials in it. If available, suction may be used.

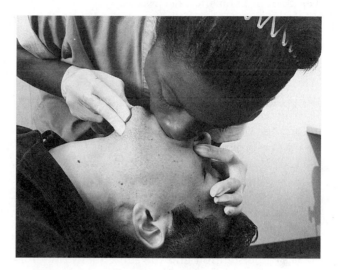

**Figure 5-15**  To perform mouth-to-mouth resuscitation, the rescuer maintains head tilt while pinching the victim's nostrils closed with the thumb and index finger, taking a deep breath, forming a tight seal around the victim's mouth, and blowing air into the mouth. Adequate ventilation is achieved when the victim's chest visibly rises with each ventilatory effort.

vascular pharyngeal mucosa); bleeding can compound airway obstruction. Suctioning should continue until all foreign material is removed from the victim's airway followed by the basic steps of airway maintenance.

Once airway patency and air exchange have been ensured, the rescuer should loosen any constricting clothing, such as belts, ties, or collars, that might interfere with breathing and circulation of blood. The rescuer should monitor the victim's vital signs and, if available, administer $O_2$.

*Step 6b:* **B**—*Artificial ventilation (if necessary).* If respiratory arrest occurs or if spontaneous ventilation is inadequate, the dental team must ventilate the victim so that adequate $O_2$ is available to the brain (see Table 5-4). The victim may receive artificial ventilation in one of three ways:

1.  Exhaled air ventilation
2.  Atmospheric (ambient) air ventilation
3.  $O_2$-enriched ventilation

*Exhaled air ventilation.*  The rescuer may deliver exhaled air to the victim's lungs as one source of $O_2$. Exhaled air can deliver 16% to 18% inspired $O_2$, yielding an arterial $O_2$ tension ($PaO_2$) of 88 torr (normal

being 75 to 100 torr) at a tidal volume of 1000 to 1500 ml and maintaining an $O_2$ saturation of 97% to 100% which is quite adequate to maintain life.[28,29]

Two basic types of exhaled air ventilation include mouth-to-mouth breathing and mouth-to-nose breathing. Because these techniques do not require adjunctive equipment, they can be carried out in any rescue situation. For this reason, they remain the basic techniques of artificial ventilation. Because of the ever-increasing concerns about the transfer of infectious diseases during ventilation, the use of devices such as the pocket mask have gained popularity.

To adequately perform mouth-to-mouth ventilation, the rescuer uses the head-tilt or head tilt–chin lift position (see step 5) to maintain the victim's head in an optimal backward tilt. The rescuer's hand on the victim's forehead continues to help maintain a backward tilt while the rescuer's thumb and index fingers pinch the victim's nostrils closed (Figure 5-15). With mouth wide open, the rescuer takes a deep breath, makes a tight seal around the victim's mouth, and blows into the mouth. A rapid and deeply inhaled breath immediately before blowing delivers expired air with the lowest carbon dioxide content.[23]

The first cycle of ventilation should consist of two full breaths, with the rescuer allowing 1½ to 2 seconds per inspiration and taking a breath after each ventilation. Exhalation occurs passively when the rescuer's mouth is removed from the victim's, allowing gravity to deflate the lungs. Artificial ventilation in the adult must be repeated once every 5 to 6 seconds (10 to 12 times per minute) for as long as necessary. The procedure must be repeated once every 3 seconds (20 times per minute) in infants and children.

The rescuer can gauge the adequacy of ventilation efforts for victim of any size or age by using the following two guides:

1. Feeling air escape as the victim passively exhales
2. Seeing the rise and fall of the victim's chest

The second sign is the more important of the two. In most adults the volume of air required to produce chest expansion is 800 ml (0.8 L). Adequate ventilation usually need not exceed 1200 ml.[30]

Gastric distention and the subsequent risk of aspiration are potentially the most serious dangers of artificial ventilation. The major cause of gastric distention is overinflation during ventilation, which is much more common in children than in adults. Other causes include ventilation against a partially or totally obstructed airway, which can force air into the esophagus and gastrointestinal tract.

Gastric distention is dangerous both because it increases the incidence of regurgitation during resuscitation and because it increases intraabdominal pressure, which may limit movement of the diaphragm thereby reducing the ability of the rescuer to ventilate the victim.[31] The rescuer can minimize gastric distention by limiting efforts at ventilation to the point at which the chest rises. Mouth-to-nose ventilation, a discussion of which follows, may prevent overventilation better; the greater resistance to the flow of ventilating gases through the nose decreases the pressure of gases reaching the pharynx. In some instances mouth-to-nose ventilation is more effective than mouth-to-mouth ventilation.[32] This is especially true when the rescuer cannot open the victim's mouth (for example, as with trismus or a fractured mandible) to ventilate or seal the mouth adequately.

In the mouth-to-nose technique the rescuer keeps the victim's head tilted backward with one hand on the victim's forehead; the other hand lifts the victim's mandible, sealing the lips (Figure 5-16). Taking a deep breath, the rescuer then seals their lips around the victim's nose and blows until feeling and seeing the victim's lungs expand. As in mouth-to-mouth ven-

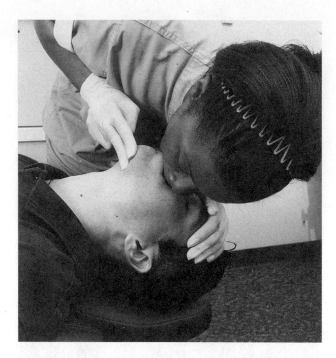

**Figure 5-16**  In mouth-to-nose ventilation, the rescuer maintains head tilt and chin lift, closes the victim's mouth, seals the lips around the victim's nose, and blows air. Adequate ventilation is achieved when the victim's chest visibly rises with each ventilatory effort.

tilation, exhalation is passive. The rescuer uses the same rates—10 to 12 breaths or 20 breaths per minute—in the mouth-to-nose technique for the adult and the child or infant, respectively, as recommended in mouth-to-mouth ventilation.

The rescuer must modify the ventilation technique if the victim is an infant or young child (see previous discussion of the head–tilt procedure). The opening of the airway and method of artificial ventilation are essentially the same in children; however, when the victim is smaller, the rescuer's mouth may cover the child's mouth and nose. The rate of respiration is increased to once every 3 seconds for children 1 year through 8 years and for infants under 1 year, using smaller breaths and less air volume. The same criteria are used for successful ventilation—feeling air escape as the victim passively exhales and seeing the rise and fall of the victim's chest with each inhalation—with infants and small children. In addition, the increased flexibility of the child's neck requires that the rescuer maintain care not to overextend the neck, which can further increase the victim's airway obstruction. When properly performed, artificial ventilation using either method may be continued for long periods without the rescuer becoming fatigued.

*Atmospheric air ventilation.* The administration of increased concentrations of $O_2$ enhances any resuscitative effort. Although exhaled air ventilation, which contains 16% to 18% $O_2$, is adequate to sustain life, greater $O_2$ concentrations provide the victim with greater benefits. The air we breathe contains approximately 21% $O_2$. Devices are available that permit the rescuer to deliver atmospheric air to the victim's lungs; however, all such devices are effective only when basic airway procedures are continually maintained.

Bag-valve-mask (BVM) devices, such as the Ambu-Bag and Pulmonary Manual Resuscitator, usually provide less ventilatory volume than mouth-to-mouth or mouth-to-nose ventilation because of the difficulty in maintaining an airtight seal (Figure 5-17). For this reason the American Heart Association recommends that manually operated, self-inflating BVM devices be used by well-trained and experienced personnel only.[24] To use these units properly, the rescuer must be positioned near the top of the victim's head, making it virtually impossible to carry out one-rescuer BLS (see Section Seven).

To be considered adequate, a BVM unit must have the following features:[24,33,34]

- Be self-refilling (no sponge rubber inside)
- Transparent, plastic face mask with an air-filled or contoured resilient cuff
- Delivers high concentrations of $O_2$ through an ancillary $O_2$ inlet at the back of the bag or by means of an $O_2$ reservoir
- Nonrebreathing valve
- Availability in adult and pediatric sizes
- Standard 15-mm/22-mm fittings (for endotracheal tubes)
- Ease in cleaning
- Minimal dead space

Before purchasing this device, the doctor should enroll in a program that teaches advanced airway management and become thoroughly trained in the proper use of this and other adjunctive equipment.

*Artificial airways.* Artificial airways (oropharyngeal, nasopharyngeal) may be used to assist in airway management but only by persons well-trained in their use (Figure 5-18). Artificial airways should be used only on deeply unconscious individuals when management of the airway with conventional (manual) techniques is difficult. If used on conscious or stuporous patients, artificial airways—especially the oropharyngeal airway—may provoke gagging, vomiting, or laryngospasm, causing a delay in providing adequate ventilation.[35] An oropharyngeal airway must be placed carefully because improper positioning can displace the tongue farther into the pharynx and increase airway obstruction.

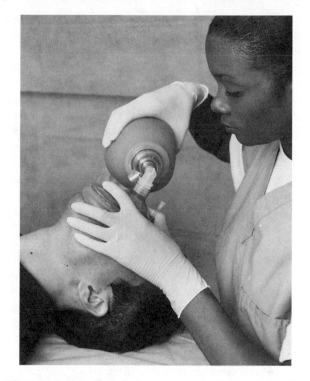

**Figure 5-17**   To administer atmospheric-air ventilation, the rescuer maintains head tilt and hold the face mask securely in place. The victim's chest must rise with each compression of the self-inflating, bag-valve-mask device.

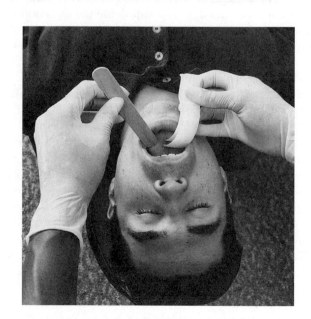

**Figure 5-18**   Insertion of an orophryngeal airway. Only persons with proper training should insert artificial airways.

The nasopharyngeal airway is used when entry into the patient's mouth is difficult. The nasopharyngeal airway is less likely to stimulate gagging or vomiting in the unconscious patient.[36] Semiconscious and conscious patients are better able to tolerate nasopharyngeal airways than they are oropharyngeal airways. However, insertion of the nasopharyngeal airway is more likely to produce bleeding because it traumatizes the delicate and highly vascular nasal mucosa.

Several studies have demonstrated that direct mouth-to-mouth ventilation provides more effective artificial ventilation than that obtained through the use of adjunctive devices.[24,37] Other devices and techniques of airway maintenance, including the esophageal obturator airway, laryngeal mask airway, and endotracheal intubation, are recommended for use by well-trained personnel only.[38-40] A pocket mask should always be available so that initial efforts at ventilation need not be through direct mouth-to-mouth contact.[41] Dentists properly trained in advanced cardiac life support or anesthesiology may use such devices safely and effectively.

*O₂-enriched ventilation.* Whenever possible, the rescuer should use artificial ventilation with supplemental $O_2$. Exhaled air ventilation delivers 16% to 18% $O_2$, whereas atmospheric air provides 21% $O_2$ (at sea level). Because the object of BLS is to provide the brain with $O_2$, the use of supplemental $O_2$ (>21%) is preferred. However, artificial ventilation must never be delayed until supplemental $O_2$ becomes available. As suggested in Chapter 3, every doctor's office should have available one E cylinder of $O_2$. In situations in which artificial ventilation is required, the E cylinder provides approximately 30 minutes of $O_2$; smaller cylinders (A, B, C, D) provide lesser amounts and are entirely inadequate.

Sources of $O_2$ available in the dental office may include the portable E cylinder with adjustable $O_2$ flow (10 to 15 L per minute) and a face mask, an E cylinder with a demand-valve mask unit (Figure 5-19), or an inhalation-sedation unit. If the inhalation-sedation unit is to be used for artificial ventilation, the nasal hood should be removed and replaced with a full-face mask. The reservoir bag on the inhalation sedation unit is squeezed to force $O_2$ into the victim's lungs. $O_2$ from sources other than compressed gas cylinders (such as from canisters that produce $O_2$ via chemical reactions) should not be considered because they are entirely inadequate for artificial ventilation.

Although $O_2$ is beneficial to the unconscious patient, the doctor should receive adequate training in airway maintenance through mouth-to-mouth and

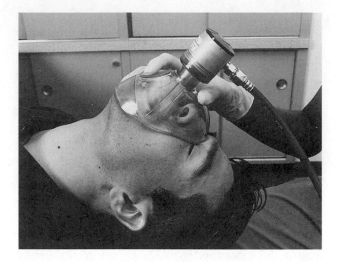

**Figure 5-19** Enriched-oxygen ventilation. The demand-valve mask unit can provide either a conscious or unconscious patient with up to 100% oxygen.

mouth-to-mask ventilation because administration of enriched $O_2$ is effective only as long as $O_2$ remains in the compressed gas cylinder. When the cylinder is empty or if one is not available at the onset of the emergency, the rescuer must revert to the basic technique of artificial respiration.

*Step 7:* **C**—*Assess circulation.* After establishing a patent airway, the rescuer must determine the adequacy of the victim's circulation. This includes monitoring of the heart rate and blood pressure. Several sites are available for the recording of heart rate, including the brachial and radial arteries in the arm and the carotid artery in the neck. In nonemergency situations either artery in the arm adequately indicates the patient's heart rate; however, when a patient is unconscious and particularly when respiratory movements are absent, the carotid artery is the most reliable indicator of cardiovascular function in the adult.

The ability of the rescuer to locate the carotid artery properly is vital (Figure 5-20). The rescuer should place the hand supporting the victim's chin onto the thyroid cartilage ("Adam's apple"). On the side on which the rescuer is positioned, the fingers should slide into the groove between the victim's thyroid cartilage and sternocleidomastoid muscle band in the neck. The carotid artery is located in this groove. The rescuer should allow 5 to 10 seconds to feel the pulse before initiating external chest compression if a pulse is absent.

If a pulse, however weak, is present, the rescuer should continue to perform steps 4 through 6 until the victim recovers or until further medical assistance

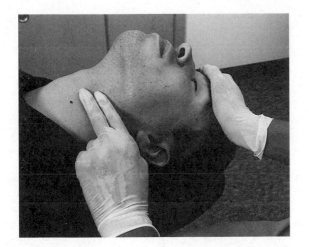

**Figure 5-20**  To locate the carotid pulse, the rescuer places two fingers (not the thumb) on the victim's thyroid cartilage ("Adam's apple") and moves them laterally into the groove formed by the sternocleidomastoid muscle.

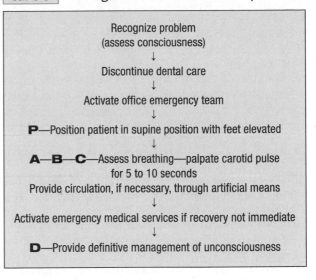

box **5-3**   *Management of unconscious patients*

Recognize problem
(assess consciousness)
↓
Discontinue dental care
↓
Activate office emergency team
↓
**P**—Position patient in supine position with feet elevated
↓
**A**—**B**—**C**—Assess breathing—palpate carotid pulse
for 5 to 10 seconds
Provide circulation, if necessary, through artificial means
↓
Activate emergency medical services if recovery not immediate
↓
**D**—Provide definitive management of unconsciousness

becomes available. If the victim is a child (1 to 8 years) the rescuer also uses the carotid artery, whereas in the infant victim (<1 year) the brachial artery in the upper arm is the recommended route.[42] If a palpable pulse is not present, the rescuer must initiate external chest compression immediately.

*Step 8:* **D**—*Definitive management.* Once a patent airway has been provided and adequate circulation ensured, the dental team can proceed with definitive management. (These specific procedures will be discussed in each of the three following chapters.) The steps described in detail in this chapter comprise the **P-A-B** segments of BLS.

In every instance in which consciousness is lost, these steps must be carried out in precisely the order in which they are described in this chapter. In most cases of unconsciousness, fulfillment of segments **P + A** alone or in fewer cases segments **P-A-B** of BLS are all the support measures required to sustain the victim's life. However, **C** (adequacy of circulation) must always be determined; if a palpable pulse is not present, the rescuer must initiate external chest compressions immediately (see Chapter 30).

Box 5-3 summarizes the management of the unconscious patient. (Additional airway management procedures will be discussed in the section on respiratory difficulty [see Section Three].) This chapter's discussion was based on the fact that hypopharyngeal obstruction by the tongue is the most common cause of airway obstruction in the unconscious patient.[18] (Lower-airway [tracheal and bronchial] obstruction are discussed in Chapter 10.)

## REFERENCES

1. Fast TB, Martin MD, Ellis TM: Emergency preparedness: a survey of dental practitioners, *J Am Dent Assoc* 112:499, 1986.
2. Malamed SF: Survey of emergencies in dental practice, Unpublished data, 1992.
3. Schultz KE: Vertigo and syncope. In Rosen P, editor: *Emergency medicine: concepts and clinical practice,* ed 3, St Louis, 1992, Mosby.
4. Huff JS: Coma. In Rosen P, editor: *Emergency medicine: concepts and clinical practice,* ed 3, St Louis, 1992, Mosby.
5. American Dental Association Council on Dental Education: *Guidelines for teaching the comprehensive control of pain and anxiety in dentistry,* Chicago, 1987, The Association.
6. Martin GJ and others: Prospective evaluation of syncope, *Ann Emerg Med* 13:499, 1984.
7. American Dental Association Council on Dental Education: Guidelines for teaching the comprehensive control of pain and anxiety in dentistry, *J Dent Educ* 36:62, 1972.
8. Selcuk E, Erturk S, Afrashi A: An adverse reaction to local anaesthesia: report of a case, *Dent Update* 23(8):345-346, 1996.
9. Boorin MR: Anxiety: its manifestation and role in the dental patient, *Dent Clin North Am* 39(3):523-539, 1995.
10. Engel GL: Psychologic stress, vasodepressor (vasovagal) syncope, and sudden death, *Ann Intern Med* 89:403, 1978.
11. Guedel AE: *Inhalation anesthesia: a fundamental guide,* ed 2, New York, 1952, Macmillan.
12. Malamed SF: Systemic complications. In Malamed SF: *Handbook of local anesthesia,* ed 4, St Louis, 1997, Mosby.
13. Aldrete JA, Johnson DA: Evaluation of intracutaneous testing for investigation of allergy to local anesthetic agents, *Anesth Analg* 49:173, 1970.

14. Corah NL, Gale EN, Illig SJ: Assessment of a dental anxiety scale, *J Am Dent Assoc* 97:816, 1981.
15. McCarthy FM: *Emergencies in dental practice,* ed 3, Philadelphia, 1979, WB Saunders.
16. Engle LL: *Fainting,* ed 2, Springfield, Ill, 1962, Charles C Thomas.
17. Safar P, Escarraga L, Change F: A study of upper airway obstruction in the unconscious patient, *J Appl Physiol* 14:760, 1961.
18. Boidin MP: Airway patency in the unconscious patient, *Br J Anaesth* 57:306, 1985.
19. Redding JS and others: Resuscitation from asphyxia, *JAMA* 182:283, 1962.
20. Salins PC and others: Hypoglycemia as a possible factor in the induction of vasovagal syncope, *Oral Surg Oral Med Oral Pathol* 74(5):544-549, 1992.
21. Rossen R, Kabat H, Anderson JP: Acute arrest of the cerebral circulation in man, *Arch Neurol Psychiatr* 50:510, 1943.
22. Goldberg AH: Cardiopulmonary arrest, *N Engl J Med* 290:381, 1974.
23. Safar P: Ventilatory efficacy of mouth-to-mouth artificial respiration, *JAMA* 182:283, 1958.
24. American Heart Association Emergency Cardiac Care Committee and Subcommittee: Guidelines for cardiopulmonary resuscitation and emergency cardiac care, *JAMA* 268(16):2171-2302, 1992.
25. Erie JK: Effect of position on ventilation. In Faust RJ, editor: *Anesthesiology review,* New York, 1991, Churchill Livingstone.
26. Wright KE Jr, McIntosh HD: Syncope: a review of pathophysiological mechanisms, *Progr Cardiovasc Dis* 13:580, 1971.
27. Guildner CW: Resuscitation: opening the airway—a comparative study of techniques for opening an airway obstructed by the tongue, *JACEP* 5:588, 1976.
28. Gordon AS and others: Mouth-to-mouth versus manual artificial respiration for children and adults, *JAMA* 167:320, 1958.
29. Safar P and others: A comparison of the mouth-to-mouth and mouth-to-airway methods of artificial respiration with the chest-pressure arm-lift methods, *N Engl J Med* 258:671, 1958.
30. Melker R: Recommendations for ventilation during cardiopulmonary resuscitation: time for change? *Crit Care Med* 13:882, 1985.
31. Zwillich CW and others: Complications of assisted ventilation, *Am J Med* 57:161, 1974.
32. Ruben H and others: Investigation of upper airway problems in resuscitation, *Anesthesiology* 22:271, 1961.
33. White RD, Gilles BP, Polk BV: Oxygen delivery by hand-operated emergency ventilation devices, *JACEP* 2:105, 1973.
34. Carden E, Friedman D: Further studies of manually operated self-inflating resuscitation bags, *Anesth Analg* 56:202, 1977.
35. Grauer K, Cavallaro D: *ACLS: certification preparation,* ed 3, St Louis, 1993, Mosby Lifeline.
36. Cummins RO, editor: *Advanced cardiac life support,* Dallas, 1997, American Heart Association Subcommittee on Advanced Cardiac Life Support.
37. Elling R, Politis J: An evaluation of emergency technicians' ability to use manual ventilation devices, *Ann Emerg Med* 12:765-768, 1983.
38. Donen N and others: The esophageal obturator airway: an appraisal, *Can Anaesth Soc J* 30:194, 1983.
39. Uhl RR: Respirator care in emergencies, *Comprehensive Therapy* 3(3):66-72, 1997 Mar.
40. Verghese C, Brimacombe JR: Survey of laryngeal mask airway usage in 11,910 patients: safety and efficacy for conventional and nonconventional usage, *Anesth Analg* 82(1):129-33, 1996.
41. Safar P: Pocket mask for emergency artificial ventilation and oxygen inhalation, *Crit Care Med* 2:273, 1974.
42. Cavallaro D, Melker R: Comparison of two techniques for determining cardiac activity in infants, *Crit Care Med* 14:397, 1983.

# 6

# Vasodepressor Syncope

**V**ASODEPRESSOR syncope—also known as *vasovagal syncope* but more often referred to as *common faint*—is a frequently observed, usually benign and self-limiting process which is potentially life threatening. In two surveys of dental office emergencies, vasodepressor syncope was the most common emergency observed, accounting for approximately 53% of all reported emergencies.[1,2] Fainting is associated with all types of dental care, including tooth extractions and other surgical procedures, local anesthetic injections, and procedures such as venipuncture. Fainting has occurred on being seated in the dental chair and even when an individual first entered the dental office.[3-5]

*Syncope* is a general term referring to a sudden, transient loss of consciousness that usually occurs secondary to a period of cerebral ischemia. Box 6-1 lists a number of the many synonyms that describe syncope. *Vasodepressor syncope,* the most descriptive and accurate of these terms, is the name by which this condition is referred throughout the text.

Ordinarily, vasodepressor syncope is a relatively harmless situation during which the victim either falls gently to the floor or is laid down by a second party. The individual regains consciousness almost immediately, and within a short period appears to have recovered completely. Statistics from Great Britain confirm the relatively benign nature of this situation. During World War II more than 25,000 blood donors fainted, and all recovered.[6] Yet despite its seemingly innocuous nature, any loss of con-

box **6-1**  *Synonyms for syncope*

| | |
|---|---|
| Atrial bradycardia | Simple faint |
| Benign faint | Swoon |
| Neurogenic syncope | Vasodepressor syncope |
| Psychogenic syncope | Vasovagal syncope |

box **6-2**  *Predisposing factors for vasodepressor syncope*

**Psychogenic factors**

Fright
Anxiety
Emotional stress
Receipt of unwelcome news
Pain, especially sudden and unexpected pain
The sight of blood or surgical or other dental instruments (for example, a local anesthetic syringe)

**Nonpsychogenic factors**

Erect sitting or standing posture
Hunger from dieting or a missed meal
Exhaustion
Poor physical condition
Hot, humid, crowded environment
Male gender
Age between 16 and 35 years

sciousness, however brief, produces physiologic changes and can place the victim's life in danger.[7] Examples include cardiopulmonary changes that occur secondary to hypoxia or anoxia, both of which are produced by airway obstruction in the unconscious patient. Although vasodepressor syncope is a fairly common emergency situation, it usually is preventable. When syncope is recognized promptly and managed properly, few individuals experience serious complications.

## Predisposing Factors

Factors that can precipitate vasodepressor syncope are classified into two groups. The first group consists of psychogenic factors, such as fright, anxiety, emotional stress, and receipt of unwelcome news. Two other factors in this group are pain—especially sudden and unexpected pain—and the sight of blood or surgical or dental instruments (for example, the local anesthetic syringe). These factors lead to the development of the "fight-or-flight" response and in the absence of muscular movement by the patient, produce the transient loss of consciousness known as *vasodepressor syncope.*

The second group consists of nonpsychogenic factors. These include sitting in an upright position or standing, which permits blood to pool in the periphery; decreasing cerebral blood flow below critical levels (for consciousness); hunger from dieting or missed meals, which decreases the glucose supply to the brain to below critical levels; exhaustion; poor physical condition; and hot, humid, crowded environments.

Although incidents of vasodepressor syncope are not limited to one age-group, young adults faint more often than other age-groups. In addition, men experience vasodepressor syncope more than women; indeed men between 16 and 35 years may be the most likely candidates for the development of vasodepressor syncope. Society's view of the male as someone who can "take it" (the pain) without exhibiting emotion may explain this gender gap.[8] The fear of injury, coupled with the expectation by peers to act courageously, sets the scene for the escape mechanism of fainting.

In a prospective study of patients who fainted, Martin and others[9] demonstrated that the average age of those who fainted was 35.5 years. On the other hand, vasodepressor syncope is rare in pediatric patients. Children do not hide their fears; they yell, cry, and move about, unlike the more mature and typically more inhibited adult male. The diagnosis of vasodepressor syncope in a pediatric patient or an adult older than 40 years (especially if it develops without prodromal symptoms) should be questioned seriously.[9]

Within dental settings the most common precipitating factors of vasodepressor syncope are the psychogenic factors (Box 6-2). The dental situation most likely to result in vasodepressor syncope is the administration of a local anesthetic by a female doctor to an anxious "macho" male patient under 35 years who is seated upright in the dental chair.

## Prevention

Prevention of vasodepressor syncope is directed at the elimination of factors that may predispose an individual to faint. Most dental offices are not hot, humid, or crowded. Adequate air conditioning eliminates the heat factor. Patient hunger, the result of dieting or a missed meal before the dental appointment also should be considered; each patient, especially those who are anxious, should be requested to eat a light snack or meal before their dental appointment to minimize the risk of developing hypoglycemia in addition to a psychogenic response (see Chapter 17). An individual classified by the American Society of Anesthesiologists' (ASA) Physical Status Classification System with impaired physical status (ASA III or greater) has a greater likelihood of developing a life-threatening situation.

Psychologic stress, which in individuals without cardiovascular problems may induce fainting, may precipitate sudden death secondary to life-threatening dysrhythmias in those with preexisting cardiac disorders.[8] Modifications in dental treatment should be seriously considered for the more medically compromised patient.

## PROPER POSITIONING

An important contributing factor in most cases of vasodepressor syncope is the patient's position in the dental chair. The risk of vasodepressor syncope is increased greatly in the apprehensive patient who is standing or is seated upright during treatment. With the introduction of the contoured dental chair and the advent of sit-down dentistry, most patients no longer are treated in upright positions. Today, patients will be placed in a supine or semisupine (30- to 45-degree) position, a practice that has reduced many instances of vasodepressor syncope in the dental chair.

The dentist who seats patients in the upright position and is unable to make the change to sit-down dentistry still may be able to minimize the risk of vasodepressor syncope. Injection of local anesthetics is *the* procedure which most often precipitates vasodepressor syncope. If the dentist can administer a local anesthetic to a patient who is in the supine position, syncope (the actual loss of consciousness) will rarely if ever occur. After administration of the local anesthetic the patient may be repositioned and dental treatment may resume in the usual manner.

## ANXIETY RELIEF

Most cases of vasodepressor syncope in the dental office involve psychogenic factors. Thus each potential patient must be evaluated carefully for the presence of dental anxiety. If the patient is overly anxious, dental treatment should be modified—to minimize or to eliminate it.

Unfortunately, adult anxiety often is difficult to recognize. The discussion in Chapter 2 established that many men and women do not consider an admission of fear as the "adult" thing to do. Corah's questionnaire[10] is a great asset in the recognition of anxiety (see Chapter 2). Although many patients do not admit their fears in oral interviews, experience with the anxiety questionnaire has shown that they will more often express their feelings honestly in writing. Therefore the inclusion of this survey or of several questions appended to the medical history questionnaire is worthwhile.

Conversely, the presence of anxiety and fear in children usually is not difficult to recognize. Children not having the inhibitions that adults do usually make their feelings quite well known to the doctor and to all others present in the office. It is for this reason that healthy children rarely develop vasodepressor syncope.

## Medical History Questionnaire

The University of Southern California's School of Dentistry medical history questionnaires (see Figures 2-1 and 2-2) provide the doctor with some information about patient anxiety. The following questions may help uncover potential problems:

**Question 2:  Do you feel very nervous about having dentistry treatment?**
**Question 3:  Have you ever had a bad experience in the dentistry office?**

> *Comment:* Such questions permit patients to provide voluntarily information about their attitudes toward dental treatment. An affirmative response to either or both questions should lead to a thorough dialogue history and to possible treatment modifications aimed at decreasing the patient's dental fears.

## DENTAL THERAPY CONSIDERATIONS

Once anxiety is recognized it should be managed. Combined with the positioning of patients in supine or reclined positions, the use of psychosedation should be considered; increased use of psychosedation has decreased the incidence of vasodepressor syncope during dental treatment. Routes of drug administration include oral, sublingual, rectal, intranasal, and intramuscular; inhalation sedation with nitrous oxide ($N_2O$) and oxygen ($O_2$); and intravenous sedation.

Psychosedation is just one of a number of stress-reducing factors discussed in Chapter 2. The concept of total patient care has led to the development of specific stress-reduction protocols and has been responsible for the decreasing number of stress-related, life-threatening situations arising in dentistry. Use of these protocols can virtually eliminate all occurrences of vasodepressor syncope in dental offices.

# Clinical Manifestations

Clinical signs and symptoms of vasodepressor syncope usually develop rapidly in the presence of an appropriate stimulus however, the actual loss of consciousness does not normally occur immediately. Thus individuals who experience vasodepressor syncope while alone rarely are injured seriously. There is usually sufficient time for them to sit or lie down before they lose consciousness. The clinical manifestations of vasodepressor syncope can be grouped into three definite phases—presyncope, syncope, and postsyncope (recovery period).

## PRESYNCOPE

The prodromal manifestations of vasodepressor syncope are well known. The patient in the erect or sitting position complains of a feeling of warmth in the neck and face, loses color (pale or ashen-gray skin color), and becomes bathed in a cold sweat (noted primarily on the forehead). During this time the patient usually complains of feeling "bad" or "faint" and may also feel nauseous. The blood pressure at this time is at the baseline level or slightly lower, whereas the heart rate increases significantly (for example, from 80 to 120 or more beats per minute).

As presyncope continues, pupillary dilation, yawning, hyperpnea (increased depth of respiration) and coldness in the hands and feet are noted. The blood pressure and heart rate become acutely depressed (hypotension and bradycardia) just before loss of consciousness.[4,7,11] At this time the patient experiences disturbed vision, becomes dizzy, and syncope occurs.

As syncope develops, the individual usually exhibits warning symptoms for several minutes before losing consciousness (Box 6-3).[9] If the patient is in an erect position, presyncope may lead to unconsciousness in a relatively short time (approximately 30 seconds), whereas if the patient is in a supine position, the presyncopal phase may never reach the point at which consciousness is lost.

## SYNCOPE

With the onset of syncope, breathing may (1) become irregular, jerky, and gasping; (2) become quiet, shallow, and scarcely perceptible; or (3) cease entirely (respiratory arrest or apnea). The pupils dilate, and the patient takes on a deathlike appearance. Convulsive movements and muscular twitching of the hands, legs, or facial muscles are common when patients lose consciousness and their brains become hypoxic, even for periods as short as 10 seconds.

box **6-3**    *Presyncopal signs and symptoms*

**Early**

Feeling of warmth
Loss of color; pale or ashen-gray skin tone
Heavy perspiration
Complaints of "feeling bad" or "feeling faint"
Nausea
Blood pressure at baseline level or slightly lower
Tachycardia

**Late**

Pupillary dilation
Yawning
Hyperpnea
Cold hands and feet
Hypotension
Bradycardia
Visual disturbances
Dizziness
Loss of consciousness

Bradycardia, which develops during the late presyncopal phase, continues. A heart rate of less than 50 beats per minute is common during syncope. In severe episodes, periods of complete ventricular asystole have been recorded—even in normally healthy individuals. The blood pressure, which falls precipitously to an extremely low level (30/15 mmHg being common), also remains low during this phase and often is difficult to obtain. The pulse becomes weak and thready. Loss of consciousness is also associated with a generalized muscular relaxation that quite commonly leads to partial or complete airway obstruction. Fecal incontinence may occur, particularly when systolic blood pressure falls below 70 mmHg.

Once the patient is placed in the supine position, the duration of syncope is extremely brief, ranging from several seconds to several minutes. If the patient remains unconscious for more than 5 minutes after proper positioning and management are achieved, or if the patient does not undergo a complete clinical recovery in 15 to 20 minutes, causes other than syncope should be considered. Such causes are important, especially if the patient is more than 40 years and does not exhibit prodromal symptoms before losing consciousness.[9]

## POSTSYNCOPE (RECOVERY)

With proper positioning, recovery (return of consciousness) is rapid. In the postsyncopal phase the patient may demonstrate pallor, nausea, weakness, and sweating, all of which can last from a few minutes to several hours. Occasionally, symptoms persist for 24 hours.[12] During the immediate postsyncopal phase the patient may experience a short period of confusion or disorientation. The arterial blood pressure begins to rise at this time; however, it may not return to the baseline level until several hours after the syncopal episode. The heart rate, which is depressed, also returns slowly toward the baseline level, and the pulse becomes stronger.

In addition, a point worth stressing is that once a patient loses consciousness, the tendency for that patient to faint again may persist for many hours if the patient assumes a sitting position or stands too soon.

# Pathophysiology

Vasodepressor syncope is most commonly precipitated by a decrease in cerebral blood flow below a critical level and usually is characterized by a sudden drop in blood pressure and a slowing of the heart rate. When such predisposing factors occur, a certain pattern of events usually develops.

## PRESYNCOPE

Stress, whether emotionally triggered (as with fear) or sensorially triggered (unexpected pain), causes the body to release into the circulatory system increased amounts of the catecholamines epinephrine and norepinephrine. Their release is part of the body's adaptation to stress, commonly called the "fight-or-flight" response. This increase in catecholamines results in changes in tissue blood perfusion designed to prepare the individual for increased muscular activity (fight or flight).

Among the many responses to catecholamine release are a decrease in peripheral vascular resistance and an increase in blood flow to many tissues, particularly the peripheral skeletal muscles. In situations in which this anticipated muscular activity occurs, the blood volume that was diverted to the muscles in preparation for this movement is pumped by the muscles back to the heart. In this case peripheral pooling of blood does not occur. The blood pressure remains at or above the baseline level, and signs and symptoms of vasodepressor syncope do not develop.

In contrast, in situations in which the preparation for muscular activity does not occur (for example, sitting still in the dental chair and "taking it like a man"), the diversion of large volumes of blood into skeletal muscles causes a significant pooling of blood in these muscles, and a decreased volume of blood returns to the heart. This leads to a relative decrease

in circulating blood volume, a drop in arterial blood pressure, and a decrease in cerebral blood flow. Presyncopal signs and symptoms are related to decreased cardiac output, diminished cerebral blood flow, and other physiologic alterations.[4]

As blood pools in peripheral vessels and the arterial blood pressure begins to fall, compensatory mechanisms are activated that attempt to maintain adequate cerebral blood flow. These mechanisms include baroreceptors, which reflexly constrict peripheral blood vessels, and the carotid and aortic arch reflexes, which increase the heart rate. These mechanisms help increased venous return to the heart, increased cardiac output, and heart rate and the maintenance of a near-normal blood pressure, all of which are noted during the early presyncopal period.

However, these compensatory mechanisms soon fatigue (decompensate) which is manifested through the development of reflex bradycardia. Slowing of the heart rate to less than 50 beats per minute is common and leads to a significant drop in cardiac output, which is associated with a precipitous fall in blood pressure to levels below those critical for maintenance of consciousness. In such cases, cerebral ischemia results and the individual loses consciousness.

## SYNCOPE

The critical level of cerebral blood flow for the maintenance of consciousness is estimated to be about 30 ml of blood per 100 g of brain tissue per minute. The human adult brain weighs approximately 1360 g (young adult male of medium stature). The normal value of cerebral blood flow is 50 to 55 ml per 100 g per minute. In a fight-or-flight situation in which muscular movement is absent with the patient maintained in the upright position, the heart's ability to pump the critical volume of blood to the brain is impaired and this minimal cerebral blood flow is not reached, leading to syncope. In a normotensive individual (systolic blood pressure below 140 mmHg), this minimal blood flow is equivalent to an approximate systolic blood pressure of 70 mmHg. For patients with atherosclerosis and/or high blood pressure, this critical level for cerebral blood flow may be reached with a systolic pressure considerably above 70 mmHg. Clinically, systolic blood pressure may descend to as low as 20 to 30 mmHg, during the syncopal episode with periods of asystole (systolic blood pressure of 0) occurring.

Convulsive movements, such as tonic or clonic contractions of the arms and legs or turning of the head, may occur with the onset of syncope. Cerebral ischemia lasting only 10 seconds can lead to seizure activity in patients with no prior histories of seizure disorders.[13] The degree to which the individual moves during the seizure usually depends on the degree and duration of the cerebral ischemia. When present, these muscular movements are usually of brief duration and are rather mild.

## RECOVERY

Recovery is usually hastened by placing the victim in the supine position with the legs elevated slightly, improving venous return to the heart and increasing blood flow to the brain so that cerebral blood flow once again exceeds the critical level necessary for consciousness. Signs and symptoms, such as weakness, sweating, and pallor, may persist for hours. The body is fatigued and may require as long as 24 hours to return to its normal functioning state after a syncopal episode.[14] In addition, the removal of the factor that precipitated the episode (for example, a syringe or blood-soaked gauze) will help speed recovery.

# Management

The method of management for syncopal patients differs, depending on the signs and symptoms the particular individual exhibits. This section deals with the management of four separate stages of syncope—presyncope, syncope, delayed recovery, and postsyncope.

## PRESYNCOPE

*Step 1: **P** (position).* As soon as presyncopal signs and symptoms appear, the procedure should be halted and the patient placed in the supine position with the legs slightly elevated. This position change usually halts the progression of symptoms. Muscle movement also helps increase the return of blood from the body's peripheral regions. If the patient can move the legs vigorously, the patient is less likely to experience significant peripheral pooling of blood, minimizing the severity of the reaction.

*Step 2: **A-B-C** (airway-breathing-circulation).* The fairly common practice (outside of medical/dental offices) of placing the victim's head between his or her legs when presyncopal signs and symptoms develop should be discontinued. Bending over to such an extreme degree may actually further impede the return of blood from the legs through partially obstructing the inferior vena cava, resulting in a greater decrease in blood flow to the brain. Furthermore, if the individual loses consciousness while placing the head between the legs, this position (for example, face down or prone) does not facilitate proper airway management. $O_2$ may be administered through use of a full-face mask, or an ammonia ampule may be crushed under the patient's nose to speed recovery (Figure 6-1).

*Step 3: **D** (definitive care).* Following management of presyncope, attempts should be made to determine the cause of the episode while the patient recovers. Modifications in future dental treatment should be considered to minimize the risk of reoccurrence. The planned dental treatment may proceed only if both the doctor and the patient feel it is appropriate. If either party remains doubtful, the treatment should be postponed.

## SYNCOPE

Proper management of vasodepressor syncope follows the basic management recommended for all unconscious patients—**P-A-B-C.**[15] This discussion presents a summary of the proper procedures.

*Step 1: assessment of consciousness.* The patient (victim) suffering vasodepressor syncope demonstrates a lack of response to sensory stimulation ("shake and shout").

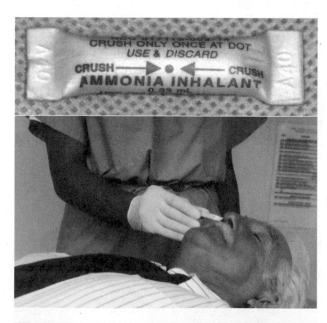

**Figure 6-1  A,** An aromatic ammonia vaporole respiratory stimulant. **B,** An aromatic ammonia vaporole is crushed between the rescuer's fingers and held near victim's nose to stimulate movement.

*Step 2: activation of the dental office emergency system.* Office team members should perform their assigned duties.

*Step 3:* **P.** The first and most important step in the management of syncope is the placement of the victim in the supine position. In addition, a slight elevation of the legs helps increase the return of blood from the periphery. This step is so vital because the majority of the observed clinical manifestations during syncope are the result of inadequate cerebral blood flow. Failure to place the victim in the supine position may result in death or permanent neurologic damage secondary to prolonged cerebral ischemia. This damage can occur in as little as 2 to 3 minutes if the victim maintains an upright position.

The ancient Roman practice of crucifixion is an example of death from vasodepressor syncope; individuals who were forced to maintain upright positions eventually died. The supine position therefore is the preferred position for the management of unconscious patients (Figure 6-2). However, females in the latter stages of pregnancy who lose consciousness are one important exception to this position (see Chapter 5). (Other possible modifications of this positioning will be discussed in later sections.)

*Step 4:* **A-B-C** *(basic life support, as needed).* The victim must be assessed immediately and a patent airway ensured. In most instances of vasodepressor syncope, the head tilt–chin lift procedure successfully establishes a patent airway (Figure 6-3).

Assessment of airway patency and adequacy of breathing constitute the next actions. An adequate airway is present when the patient's chest moves and exhaled air can be heard and felt (Figure 6-4). Spontaneous respiration usually is evident during syncope; however, artificial ventilation may be necessary on those few occasions in which spontaneous breathing ceases. Positioning of the victim and establish-

ment of a patent airway usually lead to the rapid return of consciousness.

To assess circulation, the carotid pulse must be palpated. Although rare, brief periods of ventricular asystole can develop during syncope. Though rare, brief periods of ventricular asystole may develop during syncope. In most circumstances, however, a weak, thready pulse is palpable in the neck. The heart rate is commonly quite low. More frequently, however, the victim has regained consciousness by this time.

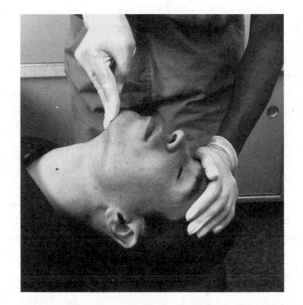

**Figure 6-3** Airway patency may be obtained through use of the head tilt–chin lift method.

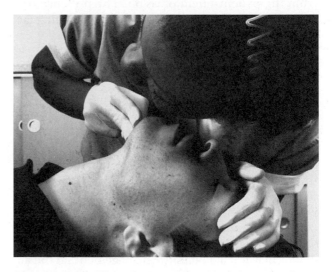

**Figure 6-4** The adequacy of an airway may be determined through use of the "look, listen, feel" technique.

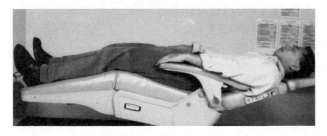

**Figure 6-2** Position of unconscious victim. The patient is placed in the supine position with the legs elevated slightly.

*Step 5:* **D:** *(definitive care)*

*Step 5a: administration of O₂.* O₂ may be administered to the syncopal or postsyncopal patient at any time during the episode.

*Step 5b: monitoring of vital signs.* Vital signs, including blood pressure, heart rate, and respiratory rate, should be monitored, recorded and compared to the patient's preoperative baseline values to determine the severity of the reaction and the degree of recovery.

*Step 5c: performance of additional procedures.* These procedures include the loosening of binding clothes such as ties, collars (which can decrease blood flow to the brain), and belts (which can decrease return of blood from the legs) and the use of a respiratory stimulant such as aromatic ammonia. The rescuer should crush an ammonia vaporole between the fingers and allow the patient to inhale it. Ammonia, which has a noxious odor, stimulates both increased breathing and muscular movement.

If the doctor keeps vaporoles handy near the dental chair, the syncopal episode may end before it requires further assistance. A cold towel may be placed on the patient's forehead or blankets provided if the victim complains of feeling cold or is shivering. If blankets are unavailable, the kind of plastic patient drape commonly found in dental offices may be used. If bradycardia persists, an anticholinergic, such as atropine, may be administered either intravenously or intramuscularly.

As the victim regains consciousness, it is important that the doctor and emergency team maintain their composure. In addition, the stimulus that precipitated the episode (for example, a syringe, an instrument, or a piece of bloody gauze) must be removed from the patient's field of vision. The presence of a terrified dental staff member or the precipitating factor may induce a second episode of syncope.

## DELAYED RECOVERY

If the victim does not regain consciousness after the steps previously described have been performed or does not recover completely in 15 to 20 minutes, a different cause for the syncopal episode should be seriously considered and the EMS system activated. Indeed the doctor may want to activate the EMS system at any time during the syncopal episode and should continue performing basic life support while awaiting the arrival of the EMS team. If another cause of unconsciousness (for example, hypoglycemia) becomes obvious, the doctor may initiate definitive management. In the absence of an obvious cause, however, the doctor should continue performing basic life support and if possible start an intravenous infusion (see Chapter 3).

## POSTSYNCOPE

After recovering from a period of syncope (of any duration), the victim should not undergo additional dental treatment the rest of that day. The possibility of a second syncopal episode is greater during the postsyncopal phase; research has demonstrated that the body requires up to 24 hours to return to its normal state.

Prior to dismissal, the doctor should determine the primary precipitating event and any other factors (for example, hunger or fear) that may have contributed to it. The doctor can use this information to formulate a plan for future treatment that can avoid additional syncopal episodes.

Arrangements must be made for a friend or family member to take the patient home. Allowing the patient to leave the office unescorted and drive a car puts that patient in danger because of the possibility of recurrent syncopal episodes. Providing an escort is especially important whenever an individual has lost consciousness.

Box 6-4 summarizes the management of vasodepressor syncope. In addition, the following items may prove helpful:

- Drugs used in management: O₂, ammonia, and atropine

box **6-4**   *Management of vasodepressor syncope*

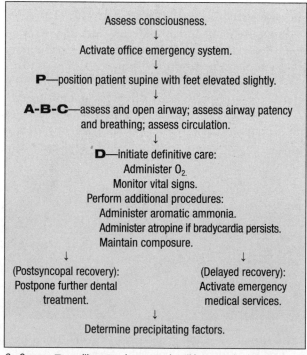

Assess consciousness.
↓
Activate office emergency system.
↓
**P**—position patient supine with feet elevated slightly.
↓
**A-B-C**—assess and open airway; assess airway patency and breathing; assess circulation.
↓
**D**—initiate definitive care:
Administer O₂.
Monitor vital signs.
Perform additional procedures:
Administer aromatic ammonia.
Administer atropine if bradycardia persists.
Maintain composure.

↓ (Postsyncopal recovery):   ↓ (Delayed recovery):
Postpone further dental treatment.   Activate emergency medical services.
↓
Determine precipitating factors.

*O₂,* Oxygen; **P,** position; **A,** airway; **B,** breathing; **C,** circulation; **D,** definitive care.

- Medical assistance: Assistance rarely is required because consciousness normally returns rapidly when the individual is positioned properly and when airway, breathing, and circulation are managed. A delayed recovery of consciousness or a delayed return to normal CNS status mandates EMS activation.

## REFERENCES

1. Fast TB, Martin MD, Ellis TM: Emergency preparedness: a survey of dental practitioners, *J Am Dent Assoc* 112(4):499-501, 1986.
2. Malamed SF: Beyond the basics: emergency medicine in dentistry, *J Am Dent Assoc* 128(7):843-854, 1997.
3. Locker D, Shapiro D, Liddell A: Overlap between dental anxiety and blood-injury fears: psychological characteristics and response to dental treatment, *Behav Res Ther* 35(7):583-590, 1997.
4. Leonard M: An approach to some dilemmas and complications of office oral surgery, *Aust Dent J* 40(3):159-163, 1995.
5. Tizes R: Cardiac arrest following routine venipuncture, *JAMA* 236:1846, 1976.
6. Ebert RV: Response of normal subjects to acute blood loss, *Arch Int Med* 68:578, 1941.
7. Wright KE, McIntosh HD: Syncope: a review of pathophysiological mechanisms, *Prog Cardiovasc Dis* 13:58, 1971.
8. Engel GL: Psychologic stress, vasodepressor (vasovagal) syncope, and sudden death, *Ann Intern Med* 89:403, 1978.
9. Martin GJ and others: Prospective evaluation of syncope, *Ann Emerg Med* 13:499, 1984.
10. Corah NL: Development of a dental anxiety scale, *J Dent Res* 48:596, 1969.
11. Glick G, Yu PN: Hemodynamic changes during spontaneous vasovagal reactions, *Am J Med* 34:42, 1963.
12. Friedberg CK: Syncope: pathological physiology, differential diagnosis, and treatment, *Mod Concepts Cardiovasc Dis* 40:55, 1971.
13. Cutino SR: Vasovagal syncope associated with seizure activity, *Gen Dent* 42(4):342-343, 1994.
14. Thomas JE, Rooke ED: Fainting, *Mayo Clin Proc* 38:397, 1963.
15. Leonard M: Syncope: treating fainting in the dental office, *Dent Today* 15(1):72-73, 1996.

# 7

# Postural Hypotension

**P**OSTURAL hypotension, also known as *orthostatic hypotension*, is the second-leading cause of transient loss of consciousness (syncope) in dental settings. *Postural hypotension* is defined as a disorder of the autonomic nervous system in which syncope occurs when the patient assumes an upright position. Postural hypotension may also be defined as a drop in systolic pressure of 20 mmHg or more that occurs on standing.[1,2] Postural hypotension is a result of a failure of the baroreceptor reflex–mediated increase in peripheral vascular resistance in response to positional changes.[3]

Postural hypotension differs in several important respects from vasodepressor syncope and is only infrequently associated with fear and anxiety. Awareness of predisposing factors allows the dentist to prevent the development of this condition, which can be dangerous. An example of injury arising as a result of postural hypotension occurring in a dental office follows:

A 45-year-old healthy male patient was placed in a semi-reclined position for the administration of a local anesthetic prior to the start of dental treatment. After administering several maxillary infiltrations (1.5 anesthetic cartridges), the doctor remained with the patient for several minutes to ensure the adequacy of the anesthesia. Then, 2 minutes after the injection the doctor left the room, leaving the patient with a dental assistant, who was busy preparing instruments and materials for the upcoming procedure.

The assistant left the room several minutes later. The patient then began to feel "funny" and called for assistance. When his calls elicited no immediate response, the patient sat up in the chair, legs dangling over the side, and leaned forward to get up out of the chair.

Seconds later, the doctor and staff members heard a crashing sound come from the room and immediately ran to help. There, they found the patient lying unconscious on the floor next to the dental chair, bleeding on the face. The patient suffered a broken nose and fractured his clavicle and forearm.

Two more examples of postural hypotension episodes that occurred in dental offices include the following:

- Syncope developed in a 76-year-old woman whose recumbent blood pressure was 180/100 mmHg and dropped to 100/50 mmHg immediately after she rose from the dental chair.
- A 35-year-old male lost consciousness after lying in the dental chair in the supine position for 1 hour. He stood up and walked to the reception desk to schedule another appointment. When he reached the front desk and stopped moving, he felt "faint" and lost consciousness.

## Predisposing Factors

Many factors have been identified as causes of postural hypotension; several have possible dental implications. These include the following:

- Administration and ingestion of drugs[4,5]
- Prolonged period of recumbency or convalescence[6]
- Inadequate postural reflex
- Late-stage pregnancy[7]
- Advanced age[2,8]
- Venous defects in the legs (for example, varicose veins)
- Recovery from sympathectomy for "essential" hypertension
- Addison's disease
- Physical exhaustion[9] and starvation
- Chronic postural hypotension (Shy-Drager syndrome)

The incidence of postural hypotension increases with age.[2,8] In a group of 100 ambulatory patients 65 years and older, 31% demonstrated decreases in systolic blood pressure of 20 mmHg or more when they stood, whereas 16% suffered diastolic drops of 10 mmHg or more. In addition, 12% experienced significant drops in both systolic pressure and diastolic pressures.[2] Although the incidence of postural hypotension increases with age, it is relatively uncommon in infants and children.[10]

## DRUG ADMINISTRATION AND INGESTION

Probably the most frequently encountered cause of postural hypotension in the dental office is in response to the use of drugs. The dentist may administer these drugs before, during, or after the dental treatment, or the patient's primary-care physician may prescribe them for the management of specific physical or psychologic disorders. These drugs fall into the broad categories of antihypertensives, especially sodium-depleting diuretics, calcium channel blockers, and ganglionic-blocking agents; psychotherapeutics (sedatives and tranquilizers); opioids; histamine-blockers; and L-dopa, which is used for the treatment of Parkinson's disease. In general, the drugs produce postural hypotension by diminishing the body's ability to maintain blood pressure (and in turn adequate cerebral perfusion) in response to the increased influence of gravity, which occurs when the patient rises suddenly. An exaggerated blood pressure response is observed.

Medications used to manage fear and anxiety are capable of inducing postural hypotension, especially with parenteral administration (via intramuscular, intravenous, or inhalation routes). Those drugs most often used in dentistry include nitrous oxide and oxygen (inhalation); diazepam and pentobarbital (intravenous); midazolam (intramuscular or intravenous); meperidine; and fentanyl and its congeners—alfentanil and sufentanil (intravenous, intramuscular). Positional changes should be made slowly and carefully in patients receiving these drugs (Box 7-1).

## PROLONGED RECUMBENCY AND CONVALESCENCE

Patients confined to bed for as little as 1 week have an increased risk of postural hypotension.[6] This is one reason hospitalized patients are encouraged to ambulate as soon as possible after undergoing surgical procedures. Although dental patients usually are not confined for periods up to a week, longer dental appointments have gained popularity in recent years. Patients may remain reclined in the dental chair undergoing treatment for 2 or 3 hours. In these circumstances, postural hypotension may develop when the dental chair is returned to the upright position or the patient stands. When the dental treatment combines long periods of recumbency with the use of psychosedative drugs, the risk of postural hypotension increases.

box **7-1** | *Drugs and drug categories producing postural hypotension*

**Category**
Adrenergic neuron blockers
$\alpha$- and $\beta$-adrenergic blockers
Amiodarone
Angiotensin-converting enzyme inhibitors
Centrally acting antihypertensives
Calcium channel blockers
Diuretics
Ganglionic blockers
Levodopa
Vasodilators

## INADEQUATE POSTURAL REFLEX

Healthy young people may faint when forced to stand motionless for prolonged periods, such as during school assemblies, religious services, or parades. Syncope also can develop when a patient is seated upright in the dental chair for a prolonged period. This situation is more likely to occur in a hot environment, which produces concomitant peripheral vasodilation. The following example, excerpted from the *Los Angeles Times*,[11] illustrates one government agency's response to this physiologic occurrence:

> *How to faint by the numbers*
> VANCOUVER (UPI)—The order has gone out: Canadian troops may no longer faint in a slovenly or unseemly way while on parade. Soldiers disobeying the order will be put on report. The memo said: "To avoid the possibility of fainting, a soldier should make sure he has had breakfast on the morning of parade day. If worse comes to worst and he must faint, a soldier should fall to the ground under control. To do so, he must turn his body approximately 45 degrees, squat down, roll to the left, and retain control of his weapon to prevent personal injury and minimize damage to the weapon. We must ensure that soldiers who have not complied with the above instructions be charged."

## PREGNANCY

Pregnant women may demonstrate two forms of hypotension. In the first, the woman experiences postural hypotension during the first trimester, usually when she rises from bed in the morning but not recurring again during the day. The precise cause of this phenomenon is not known.

The second form, known as the *supine hypotensive syndrome of pregnancy*, occurs late in the third trimester if the woman remains in the supine position for more than 3 to 7 minutes.[12] Signs and symptoms of syncope become evident during this period, and the woman loses consciousness shortly thereafter. It has been demonstrated that the flaccid, gravid uterus compresses the inferior vena cava, decreasing venous return from the legs. If the woman alters her position to the lateral seated, or standing position, the weight of the uterus no longer creates this pressure on the vena cava and the clinical symptoms of syncope rapidly reverse.

## AGE

The incidence of postural hypotension shows a very definite increase with increasing age and proves to be a major problem in the aging population.[1,2,8,13,14] Patients who demonstrated a drop in both diastolic and systolic pressures were more likely to have had a fall during the year before the evaluation and decreased functional abilities, compared with those patients who did not experience postural hypotension.[2] The mean incidence of falls in nursing homes is 1.5 falls per bed per year (range being 0.2 to 3.6 falls).[15]

Campbell[16] studied 761 individuals 70 years or older and discovered that 507 had fallen during the year before monitoring began. Although many patients had multiple risk factors for falls, postural hypotension was frequently present. Macrae[8] evaluated blood pressure changes in older patients in the morning and afternoon. Elderly patients experienced the greatest decrease—9.3 mmHg—in systolic pressure in the morning, approximately 30 seconds after first standing, and returned to normal within 2 minutes. In contrast, diastolic pressure rose a maximum of 9.7 mmHg in those 2 minutes. When doctors measured these individuals' blood pressures in the afternoon after lunch, the decrease ($n=13$) was significantly greater across the board—20.8 mmHg $\pm$ 3.6 mmHg—compared with 7.1 mmHg $\pm$ 2.0 mmHg in the morning ($p = 0.01$).

## VENOUS DEFECTS IN THE LEGS

Postural hypotension also occurs in patients with varicose veins and other vascular disorders of the legs. These disorders permit excessive pooling of blood in these patients' legs.

## RECOVERY FROM SYMPATHECTOMY FOR HIGH BLOOD PRESSURE

Surgical procedures designed to lower blood pressure and improve circulation to the legs may result in a greater incidence of postural hypotension. Such cases usually occur immediately after surgery, with the symptoms usually declining spontaneously with time.

## ADDISON'S DISEASE

Postural hypotension frequently occurs in patients with chronic adrenocortical insufficiency. The doctor may manage this condition through the administration of corticosteroids (see Chapter 8).

## PHYSICAL EXHAUSTION AND STARVATION

When syncope occurs during a period of physical exhaustion or starvation, the cause is usually postural hypotension. Such causes are rarely the case in dental offices. Patients should be advised to eat before their dental appointments to reduce the possibility of postural hypotension.

## CHRONIC POSTURAL HYPOTENSION (SHY-DRAGER SYNDROME)

Shy-Drager syndrome, also known as *idiopathic postural hypotension* or *multiple systems atrophy,* is an uncommon disorder, the cause of which is unknown.[17] Its course is progressive; severe disability or death usually occurs within 5 to 10 years of onset. Patients who suffer from Shy-Drager syndrome are usually in their 50s and initially experience postural hypotension, urinary and fecal incontinence, sexual impotence (males), and anhidrosis (lack of sweating) in the lower trunk.

# Prevention

Awareness of a patient's medical history may help the doctor prevent postural hypotension. Prevention is based on the (1) medical history, (2) physical examination, and (3) dental treatment modifications. The first two steps are designed to identify patients with potential problems, whereas the third factor helps ensure that those patients do not lose consciousness.

## Medical History Questionnaire

**Question 6:  Have you taken any medicine or drugs during the past 2 years?**

*Comment:* Postural hypotension is a side effect of some medications. The drug-package insert or an appropriate pharmacology text such as Mosby's GenRx should be consulted (see Box 7-1).

**Question 9:  Circle any of the following that you have had or have at present:**

Fainting or dizzy spells
Epilepsy or seizures

*Comment:* A history of frequent fainting spells may indicate postural hypotension. A thorough dialogue history should be conducted to determine what factors are involved and whether prodromal signs and symptoms are associated with these syncopal episodes.

For patients with postural hypotension, the names of any medications the patient may be taking to assist in the maintenance of adequate blood pressure should be obtained. Patients often take ephedrine, up to 75 mg orally per day. Fludrocortisone acetate in doses of 0.1 mg or more daily is also effective.[18] If the patient does not know the name of a drug prescribed, the doctor should have a text available that contains illustrations of many common medications, such as *Mosby's GenRx,* so that the patient can identify the medication causing a delay in treatment.

## PHYSICAL EXAMINATION

An integral part of the pretreatment evaluation for all potential patients is the recording of vital signs, including blood pressure, heart rate and rhythm (pulse), respiratory rate, temperature, height, and weight. Postural hypotension may be detectable if the patient's blood pressure and heart rate are recorded in both the supine and standing positions. The doctor should record the first blood pressure reading after the patient has been in a supine position for 2 to 3 minutes and the second after the patient has been standing for 1 minute.[19] The normal response of this type of two-prong reading is a standing systolic blood pressure within 10 mmHg (higher or lower, but usually higher) of the supine blood pressure. The heart rate normally accelerates when the individual stands and generally remains about 5 to 20 beats per minute faster than in the supine position.

If severe clinical symptoms develop, the test for postural hypotension is positive and the patient should lie down immediately. Other criteria that indicate postural hypotension include a rise in the standing pulse of at least 30 beats per minute or a decrease of more than 25 mmHg systolic and 10 mmHg diastolic blood pressure simultaneous with the appearance of symptoms (Box 7-2). The doctor should recheck the patient's blood pressure in each position; if the patient still exhibits this differential,

| box **7-2** | *Clinical criteria for postural hypotension* |

Symptoms develop when individual stands.
Standing pulse increases at least 30 beats per minute.
Standing systolic blood pressure decreases at least 25 mmHg.
Standing diastolic blood pressure decreases at least 10 mmHg.

medical consultation should be considered before dental treatment is initiated.

## DENTAL THERAPY CONSIDERATIONS

Certain basic precautions should be observed to prevent hypotensive episodes during or after positional changes in the following types of dental patients:

- Patients with histories of postural hypotension
- Patients receiving sedation (inhalation, intravenous, or intramuscular) during dental treatment
- Patients who have been reclined in the dental chair for long periods

Patients who have been in a supine or semisupine position throughout long appointments should be cautioned against rising too rapidly. These patients should resume upright positions slowly after treatment. Changing the patient's chair position two or three times within 1 minute or so before moving the chair into the upright position and allowing the patient to remain at each incremental level until any potential dizziness abates is suggested.

As the patient moves to stand, the doctor may want to stand in front of the chair until the patient is able to stand without feeling dizzy. If the patient does become weak or faint, however, dental staff members are there to prevent the patient from falling and becoming injured. These precautions, restated in the following list, are especially important when patients lie reclined for long periods.

*Dental therapy considerations—*
*postural hypotension*
- Slowly reposition patient upright.
- Stand nearby as the patient stands after treatment.

## Clinical Manifestations

Patients who suffer chronic postural hypotension can experience precipitous drops in blood pressure and lose consciousness when they stand or sit upright; these patients often do not exhibit the prodromal signs and symptoms of vasodepressor syncope—lightheadedness, pallor, dizziness, blurred vision, nausea, and diaphoresis. The patients also may lose consciousness rapidly, or may merely become lightheaded, or develop blurred vision but not actually lose consciousness. Clinical signs and symptoms more often are seen in patients with other predisposing factors for postural hypotension, such as the administration of drugs, and may include some or all of the usual prodromal signs and symptoms of vasodepressor syncope before consciousness is lost.

Blood pressure during the syncopal period of postural hypotension is quite low, as it is during vasodepressor syncope. Unlike vasodepressor syncope, during which individuals exhibit bradycardia, the heart rate during postural hypotension remains at the baseline level or somewhat higher (>30 beats per minute above baseline). The patient with postural hypotension exhibits all the clinical manifestations of unconscious patients (see Chapters 5 and 6). If unconsciousness persists for 10 or more seconds, the patient may exhibit minor convulsive movements.[20] Consciousness returns rapidly once the patient is returned to the supine position.

## Pathophysiology

### NORMAL REGULATORY MECHANISMS

When the patient moves from a supine into an upright position, gravity's effect on the cardiovascular system intensifies. Blood pumped from the heart must now move upward, against the force of gravity, to reach the cerebral circulation and supply the brain with the $O_2$ and glucose it needs to maintain consciousness. On the other hand, when the patient is in the supine position, the force of gravity is distributed equally over the entire body and blood flows more readily from the heart to the brain. In other positions (for example, semisupine, Trendelenburg), gravity's effect is such that systolic blood pressure decreases by 2 mmHg for each inch that the patient's head is situated above the level of the heart; while for each inch that the head is situated below the level of the heart, blood pressure increases by 2 mmHg (Figure 7-1).

A number of intricate mechanisms have evolved to protect the brain and ensure that it receives an adequate supply of $O_2$ and glucose.[21] These include:

- A reflex arteriolar constriction mediated through baroreceptors (pressure receptors) located in the carotid sinus and aortic arch

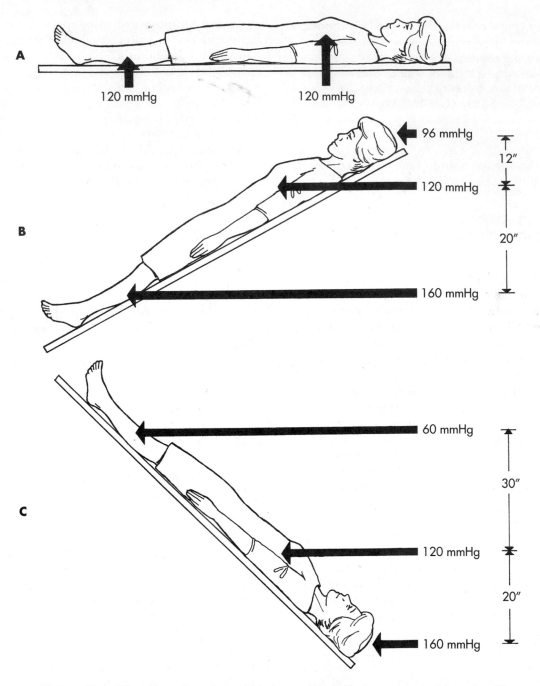

**Figure 7-1**   The effect of gravity on blood pressure. **A,** In the supine position, the effect of gravity is equalized over the entire body. The blood pressures in the legs, heart, and brain are approximately equal. **B,** In the semiupright position, pressure is decreased by 2 mmHg for each inch the individual remains above the level of the heart. **C,** In the Trendelenburg (head down) position, blood pressure increases 2 mmHg for each inch the individual is situated below the level of the heart. (Modified from Enderby GEH: *Lancet* 1:185, 1954.)

- A reflex increase in heart rate, which occurs simultaneously with the increase in arteriolar tone and is mediated through the same mechanisms
- A reflex venous constriction that increases the return of venous blood to the heart, mediated both intrinsically and sympathetically
- An increase in muscle tone and contraction in the legs and abdomen—the so-called venous pump—that facilitates the venous return of blood (of vital importance because at least 60% of circulating blood volume at any given moment is in venous circulation)
- A reflex increase in respiration, which also aids in the return of blood to the right side of the heart via changes in intraabdominal and intrathoracic pressures
- The release into the blood of various neurohumoral substances, such as norepinephrine, antidiuretic hormone, renin, and angiotensin

The usual (normal) reaction of the cardiovascular system when an individual is tilted from the supine into the upright sitting position is an immediate drop in systolic blood pressure from 5 to 40 mmHg; this drop is followed by an equally rapid rise so that within 30 seconds to 1 minute the systolic blood pressure is equal to or slightly higher than that recorded in the supine position. Thereafter the systolic blood pressure tends to remain within 10 mmHg higher or lower (usually higher) of the supine recording. The diastolic blood pressure rises approximately 10 to 20 mmHg. Heart rate (pulse) increases approximately 5 to 20 beats per minute when the patient is standing.

## POSTURAL HYPOTENSION

One or more of the adaptive mechanisms fails in the patient with postural hypotension, and the body cannot adapt adequately to gravity's effects. Dramatic blood pressure changes accompany positional changes. Blood pressure drops rapidly when the patient moves into an upright position with systolic pressure sometimes approaches 60 mmHg in less than 1 minute. Diastolic blood pressure also drops precipitously. The heart rate, however, changes only slightly or not at all; the cardiovascular system is unable to respond normally to the blood pressure depression. This combination of signs (rapid decrease in blood pressure, no change in heart rate) is pathognomonic of postural hypotension.

In addition, many patients do not exhibit any of the usual prodromal signs of vasodepressor syncope. These patients may lose consciousness when cerebral

table **7-1**    *Cardiovascular response to positional change*

| CHANGE (AT 60 SECONDS) AFTER SUDDEN ELEVATION | NORMAL | POSTURAL HYPOTENSION |
|---|---|---|
| Systolic blood pressure | Baseline or ± 10 mmHg | Decrease of >25 mmHg |
| Diastolic blood pressure | Increase of 10-20 mmHg | Decrease of >10 mmHg |
| Heart rate | 5-20 beats per minute above baseline | Baseline or higher (>30 beats per minute) |

blood flow drops below the critical level (approximately 30 ml of blood per minute per 100 g of brain), equivalent to a systolic blood pressure at heart level of approximately 70 mm Hg in a normotensive person. Syncope is short-lived once the patient is placed into the supine position because of reestablishment of adequate cerebral blood flow. Table 7-1 compares the postural responses in blood pressure and heart rate of individuals with postural hypotension with normal individuals.

## Management

Management of postural hypotension mimics that of vasodepressor syncope.

*Step 1: assessment of consciousness.* The patient may or may not demonstrate a lack of response to sensory stimulation.

*Step 2: activation of the office emergency system.*

*Step 3: P (position).* The unresponsive patient should be placed into the supine position with the feet slightly elevated. This position immediately enhances cerebral perfusion, and in most instances the individual regains consciousness within a few seconds.

*Step 4: A-B-C (airway-breathing-circulation).* In the unlikely situation in which the patient has not immediately regained consciousness after positioning, a patent airway must be established. The head tilt–chin lift procedure usually establishes a patent airway. In addition, the "look, listen, feel" technique should be used to detect any obstruction to breathing, and the carotid pulse palpated to determine adequacy of circulation.

### Step 5: D (definitive care):

*Step 5a: administration of O$_2$.* The syncopal patient may receive O$_2$ at any time during or after the episode.

*Step 5b: monitoring of vital signs.* The patient's vital signs—blood pressure, heart rate, and respiratory rate—should be monitored and compared with preoperative baseline values to determine the severity of the hypotensive reaction and the degree of recovery. The patient's position also should be noted with each recording of vital signs.

**Step 6: subsequent management.** After an episode of postural hypotension, the now-supine patient usually feels almost normal, experiencing little or no postsyncopal feelings of exhaustion or malaise; these feelings frequently occur in patients after episodes of vasodepressor syncope.

Most importantly, changes in position from supine to upright must occur slowly. The patient should be repositioned approximately 22.5 degrees, with sufficient time for accomodation before being raised to approximately 45 degrees. After making this height adjustment, the patient then should be raised to about 67.5 degrees, allowed to accomodate, and finally raised to the fully erect position of 90 degrees. All signs and symptoms of hypotension must be resolved before the patient assumes the upright position. As a final precaution, the blood pressure should be checked and compared with the baseline level before the patient stands. Finally, the doctor or assistant should help the patient rise from the chair and be available for support, if necessary.

*Step 6a: delayed recovery.* If hypotensive episodes continue to occur when the patient assumes the upright position (an unlikely event), the doctor should consider seeking outside medical assistance to definitively manage the problem.

**Step 7: discharge.** A patient with chronic postural hypotension or postural hypotension resulting from a prescribed medication (for example, an antihypertensive) may leave the dental office and drive a motor vehicle only if the doctor deems that the patient has recovered sufficiently from the incident. This judgment may be based on a return of vital signs to approximately baseline levels and the ability of the patient to walk freely without experiencing any clinical signs and symptoms of hypotension (for example, lightheadedness, pallor, or dizziness). When the

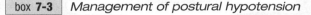

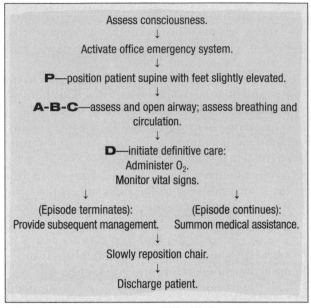

box **7-3**   *Management of postural hypotension*

> Assess consciousness.
> ↓
> Activate office emergency system.
> ↓
> **P**—position patient supine with feet slightly elevated.
> ↓
> **A-B-C**—assess and open airway; assess breathing and circulation.
> ↓
> **D**—initiate definitive care:
> Administer O$_2$.
> Monitor vital signs.
> ↓                              ↓
> (Episode terminates):          (Episode continues):
> Provide subsequent management.  Summon medical assistance.
> ↓
> Slowly reposition chair.
> ↓
> Discharge patient.

*O$_2$,* Oxygen; **P,** position; **A,** airway; **B,** breathing; **C,** circulation; **D,** definitive care.

patient's history suggests that a prescribed drug may have been responsible for the hypotensive episode, the doctor should consider consulting the patient's primary-care physician if episodes recur.

Patients experiencing postural hypotensive episodes who do not have prior histories of such occurrences or patients who experience such episodes after the administration of drugs should recover in the dental office while arrangements are made for a responsible adult to escort the patient home or for emergency personnel to escort the patient to an acute-care facility. Consultation with the patient's primary-care physician should be considered in those cases in which the patient has no prior history of postural hypotension.

Box 7-3 summarizes the proper management of postural hypotension.

- **Drugs used in management:** Oxygen
- **Medical assistance required:** Such assistance usually is not required. Most individuals regain consciousness rapidly after proper positioning. When consciousness does not return promptly or recurrent hypotensive episodes develop after repositioning, further medical assistance should be considered.

## REFERENCES

1. Consensus statement on the definition of orthostatic hypotension, pure autonomic failure, and multiple system atrophy, *J Neurol Sci* 144(1-2):218-219, 1996.

2. Susman J: Postural hypotension in elderly family practice patients, *J Am Board Fam Pract* 2(4):234, 1989.
3. Hickler RB: Orthostatic hypotension and syncope, *N Engl J Med* 296:336, 1977.
4. Atkins D and others: Syncope and orthostatic hypotension, *Am J Med* 91(2):179-185, 1991.
5. Coperchini ML, Kreeger LC: Postural hypotension from topical glyceryl trinitrate ointment for anal pain, *J Pain Symptom Manage* 14(5):263-264, 1997.
6. Akhtar M, Jazayeri M, Sra J: Cardiovascular causes of syncope: identifying and controlling trigger mechanisms, *Postgrad Med* 90(2):87-94, 1991.
7. Ikeda T and others: Maternal cerebral hemodynamics in the supine hypotensive syndrome, *Obstet Gynecol* 79(1):27-31, 1992.
8. Macrae AD, Bulpitt CJ: Assessment of postural hypotension in elderly patients, *Age Ageing* 18(2):110, 1989.
9. Yang TM, Chang MS: The mechanism of symptomatic postural hypotension in the elderly, *Chung Hua I Hsueh Tsa Chih* 46(3):147-155, 1990.
10. de Jong-de Vos van Steenwijk CC and others: Variability of near-fainting responses in healthy 6–16-year-old subjects, *Clin Sci (Colch)* 93(3):205-211, 1997.
11. United Press International: How to faint by the numbers, *Los Angeles Times,* Feb 23, 1975.
12. Ikeda T and others: Maternal cerebral hemodynamics in the supine hypotensive syndrome, *Obstet Gynecol* 79(1):27-31, 1992.
13. Mader SL: Aging and postural hypotension: an update, *J Am Geriatr Soc* 37(2):129, 1989.
14. Wing LM, Tonkin AL: Orthostatic blood pressure control and aging, *Aust N Z J Med* 27(4):462-466, 1997.
15. Rubenstein LZ, Josephson KR, Osterweil D: Falls and fall prevention in the nursing home, *Clin Geriatr Med* 12(4):881-902, 1996.
16. Campbell AJ, Borrie MJ, Spears GF: Risk factors for falls in a community-based prospective study of people 70 years and older, *J Gerontol* 44(4):M112, 1989.
17. Mathias CJ and others: The influence of food on postural hypotension in three groups with chronic autonomic failure—clinical and therapeutic implications, *J Neurol Neurosurg Psychiatry* 54(8):726-730, 1991.
18. Perdue C: Treating postural hypotension, *Nurs Times* 94(14):54-56, 1998.
19. Williams TM: Orthostatic hypotension. In Callaham ML, Barton CW, Schumaker HM, editors, *Decision making in emergency medicine,* Philadelphia, 1990, BC Decker.
20. Cutino SR: Vasovagal syncope associated with seizure activity, *Gen Dent* 42(4):342-343, 1994.
21. Petrella RJ, Cunningham DA, Smith JJ: Influence of age and physical training on postural adaptation, *Can J Sport Sci* 14(1):4, 1989.

# 8

# Acute Adrenal Insufficiency

**A** *THIRD* type of potentially life-threatening situation that may result in the loss of consciousness is *acute adrenal insufficiency,* or *adrenal crisis.* Of the three conditions discussed in this section—vasodepressor syncope, postural hypotension, and acute adrenal insufficiency—the latter is by far the least likely to occur in the dental office. The condition is uncommon and potentially life threatening but readily treatable.

The adrenal gland is an endocrine gland that is actually a combination of two glands—the cortex and the medulla, which are fused together yet remain distinct and identifiable entities. The adrenal cortex produces and secretes more than 30 steroid hormones, most of which do not aid in the performance of any important, currently identifiable biologic activity.[1] Cortisol, a glucocorticoid, is widely considered the most important product of the adrenal cortex; cortisol helps the body adapt to stress, and is thereby extremely vital to survival.

Hypersecretion of cortisol leads to increased fat deposition in certain areas, such as the face and back (often called a "buffalo hump"); elevates blood pressure; and alters blood cell distribution (eosinopenia and lymphopenia).[2] Hypersecretion of cortisol usually does not result in the acute, life-threatening situation that is noted with acute cortisol deficiency. Clinically, cortisol hypersecretion is referred to as *Cushing's syndrome,*[3] a condition that can normally be corrected through surgical removal of part or all of the adrenal gland.[4] Today, renal and adrenal surgery are important factors in the development of primary adrenocortical insufficiency.[5]

box **8-1** *Clinical indications for glucocorticosteroid use*

**Allergic diseases**
Angioedema
Asthma, acute and chronic
Dermatitis, contact
Dermatitis venenata
Insect bites
Pollinosis (hay fever)
Rhinitis, allergic
Serum reaction, drug and
  foreign, acute and delayed
Status asthmaticus
Transfusion reactions
Urticaria

**Cardiovascular diseases**
Postpericardiotomy syndrome
Shock, toxic (septic)

**Eye diseases**
Blepharoconjunctivitis
Burns, chemical and thermal
Conjunctivitis, allergic,
  catarrhal
Corneal injuries
Glaucoma, secondary
Herpes zoster
Iritis
Keratitis
Neuritis, optic, acute
Retinitis, centralis
Scleritis; episcleritis

**Gastrointestinal diseases**
Colitis, ulcerative
Enteritis, regional
Hepatitis, viral
Sprue

**Genitourinary diseases**
Hunner's ulcer
Nephrotic syndrome

**Hematopoietic disorders**
Anemia, acquired hemolytic
Leukemia, acute and chronic
Lymphoma
Purpura, idiopathic thrombo-
  cytopenic

**Infections and inflammations**
Meningitis
Thyroiditis, acute
Typhoid fever
Waterhouse-Friderichsen
  syndrome

**Injected locally**
Arthritis, traumatic
Bursitis
Osteoarthritis
Tendinitis

**Mesenchymal diseases**
Arthritis, rheumatoid
Dermatomyositis
Lupus erythematosus,
  systemic
Polyarteritis
Rheumatic fever, acute

**Metabolic diseases**
Arthritis, gouty acute
Thyroid crisis, acute

**Miscellaneous conditions**
Bell's palsy
Dental surgical procedures

**Pulmonary diseases**
Emphysema, pulmonary
Fibrosis, pulmonary
Sarcoidosis
Silicosis

**Skin diseases**
Dermatitis
Drug eruptions
Eczema, chronic
Erythema multiforme
Herpes zoster
Lichen planus
Pemphigus vulgaris
Pityriasis rosea
Purpura, allergic
Sunburn, severe

On the other hand, cortisol deficiency can lead to a relatively rapid onset of clinical symptoms, including loss of consciousness and possible death. Adrenal insufficiency first was recognized by Addison in 1844; thus primary adrenocortical insufficiency is called *Addison's disease,* an insidious and usually progressive condition.[6] The incidence of Addison's disease, estimated between 0.3 and 1 case per 100,000 individuals, occurs equally in both sexes and among all age groups, including infants and children.[7] Although all corticosteroids may be deficient in this disease state, administration of physiologic doses of exogenous cortisol can correct most pathophysiologic effects associated with Addison's disease.[8]

Clinical manifestations of adrenocortical insufficiency usually do not develop until at least 90% of the adrenal cortex is destroyed.[9] Because this destruction usually progresses slowly, several months may pass before a diagnosis of adrenocortical insufficiency is made and therapy (exogenous cortisol) is instituted. During this time the patient will remain in constant jeopardy of developing acute adrenal insufficiency. The patient is capable of maintaining levels of endogenous cortisol adequate to meet the requirements of day-to-day living; however, in stressful situations (for example, a dental appointment for a fearful patient), the adrenal cortex cannot produce the additional cortisol required to adapt to the stress, and signs and symptoms of acute adrenal insufficiency develop.

The administration of exogenous glucocorticosteroids to a patient with functional adrenal cortices may produce a second form of adrenocortical hypofunction. Glucocorticosteroid drugs are widely prescribed in pharmacologic doses for the symptomatic relief of a wide variety of disorders (Box 8-1). When used in this manner, exogenous glucocorticosteroid administration produces a disuse atrophy of the adrenal cortex, decreasing the ability of the adrenal cortex to increase corticosteroid levels in response to stressful situations. This in turn leads to the development of signs and symptoms associated with acute adrenal insufficiency. Today, secondary adrenal insufficiency is a greater potential threat than Addison's disease in the development of acute adrenal crisis.[10] Acute adrenal insufficiency is a true medical emergency in which the victim is in immediate danger due to glucocorticoid (cortisol) insufficiency. Peripheral vascular collapse (shock) and ventricular asystole (cardiac arrest) are the usual cause of death.[11,12]

The dentist is in the unenviable position of being a major stress factor in the lives of many patients. Therefore all dental office personnel must become capable of recognizing and managing acute adrenal

crises; even more importantly, staff members must be able to prevent this situation from developing.

## Predisposing Factors

Before the availability of glucocorticosteroid therapy, acute adrenal insufficiency was the terminal stage of Addison's disease. With exogenous glucocorticosteroid therapy, however, addisonian patients can lead relatively normal lives. Unusually stressful situations require that the patient modify the steroid dose to prevent the development of acute adrenal insufficiency. The lack of glucocorticosteroid hormones is the major predisposing factor in all cases of acute adrenal insufficiency; this deficiency develops through the following six mechanisms:

*Mechanism 1:* After the sudden withdrawal of steroid hormones in a patient who suffers primary adrenal insufficiency (Addison's disease)

*Mechanism 2:* After the sudden withdrawal of steroid hormones from a patient with normal adrenal cortices but with a temporary insufficiency resulting from cortical suppression through prolonged exogenous glucocorticosteroid administration (secondary insufficiency)

Patients with primary and secondary adrenocortical insufficiency are dependent on exogenous steroids. Abrupt withdrawal from therapy leaves patients with a deficiency of glucocorticosteroid hormones, making them unable to adapt normally to stress (they become stress-intolerant). Evidence indicates that it may take up to 9 months to achieve full recovery of adrenal function following prolonged exogenous steroid therapy in patients with normal cortices.[13] Others have estimated that normal function may not return for as long as 2 years.[14]

Patients with Addison's disease require the administration of glucocorticosteroids as long as they live. Withdrawal from exogenous steroid therapy of patients who do not suffer Addison's disease should occur gradually; in this way the adrenal glands can increase production of endogenous glucocorticoids as the levels of exogenously administered steroids decrease. The time required for the return to normal adrenocortical functioning varies and is influenced by a number of factors (Box 8-2). Predesigned protocols help withdraw patients from long-term glucocorticosteroid therapy with a minimum of side effects and with relative convenience and safety.[15]

The widespread use of glucocorticosteroids in patients who do not have Addison's disease has become

---

box **8-2**    *Factors influencing the return of adrenocortical function after exogenous glucocorticosteroid therapy*

Dose of glucocorticosteroid administered
Duration of course of therapy
Frequency of administration
Time of administration
Route of administration

---

the most common cause of adrenal insufficiency. The hypothalamic-pituitary-adrenocortical axis generally is not suppressed unless exogenous steroid therapy has continued over long periods, in nonphysiologic doses, or both. Most of the indications for glucocorticosteroids in Box 8-1 require pharmacologic doses; these generally are much greater than physiologic doses.*

*Mechanism 3:* After stress, either physiologic or psychologic

Physiologic stress can include traumatic injuries, surgery (including oral, periodontal, or endodontic), extensive dental procedures, infection, acute changes in environmental temperature, severe muscular exercise, or burns. Psychologic stress, such as that seen in the fearful dental patient, may also precipitate adrenal crisis.

In stressful situations there is normally an increased release of glucocorticoids from the adrenal cortices. The hypothalamic-pituitary-adrenocortical axis mediates this increase, which normally results in a rapid elevation of glucocorticosteroid blood levels. If the adrenal gland cannot meet this increased demand, clinical signs and symptoms of adrenal insufficiency develop. In dental settings, stress is the most common immediate precipitating factor producing acute adrenal insufficiency.

*Mechanism 4:* After bilateral adrenalectomy or removal of a functioning adrenal tumor that was suppressing the other adrenal gland

*Mechanism 5:* After the sudden destruction of the pituitary gland

*Mechanism 6:* After both adrenal glands are injured through trauma, hemorrhage, infection, thrombosis, or tumor

The last three causes of adrenal crisis occur most commonly in hospitalized patients and therefore are

---

*Physiolgic, or replacement, doses equal the normal daily production of functioning adrenal cortex—approximately 20 mg cortisol. Pharmacologic doses are commonly four or five times greater.

not of immediate concern in most dental offices. The first three precipitating factors, however, are primary factors in the development of acute adrenal insufficiency in dental settings. (These factors will be discussed more fully in later sections of this chapter.)

Stress is a precipitating factor in a majority of cases of acute adrenal insufficiency. Factors that may precipitate stress include surgery, anesthesia, psychologic stress, alcohol intoxication, hypothermia, myocardial infarction, diabetes mellitus, intercurrent infection, asthma, pyrogens, and hypoglycemia.[16-19]

## Prevention

Acute adrenal insufficiency can best be managed through its prevention, which is based on the medical history questionnaire and ensuing dialogue history between the doctor and patient. In many instances, specific dental therapy modifications will be necessary for the patient at risk for acute adrenal insufficiency.

### Medical History Questionnaire

**Question 6: Have you taken any medicine or drugs during the past 2 years?**

*Comment:* The phrase "during the past 2 years" was added to this question because of the probability that an individual may develop varying degrees of adrenocortical suppression with long-term pharmacologic doses of glucocorticosteroids. Table 8-1 lists many of the generic and proprietary names of commonly prescribed corticosteroid drugs. In many instances the patient may know only the proprietary name of the drug. In such cases the doctor must have available a list such as this or an appropriate drug reference[20,21]; these texts can aid in identification of the drug and help the doctor minimize potential problems.

**Question 9: Circle any of the following that you have had or have at present:**

Rheumatic fever
Asthma
Hay fever
Allergies or hives
Arthritis
Rheumatism
Cortisone medicine

*Comment:* The specific diseases or medications listed in Question 9 represent only a small number of the clinical uses of glucocorticosteroids (see Box 8-1). With each of these drugs, pharmacologic doses—doses many times greater than the adrenal gland's normal daily output—are administered.

## DIALOGUE HISTORY

If the patient responds positively to any of the preceding questions, the doctor must vigorously pursue a dialogue history for additional facts, including the following vital drug information:

- Drugs used to manage the disorder

**table 8-1** *Systemic corticosteroids*

| GENERIC NAME | PROPRIETARY NAME |
|---|---|
| Hydrocortisone | A-HydroCort |
| | Cortef |
| | Hydrocortone |
| | Solu-Cortef |
| Cortisone | Cortone |
| | Cortone |
| Prenisolone | Articulose |
| | Cortalone |
| | Deltasolone |
| | Hydeltra |
| | Key-Pred |
| | Medicortelone |
| | Predaject |
| | Predcor-50 |
| Prednisone | Apo-Presnisone |
| | Deltasone Liquid Pred |
| | Fernisone |
| | Innpred |
| | Meticorten |
| | Orasone |
| | Prednicen-M |
| | Prednisone Intensol |
| | Sterapred |
| Methylprednisolone | Depoject |
| | Depo-Medrol |
| | Depopred |
| | Duralone |
| | Medrol |
| | Solu-Medrol |
| Traimcinolone | Aristocort |
| | Aristospan |
| | Articulose L.A. |
| | Cenocort |
| | Kenacort |
| | Kenalog |
| | Trilog |
| | Trilone |
| Paramethasone | Haldrone |
| Dexamethasone | Dalalone |
| | Decadron |
| | Dexone |
| | Hexadrol |
| | Solurex |
| Betamethasone | Betaclan |
| | Celestone |
| Fludrocortisone | Florinef |

- Drug dose
- Route of administration
- Duration of drug therapy
- Length of time elapsed since drug therapy ended

### What drugs did you use to manage the disorder?

*Comment:* Physicians frequently manage the conditions listed in Question 9 in part through the administration of glucocorticosteroids. However, the doctor first must determine the name of the specific drugs involved in the patient's treatment (see Box 8-1 and Table 8-1).

### What was your daily drug dose?

*Comment:* The specific dose of glucocorticosteroid is an important measure of the degree of cortical suppression. The equivalent therapeutic doses of glucocorticosteroids vary from drug to drug (Table 8-2). For example, 20 mg hydrocortisone is equivalent to 5 mg prednisolone, prednisone, and methylprednisone; to 4 mg methylprednisolone and triamcinolone; and to 0.75 mg dexamethasone.

Patients with primary adrenocortical insufficiency (Addison's disease) receive physiologic (replacement) doses of glucocorticosteroids. Such doses usually mandate daily administration of approximately 15 to 25 mg hydrocortisone orally in two divided doses—two thirds in the morning and the remaining third in the late afternoon or early evening. Many patients, however, do not retain salt sufficiently and require 0.05 to 0.3 mg oral fludrocortisone supplementation daily or every other day.[22] These doses satisfactorily replace the normal output of the adrenal cortex (approximately 20 mg cortisol daily).

Patients receiving glucocorticosteroid therapy for symptomatic treatment of disorders (see Box 8-1) commonly receive large pharmacologic, or therapeutic, doses. For example, patients suffering from rheumatoid arthritis frequently receive daily oral doses of 10 mg prednisone[23]; this dose is equivalent to approximately 50 mg cortisone. Increasingly, individuals whose acute asthmatic attacks do not respond readily to bronchodilator therapy receive prednisone orally.[24] These doses are divided and total 40 to 60 mg per day; this is equivalent to 200

to 300 mg cortisone. Doses such as these may cause suppression of the normal adrenal cortex if continued for long periods. Although admittedly conservative, the "rule of twos" (Box 8-3) is helpful in determining the risk factors for patients who are taking or recently have taken a course of glucocorticosteroid therapy.[25] The first of the three factors in the rule of twos is the daily administration of 20 mg or more of cortisone or its equivalent.

### By what route did you take the drug?

*Comment:* Glucocorticosteroids may be administered via a variety of routes. Parenteral (intramuscular [IM], intravenous [IV], or subcutaneous [SQ]) or enteral administration (oral) may result in the suppression of a normal adrenal cortex with a decrease in production of endogenous corticosteroids. Drugs administered topically (ophthalmic, dermatologic, intranasal, tracheobronchial, vaginal, or rectal administration) and via intraarticular application normally do not result in clinically significant cortical suppression because these routes provide relatively poor systemic absorption.

### How long did your glucocorticosteroid therapy last?

*Comment:* Although the exact length of time required for the development of significant cortical suppression varies from patient to patient, it has been demonstrated that uninterrupted glucocorticosteroid therapy for as little as 2 weeks may induce suppression.[26] Any patient who has received glucocorticosteroid therapy continuously for 2 weeks or longer risks developing adrenal insufficiency. This is the second important factor in the rule of twos.

### How long ago did you stop receiving glucocorticosteroid therapy?

*Comment:* This question is applicable to patients who had normal, functional adrenal cortices at the onset of glucocorticosteroid therapy, underwent therapy (probably at pharmacologic dose levels) until the underlying disorder was controlled, and then were gradually withdrawn from the drugs. The atrophic adrenal cortex does not function normally for a variable period after withdrawal from exogenous glucocorticosteroid therapy. During this time the cortex usually can produce minimal daily levels of endogenous corticosteroids; however, in stressful situations, it may be incapable of meeting the increased demand, thus inducing signs and symptoms of acute adrenal insufficiency.

---

**table 8-2** *Equivalent doses of glucocorticosteroids*

| AGENT | EQUIVALENT DOSE (mg) |
| --- | --- |
| Cortisone | 25 |
| Hydrocortisone | 20 |
| Prednisolone | 5 |
| Prednisone | 5 |
| Methylprednisone | 5 |
| Methylprednisolone | 4 |
| Triamcinolone | 4 |
| Dexamethasone | 0.75 |
| Betamethasone | 0.6 |

**box 8-3** *Rule of twos*

Adrenocortical suppression should be suspected if a patient has received glucocorticosteroid therapy through two of the following methods:
1. In a dose of 20 mg or more of cortisone or its equivalent
2. Via the oral or parenteral route for a continuous period of 2 weeks or longer
3. Within 2 years of dental therapy

The length of time required for full regeneration of normal cortical function varies according to the dosage and length of therapy but is normally at least 9 to 12 months.[11] Instances of acute adrenal insufficiency lasting as long as 2 years after termination of therapy have been reported. The third factor in the rule of twos relates to patients who have received glucocorticosteroid therapy with 2 years of dental treatment. The rule of twos allows the doctor to predict with a degree of reliability those patients at increased risk for acute adrenal insufficiency.

## DENTAL THERAPY CONSIDERATIONS

Patients who are currently receiving glucocorticosteroid therapy or recently have received such therapy and meet the criteria of the rule of twos may require dental treatment modifications. In such circumstances a complete medical and dental evaluation should be completed, a provisional treatment plan established, and the patient's primary-care physician consulted before dental treatment begins. A patient with Addison's disease or a patient receiving long-term pharmacologic doses of glucocorticosteroid therapy usually is classified as an ASA II or III risk.

**Glucocorticosteroid coverage**    Because patients with adrenocortical insufficiency physically are less able to adapt to stress in a normal manner, they require administration of glucocorticosteroids before, during, and possibly after the stressful situation to in-crease their blood steroid levels. The choice of a therapeutic regimen depends on the primary-care physician's evaluation of the patient's physical status and on the dentist's evaluation of the stress involved in the planned treatment.

Many primary-care physicians underestimate the degree of stress associated with nonsurgical dental treatment. Thus the dentist must evaluate this factor carefully. In an extreme instance, such as a fearful patient with Addison's disease, the patient may be hospitalized and receive 200 to 500 mg cortisone per day, which is equivalent to the maximal response of the normal pituitary-adrenal system to extreme stress.

The requirement for increased glucocorticosteroid therapy decreases in individuals who are only moderately fearful and undergoing dental procedures that are only mildly stressful (as most dental procedures are classified). Usually a twofold or fourfold increase in glucocorticosteroid dosage on the day of the dental treatment prepares the patient adequately. The adrenal cortices of normal adults secrete about 20 mg cortisol daily, the daily maintenance level that most patients with Addison's disease require. The dentist also may administer or prescribe oral medications. Figure 8-1 is a sample of a corticosteroid coverage protocol.

**Stress-reduction protocol**    In addition to medical consultation and the possible use of glucocorticosteroids during dental treatment, the stress-reduction protocol (see Chapter 2) is an extremely

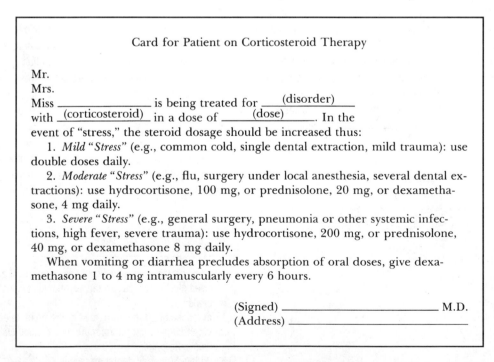

Card for Patient on Corticosteroid Therapy

Mr.
Mrs.
Miss _____ is being treated for ____(disorder)____
with __(corticosteroid)__ in a dose of _____(dose)_____. In the
event of "stress," the steroid dosage should be increased thus:
   1. *Mild "Stress"* (e.g., common cold, single dental extraction, mild trauma): use double doses daily.
   2. *Moderate "Stress"* (e.g., flu, surgery under local anesthesia, several dental extractions): use hydrocortisone, 100 mg, or prednisolone, 20 mg, or dexamethasone, 4 mg daily.
   3. *Severe "Stress"* (e.g., general surgery, pneumonia or other systemic infections, high fever, severe trauma): use hydrocortisone, 200 mg, or prednisolone, 40 mg, or dexamethasone 8 mg daily.
   When vomiting or diarrhea precludes absorption of oral doses, give dexamethasone 1 to 4 mg intramuscularly every 6 hours.

(Signed) _____ M.D.
(Address) _____

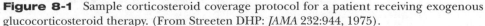

**Figure 8-1**    Sample corticosteroid coverage protocol for a patient receiving exogenous glucocorticosteroid therapy. (From Streeten DHP: *JAMA* 232:944, 1975).

valuable tool in the proper management of patients with adrenocortical insufficiency.

**Additional considerations**    The patient with Addison's disease also may wear an identification bracelet that states the patient's name, the name and telephone number of a close relative, and the primary-care physician's name and telephone number. Each bracelet also states, "I have adrenal insufficiency. In any emergency involving injury, vomiting, or loss of consciousness, the hydrocortisone in my possession should be injected under my skin, and my physician should be notified." Such patients carry small, clearly labeled kits containing 100 mg hydrocortisone phosphate solution in a sterile syringe ready for use. These kits constantly remind patients that their survival may depend on the timely administration of this drug. During dental treatment the doctor should take the kit from the patient and place it on the instrument tray or another easily accessible location.

# Clinical Manifestations

In stressful situations like dental procedures, patients with hypofunctioning adrenal cortices may exhibit clinical signs and symptoms of acute glucocorticosteroid insufficiency. The end result of this acute insufficiency may be the loss of consciousness and possible coma. Table 8-3 lists the clinical signs and symptoms of adrenal insufficiency.

Individuals suffering acute adrenal insufficiency almost universally exhibit lethargy, extreme fatigue, and weakness. In extreme cases the weakness may be so pronounced that even speaking can be difficult.[27] Hyperkalemia may also develop; if severe, this condition can lead to skeletal muscle paralysis.[28] Most cases of mortality and major morbidity that accompany adrenal insufficiency are usually secondary to hypotension or hypoglycemia.

In addition, most patients with Addison's disease demonstrate hypotension with systolic blood pressures of less than 110 mmHg. Of 108 patients with Addison's disease studied only 3% had systolic blood pressures greater than 125 mmHg.[29] Mucocutaneous hyperpigmentation is present in more than three fourths of patients with Addison's disease.[29,30] Melanin deposits usually occur in areas of trauma or friction, such as the palms, soles, elbows, knees, buccal mucosa, and old scars.[31]

Patients with adrenal insufficiency may also suffer orthostatic hypotension with episodes of postural syncope. More than half of such patients also exhibit nausea, vomiting, and other nonspecific gastrointestinal symptoms.[30] Anorexia is present almost universally and results in the weight loss that inevitably accompanies chronic adrenal insufficiency.[31] Two thirds of patients with adrenal insufficiency have hypoglycemia.[29,30] Symptoms are those normally associated with hypoglycemia (see Chapter 17), including tachycardia, perspiration, weakness, nausea, vomiting, headache, convulsions, and coma.[32] Electrolyte disturbances are almost always evident in these patients, including hyponatremia in 88% of cases, hyperkalemia in 64% of cases, and hypercalcemia in 6% to 33% of cases.[29,30,33,34]

In the dental setting the acute episode will be marked most notably by a progressively severe mental confusion. The individual also experiences intense pain in the abdomen, lower back, and legs, and the cardiovascular system progressively deteriorates. This latter symptom may result in a loss of consciousness and onset of coma. (Coma is a state in which a patient is totally unresponsive or is unresponsive to all except very painful stimuli; the patient in such a state immediately returns to the state of unresponsiveness when the stimulus is removed.)

If not managed properly, acute adrenal insufficiency may result in death. Mortality is usually secondary to hypoglycemia or hypotension. Most individuals do not lose consciousness immediately. The progressive mental confusion and other clinical symptoms usually permit the prompt recognition of the problem and the immediate initiation of proper management.

table **8-3**    *Clinical manifestations of adrenal insufficiency*

| SYMPTOMS | FREQUENCY (%) |
|---|---|
| Weakness and fatigue | 99-100 |
| Anorexia | 98-100 |
| Weight loss | 97-100 |
| Hyperpigmentation (skin) | 92-97 |
| Hypotension (110/70 mmHg) | 82-91 |
| Hyperpigmentation (mucous membranes) | 71-82 |
| Nausea, vomiting | 56-87 |
| Abdominal pain | 34 |
| Salt craving | 22 |
| Diarrhea | 20 |
| Constipation | 19 |
| Syncope | 12-16 |
| Musculoskeletal complaints | 6 |
| Vitiligo | 4-9 |
| Lethargy | Minimal |
| Confusion | Minimal |
| Psychosis | Minimal |
| Auricular calcification | Minimal |

Modified from Wogan JM: Endocrine disorders. In Rosen P, editor: *Emergency medicine,* ed 2, St Louis, 1988, Mosby.

# Pathophysiology

## NORMAL ADRENAL FUNCTION

The actions of adrenocortical steroid hormones affect all bodily tissues and organs and help keep the body's internal environment constant (a condition known as *homeostasis*) through their actions on the metabolism of carbohydrates, fats, proteins, water, and electrolytes. The body provides a minimal supply of corticosteroid hormones (approximately 20 mg cortisol daily in nonstressed adults[35]) through the actions of adrenocorticotropic hormone (ACTH), which is released by the anterior portion of the pituitary gland. ACTH levels in the blood control the adrenal cortex and the production of all steroids except aldosterone.

In nonstressed situations the level of circulating cortisol regulates the rate of ACTH secretion; a high level suppresses ACTH secretion, whereas a low circulating cortisol level permits its more rapid secretion (Figure 8-2, *A* and *B*). The mechanism is relatively slow acting and does not account for the rapid increase in blood ACTH levels during stressful situations. A second factor regulating the secretion of ACTH is the individual's sleep schedule. Plasma ACTH levels begin to rise at 2 AM in individuals who sleep at night, reaching peak levels at the time of awakening. They fall during the day, reaching their ebb during the evening. These fluctuations in cortisol blood levels, a process known as *diurnal variation,* is reversed in individuals who work at night and sleep during the day.

In stressful situations the pituitary gland rapidly increases the release of ACTH, and the adrenal cortex responds within minutes by synthesizing and secreting increased amounts of various corticosteroids. This increased steroid production prepares the body to successfully manage the stressful situation; it increases the metabolic rate and the retention of sodium and water, while making small blood vessels increasingly responsive to the actions of norepinephrine.

To rapidly raise the levels of corticosteroids in the blood, a third mechanism must be activated (Figure 8-2, *C*). When the central nervous system receives stressful stimuli, these stimuli reach the level of the hypothalamus, which releases a substance known as *corticotrophin-releasing hormone (CRH)*. The hypothalamic-hypophyseal portal venous system transports CRH to the anterior lobes of the pituitary gland, where it stimulates the secretion of ACTH into the circulation, which then allows the adrenal cortex to increase its secretion of corticosteroids. Cortisol secretion begins within minutes and continues as long as the plasma ACTH level is maintained. Once ACTH secretion ceases (for exam-

ple, when the stress is removed), plasma ACTH concentration has a half-life of 10 minutes; once cortisol secretion ceases, the plasma cortisol level drops during a half-life of 1 to 2 hours.

## ADRENAL INSUFFICIENCY

Patients with primary adrenocortical insufficiency (Addison's disease) have hypofunctioning adrenal cortices and cannot produce the blood levels of corticosteroids required to maintain life even at nonstressful levels. For this reason either oral or parenteral glucocorticosteroid replacement therapy is required.

Figure 8-3 shows the feedback mechanisms operating in the patient with Addison's disease. Corticosteroid blood levels are fixed, depending on the total milligram dose administered during the day. As a general rule a normal adult secretes 20 mg cortisol per day; thus replacement therapy for patients with Addison's disease is approximately 20 mg exogenous cortisol (hydrocortisone) daily. The drug may be administered either orally or parenterally, in single or more commonly in divided doses. The hypofunctioning adrenal cortex cannot respond to increases or decreases in blood levels of ACTH, which the anterior pituitary continues to secrete.

In the patient with a normal adrenal cortex who is receiving glucocorticosteroid therapy for a non–endocrine-related disorder, the total amount of endogenous and exogenous steroids determines the blood level of cortisol. Initially, the adrenal cortex continues to secrete approximately 20 mg cortisol daily, to which may be added doses of more than 50 mg exogenous glucocorticosteroids. The effect of this elevation of glucocorticosteroid levels in the blood is to inhibit ACTH secretion, which in turn inhibits the adrenal cortex from secreting cortisol.

As glucocorticosteroid therapy continues, the ability of the adrenal glands to produce endogenous glucocorticoids decreases and a variable degree of disuse atrophy develops (Figure 8-4, *A*). If exogenous therapy is stopped abruptly, or on rare occasions even after a gradual withdrawal, the blood level of cortisol falls; this stimulates the anterior pituitary to produce increased blood levels of ACTH, which in turn stimulates production of cortisol by the adrenal cortex.

At this time ACTH and endogenous corticosteroid levels may prove deficient (see Figure 8-4, *B*). The adrenal cortex cannot produce the required cortisol levels, and a hypoadrenal state ensues. Any increased requirement for cortisol, such as occurs in a stressful situation, may provoke acute adrenal insufficiency. Although the adrenal cortex usually returns to normal function within 2 to 4 weeks of cessation of glu-

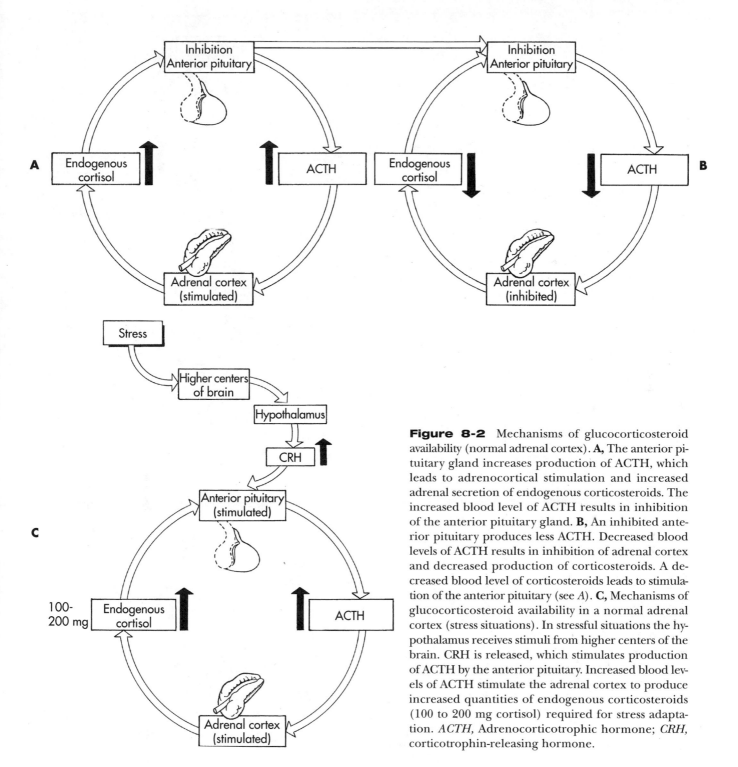

**Figure 8-2** Mechanisms of glucocorticosteroid availability (normal adrenal cortex). **A,** The anterior pituitary gland increases production of ACTH, which leads to adrenocortical stimulation and increased adrenal secretion of endogenous corticosteroids. The increased blood level of ACTH results in inhibition of the anterior pituitary gland. **B,** An inhibited anterior pituitary produces less ACTH. Decreased blood levels of ACTH results in inhibition of adrenal cortex and decreased production of corticosteroids. A decreased blood level of corticosteroids leads to stimulation of the anterior pituitary (see *A*). **C,** Mechanisms of glucocorticosteroid availability in a normal adrenal cortex (stress situations). In stressful situations the hypothalamus receives stimuli from higher centers of the brain. CRH is released, which stimulates production of ACTH by the anterior pituitary. Increased blood levels of ACTH stimulate the adrenal cortex to produce increased quantities of endogenous corticosteroids (100 to 200 mg cortisol) required for stress adaptation. *ACTH,* Adrenocorticotrophic hormone; *CRH,* corticotrophin-releasing hormone.

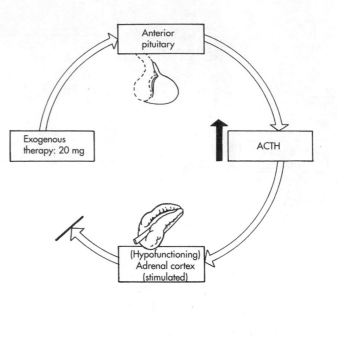

**Figure 8-3** Corticosteroid levels in an individual with primary insufficiency (Addison's disease). The anterior pituitary gland secretes ACTH, which stimulates the adrenal cortex. A hypofunctioning adrenal cortex cannot synthesize and secrete the required level of cortisol. Blood levels of corticosteroids do not fluctuate in response to ACTH levels; they are fixed by exogenous doses of approximately 20 mg cortisol daily. *ACTH,* Adrenocorticotrophic hormone.

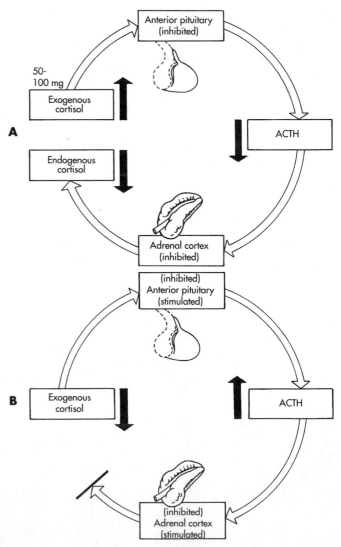

**Figure 8-4** Glucocorticosteroid levels in an individual with secondary insufficiency due to exogenous therapy. **A,** If additional exogenous glucocorticosteroids are administered to an individual with a normal adrenal cortex, blood levels are increased significantly. ACTH production by the anterior pituitary is inhibited, resulting in inhibition of adrenal cortical function. Inhibition of both ACTH and corticosteroid production continues for the duration of the exogenous therapy. **B,** After a prolonged period of exogenous therapy (2 weeks or longer), disuse atrophy of the adrenal cortex and anterior pituitary develops. After therapy is terminated, blood levels of corticosteroids fall, stimulating the anterior pituitary to produce ACTH. ACTH production may be subnormal, and even if it is normal, the adrenal cortex's response may be inadequate. Blood cortisol levels are inadequate, and the patient enters a stress-intolerant state. *ACTH,* Adrenocorticotrophic hormone.

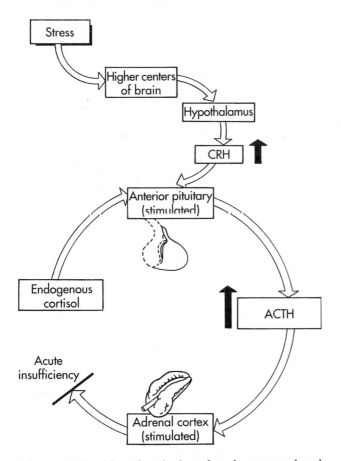

**Figure 8-5** A hypofunctioning adrenal cortex produced by exogenous cortisol (Addison's disease and nonendocrine cortisol). The blood level of glucocorticosteroids is fixed by daily cortisol doses. In a stressful situation, the CRH secreted by the hypothalamus induces ACTH secretion by the anterior pituitary, which in turn stimulates the adrenal cortex. The anterior pituitary and/or the adrenal cortex may not be able to function properly, leading to inadequate cortisol blood levels for stress adaptation. Acute insufficiency results. *ACTH,* Adrenocorticotrophic hormone; *CRH* corticotrophin-releasing hormone.

cocorticosteroid therapy, in some instances it may require more than a year.[13] As a general rule, the longer the duration of glucocorticosteroid therapy and the larger the doses during therapy, the longer is the recovery period.

A patient with adrenal hypofunction—either primary (Addison's disease) or secondary (exogenous glucocorticosteroid therapy)—receives a fixed level of glucocorticosteroids during therapy (Figure 8-5). In stressful situations the patient cannot increase this level in response to the increasing ACTH levels in the blood, produced as a result of CRH released from the hypothalamus; thus the clinical manifestations of acute adrenal insufficiency develop. Management of this situation requires replacement and augmentation of low blood levels of steroids.

Hypotension observed in patients with adrenal insufficiency is the result of several mechanisms. A deficiency in cortisol can lead to hypotension even in patients who have normal volumes of circulating blood. Direct depression of myocardial contractility and reduction in myocardial responsiveness to catecholamines together produce hypotension.[36,37]

About two thirds of individuals who demonstrate adrenal insufficiency become hypoglycemic. Glucose levels are less than 45 mg/dl. Hypoglycemia is the result of a decrease in gluconeogenesis and increased peripheral use of glucose secondary to lipolysis.[38,39]

In addition, hyperpigmentation is common in patients with chronic primary adrenal insufficiency and is produced by compensatory secretion of ACTH and melanin-stimulating hormone.[29,30] The condition develops over a period of several months when relative adrenal insufficiency is present; individuals with secondary adrenal insufficiency do not exhibit hyperpigmentation.

# Management

Acute adrenal insufficiency is a life-threatening situation. Effective management requires that the doctor follow the steps of basic life support (BLS) and administer glucocorticosteroids. Glucocorticoid deficiency, depletion of extracellular fluid, and hyperkalemia place the patient in immediate danger. Treatment is predicated on the prompt correction of these conditions.

## CONSCIOUS PATIENT

*Step 1: termination of dental treatment.* As soon as the individual exhibits signs and symptoms of possible acute adrenal insufficiency, dental treatment should cease. Acute adrenal insufficiency should be suspected in patients who exhibit mental confusion, nausea, vomiting, and abdominal pain and who currently are receiving glucocorticosteroids or have received 20 mg or more cortisone (or its equivalent) via oral or parenteral administration for 2 weeks or longer within the past 2 years (Box 8-4).

*Step 2: **P** (position).* If the patient appears mentally confused, wet, and clammy (signs and symptoms of hypotension), that individual should be placed in the supine position with the legs elevated slightly. If the patient does not exhibit any of these signs and symptoms, comfort should determine the position.

*Step 3: **A-B-C** (airway-breathing-circulation), or BLS, as needed.* In the conscious patient, **A-B-C** are assessed but need not be employed.

*Step 4: **D** (definitive care):*

*Step 4a: monitoring of vital signs.* The blood pressure and heart rate should be monitored in 5-minute intervals throughout the episode. The individual usually exhibits hypotension with an increased heart rate (tachycardia).

*Step 4b: summoning of medical assistance.* The appropriate team member should seek medical assistance as soon as possible. Because the victim is still conscious, it may be wise to contact the patient's primary-care physician. In most cases emergency personnel will transport the patient immediately to the emergency department of a hospital, where more definitive management may be instituted. If hospitalization is required, the doctor should accompany the patient.

*Step 4c: emergency kit and oxygen (O₂).* The appropriate team member should obtain the emergency kit and portable $O_2$ immediately. $O_2$ may be administered via a full-face mask or nasal hood at a flow of approximately 5 to 10 L per minute.

*Step 4d: administration of glucocorticosteroid.* The corticosteroid (if available) and a plastic disposable syringe should be removed from the emergency kit. If the patient has a history of chronic adrenal insufficiency, the doctor may administer the patient's own corticosteroid medication. A corticosteroid is not

considered a critical (essential) emergency drug because the incidence of acute adrenal insufficiency is low, and medical assistance is usually available within a relatively short period.

If the patient is known to suffer chronic adrenal insufficiency, the administration of 100 mg hydrocortisone sodium succinate is the next immediate step. The drug should be readministered every 6 to 8 hours.[40] Hydrocortisone sodium succinate (Solu-Cortef) is available as an unmixed powder and liquid in a 2-ml Mix-o-vial (Figure 8-6). When the solution is mixed, each milliliter contains 50 mg hydrocortisone. To mix the solution, the top plastic cap is removed and the rubber plunger is depressed. This combines the powder and liquid. The vial is then mixed until a clear solution forms. The syringe then is inserted through the rubber stopper and 2 milliliters of solution withdrawn. If possible, the 100 mg hydrocortisone should be administered intravenously over a period of 30 seconds. However, the IM route also may be used and 100 mg (2 ml) injected into the vastus lateralis or middeltoid areas.

If the patient does not have a prior history of adrenal insufficiency or glucocorticosteroid use, the dentist should manage the patient as described in steps 1 through 4b and await the arrival of emergency personnel.

However, as the immediate diagnosis of acute adrenal insufficiency is empiric (based on the presenting signs and symptoms), it is often recommended that corticosteroid therapy be initiated immediately, even before the diagnosis is confirmed by laboratory testing (ACTH stimulation test).* In the office of a doctor with

---

| box **8-4** | *Criteria for a determination of adrenal insufficiency* |
|---|---|

History of current or recent long-term steroid use
Mental confusion
Nausea and vomiting
Abdominal pain
Hypotension

---

*In the ATCH stimulation test, 0.25 mg cosyntropin, a synthetic ACTH, is administered at time 0. To measure the patient's cortisol level, serum samples are drawn at time 0, then in 1 hour, and finally in 6 to 8 hours. Normal adrenal glands respond with increases in cortisol of at least 10 mg/fl, or three times the baseline level.

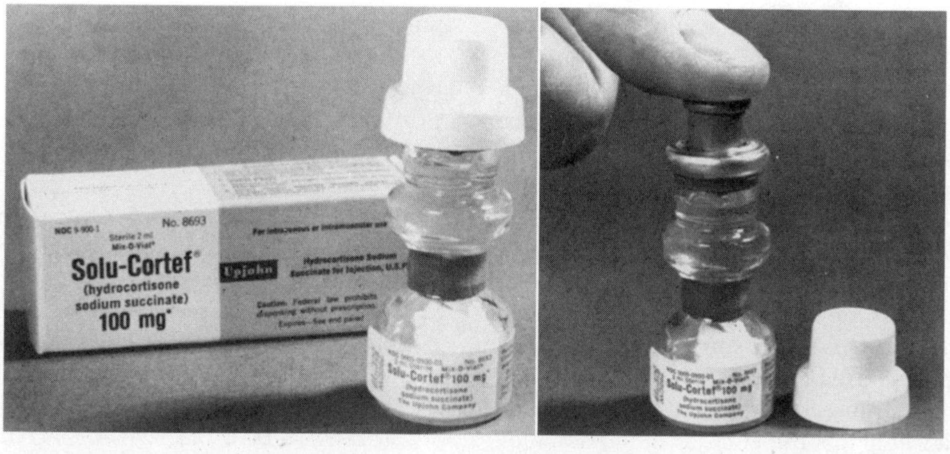

**Figure 8-6** **A,** Corticosteroid. **B,** Preparation of corticosteroid for use. Depression of the plunger mixes the powder and liquid so that fresh solution is immediately available for use.

proper training and experience, 4 mg dexamethasone phosphate should be administered IV every 6 to 8 hours while awaiting the ACTH stimulation test.[41] Dexamethasone is approximately 100 times more potent than cortisol.

*Step 5: additional management.* In most cases of adrenal insufficiency in which the patient retains consciousness, the administration of BLS as needed, $O_2$, and glucocorticosteroids is adequate to stabilize the patient. Emergency medical personnel will establish an IV line when they arrive and administer additional drugs after confirming the diagnosis. These additional drugs include IV fluids to counteract depletion of the body's circulating fluid (hypovolemia) and hypotension, which are usually present in adrenal insufficiency. A patient with Addison's disease may be up to 20% volume depleted.[41]

Unless it is contraindicated by the patient's cardiovascular condition, 1 L of normal saline should be infused in the first hour. A 5% dextrose solution usually is added next to help combat the hypoglycemia. The individual may require up to 3 L of fluid over the first 8 hours. Hypoglycemia also must be treated immediately and aggressively. If the individual is symptomatic or if a finger-stick blood glucose test demonstrates low glucose levels (45 mg/dl), 50 to 100 ml of a 50% dextrose solution should be administered. If an IV line is unavailable, 1 to 2 mg glucagon may be administered IM.

## UNCONSCIOUS PATIENT

When a patient loses consciousness, the doctor may not at the outset be aware of the patient's medical history of adrenal insufficiency or glucocorticosteroid therapy.

*Step 1: recognition of unconsciousness.* The shake-and-shout method—yelling "Are you all right?"—should be used to determine the individual's level of consciousness. Lack of response is unconsciousness.

*Step 2:* **P.** The patient should be placed in the supine position with the legs elevated slightly.

*Step 3:* **A-B-C** *(BLS).* Immediate application of the steps of BLS (see Chapter 5) is essential. These include use of head tilt–chin lift, assessment of the airway and breathing, artificial ventilation (if necessary), and assessment of circulation.

In most instances of acute adrenal insufficiency, the individual demonstrates depressed respiration and blood pressure and a rapid but weak (thready) heart rate. Airway maintenance and $O_2$ administration are necessary in virtually all cases. In the unlikely occurrence that a pulse is absent, external chest compression should be initiated immediately and continued until assistance arrives.

*Step 4:* **D:**
*Step 4a: emergency kit and $O_2$.* The designated team member should bring the office kit and $O_2$ to the site of the emergency. $O_2$ may be administered through a positive-pressure face mask or nasal hood. Aromatic spirits of ammonia also may be used because differentiation between acute adrenal insufficiency and other, more common causes of unconsciousness (for example, vasodepressor syncope) may be difficult at this early stage. The patient with adrenal insufficiency will not respond to the inhalation of aromatic ammonia.

Positioning of the patient, maintenance of an adequate airway, and use of aromatic ammonia and $O_2$ will not lead to a noticeable improvement of the patient suffering acute adrenal insufficiency. If the patient's condition does not improve, additional steps should be considered.

*Step 4b: summoning of emergency medical assistance.* If the patient remains unconscious after the preceding steps are completed, the unconsciousness most likely is not due to one of the more commonly encountered conditions, such as vasodepressor syncope or orthostatic hypotension. At this point the appropriate team member should summon emergency medical assistance.

*Step 4c: evaluation of medical history.* While BLS is being administered and emergency assistance is on the way, a member of the emergency team should review the patient's medical history for evidence of a possible cause. If the cause is not obvious, the dental office team should continue to implement the steps of BLS until emergency assistance arrives. If evidence exists that glucocorticosteroid insufficiency may be the cause of unconsciousness, treatment should proceed to step 4d.

*Step 4d: administration of glucocorticosteroid.* Individuals with suspected adrenal insufficiency should receive 100 mg hydrocortisone via IV or IM administration. If possible, 100 mg should be injected IV over a period of 30 seconds. An IV infusion should be started, and an IV solution to which 100 mg of hydrocortisone is added should be administered over 2 hours. If the IV route is unavailable, the individual may receive 100 mg hydrocortisone IM.

*Step 4e: additional drug therapy.* If hypotension also is present, an IV infusion of 1 L of normal saline or a 5% dextrose solution should be administered over 1 hour while awaiting emergency assistance.

| box **8-5** | *Management of adrenal insufficiency* |

**Conscious patient**

Terminate dental treatment.

↓

**P**—position patient comfortably, if asymptomatic, supine with feet elevated slightly, if symptomatic.

↓

**A-B-C**—provide BLS, as needed.

↓

**D**—definitive care:
Monitor vital signs.
Summon medical assistance.
Obtain emergency kit and $O_2$.
Administer glucocorticosteroid, if available, and if history of adrenal insufficiency exists.

↓

Consider additional management:
Provide BLS, as needed.
Provide $O_2$, as needed.
Provide glucocorticosteroid, as needed.
Establish IV line.

**Unconscious patient**

Recognize unconsciousness.

↓

**P**—position patient supine with feet elevated slightly.

↓

**A-B-C**—provide BLS, as needed.

↓

**D**—definitive care:
Obtain emergency kit and $O_2$.
Summon medical assistance.
Evaluate medical history.
Administer glucocorticosteroid.
Establish IV line, if possible.

↓

Transfer to hospital.

*BLS,* Basic life support; *IV,* intravenous; *$O_2$,* oxygen; **P,** position; **A,** airway; **B,** breathing; **C,** circulation; **D,** definitive care.

*Step 5: transfer to hospital.* After emergency personnel arrive, they will stabilize the patient for transfer to an emergency medical facility, where emergency physicians obtain blood specimens and correct existing electrolyte imbalances, such as hyperkalemia.

Definitive therapy is designed to meet the needs of the individual patient but consists initially of large IV doses of glucocorticosteroids followed by additional doses of oral or IM steroids, or both. Again, if the possibility exists that the loss of consciousness is related in any way to corticosteroid deficiency, the immediate administration of 100 mg hydrocortisone succinate may save the patient's life. If no such indi-

cations exist, the doctor should continue to maintain the steps of BLS until emergency personnel arrive.

Box 8-5 summarizes the management of acute adrenal insufficiency. In addition, the following facts may prove helpful:

- **Drugs used in management:** $O_2$ and glucocorticosteroids
- **Medical assistance required: Yes,** if patient is unconscious; **yes,** if conscious patient with history of adrenal insufficiency shows clinical signs and symptoms of acute insufficiency

## REFERENCES

1. Guyton AC: The adrenocortical hormones. In *Human physiology and mechanisms of disease,* ed 5, Philadelphia, 1992, WB Saunders.
2. Findling JW: Cushing's syndromes: an enlarged clinical spectrum, *N Engl J Med* 321:1677, 1989.
3. O'Riordain DS and others: Long-term outcome of bilateral adrenalectomy in patients with Cushing's syndrome, *Surgery* 116(6):1088-1093, 1994.
4. Zeiger MA and others: Primary bilateral adrenocortical causes of Cushing's syndrome, *Surgery* 110(6):1106-1115, 1991.
5. Dahlberg PJ, Goellner MH, Pehling GB: Adrenal insufficiency secondary to adrenal hemorrhage: two case reports and a review of cases confirmed by computed tomography, *Arch Intern Med* 150(4):905-909, 1990.
6. Vallotton MB: Endocrine emergencies: disorders of the adrenal cortex, *Baillieres Clin Endocrinol Metab* 6(1):41-56, 1992.
7. Oelkers W: Adrenal insufficiency, *N Engl J Med* 335(16): 1206-1212, 1996.
8. Streeten DHP: Corticosteroid therapy. I. Pharmacological properties and principles of corticosteroid use, *JAMA* 232:944, 1975.
9. Burke CW: Adrenocortical insufficiency, *Clin Endocrinol Metab* 14:947, 1985.
10. Cronin CC and others: Addison disease in patients treated with glucocorticoid therapy, *Arch Intern Med* 157(4):456-458, 1997.
11. O'Donnell M: Emergency! addisonian crisis, *Am J Nurs* 97(3):41, 1997.
12. Bruton-Maree N, Maree SM: Acute adrenal insufficiency: a case report, *CRNA* 4(3):128-132, 1993.
13. Graber AL and others: Natural history of pituitary-adrenal recovery following long-term suppression with corticosteroids, *J Clin Endocrinol Metab* 25:11, 1965.
14. Streeten DHP: Corticosteroid therapy. II. Complications and therapeutic indications, JAMA 232:1046, 1975.
15. Byyny R: Withdrawal from glucocorticoid therapy, *N Engl J Med* 295:30, 1976.
16. von Werder K and others: Adrenal function during long-term anesthesia in man, *Proc Soc Exp Biol Med* 135: 854, 1970.

17. Sachar EJ: Hormonal changes in stress and mental illness, *Hosp Pract* 10:49, 1970.
18. Bellet S and others: Effect of acute ethanol intake on plasma 11-hydroxycorticosteroid levels in accidental hypothermia, *Lancet* 1:324, 1970.
19. Jacobs HS, Nabarro JDN: Plasma 11-hydroxycorticosteroid and growth hormone levels in acute medical illnesses, *Br Med J* 2:595, 1969.
20. *Physicians' desk reference,* ed 52, Oradell, NJ, 1998, Medical Economics.
21. American Dental Association: *ADA guide to dental therapeutics,* Chicago, 1998, The Association.
22. Fitzgerald PA, Camargo CA: Endocrine disorders. In Schroeder SA and others, editors: *Current medical diagnosis & treatment 1996,* Stamford, Conn, 1996, Appleton & Lange.
23. Hellmann DB: Arthritis and musculoskeletal disorders. In Schroeder SA and others, editors, *Current medical diagnosis & treatment 1996,* Stamford, Conn, 1996, Appleton & Lange.
24. Sertl K, Clark T, Kaliner M, editors: Corticosteroids: their biologic mechanisms and application to the treatment of asthma (symposium) *Am Rev Respir Dis* 141(suppl:1S, entire issue), 1990.
25. McCarthy FM: Adrenal insufficiency. In McCarthy FM, editor: *Essentials of safe dentistry for the medically compromised patient,* Philadelphia, 1989, WB Saunders.
26. Melby J: Systemic corticosteroid therapy: pharmacology and endocrine considerations, *Ann Intern Med* 81:505, 1974.
27. Tzagournis M: Acute adrenal insufficiency, *Heart Lung* 7:603, 1978.
28. Bell H, Hayes W, Vosbrugh J: Hyperkalemic paralysis due to adrenal insufficiency, *Arch Intern Med* 115:418, 1965.
29. Nerup J: Addison's disease—clinical studies: a report of 108 cases, *Acta Endocrinol* 76:127, 1974.
30. Dunlop D: Eighty-six cases of Addison's disease, *Br Med J* 2:887, 1963.
31. Kozak G: Primary adrenocortical insufficiency (Addison's disease), *Am Fam Physician* 15(5):124, 1977.
32. Vesely DL: Hypoglycemic coma: don't overlook adrenal crisis, *Geriatrics* 37:71, 1982.
33. Jorgensen H: Hypercalcemia in adrenocortical insufficiency, *Acta Med Scand* 193:175, 1973.
34. Walser M, Robinson BHB, Duckett JWL: The hypercalcemia of adrenal insufficiency, *J Clin Invest* 42:456, 1963.
35. Bondy PK: Disorders of the adrenal cortex. In Wilson JD, Foster DW, editors: *William's textbook of endocrinology,* ed 7, Philadelphia, 1985, WB Saunders.
36. Webb WR and others: Cardiovascular responses in acute adrenal insufficiency, *Surgery* 58:273, 1965.
37. Ramey ER, Goldstein MS: The adrenal cortex and the sympathetic nervous system, *Physiol Rev* 37:155, 1957.
38. Liddle G: The adrenals. In *Williams' textbook of endocrinology,* Philadelphia, 1981, WB Saunders.
39. Szwed JJ, White C: Normokalemic nonazotemic adrenal insufficiency, *South Med J* 76:919, 1983.
40. Leshin M: Acute adrenal insufficiency: recognition, management and prevention, *Urol Clin North Am* 9:229, 1982.
41. Wogan JM: Endocrine disorders. In Rosen P, editor: *Emergency medicine,* ed 2, St Louis, 1988, Mosby.

# 9

# Unconsciousness

## Differential Diagnosis

UNCONSCIOUSNESS, whatever its cause, must be recognized quickly and managed effectively. When unconsciousness occurs, the proximate cause may not always be obvious; and indeed, at the onset of unconsciousness the cause is not the primary concern. In all cases in which loss of consciousness occurs, several basic steps—those described in the preceding chapters on vasodepressor syncope, postural hypotension, and acute adrenal insufficiency—must be implemented as soon as possible. These steps comprise the primary phase of assessment and management (Box 9-1).

After these steps are completed successfully and while awaiting the arrival of emergency personnel (if necessary), dental office team members should proceed to the secondary steps of assessment and management, also termed *definitive management*. The information in this chapter will aid the team in the differential diagnosis of the cause of unconsciousness. Several clinical factors presented here may help establish a diagnosis (see Table 5-1 for common causes of loss of consciousness).

## Age of Patient

The age of the patient may assist in the differential diagnosis of unconsciousness. Unconsciousness occurring in the dental office in normal healthy patients in their mid- to late teens to late thirties will in almost all instances be most likely related to psychogenic re-box **9-1**  *Management of unconsciousness*

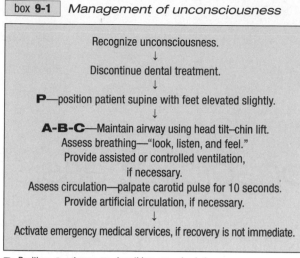

Recognize unconsciousness.

↓

Discontinue dental treatment.

↓

**P**—position patient supine with feet elevated slightly.

↓

**A-B-C**—Maintain airway using head tilt–chin lift.
Assess breathing—"look, listen, and feel."
Provide assisted or controlled ventilation,
if necessary.
Assess circulation—palpate carotid pulse for 10 seconds.
Provide artificial circulation, if necessary.

↓

Activate emergency medical services, if recovery is not immediate.

**P,** Position; **A,** airway; **B,** breathing; **C,** circulation.

table **9-1**  *Causes of unconsciousness*

| | AGE OF PATIENT | |
|---|---|---|
| CHILD | TEEN TO MID-30S | MORE THAN 40 YEARS |
| Hypoglycemia Epilepsy Congenital heart lesions | Psychogenic reactions Hypoglycemia Epilepsy | Cardiovascular causes |

table **9-2**  *Circumstances associated with the loss of consciousness*

| STRESS PRESENT | STRESS ABSENT |
|---|---|
| Vasodepressor syncope Hypoglycemia Epilepsy Myocardial infarction Cerebrovascular accident Adrenal insufficiency | Postural hypotension Ingestion of drugs Allergic reactions Hyperglycemic reactions |

sponses such as vasodopressor syncope. Two other possible causes of unconsciousness in patients under 40 years include hypoglycemia and epilepsy. These conditions normally are easy to differentiate from the more common causes of unconsciousness. (Other sections of this text will discuss these conditions in detail.)

In patients older than 40 years, cardiovascular complications, such as acute myocardial infarction, cerebrovascular accident, valvular lesions (for example, aortic stenosis), or acute cardiac dysrhythmias, are more likely to precipitate unconsciousness (see Section 7). Patients in this age-group experience psychogenic reactions much less frequently because they are more likely to have adapted to their dental fears.

Unconsciousness rarely occurs in younger children, except in the presence of specific disease states, including diabetes mellitus (hypoglycemia), epilepsy, and congenital heart lesions. Psychogenic reactions (vasodepressor syncope) in children are infrequent because children are extremely vocal in expressing their feelings toward dentistry, releasing their tensions, and producing muscular movements: in short, they just act like children! (Table 9-1).

## Circumstances Associated with Loss of Consciousness

Stress, whether psychologic (anxiety) or physiologic (pain), is a precipitating factor in most cases of unconsciousness that occur in dental offices. Instances in which stress may be a precipitating factor in the

loss of consciousness include vasodepressor syncope, adrenal insufficiency, cerebrovascular accident, hypoglycemia, epilepsy, and myocardial infarction. However, patients may still lose consciousness in the absence of obvious stress. Postural hypotension is the most common non–stress-related cause of unconsciousness; other nonstress leading to the loss of consciousness include allergic reactions, hyperglycemic reactions (diabetic coma), and the administration or ingestion of drugs (Table 9-2).

## Position of Patient

The patient's position at the time unconsciousness occurs may aid in the differential diagnosis. Syncope, or the transient loss of consciousness, rarely develops when the patient is in the supine position.

However, certain instances do exist in which a patient in the supine position may lose consciousness. These include unconsciousness that occurs secondary to (1) the administration of drugs; (2) seizures in epileptic patients; (3) seizures that develop with hypoglycemic reactions; (4) hyperglycemia; (5) acute adrenal insufficiency; (6) cardiovascular disorders, including valvular disorders, dysrhythmias, and myocardial infarction; and (7) cerebral vascular accident. In such circumstances placement of the patient in

| table **9-3** | Position of patient at time syncope occurs | | |
|---|---|---|

| UPRIGHT | SUPINE INTO UPRIGHT | SUPINE |
|---|---|---|
| Vasodepressor syncope Hyperventilation (unlikely) | Postural hypotension | Drug administration Seizures Hypoglycemia or hyperglycemia Cardiovascular causes |

the supine position does not always help the patient regain consciousness because the primary causative factor is not related to a deficit in cerebral blood flow. Definitive management is required in all such cases.

Patients suffering from postural hypotension do not experience syncopal episodes in the supine position; however, signs and symptoms of hypotension develop rapidly when they assume a more upright position and reverse just as rapidly when they are returned to the supine position. Hyperventilation only rarely progresses to the loss of consciousness—and then only when the patient remains untreated in the upright position for an extended period. More commonly, hyperventilation produces a state of mental confusion, often characterized as lightheadedness and dizziness (Table 9-3).

# Presyncopal Signs and Symptoms

## NO CLINICAL SYMPTOMS

Rapid loss of consciousness without prodromal symptoms leads to a presumptive diagnosis of postural hypotension if the episode occurs immediately after a change in the patient's position (supine to upright). Certain drugs used in dentistry can increase the likelihood of postural hypotension (see Box 7-1). In addition, syncope secondary to cardiac dysrhythmias and heart block is usually of sudden onset and may occur without warning signs or symptoms. It may develop when the patient is either sitting or standing. On rare occasions, cardiac arrest may lead to a patient's unconsciousness without prodromal signs and symptoms (instantaneous death); diagnosis of this situation will be established during implementation of the steps of basic life support.

## PALLOR AND COLD, CLAMMY SKIN

Restlessness, pallor (loss of normal skin color), clammy (moist) skin, nausea, and vomiting are classic warning signs of fainting. They usually are present in cases of vasodepressor syncope; however, individuals experiencing hypoglycemic reactions, adrenal insufficiency, and myocardial infarction also may exhibit these signs.

## TINGLING AND NUMBNESS OF THE EXTREMITIES

Hyperventilation, although it rarely leads to syncope, may do so if the patient remains untreated and seated upright for an extended period during the episode. Hyperventilation is recognized readily through alterations in the rate (increased) and depth (increased) of breathing as well as by the clinical symptoms of tingling and numbness of the fingers, toes, and perioral areas.

## HEADACHE

Many patients develop an intense headache at the outset of a cerebrovascular accident, especially of the hemorrhagic type.

## CHEST PAIN

Chest pain or discomfort may precede the loss of consciousness in cases of angina pectoris (in which unconsciousness rarely occurs), myocardial infarction (in which cardiac arrest and loss of consciousness are more likely), or hyperventilation (rarely).

## BREATH ODOR

The smell of alcohol on the dental patient's breath is not uncommon; alcohol is probably the most frequently self-administered drug among patients trying to reduce dental stress. The presence of alcohol on the breath should prompt the doctor to evaluate the patient for dental fears and anxieties; the doctor also should exercise caution in the use of drugs known to produce further central nervous system depression, including local anesthetics.

Unconsciousness under such situations may be due to psychogenic factors or to profound central nervous system depression produced by one drug or a combination of various drugs. In addition, the sweet, fruity odor of acetone is noticeable on the breath of patients who are hyperglycemic and ketoacidotic. In most instances, these patients will be known (medical history) type I, insulin-dependent diabetics.

## TONIC-CLONIC MOVEMENTS AND INCONTINENCE

All individuals who lose consciousness may exhibit tonic-clonic movements of the upper and lower extremities. This is especially likely to occur in patients who are maintained in an upright position during the period of unconsciousness. Seizure-like movements in such situations are due to decreased cerebral perfusion. Inadequate airway management, regardless of the patient's position, also produces tonic-clonic movements secondary to cerebral hypoxia (or anoxia).

Although tonic-clonic movements can occur during vasodepressor syncope, they occur only rarely if proper positioning and airway management are provided. Patients with hypoglycemia also may exhibit tonic-clonic movements; in this situation, the movements are secondary to inadequacies in cerebral blood glucose levels. Seizures caused by nonepileptic factors are usually mild and are rarely associated with sphincter-muscle relaxation. However, a diagnosis of epilepsy is strongly suggested in most cases of seizure activity in which the patient exhibits urinary or fecal incontinence and tongue biting.

## HEART RATE AND BLOOD PRESSURE

In most instances of unconsciousness the heart rate rises above its baseline level while the blood pressure decreases. For example, the blood pressure may be quite low during a hypoglycemic or hyperglycemic reaction while the heart, attempting to compensate for the decrease in blood pressure, accelerates its rate of contraction. However, vasodepressor syncope, postural hypotension, and cerebrovascular accident are exceptions to these changes in vital signs.

In vasodepressor syncope both the blood pressure and the heart rate usually decrease. A heart rate of 50 beats per minute or less is common during the syncopal phase of vasodepressor syncope. The heart rate during postural hypotension remains at approximately the baseline level, although the blood pressure drops precipitously. The pulse, as monitored in the radial, brachial, or carotid artery, is usually described as weak or thready in persons whose blood pressures are low. On the other hand, the blood pressure in the case of a hemorrhagic cerebrovascular accident may be elevated significantly (systolic pressure elevated more than diastolic pressure) and the pulse strong, or bounding.

In cases of clinically significant dysrhythmias, the heart rate may be variable (bradycardic, tachycardic, or baseline), but the functional output of the heart decreases to a level at which it adversely affects peripheral perfusion. The blood pressure is almost always depressed in such situations (Table 9-4).

## DURATION OF UNCONSCIOUSNESS AND RECOVERY

The response or lack of response of the patient to the basic steps (**P-A-B-C** [position-airway-breathing-circulation]) of management can provide a wealth of significant diagnostic information. Unconsciousness produced by vasodepressor syncope is usually reversed within a few seconds once the patient is placed in the supine position (Table 9-5). In the recovery period the patient does not return to a normal state rapidly. More frequently, signs and symptoms of shivering, sweating, headache, and fatigue are present.

Patients who suffer postural hypotension normally regain consciousness rapidly after assuming the supine position. Recovery from postural hypotension is more complete and rapid than recovery from vasodepressor syncope; residual signs and symptoms are absent or less intense.

Syncope secondary to cardiac dysrhythmias also reverses quickly following correction of the underlying rhythm disturbance; the patient usually is alert on recovery. The duration of syncope is related to the duration of the dysrhythmia.

table **9-4** *Vital signs during unconsciousness*

| CAUSES OF UNCONSCIOUSNESS | HEART RATE | BLOOD PRESSURE |
|---|---|---|
| Hypoglycemia or hyperglycemia | Increases | Decreases |
| Vasodepressor syncope | Decreases | Decreases |
| Postural hypotension | Baseline | Decreases |
| Cerebrovascular accident (hemorrhagic) | Variable | Increases |
| Clinically significant dysrhythmias | Variable | Decreases |

table **9-5** *Duration of syncope with basic life support*

| SHORT | PROLONGED |
|---|---|
| Postural hypotension | Hypoglycemia |
| Vasodepressor syncope | Hyperglycemia |
| Cardiac dysrhythmias | Adrenal insufficiency |
| | Cardiac dysrhythmias |

Syncope produced through a mechanism other than a lack of adequate cerebral blood flow is not readily reversed with changes. Epileptic patients' seizures usually terminate after a few moments; however, these patients may remain somnolent and often develop intense headaches during recovery. Significant tonic-clonic seizure activity does not usually occur during vasodepressor syncope or postural hypotension, although this may occur in isolated instances.

Basic life support alone will not reverse unconsciousness secondary to alterations in the blood's composition, such as that after drug administration, hypoglycemia, hyperglycemia, or adrenal insufficiency (see Table 9-5). Although proper implementation of these steps is absolutely critical to the patient's survival, definitive management involving specific drug therapy is necessary in each case for the patient to regain consciousness. (These situations will be described in detail in subsequent chapters.)

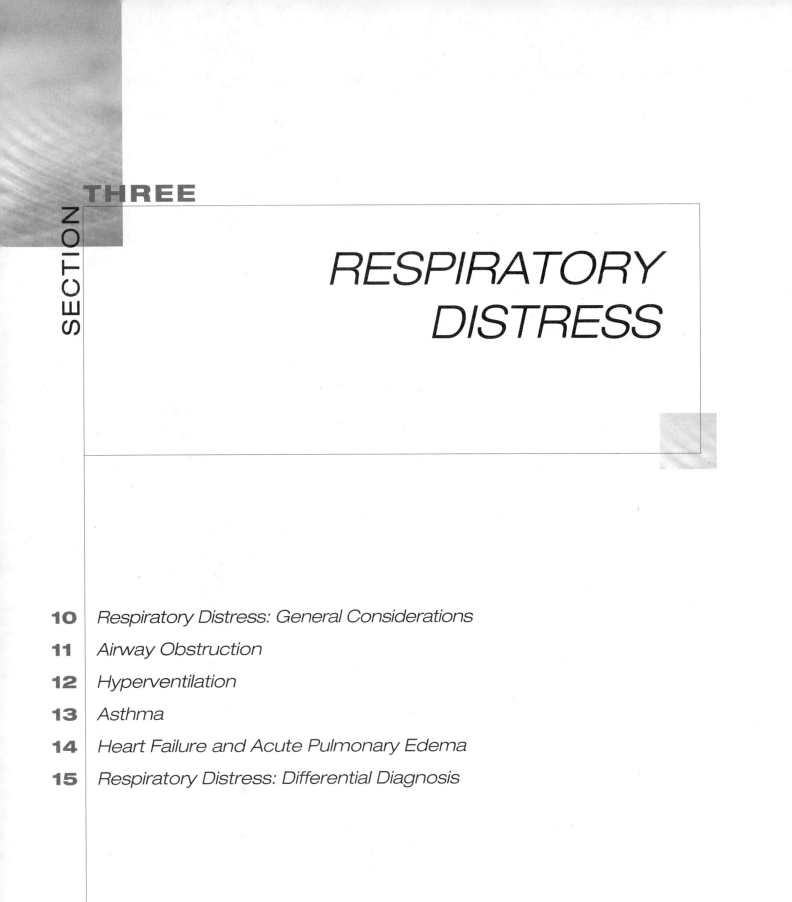

SECTION

**THREE**

*RESPIRATORY
DISTRESS*

# 10

# Respiratory Distress

## General Considerations

**B**REATHING difficulty can be very disconcerting to a conscious patient. This section focuses on several of the more common causes of respiratory distress, including hyperventilation, asthma (bronchospasm), and pulmonary edema. Because the patient in respiratory distress usually remains conscious throughout the episode, this section also discusses the extremely important psychologic aspects of patient management. Box 10-1 lists some terms and definitions relevant to cases of respiratory distress.[1]

In almost all medical emergencies involving the loss of consciousness, some degree of airway obstruction is present. The primary cause of airway obstruction is mechanical; the tongue falls into the hypopharynx as skeletal muscle tone is lost. Two steps of basic life support—**A** (airway) and **B** (breathing)—are designed to eliminate this problem. (Chapter 11 will expand on the management of airway obstruction.)

## Predisposing Factors

Table 10-1 lists potential causes of acute respiratory distress. In most of these situations the patient does not exhibit respiratory distress unless an underlying medical disorder becomes acutely exacerbated; acute myocardial infarction, anaphylaxis, cerebrovascular accident, hyperglycemia, and hypoglycemia are examples.

Awareness of any medical disorders the patient suffers helps in the modification of treatment to prevent

169

or minimize the risk that the underlying condition will be exacerbated. However, there are situations, asthma and heart failure, in which the patient suffers from chronic respiratory problems. Patients with these disorders may experience difficulty breathing at all times, particularly those with heart failure. In such cases the doctor's role in preventing the worsening of these disorders during dental treatment becomes vitally important.

A major factor that can exacerbate respiratory disorders is undue stress, either physiologic or psychologic. Indeed hyperventilation and vasodepressor syncope—the most frequently encountered emergency situations in dentistry—are almost exclusively manifestations of psychologic stress. Psychologic stress associated with dental treatment is the primary factor in the exacerbation of preexisting medical problems. Although respiratory distress in pediatric patients rarely is attributable to hyperventilation or vasodepressor syncope, children with asthma may exhibit acute episodes of bronchospasm when they are faced with stressful situations such as dental treatment.

## Prevention

Adequate pretreatment medical and dental evaluations often can prevent the development of some respiratory problems. If the doctor is aware of existing medical disorders that may result in respiratory distress, modifications in patient management can minimize the risk that these conditions may worsen. For example, when dental anxiety is a major factor, psychosedative procedures and other stress-reduction techniques should be considered.

## Clinical Manifestations

Clinical manifestations of respiratory distress vary according to the degree of breathing difficulty present. In most cases the patient remains conscious through-

---

### box 10-1 Terms related to respiratory distress

**anoxia** Absence of oxygen ($O_2$)

**apnea** Absence of respiratory movement

**dyspnea** A subjective sense of shortness of breath; a difficulty in breathing often referred to as "air hunger"

**hyperpnea** Greater-than-normal, per-minute ventilation that just meets metabolic demands

**hyperventilation** Ventilation that exceeds metabolic demands; $PaCO_2$ less than 35 torr

**hypoventilation** Ventilation that does not meet metabolic demands; $PaCO_2$ more than 45 torr

**hypoxia** Deficiency of $O_2$ in inspired air

**orthopnea** Inability to breathe except in the upright position

**$PaCO_2$** Arterial carbon dioxide tension (normal being 35 to 45 torr)

**$PaO_2$** Arterial $O_2$ tension (normal [air] being 75 to 100 torr)

**respiration** Process of gas exchange whereby the body gains $O_2$ and loses carbon dioxide

**tachypnea** Greater-than-normal respiratory rate

**torr** Unit of pressure equal to 1 mmHg (named for Torricelli)

**ventilation, alveolar** Volume of air exchanged per minute

$$\frac{\text{Volume}}{\text{Breath}} - \text{Dead space} \times \text{Respiratory rate}$$

---

### table 10-1 Potential causes of respiratory distress

| CAUSE | FREQUENCY | TEXT DISCUSSION |
| --- | --- | --- |
| Hyperventilation | Most common | Respiratory distress (Section Three) |
| Vasodepressor syncope | Most common | Unconsciousness (Section Two) |
| Asthma | Common | Respiratory distress (Section Three) |
| Heart failure | Common | Respiratory distress (Section Three |
| Hypoglycemia | Common | Altered consciousness (Section Four) |
| Overdose reaction | Less common | Drug-related emergencies (Section Six) |
| Acute myocardial infarction | Rare | Chest pain (Section Seven) |
| Anaphylaxis | Rare | Allergy (Chapter 24) |
| Angioneurotic edema | Rare | Allergy (Chapter 24) |
| Cerebrovascular accident | Rare | Altered consciousness (Section Four) |
| Epilepsy | Rare | Seizures (Chapter 21) |
| Hyperglycemic reaction | Rare | Altered consciousness (Section Four) |

out the acute episode. Although retention of consciousness is a positive sign, indicating that the patient is receiving at least the minimum amount of blood and $O_2$ required for normal cerebral function, it does create an additional problem—acute anxiety. For this reason the doctor managing the situation must appear calm and in control of the situation at all times.

The clinical symptomatology of distressed breathing and the sounds associated with it depend on the cause of the problem. Asthmatics often exhibit characteristic wheezing sounds produced by turbulent airflow through partially occluded bronchioles. Individuals suffering heart failure often cough and produce other sounds associated with pulmonary venous congestion. (A more detailed discussion and a differential diagnosis will be discussed in later chapters.)

## Pathophysiology

The syndromes responsible for respiratory distress involve various parts of the respiratory system. Bronchioles are the primary site of asthma. In asthmatic patients the bronchi become highly reactive, demonstrating significant smooth muscle reactivity (bronchospasm) in response to various stimuli. Clinical signs and symptoms exhibited during an acute asthmatic attack are related in large part to the restricted exchange of $O_2$ and carbon dioxide in the lungs.

Patients with heart failure usually report respiratory distress as one of their first symptoms. The chronic inability of the lungs to adequately oxygenate venous blood and the accompanying overuse of the $O_2$ already present in the blood that is available to tissues produces respiratory distress during heart failure. This type of respiratory distress is related to an engorgement of the pulmonary veins with fluid exuding into alveolar air sacs. This excess fluid prevents portions of the lung from participating in ventilation (removal of carbon dioxide and absorption of $O_2$), which produces many of the signs and symptoms associated with heart failure.

Hyperventilation is a more generalized problem. The primary site of this disorder is in the mind (brain) of the patient, and its clinical signs and symptoms are produced by an alteration in the chemical composition of the blood. The rapid breathing associated with hyperventilation results in the elimination of an excessive amount of carbon dioxide, leading to the development of respiratory alkalosis. This condition in turn produces many of the clinical signs and symptoms that hyperventilating patients exhibit. Successfully managed hyperventilation pro-

duces no residual effects. However, heart failure and asthma, which are chronic disorders, may induce permanent changes in the respiratory system.[2,3] Therefore patients who are at risk for acute exacerbations of asthma (bronchospasm) or heart failure (pulmonary edema) usually require special management considerations during all phases of dental treatment.

Acute lower-airway obstruction is a life-threatening situation in which a foreign object becomes impacted in the respiratory tract. The level at which the airway is occluded determines the severity of the situation and to some degree the manner in which it is managed. If an object enters either the right or left main-stem bronchus, the resulting situation is critical but not immediately life threatening. The foreign body most often enters the right main-stem bronchus because of the angle at which this bronchus branches off the trachea.[4] In this situation all or part of the right lung is excluded from ventilation, but the patient still maintains adequate ventilation with the left lung. The patient requires hospitalization, but the condition usually is not acutely life threatening.

In contrast, if the foreign object becomes impacted in the trachea, total airway obstruction ensues—an acutely life-threatening situation.[5] Immediate recognition and management are essential to prevent permanent neurologic damage or death. (The management of acute airway obstruction will be discussed more fully in Chapter 11.) Figure 10-1 illustrates the sites of origin of the various respiratory disorders.

## Management

Definitive management of respiratory distress depends on the doctor's prompt recognition of the problem and a determination of its probable cause (Box 10-2). This chapter focuses on the basic steps common to the management of most cases of respiratory distress.

*Step 1: recognition of respiratory distress.* Many respiratory disorders are associated with characteristic sounds, such as the wheezing of bronchospasm and the cough and moist respirations (rales) of pulmonary edema. In contrast, hyperventilation usually does not produce a characteristic sound; however, hyperventilating patients appear—and actually are—acutely anxious and unable to control their breathing.

*Step 2: termination of the dental procedure.* Dental treatment should cease as soon as respiratory distress is recognized. Because stress is a primary pre-

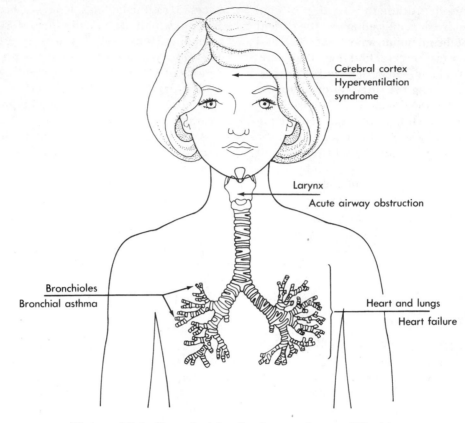

Cerebral cortex
Hyperventilation
syndrome

Larynx
Acute airway obstruction

Bronchioles
Bronchial asthma

Heart and lungs
Heart failure

**Figure 10-1**  Sites of origin of various respiratory difficulties.

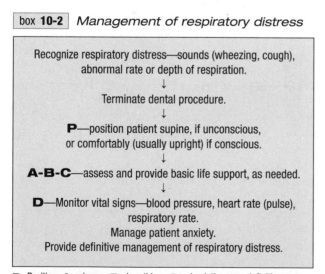

box **10-2**    *Management of respiratory distress*

Recognize respiratory distress—sounds (wheezing, cough),
abnormal rate or depth of respiration.
↓
Terminate dental procedure.
↓
**P**—position patient supine, if unconscious,
or comfortably (usually upright) if conscious.
↓
**A-B-C**—assess and provide basic life support, as needed.
↓
**D**—Monitor vital signs—blood pressure, heart rate (pulse),
respiratory rate.
Manage patient anxiety.
Provide definitive management of respiratory distress.

**P,** Position; **A,** airway; **B,** breathing; **C,** circulation; **D,** definitive care.

cipitating factor in most respiratory-related situations, the cessation of treatment may improve the patient's clinical signs and symptoms significantly.

*Step 3:* **P** *(position) the patient.* In conscious patients experiencing respiratory distress, positioning is based on the comfort of the patient. In the presence of a near-normal or slightly elevated blood pressure (as is almost always the case in situations of respiratory distress), most patients feel more in control of their breathing in an upright (sitting or standing) position. However, patients can be maintained in these positions only as long as they remain conscious.

*Step 4:* **A-B-C** *(airway-breathing-circulation), basic life support, as needed.* Patients in respiratory distress often experience two major problems—the primary breathing difficulty initially induced by their fear of dentistry and the added problem of increased anxiety produced by their inability to breathe normally. In the unlikely event that respiratory distress leads to unconsciousness, the patient must be placed immediately into the supine position and the steps in the management of unconsciousness followed.

*Step 5:* **D** *(definitive care).* Response of the victim to the steps of basic life support determines additional management.

*Step 5a: monitoring of vital signs.* The individual's blood pressure, heart rate (pulse), and respiratory rate should be measured at frequent intervals (every 5 minutes, if possible) throughout the episode and recorded in a permanent record.

*Step 5b: definitive management of anxiety.* The doctor should keep the patient in respiratory distress as comfortable as possible and begin to manage the anxiety by speaking calmly but firmly to the patient. The patient's collar or other tight garments also should be loosened, enabling the patient to breathe easier (even if the "ease" in breathing is psychologic).

*Step 5c: definitive management of respiratory distress.* After assessing the patient's cardiovascular status, the doctor may begin to manage the cause of the patient's breathing problem. (The following chapters will focus in large part on such management procedures and on the most common causes of respiratory distress.)

## REFERENCES

1. Anderson KN, editor: *Mosby's medical, nursing, & allied health dictionary,* ed 5, St Louis, 1998, Mosby.
2. Apstein CS, Lorell BH: The physiological basis of left ventricular diastolic dysfunction, *J Card Surg* 3(4):475-485, 1988.
3. Djukanovic R and others: Mucosal inflammation in asthma, *Am Rev Respir Dis* 142(2):434-457, 1990.
4. Bhatia PL: Problems in the management of aspirated foreign bodies, *West Afr J Med* 10(2):158-167, 1991.
5. Heimlich HJ, Patrick EA: The Heimlich maneuver: best technique for saving any choking victim's life, *Postgrad Med* 87(6):38-48, 53, 1990.

# 11

# *Airway Obstruction*

**B**ECAUSE of its frequently sudden and critical nature, acute obstruction of the airway must be recognized and managed as quickly as possible. For this reason an immediate diagnosis of complete or partial airway obstruction must be made and treatment initiated as quickly as possible.

During dental treatment the potential is great that objects may fall into the posterior portion of the oral cavity and subsequently into the pharynx. Indeed a variety of devices and objects are recovered from the throats of patients each year.[1] I am aware of the recovery of the head of a pedodontic handpiece, mouth mirror heads, and gold crowns—either orally or from stool specimens—after they had been swallowed accidentally. Published reports have documented the retrieval of rubber dam clamps, endodontic instruments, a post and core, and a crucifix.[1-4]

In the conscious dental patient the chances are excellent that any object lost in the pharynx will be swallowed by the patient and enter into the esophagus or will be retrieved after being coughed up, so that the actual incidence of acute airway obstruction or aspiration into the trachea and lung is quite low. A high probability also exists that any object that enters into the airway is small enough in diameter to pass through the larynx (the narrowest portion of the upper airway) without causing an obstruction. In this situation the object usually continues through the trachea (if gravity assists) and comes to rest in a portion of one of the main-stem bronchi or smaller bronchioles in the lung.

While an acutely life-threatening situation does not exist at the time, certain important steps must be performed immediately to ensure the removal of the object within a reasonable period to avoid serious consequences. However, the possibility that a foreign object may lodge in the larynx and obstruct the trachea does exist; thus all dental office personnel must become familiar with proper management of acute upper-airway obstruction.

The National Safety Council estimated that approximately 3100 individuals in the United States died as a result of acute airway obstruction in 1984.[5] More than 90% of deaths from foreign body aspiration in the pediatric age-group occur in children younger than 5 years; 65% of those deaths are infants.[6] Commonly aspirated items include hot dogs, rounded candies, nuts, grapes, coins, toys, and other hard, colorful objects.[7,8] Baby aspirin, with a diameter of 7.5 mm, has obstructed airways and caused subsequent deaths in several young children.[9] (The diameter of the glottic opening is about 6.5 mm in a 2-year-old.[10])

After evaluating newer clinical research findings, the American Heart Association implemented changes in the recommended techniques for the management of obstructed airway in infants, children, and adults.[6] This chapter outlines such techniques.

In most cases the object causing the acute airway obstruction is lodged firmly in the airway where it can neither be seen nor felt through the mouth without the use of special equipment, such as a laryngoscope or a pair of Magill forceps, items that are not normally available. The doctor therefore must be able to recognize the problem instantly and act rapidly to dislodge the object.

# Prevention

In spite of the best efforts at prevention, small objects, such as inlays, alloy, burs, or pieces of debris, may fall into the oropharynx of a patient who may subsequently swallow or aspirate them. The introduction of sit-down dentistry, in which the patient is placed in a semisupine or supine position during treatment, has increased the possibility that such an accident may occur.

When objects are swallowed, they usually enter the gastrointestinal (GI) tract. During the act of swallowing, the epiglottis seals the tracheal opening so that liquid and solid materials do not enter the trachea. The esophagus is the most likely site in the GI tract for objects to become obstructed because of the nature of the esophagus—a collapsed tube through which liquids and solids are forced (Figure 11-1).[11] More than 90% of swallowed foreign objects that suc-

cessfully pass through the esophagus into the stomach and intestines pass completely through the GI tract without complications.[12]

However, complications are associated with both swallowed and aspirated objects. Swallowed objects entering the GI tract have produced GI blockage, peritoneal abscess, perforation, and peritonitis.[13] Objects aspirated into either the right or left mainstem bronchus can produce infection, lung abscess, pneumonia, and atelectasis.[14] In a discussion of prevention of aspiration, Barkmeier[15] urged the use of two major preventive measures—rubber dam and oral packing. These measures can minimize significantly the occurrence of swallowed foreign objects. Other preventive measures include patient positioning, the dental assistant, suction, Magill intubation forceps, and ligature (Box 11-1).

## RUBBER DAM

Rubber dam effectively isolates the operative field from the oral cavity and airway and prevents the swallowing of objects (Figure 11-2). The use of rubber dams is recommended in all possible situations. Unfortunately, use of the rubber dam during many dental procedures, such as periodontics and surgery, is not feasible.

## ORAL PACKING

A pharyngeal curtain, created by the spreading of 3-inch by 3-inch gauze pads across the posterior portion of the oral cavity, effectively prevents small particles or liquids from entering the airway (Figure 11-3). The pharyngeal curtain is especially useful for patients who are receiving intramuscular or intravenous sedation or general anesthesia for whom protective airway reflexes may be compromised. The nonsedated patient does not normally tolerate oral packing because it may interfere with swallowing or restrict the volume of air that can be inhaled through the mouth.

box **11-1**  *Instruments and techniques used to prevent aspiration and swallowing of objects*

Rubber dam
Oral packing
Chair position
Dental assistant
Suction
Magill intubation forceps
Ligature

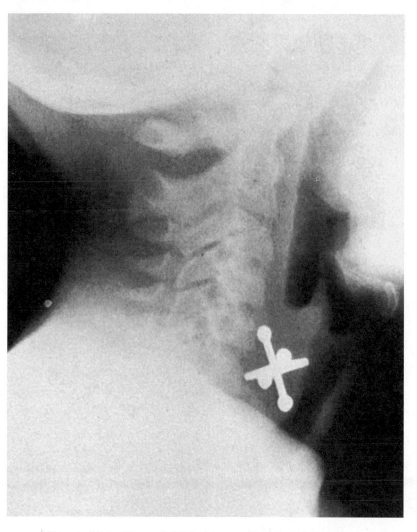

**Figure 11-1**    X-ray of child with metal jack in the esophagus.

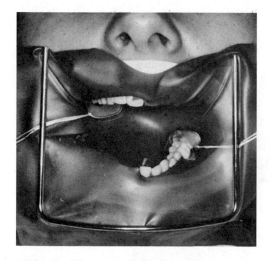

**Figure 11-2**    The use of rubber dam helps prevent foreign objects from entering the airway. (From Chasteen J: *Four-handed dentistry in clinical practice,* ed 3, St Louis, 1984, Mosby.)

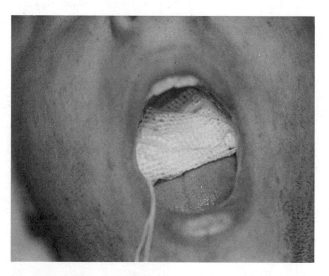

**Figure 11-3**    A pharyngeal curtain, created by the spreading 3-inch by 3-inch gauze pads across the posterior portion of the oral cavity effectively prevents small particles or liquids from entering the airway.

## CHAIR POSITION

The supine position, which serves to prevent the development of syncope, becomes detrimental to the patient who must use the body of the tongue when a foreign object is being held tenuously by the body of the tongue against the roof of the mouth. Gravity acts to force the object posteriorly into the pharynx. If equipment is not readily available to aid in the retrieval of the object, the patient should be turned onto the side and leaned into a head-down position

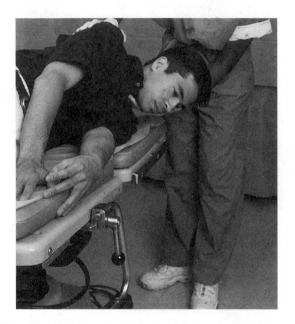

**Figure 11-4** The patient should turn to the side and bend into a head-down position with the upper body over the side of the dental chair in cases of a swallowed object.

with the upper body over the side of the dental chair (Figure 11-4). This position uses gravity to the patient's advantage, allowing the object to fall from the patient's mouth.

## DENTAL ASSISTANT AND SUCTION

A dental assistant is seated across from the doctor in most situations. When an object becomes free and is in danger of being swallowed, the assistant has available one or more devices to aid in its immediate retrieval. If such a device is not readily available, a high-volume, large-diameter suction tip may be used to remove the object from the patient's mouth. A trap on the suction line allows for quick retrieval of the object.

Saliva ejectors are not always beneficial in the removal of objects because the force of the suction is not great enough to permit removal of the object. When it is present, a Magill intubation forceps allows the assistant to retrieve objects easily from the posterior part of the oral cavity.

## MAGILL INTUBATION FORCEPS

The Magill intubation forceps (Figure 11-5), which is included in the basic emergency kit, is designed to permit retrieval of large and small objects from the distal regions of the oral cavity and pharynx (Figure 11-6). The right-angled bend in the Magill forceps permits a comfortable hand position for the user while the blunt-ended beaks permit easy grasping of the object. No other device, including pick-up forceps (cotton pliers) or hemostats, are designed for this purpose (Figure 11-7).

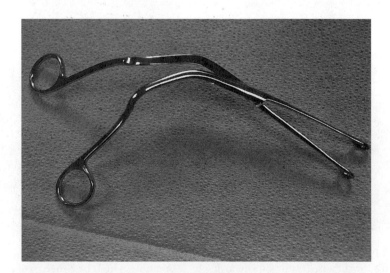

**Figure 11-5** Magill intubation forceps should be included in the office emergency kit.

## LIGATURE

The use of ligature or dental floss can aid in both the prevention or loss of objects and their retrieval from the distal regions of the oral cavity and pharynx. Dental floss should be secured to rubber dam clamps, endodontic instruments, cotton rolls, gauze pads, around pontics in fixed bridges, or to other small objects placed in the oral cavity during dental treatment (Figures 11-8 and 11-9). The presence of dental floss lessens the possibility that a patient may swallow an object or inadvertently leave the dental office with a cotton roll remaining in the buccal fold.

## Management

When an object enters the oropharynx of a patient seated in the supine or semisupine position, do not allow the patient to sit up. The chair should be moved into a more reclined position (for example, into the Trendelenburg position,* if possible) while the assistant picks up the Magill intubation forceps. Placing the patient into the Trendelenburg position may allow gravity to move the object closer to the oral cavity where it may become more visible and easier to retrieve with the Magill intubation forceps (Box 11-2).

If the object is irretrievable (that is, if the patient swallows it), radiographs are warranted to determine its location; the patient should not leave the office before these radiographs are obtained. Because clinical signs and symptoms do not always indicate whether the object has entered the GI or respiratory tract, the doctor must escort the patient (if possible)

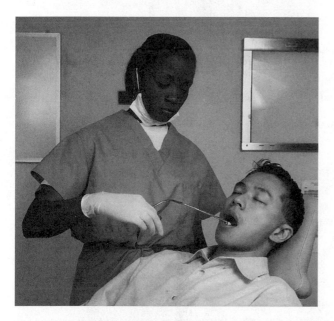

**Figure 11-6**  Proper use of the Magill intubation forceps.

---

*The Trendelenburg position is a position in which the patient's head is placed low and the body and legs are placed on an elevated or inclined plane.

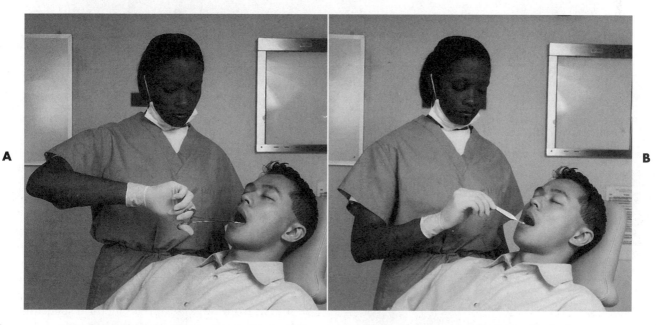

**Figure 11-7**  Hemostats and cotton pliers are not designed for easy use in the retrieval of objects.

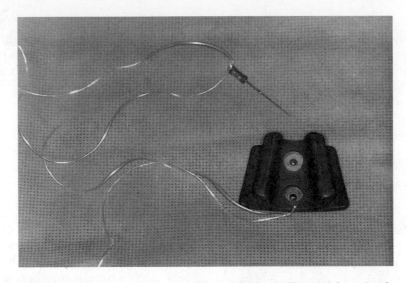

**Figure 11-8**  Dental floss is tied to an object to allow quick retrieval.

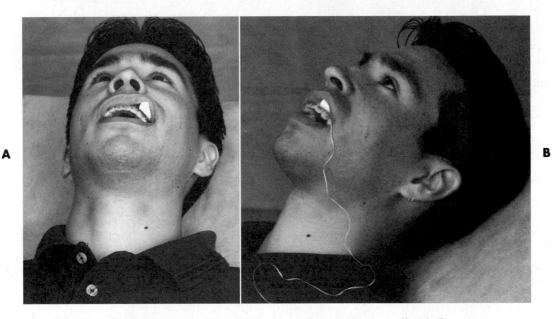

**Figure 11-9**  **A,** Cotton roll without floss. **B,** Cotton roll with floss.

box **11-2**  *Management of visible objects*

**If assistant is present:**
Place patient in supine or Trendelenburg position.
↓
Use Magill intubation forceps or suction.

**If assistant is not present:**
Instruct patient to bend over arm of chair with head down.
↓
Encourage patient to cough.

to the emergency department of a local hospital or to a radiology laboratory. In most instances the radiologist recommends (1) a flat plate of the abdomen, and/or (2) an anteroposterior view of the chest (Figure 11-10), or (3) a lateral view of the chest.

It is hoped that if the object is found, it will be seen on the abdominal radiograph rather than on the chest radiographs within, for example, a bronchus. In any situation in which a foreign object is located within either the GI or respiratory tracts, assistance must be sought from the appropriate medical specialty—gastroenterology, pulmonology, or anesthesiology. Further management of the situation will usually be

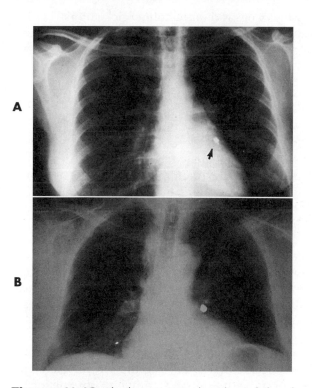

**Figure 11-10** **A,** Anteroposterior view of the chest demonstrating a rubber prophylaxis cup *(arrow).* **B,** Gold crown that was aspirated into the left lung of the patient.

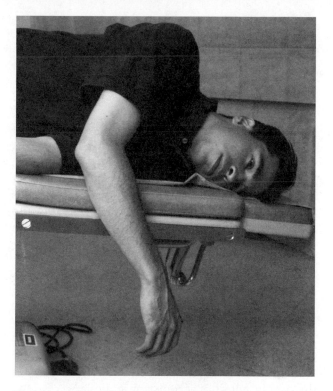

**Figure 11-11** The patient should be placed in the left lateral decubitus position with the head down when an object enters the trachea.

---

box **11-3**  *Management of swallowed objects*

Consult radiologist.
↓
Obtain appropriate radiographs to determine location of object.
↓
Initiate medical consultation with appropriate specialist.

---

directed by the physician. If the object's location is not apparent in the radiograph or if any question exists as to its location or any potential complications, immediate medical consultation is warranted (Box 11-3).

Usually, the signs and symptoms that the patient exhibits help determine whether an object has entered into the trachea. Signs and symptoms include the sudden onset of coughing, choking, wheezing, and shortness of breath. More than 90% of patients who aspirate exhibit these signs and symptoms within 1 hour of aspiration. A few patients may experience a time lag as long as 6 hours before symptoms become evident.[16] Depending on the seriousness of the episode, immediate apnea may follow in

as many as one third of these patients. These symptoms may progress to cyanosis and other signs of serious hypoxemia.[17]

In situations in which a foreign body presumably enters the trachea, a well-defined protocol should be followed, beginning with ensuring that the patient does not sit up, an action that may propel the object deeper into the trachea or bronchi. The patient should be placed into the left lateral decubitus position with the head down (Figure 11-11). The patient may cough spontaneously; if not, coughing should be encouraged to aid in retrieval of the object. The normal cough reflex is powerful and in many cases may be adequate to remove the aspirated object.

Should the patient cease coughing and state that the object has been swallowed, that patient should not be permitted to leave the office until a physician or radiographer can locate the object to ensure that it is not located in the lungs. Only if the object is recovered should the patient be discharged before a radiograph has been obtained.

In addition, before the patient leaves the office, medical consultation should be sought from an appropriate specialist (for example, a pulmonologist) to discuss the prevention, recognition, and management of postaspiration complications. If the object is not recovered, the doctor should accompany the patient to the emergency department of an acute-care facility for definitive diagnosis and management (Box 11-4).

If it is determined that the object is in the tracheobronchial tree, the most common location is in the right bronchus. Compared with the left bronchus, the right main-stem bronchus takes a more direct path at the bifurcation of the trachea. The right main bronchus branches off the trachea at a 25-degree angle, whereas the left main bronchus branches off at a 45-degree angle. Retrieval of the object from the bronchus may involve the use of a fiberoptic bronchoscope to locate (visualize) the object and bronchoscopy to retrieve it. If bronchoscopy is unsuccessful (a rare occurrence), a surgical procedure known as *thoracotomy* may be necessary.

An immediate life-threatening emergency does not exist in the situations just described. However, the patient should not be allowed to leave the office unless the aspirated object is retrieved. Additional medical management will be necessary to prevent the development of serious consequences.

## RECOGNITION OF AIRWAY OBSTRUCTION

Acute upper-airway obstruction in the conscious patient occurs most often while the patient is eating. In adults, meat is the most common cause of obstruction.[18] Several common factors are identified in cases of the so-called cafe coronary syndrome, including (1) large, poorly chewed pieces of food; (2) elevated blood-alcohol levels; (3) laughing or talking while eating; and (4) upper or lower dentures.[18] A higher incidence of cafe coronaries is noted in patients re-

---

box **11-4**    *Management of aspirated objects*

Place patient in left lateral decubitus position.
↓
Encourage patient to cough.
↓                    ↓
Object is retrieved.    Object is not retrieved.
↓                    ↓
Initiate medical        Consult with radiologist or emergency
consultation before     department. Obtain appropriate radio-
discharge.              graphs to determine location of object.
                       ↓
                       Perform bronchoscopy to visualize and
                       retrieve object.

---

ceiving drugs with anticholinergic actions.[19] Other causes of airway obstruction include the following:

- Congenital structural abnormalities of the airway[20]
- Infections, such as acute epiglottitis[21,22]
- Tonsillitis[23-25]
- Retropharyngeal abscesses[26]
- Ludwig's angina[27] and laryngitis[7]
- Trauma[28]
- Tumors and hematomas[29,30]
- Vocal cord pathologic processes, including laryngospasm and paralysis
- Inflammatory processes, such as angioneurotic edema and anaphylaxis,[7] ingestion of corrosives and toxins,[23] and thermal burns[31]
- Sleep apnea[7]

Airway obstruction is divided into complete and partial obstruction. For management purposes, partial obstruction is subdivided into two categories—good air exchange or poor air exchange.

**Complete airway obstruction**    Researchers have documented in the dog the physiologic events that occur with asphyxia (complete obstruction).[32] Several phases of physiologic changes are noted before death occurs as a result of acute airway obstruction. Initially, sympathetic outflow increases markedly, resulting in increased blood pressure, heart rate, and respiratory rate. As a result of the increased work of breathing, $PaO_2$ (arterial oxygen [$O_2$] tension) decreases, $PaCO_2$ (arterial carbon dioxide [$CO_2$] tension) increases, and pH falls. At 3 to 4 minutes, blood pressure and heart rate drop precipitously and respiratory efforts diminish. Blood gases deteriorate even further. At 8 to 10 minutes, vital signs disappear as the electrocardiogram degenerates from a sinus to a nodal bradycardia, then to idioventricular rhythms; the electrocardiogram then terminates in ventricular fibrillation or asystole.[32]

If the obstruction can be relieved within the initial 4 to 5 minutes, all monitored parameters usually return to normal quickly along with a return of consciousness. However, humans, especially medically compromised humans, do not appear to tolerate asphyxia as well as the dog model described in the aforementioned findings. Dailey[33] divided the clinical features of acute upper-airway obstruction in humans into three phases (Table 11-1).

The first 3 minutes of obstruction comprise the first phase. The patient is conscious but obviously in distress and demonstrates struggling paradoxical respirations and increased blood pressure and heart rate. The patient often grasps the throat in the so-called choking sign (Figure 11-12). Although respiratory movements are evident, no air is exchanged and no voice sounds produced. Supraclavicular and intercostal retraction is evident, breath sounds are absent in the chest, and the patient becomes cyanotic.

| table **11-1** | *Assessment of complete upper-airway obstruction* |

| PHASE | SIGNS AND SYMPTOMS |
|---|---|
| First phase (1-3 min) | Conscious; universal choking sign; struggling paradoxical respirations without air movement or voice; increased blood pressure and pulse |
| Second phase (2-5 min) | Loss of consciousness; decreased respiration, blood pressure, and pulse |
| Third phase (>4-5 min) | Coma; absent vital signs; dilated pupils |

Modified from Dailey RH: Acute upper airway obstruction, *Emerg Med Clin North Am* 1:261, 1983.

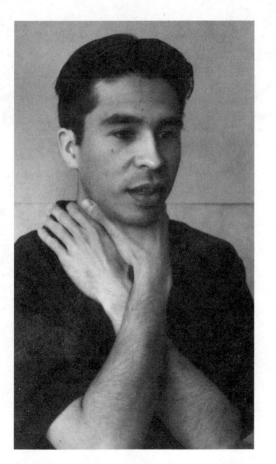

**Figure 11-12**  The victim clutches the neck, demonstrating the recommended universal distress signal for an obstructed airway.

Minutes 2 through 5 comprise the second phase. The victim loses consciousness, and respiratory efforts cease. Initially, blood pressure and pulse are present.

Phase three begins at more than 4 or 5 minutes. After a short period the blood pressure and pulse disappear as electromechanical dissociation leads to full cardiac arrest (Box 11-5).

**Partial airway obstruction**  A forceful cough often may be elicited from a victim with good air exchange. Wheezing may be noted between coughs. The victim with partial obstruction and good air exchange should be allowed to continue coughing and to breathe without any physical intervention by rescuers.[5]

Those with poor air exchange exhibit weak, ineffectual cough reflexes and a characteristic "crowing" sound during inspiration. The degree of paradoxical respiration is related to the degree of airway obstruction. Voice sounds may be absent or altered because the vocal cords cannot appose normally. The inspiratory phase of breathing is markedly prolonged. Patients with poor air exchange exhibit cyanosis, lethargy, and disorientation if severe hypoxia and hypercarbia are present; these victims must be treated as though their airways were completely obstructed (Box 11-6).[5]

| box **11-5** | *Signs of complete airway obstruction* |

Inability to speak
Inability to breathe
Inability to cough
Universal sign for choking
Panic

| box **11-6** | *Signs of partial airway obstruction* |

**Individuals with good air flow:**
Forceful cough
Wheezing between coughs
Ability to breathe

**Individuals with poor air exchange:**
Weak, ineffectual cough
"Crowing" sound on inspiration
Paradoxical respiration
Absent or altered voice sounds
Possible cyanosis
Possible lethargy
Possible disorientation

## BASIC AIRWAY MANEUVERS

Once the patient with an obstructed airway loses consciousness, basic life support, including airway maintenance, must be initiated promptly (see Chapter 5). These steps are designed to eliminate the most common cause of airway obstruction—the tongue. Performance of these steps permits the rescuer to determine whether the tongue is the cause of the airway problem and whether additional steps of airway management are required. In those instances in which a lower-airway obstruction is obvious (for example, an obstruction that develops immediately after the individual swallows a crown or dental instrument), the basic steps of life support are bypassed and the rescuer immediately proceeds to establish an emergency airway.

*Step 1:* **P** *(position).* The patient should be placed in the supine position with the feet elevated slightly (Figure 11-13).

*Step 2: head tilt–chin lift.* Extension of the patient's neck tissues is achieved through the head tilt–chin lift technique (Figure 11-14). In 80% of instances in which the tongue is the cause of the airway obstruction, this procedure effectively opens the airway.[34]

*Step 3:* **A + B.** The rescuer's ear is placed 1 inch from the victim's mouth and nose; the rescuer listens and feels for the passage of air while looking toward the victim's chest and watching for spontaneous respiratory movement (Figure 11-15).

*Step 4: jaw-thrust maneuver, if indicated.* The rescuer places the fingers behind the posterior border of the ramus of the victim's mandible and anteriorly displaces the mandible while tilting the victim's head backward and opening the mouth (Figure 11-16).

Dislocation of the mandible is a painful procedure. Therefore the jaw-thrust maneuver gives the rescuer a sense of the depth of the victim's unconsciousness. If the patient does not respond to this maneuver, the level of unconsciousness is fairly deep, whereas if the victim does respond (for example, by grimacing, phonating, or moving), the level of unconsciousness is not as deep.

*Step 5:* **A + B.** Step 3 (look, listen, and feel) should be repeated, if necessary.

*Step 6: artificial ventilation, if indicated.* When the tongue is the cause of airway obstruction, performance of the previous steps will usually reestablish the airway. When these steps are performed properly but the airway remains obstructed (diagnosed by aphonia,

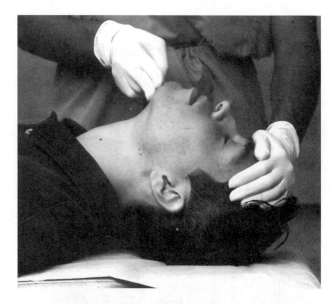

**Figure 11-14**   The head tilt–chin lift technique.

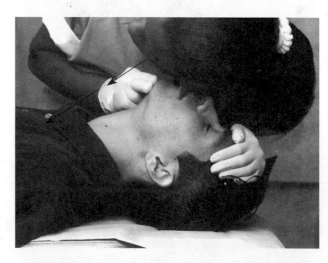

**Figure 11-15**   The "look, listen, feel" technique.

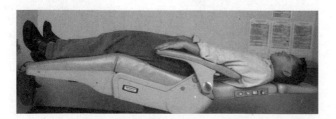

**Figure 11-13**   The patient who loses consciousness should be placed in the supine position with the feet slightly elevated.

and suprasternal retraction, and continued absence of "hearing and seeing"), the rescuer should consider the possibility that the obstruction is located within the larynx or trachea and proceed immediately to establish an emergency airway.

## ESTABLISHMENT OF AN EMERGENCY AIRWAY

When a patient's airway is obstructed, establishment of a patent airway becomes the immediate goal of treatment. A variety of procedures, some controver-

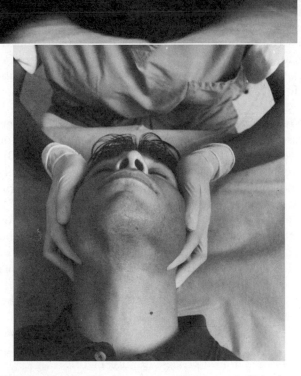

**Figure 11-16**  The jaw-thrust maneuver: **A,** Side view. **B,** Front view. Mandible is displaced anteriorly (arrows).

sial, exist to accomplish this goal. Two procedures-tracheostomy[35-37] and cricothyrotomy[38-40]—require surgical intervention and thus considerable knowledge and technical skill to be carried out effectively. A third procedure, which is nonsurgical, is the procedure of choice for the initial management of all obstructed airways when basic life support techniques prove inadequate. This is the external subdiaphragmatic compression technique, known as the *abdominal thrust,* or the *Heimlich maneuver.* [41-47] Because this procedure is nonsurgical, serious complications are, though possible, less likely to occur, which makes the maneuver particularly attractive for use in the dental office.[48,49] The American Heart Association and American Red Cross recommend the abdominal thrust when lower-airway obstruction is a possibility,[6] a situation responsible for 3100 deaths in 1984.[5]

### Noninvasive procedures

When foreign objects enter the tracheobronchial tree, a potentially life-threatening situation exists. Airway obstruction may be either partial or complete. Management of the situation varies according to the degree of obstruction present and the effectiveness of the patient's cough reflex. Manual, noninvasive procedures are used whenever possible. Surgical procedures, used as a last resort, are also within the doctor's expertise. (These techniques will be described later in the chapter.)

A victim of a partial airway obstruction who is capable of forceful coughing and is breathing adequately (that is, with no evidence of cyanosis or duskiness) should be left alone. Although wheezing may be evident between coughs, a forceful cough is highly effective in removing foreign objects. This victim should be left alone. If the victim of partial airway obstruction initially demonstrates poor air exchange or if previously good air exchange becomes ineffective, the victim must be managed as if the airway were completely obstructed.

Victims of complete airway obstructions are unable to speak or make any sounds, to breathe, or to cough. The victim remains conscious as long as the cerebral $O_2$ level of the blood is sufficiently high. Such victims may remain conscious from 10 seconds to 2 minutes, depending on whether the obstruction occurred during inspiration (when the blood has more $O_2$) or expiration (when the blood has less $O_2$). Fortunately, most airway obstruction occurs during inhalation; in this way the lungs are inflated and filled with $O_2$, and the patient can remain conscious longer. The victim also may clutch the neck (see Figure 11-12), demonstrating the universal choking sign. Prompt management is critical because the victim will lose consciousness and die unless a patent airway is reestablished immediately.

Several manual, noninvasive procedures are available for use in acute airway obstruction. Each technique will be described, followed by the recommended sequencing of these techniques in actual situations. The techniques are as follows:

- Back blows
- Manual thrust
- Heimlich maneuver (abdominal thrust)
- Chest thrust
- Finger sweep

**Back blows**  Back blows have formed an integral part of previous regimens for the removal of foreign objects from the airway.[50] However, data presented at the 1985 National Conference on Cardiopulmonary Resuscitation and Emergency Cardiac Care suggested that back blows used as the sole method of treatment may not be as effective in adults as the Heimlich maneuver.[43] For this reason the Heimlich maneuver now is the only technique recommended in the management of an obstructed airway in adults or children.

However, back blows still remain an integral part of the protocol for obstructed-airway management in the infant. When back blows are performed on the infant, the infant is straddled over the rescuer's arm with the head lower than the trunk and with the head supported by the rescuer's firm hold on the infant's jaw. Using the heel of the hand, the rescuer delivers four back blows forcefully between the infant's shoulder blades while resting the other hand on the thigh (Figure 11-17).

**Manual thrusts**  Manual thrusts consist of a series of 6 to 10 thrusts to the upper abdomen

(Heimlich maneuver or abdominal thrust) or to the lower chest (chest thrust). They produce a rapid increase in intrathoracic pressure, acting as an artificial cough that can help dislodge a foreign body. The objective of each single thrust should be to relieve the obstruction without having to complete the full series. Studies have demonstrated that no significant differences exist between abdominal and chest thrusts in the amount of air flow, pressure, and volume.[51,52]

Special situations do exist in which one technique is preferable. The chest thrust is recommended for patients in advanced stages of pregnancy and for those who are markedly obese. The chest thrust also is less likely to cause regurgitation than the abdominal thrust. In addition, chest thrusts are recommended for infants because abdominal thrusts are more likely to cause organ damage (for example, to the liver or spleen). The Heimlich maneuver is recommended especially for older patients, whose more brittle ribs are more likely to be fractured in the chest thrust, and for children.

Internal injuries are always possible whenever an abdominal or chest thrust is used. Injuries to the thoracic and abdominal organs, including the liver, spleen, and stomach, have been documented.[48,49] Proper hand placement can minimize these potential side effects. The rescuer must never place the hands over the xiphoid process or the lower margins of the rib cage. In the Heimlich maneuver the rescuer places the hands below this area, whereas in chest thrusts the hands are placed above it.

After successful application of any manual thrust technique to relieve acute airway obstruction, medical or paramedical personnel should evaluate the patient for evidence of secondary injury, such as abdominal bleeding, before discharging the patient.

**Heimlich maneuver**  The Heimlich maneuver, also known as the *subdiaphragmatic abdominal thrust* or *abdominal thrust,* was first described in 1975 by Dr. Henry J. Heimlich.[41] Today this maneuver is the recommended primary technique for relief of foreign-body airway obstruction in adults and children.[6]

If the patient is conscious and either standing or sitting, the following recommended steps should be performed:

1. Stand behind the victim and wrap your arms around the waist and under the arms.
2. Grasp one fist with the other hand, placing the thumb side of the fist against the victim's abdomen. The hand should rest in the midline, slightly above the umbilicus and well below the tip of the xiphoid process (Figure 11-18).
3. Perform repeated inward and upward thrusts until either the foreign body is expelled or the victim loses consciousness (Figure 11-19).

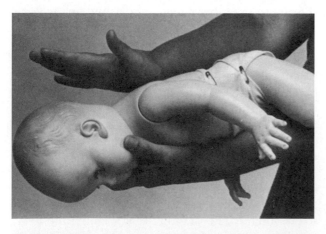

**Figure 11-17**  The rescuer uses the heel of hand to deliver four blows forcefully between the shoulder blades of an infant.

The successfully treated victim should be evaluated for the possibility of complications before dismissal from the office.

If the victim is unconscious, however, the following protocol should be performed:

1. Place the victim in the supine position.
2. Open the victim's airway using the head tilt–chin lift technique and turn the head up into the so-called neutral position. The head is turned into the neutral position to avoid airway obstruction, facilitate foreign body movement up the airway, and allow the foreign body to be visualized.
3. Whenever possible, the rescuer should straddle the victim's legs or thighs (Figure 11-20). Unfortunately, this position is virtually impossible to achieve when the patient is in the dental chair. An alternative to the straddle position places the rescuer alongside the victim. The rescuer's knees rest close to the victim's hips on either the right or left side (Figure 11-21). This position is useful when the victim is in the dental chair (Figure 11-22).
4. Place the heel of one hand against the victim's abdomen, in the midline slightly above the umbilicus and well below the tip of the xiphoid process.
5. Place the second hand directly on top of the first hand.

6. Press into the victim's abdomen with a quick inward and upward thrust. (Do not direct the force laterally.)
7. Perform up to five abdominal thrusts.
8. Open the victim's mouth and perform the finger sweep.

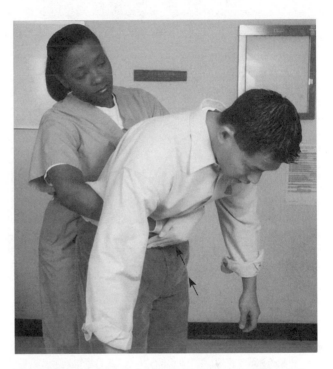

**Figure 11-19**  An abdominal thrust in a conscious victim.

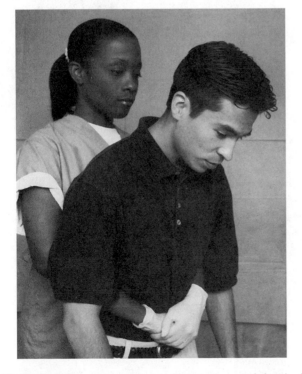

**Figure 11-18**  The proper technique for an abdominal thrust.

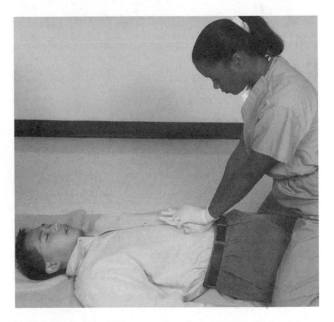

**Figure 11-20**  When performing the Heimlich maneuver on the floor, the rescuer should straddle the victim's legs.

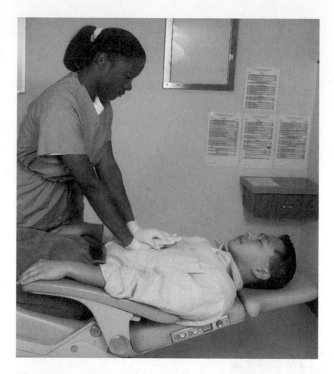

**Figure 11-21** As an alternative to the straddle position during an abdominal thrust, the rescuer may stand astride the victim in the dental chair. The victim's head should be in the neutral position.

9. Repeat steps 2 through 8 until the obstruction is dislodged.

When properly performed, the Heimlich maneuver is exclusively a soft tissue procedure. No bony structures, such as the ribs or sternum, are involved. In all cases the rescuer must apply pressure with the heel of the hand below the rib cage. The maneuver is not a bear hug; if it is performed this way, intraabdominal organs, such as the liver and spleen or to the sternum and ribs, could occur. After successful completion of the procedure, the appropriate team member should summon emergency personnel to evaluate the patient before discharge from the office.

**Chest thrust** The chest thrust is an alternative—in special situations only—to the Heimlich maneuver as a technique for opening an obstructed airway. There is no substantial difference in the effectiveness of these techniques when performed properly. Table 11-2 lists the indications and contraindications for the chest thrust.

If the victim is conscious and either standing or sitting, the following steps should be performed:
1. Stand behind the victim and place the arms directly under the armpits, encircling the chest (Figure 11-23).

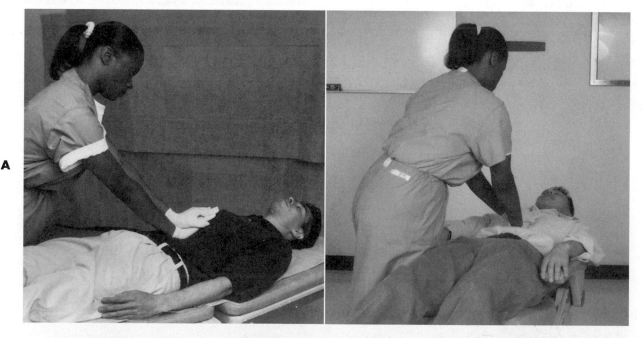

A    B

**Figure 11-22** **A,** The rescuer performs an abdominal thrust while astride the victim, who is in the dental chair. **B,** The force of the compression must be in an upward, not a lateral, direction. The victim's head remains in the neutral position.

2. Grasp one fist with the other hand, placing the thumb side of the fist on the middle of the sternum, not on the xiphoid process or the margins of the rib cage.

3. Perform backward thrusts until the foreign body is expelled or the victim loses consciousness.

If the victim is unconscious, the following steps should be performed:

1. Place the victim in the supine position.

2. Using the head tilt–chin lift maneuver, open the victim's airway and place the head into the neutral position.

3. Either straddle or stand astride the victim, as described in the Heimlich maneuver.

4. Place the heel of one hand on the lower half of the sternum with the second hand on top of it, but not on the xiphoid process (Figure 11-24). (The hand position and technique for chest thrust are identi-

cal to those of closed-chest cardiac compression [see Chapter 30]).

5. Perform up to five quick, downward thrusts to compress the chest cavity.

6. Open the victim's mouth and perform the finger sweep.

**Finger sweep**   In the conscious victim it is quite difficult for the rescuer to remove foreign bodies from the airway with the fingers. When the victim loses consciousness, muscles relax and it is considerably easier to open the victim's mouth to seek and remove foreign objects with the fingers. The rescuer must observe special care when probing an infant's or small child's airway with a finger, so as not to inadvertently force the foreign body deeper into the airway. Therefore blind finger sweeps are not recommended in the infant and child. The rescuer may, however, remove foreign bodies from the airway by this technique if the object is located above the level of the epiglottis. Finger sweeps should be performed in unconscious victims only.

A Magill intubation forceps is an integral part of

| table **11-2** | *Chest thrust* |
|---|---|
| **INDICATIONS** | **CONTRAINDICATIONS** |
| Infant (<1 year) Pregnant victim Extremely obese victim | Older victim |

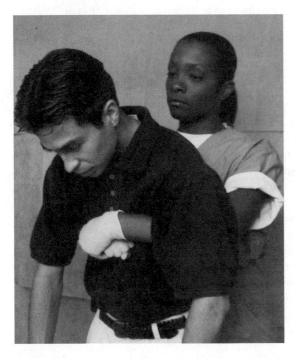

**Figure 11-23**   A chest thrust on a conscious victim.

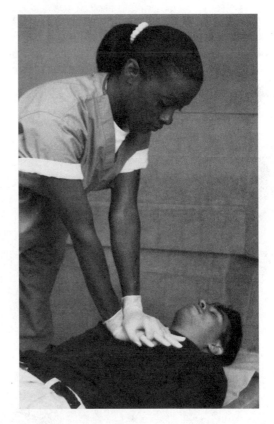

**Figure 11-24**   A chest thrust on an unconscious victim.

the dental office emergency kit (Figure 11-25). This instrument can aid in the removal of foreign objects from the airway. However, use of the Magill intubation forceps should be limited to situations in which the object is visible to the rescuer.

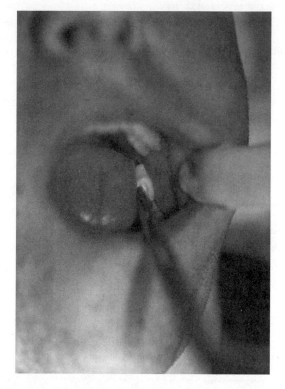

**Figure 11-25**    Clinical use of a Magill intubation forceps.

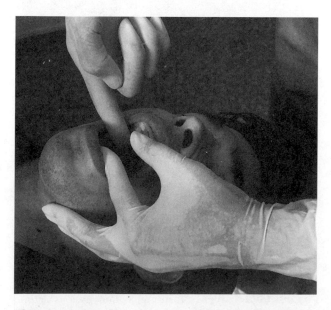

**Figure 11-26**    Use of the crossed-finger technique aids in opening the unconscious victim's mouth.

The finger sweep is performed as follows:
1. Place the victim in the supine position with the head in the neutral position.
2. Grasp the tongue and the anterior portion of the mandible. This technique is called the *tongue-jaw lift;* it pulls the tongue off the posterior wall of the pharynx, away from a foreign object that may be lodged there.

If the tongue-jaw lift is ineffective, the rescuer should use the crossed-finger technique (Figure 11-26). Open the victim's mouth by crossing the index finger and thumb between the teeth and forcing the teeth apart.

3. To perform the finger sweep, place the index finger of the other hand along the inside of the victim's cheek and advance it deeply into the pharynx at the base of the tongue. Using a hooking movement, try to dislodge the foreign body and move it into the mouth, where either suction or the Magill intubation forceps can remove it. Take care not to force the object more deeply into the airway.

Box 11-7 outlines the American Heart Association's recommended sequence for the removal of airway obstruction.[6]

## Procedures for obstructed airways in infants and children

Airway obstruction in children 1 to 8 years should be managed similar to adults—use of the Heimlich maneuver as the primary technique. However, the combination of back blows and chest thrusts is still the recommended protocol for the infant under 1 year. Box 11-8 reviews the basic rescue procedures for infants and children.

The rescuer should repeat the sequences presented in this chapter for an infant or a child with an upper-airway obstruction until the foreign matter is successfully removed or until the rescuer judges that time has been exhausted. At this time a cricothyrotomy should be considered seriously if the rescuer possesses the proper knowledge and training and has the necessary equipment available.

## Invasive procedures: tracheostomy versus cricothyrotomy

The previously described noninvasive techniques are highly successful in the removal of foreign objects from the airways of most victims. However, situations develop in which these noninvasive techniques prove ineffective (for example, in the removal of a dental cotton roll from a victim's airway). In this situation and in others, in which the airway is obstructed by the swelling of tissues such as laryngeal edema or epiglottis caused by allergy or illness, invasive procedures may be required if the victim is to survive.

| box 11-7 | *Recommended sequences for removing airway obstruction* |

---

### For adult conscious victim with obstructed airway

Identify complete airway obstruction: Ask, "Are you choking?"
↓
Identify yourself as someone who will help the victim: Say, "I can help you."
↓
Apply the Heimlich maneuver until foreign body is expelled or the victim becomes unconscious.
↓
Have medical or paramedical personnel evaluate patient for complications before dismissal.

### For adult conscious victim with known obstructed airway, who loses consciousness

Place victim in supine position with head in neutral position; call for help.
↓
Activate the EMS system (i.e., call 9-1-1) if a second person is available.
↓
Open the victim's mouth using tongue-jaw lift.
↓
Perform finger sweep.
↓
Attempt to ventilate the patient; if ineffective.
↓
Perform six to ten abdominal thrusts.
↓
Check for foreign body with finger sweep.
↓
Attempt to ventilate the patient; if ineffective:
↓

### For adult conscious victim with known obstructed airway, who loses consciousness—cont'd

Repeat abdominal thrusts, finger sweeps, and attempted ventilations until effective.
↓
Have medical or paramedical personnel evaluate patient for complications before dismissal.

### For adult unconscious victim, cause unknown

Rescuer manages unconscious victim in usual manner: Assess unresponsiveness.
↓
**P**—Position victim in supine position with feet elevated.
↓
Call for help (office emergency team).
↓
**A**—Open airway (head tilt-chin lift).
↓
**B**—Assess breathing (look, listen, feel), and
↓
Attempt to ventilate. If unsuccessful,
↓
Reposition head and attempt to ventilate; if still unsuccessful,
↓
Activate EMS system (call 9-1-1) and
↓
Perform Heimlich maneuver: six to ten abdominal thrusts.
↓
Perform foreign body check: finger sweep.
↓
Attempt to ventilate; if ineffective,
↓
Repeat Heimlich maneuver, finger sweeps, and ventilation, until successful.

---

Surgical opening of the airway may be performed in several ways. Two of the most commonly used are tracheostomy[35-37] and cricothyrotomy.[38-40] Each technique has its advocates and its critics within the medical community, but each is equally important for they ensure that the victim's lungs receive $O_2$. Invasive procedures should be performed only by persons trained in the techniques and only when proper equipment is available.

Tracheostomy has been performed for more than 2000 years, yet its role in the management of acute airway obstruction has undergone change in recent decades.[53] Tracheostomy once was considered the primary technique for the relief of acute airway obstruction. For a variety of reasons, cricothyrotomy is now considered by many to be the surgical procedure of choice for sudden airway obstruction.[39,54] In the typical dental setting almost no indications exist for the use of tracheostomy.

Tracheostomy is a surgical procedure currently used most often for long-term airway management and—with a few exceptions, such as direct laryngeal fracture[55] and emergency airway management of infants—is not well suited for emergency airway management. The tracheostomy site contains numerous important anatomic structures, such as the isthmus of the thyroid gland and several large and important blood vessels and nerves.[56] The potential also exists for accidental perforation of the esophagus.

Complications occur more commonly with tracheostomy even when it is performed slowly and meticulously under controlled conditions, such as in

box **11-8**    *Rescue procedures for infants and children*

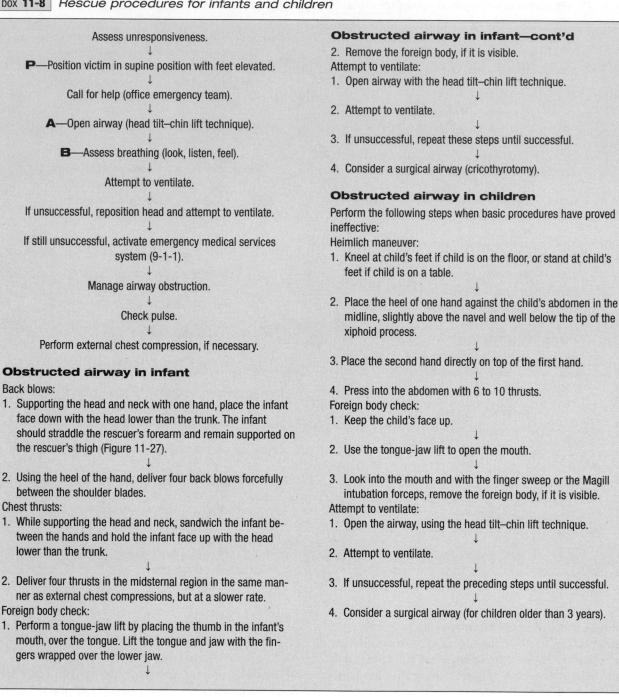

Assess unresponsiveness.
↓
**P**—Position victim in supine position with feet elevated.
↓
Call for help (office emergency team).
↓
**A**—Open airway (head tilt–chin lift technique).
↓
**B**—Assess breathing (look, listen, feel).
↓
Attempt to ventilate.
↓
If unsuccessful, reposition head and attempt to ventilate.
↓
If still unsuccessful, activate emergency medical services system (9-1-1).
↓
Manage airway obstruction.
↓
Check pulse.
↓
Perform external chest compression, if necessary.

**Obstructed airway in infant**
Back blows:
1. Supporting the head and neck with one hand, place the infant face down with the head lower than the trunk. The infant should straddle the rescuer's forearm and remain supported on the rescuer's thigh (Figure 11-27).
↓
2. Using the heel of the hand, deliver four back blows forcefully between the shoulder blades.
Chest thrusts:
1. While supporting the head and neck, sandwich the infant between the hands and hold the infant face up with the head lower than the trunk.
↓
2. Deliver four thrusts in the midsternal region in the same manner as external chest compressions, but at a slower rate.
Foreign body check:
1. Perform a tongue-jaw lift by placing the thumb in the infant's mouth, over the tongue. Lift the tongue and jaw with the fingers wrapped over the lower jaw.
↓

**Obstructed airway in infant—cont'd**
2. Remove the foreign body, if it is visible.
Attempt to ventilate:
1. Open airway with the head tilt–chin lift technique.
↓
2. Attempt to ventilate.
↓
3. If unsuccessful, repeat these steps until successful.
↓
4. Consider a surgical airway (cricothyrotomy).

**Obstructed airway in children**
Perform the following steps when basic procedures have proved ineffective:
Heimlich maneuver:
1. Kneel at child's feet if child is on the floor, or stand at child's feet if child is on a table.
↓
2. Place the heel of one hand against the child's abdomen in the midline, slightly above the navel and well below the tip of the xiphoid process.
↓
3. Place the second hand directly on top of the first hand.
↓
4. Press into the abdomen with 6 to 10 thrusts.
Foreign body check:
1. Keep the child's face up.
↓
2. Use the tongue-jaw lift to open the mouth.
↓
3. Look into the mouth and with the finger sweep or the Magill intubation forceps, remove the foreign body, if it is visible.
Attempt to ventilate:
1. Open the airway, using the head tilt–chin lift technique.
↓
2. Attempt to ventilate.
↓
3. If unsuccessful, repeat the preceding steps until successful.
↓
4. Consider a surgical airway (for children older than 3 years).

an oxygenated, well-ventilated patient in an operating theater, than occur with cricothyrotomy.[55] Hemorrhage and pneumothorax are major complications of tracheostomy. In addition, there is a risk of accidental penetration of the isthmus of the thyroid gland.[57] In most cases the bleeding that occurs with tracheostomy is a major surgical complication that the dental office may not be equipped to handle satisfactorily.

Cricothyroid membrane puncture (cricothyrotomy) involves establishment of an opening in the airway at the level of the cricothyroid membrane and is accepted as a means of emergency airway access. Cricothyrotomy is easier and quicker than tracheostomy, and the incidence of complications is significantly lower.[54] In addition, no significant anatomic structures are found near the cricothyroid membrane.

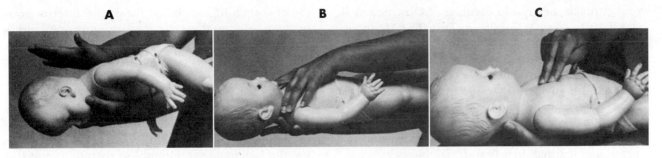

**Figure 11-27** Technique for an infant with an obstructed airway. **A,** The infant should be supported by the rescuer's forearm with the head lower than the rest of the body for performance of back blows. **B,** The infant is turned over, supported by the rescuer's arms. **C,** Using two fingers, the rescuer applies chest thrusts to the victim's.

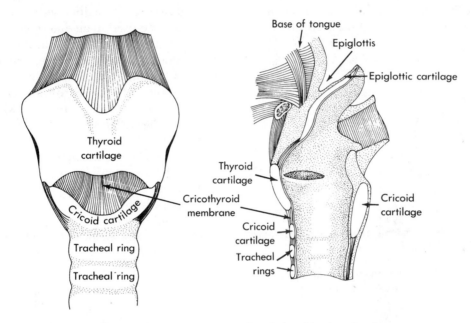

**Figure 11-28** Important anatomic relationships in cricothyrotomy.

Cricothyrotomy has been said to provide the most accessible point of entry into the respiratory tree inferior to the glottis.[58] The incision is made through skin, adipose tissue, and fascia. Aside from minor bleeding from the skin incision, major blood loss is seldom associated with cricothyrotomy. Because the cricoid cartilage has an intact posterior segment, inadvertent perforation of the posterior wall of the trachea and laceration of the underlying esophagus are not risks (Figure 11-28). An incision into the cricothyroid membrane begins to heal within a few days of removal of the airway.

The ability to rapidly locate the proper site for cricothyrotomy is important. The rationale behind any emergency surgical airway procedure is that the opening being made must lie below the obstruction in order for the procedure to be effective. Thus a vital consideration is where the foreign material is most likely to affect the trachea.

**Anatomy**    The narrowest portion of the adult trachea is located at the larynx. Most objects capable of producing obstruction come to rest in this area. Objects small enough to pass through the larynx and enter into the trachea usually pass into one of the main-stem bronchi (usually the right), creating an occlusion of one lung or a significant portion of the lung. As discussed previously, this is not an acute threat to the victim's life, although the victim may require hospitalization and surgery to remove the foreign object.

The narrowest portion of the trachea in children under 3 to 5 years occurs a short distance below the vocal cords at the cricoid cartilage.[59] Obstruction is most likely to occur at this site, making the cricothyrotomy ineffective. Thus tracheostomy is the preferred emergency surgical airway procedure in this age group, but only individuals experienced in performing the procedure on infants and children should attempt it.[59] (Immediate management of this situation in other clinical circumstances requires nonsurgical methods, such as inverting the infant and application of manual thrusts and back blows.)

The thyroid cartilage, the largest of the tracheal cartilages, and the cricoid cartilage (the second tracheal cartilage) represent the anatomic landmarks for cricothyrotomy (Figure 11-29). The thyroid and cricoid are the only two tracheal cartilages that are complete rings; the other tracheal "rings" being open on their posterior aspects. A membranous structure,

the cricothyroid membrane forms the anterior connection between these two cartilaginous rings and is the precise site for cricothyrotomy. The membrane is approximately 10 mm high and 22 mm wide.[60] It may be readily located by placing a finger on the laryngeal prominence (Adam's apple) of the thyroid cartilage and moving the finger inferiorly until reaching a slight depression. The cricothyroid membrane is approximately one to one-half of a finger breadth below the laryngeal prominence in the midline of the neck.[38] The prominence of the cricoid cartilage is inferior to this depression. The cricoid cartilage lies inferior to the incision site, whereas the thyroid cartilage and vocal cords lie superior to it.

**Equipment**    A scalpel with a straight (no. 11) blade may be used in an emergency cricothyrotomy for both the skin incision and the membrane incision. Alternatively, a 13-gauge, 12-inch needle may be used. In addition, many devices exist to aid in the performance of cricothyrotomy. One such device, the Nu-Trake,* contains the following sterile components (Figure 11-30):

- A knife blade
- A puncturing mechanism—a two-part needle with a needle stylet
- An arcuate point at one end of the stylet (facilitates initial penetration of the cricothyroid membrane)
- Several airways of 4-, 6-, and 8-mm diameters
- Obturators for the airways

---

*Nu-Trake is manufactured by International Medical Devices, 19205 Parthenia, Northridge, Calif. 91324.

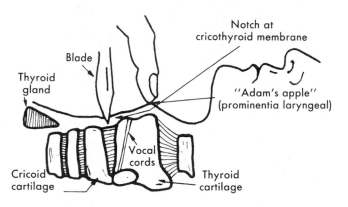

**Figure 11-29**  During cricothyrotomy, an incision is made inferior to the thyroid cartilage and superior to cricoid cartilage.

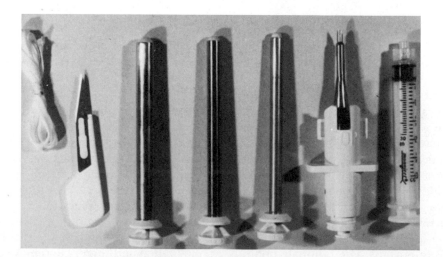

**Figure 11-30**    From left, a cricothyrotomy device contains a cord to secure the airway, a knife blade, various airways in different sizes (3), a puncturing mechanism, and a syringe.

Although any of these instruments and devices, when used properly, is effective in creating an emergency airway, only those devices with which the doctor is intimately familiar should be included in the office emergency kit.

### Use of a scalpel

*Step 1: preparation of the neck.* If enough time exists (which it usually does not), the patient's neck should be prepared surgically. However, in emergency situations, antiseptic may be poured over the neck before the incision is made.

The patient's neck should be hyperextended (head tilt) to allow easy identification of the thyroid and cricoid cartilages and cricothyroid membrane. A roll of towels or other material placed under the neck may aid hyperextension.

*Step 2: identification of landmarks.* The right-handed operator should stand on the patient's right side so that the left hand can immobilize the larynx and help identify landmarks while the right hand is used to perform the cricothyrotomy. In clinical practice the right hand often is used initially to identify landmarks, after which the index finger of the left hand should be placed on the cricothyroid membrane.

*Step 3: immobilization of the larynx.* Walls[38] wrote that the importance of this step cannot be overstated. The larynx must be immobilized so that the landmarks are not lost during the actual procedure. Immobilization of the larynx is easy to accomplish; it must be done before the incision is made

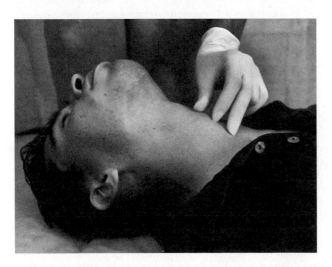

**Figure 11-31**   To stabilize the larynx, the thumb and middle finger stabilize the cartilage while the index finger rests in the cricothyroid membrane.

and maintained until the airway is obtained successfully. The right-handed operator uses the thumb and middle finger of the left hand to grasp the upper poles of the thyroid cartilage, allowing the index finger of the left hand to rest on the membrane (Figure 11-31). Once the larynx is immobilized, the index finger of the left hand can be used again to palpate the thyroid cartilage, membrane, and cricoid cartilage.

*Step 4: incision of the skin.* The skin incision must be vertical and in the midline; it should be approximately 2 to 3 cm long. The vertical incision minimizes the possibility of significant vascular problems during the procedure,[61] whereas a horizontal incision is more likely to result in bleeding. The vertical incision should be made to the depth of the thyroid cartilage, membrane, and cricoid cartilage. Minor bleeding as a result of the skin incision may result and can be ignored. The establishment of a patent airway is the primary concern; once this task is accomplished, any bleeding can be managed.

*Step 5: reidentification of the membrane.* The index finger of the left hand should be reinserted into the incision to reidentify the membrane, then the finger quickly moved up to the thyroid and down to the cricoid cartilages to ensure proper identification of the cricothyroid membrane. The fingertip may remain in the incision, but should rest on the most inferior border of the thyroid cartilage to provide a point of reference without interfering with the incision into the membrane.

*Step 6: incision of the membrane.* The incision into the membrane should be horizontal, using the no. 11 scalpel blade in the lower third of the cricothyroid space. This area is the least vascular part of the membrane. The horizontal incision in the midline should be at least 1.5 cm long to facilitate airway placement.

Upon entry into the airway, bubbling is visible. The scalpel should be withdrawn and the index finger of the left hand reinserted into the cricothyroid space to identify the incision and verify its correct placement. This finger is again moved to the inferior portion of the thyroid cartilage as a guide in airway insertion.

*Step 7: dilation of the incision.* At this point the cricothyroid space should be enlarged. The handle of the scalpel should be inserted into the horizontal incision and rotated 90 degrees to open the airway (Figure 11-32).

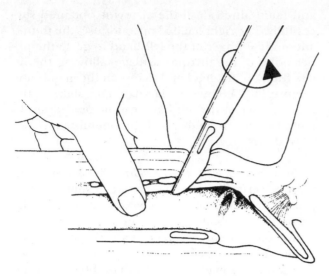

**Figure 11-32** The handle of the scalpel is inserted into the incision and rotated 90 degrees to enlarge the airway opening.

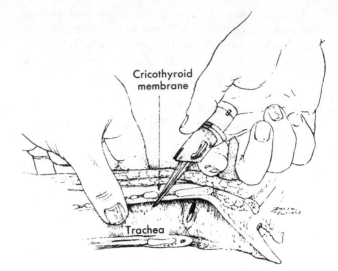

**Figure 11-33** The needle and housing unit are inserted into the cricothyroid membrane with a downward thrust toward the chest.

*Step 8: insertion of the tube.* A cricothyroid or tracheotomy tube may be inserted temporarily, if one is available.

A properly performed cricothyrotomy can be completed in 15 to 30 seconds. Anesthesia is unecessary because the patient is unconscious and thus unable to react to the stimulus of the scalpel incision.

NOTE: The patient may suffer a coughing episode once the trachea is entered.

## Use of a 13-gauge needle for cricothyrotomy

When a 13-gauge, 12-inch needle is used, the tissue is prepared and the thyroid cartilage stabilized the same as with the scalpel, using the index finger to identify the cricothyroid membrane. The needle is inserted through this area and directed toward the chest until it enters the tracheal lumen. Entry into the trachea is confirmed by the sound and feel of air entering and leaving, coughing, and bubbling of fluids. The cartilaginous posterior wall of the cricoid cartilage helps prevent overinsertion of the needle and perforation of the tracheoesophageal wall.

## Use of a cricothyrotomy device

After the 2- to 3-cm vertical skin incision with the scalpel, the needle is used to puncture the cricothyroid membrane in the midline.[62] This task is accomplished with a downward thrust toward the chest (Figure 11-33). A rush of air indicates successful entry into the trachea, and the obturator/airway unit inserted (Figure 11-34).

The blunt-edged needle is gently advancing farther into the trachea until its plastic hub rests on the skin. Gently rock the instrument; free movement indicates that overpenetration has not occurred.

In addition, an airway and obturators are now inserted into the distal end of the housing unit (Figure 11-35). The split end of the needle, within the trachea, is opened by the airway and obturator, after which the obturator is removed, leaving a clear passage for the exchange of air in the lungs. This device is available in both pediatric and adult sizes. Its use, like that of all other emergency airway equipment, is recommended only for those trained in cricothyrotomy technique.

If spontaneous respiratory movements are present, the victim may regain consciousness but still be unable to speak because of the continued presence of an obstruction at the larynx. Once consciousness returns, the opening into the trachea cannot be closed before the object producing the obstruction is removed. If spontaneous respiratory movements are absent, artificial ventilation via the cricothyrotomy should be performed to ensure adequate oxygenation of the blood. Circulatory adequacy then may be determined through palpation of the carotid artery.

Once a patent airway is established, the victim may receive $O_2$. A cannula or face mask may be placed over the tracheal opening. In addition, the appropriate team member must summon medical assistance to transfer the patient to an emergency medical facility for follow-up management (for example, removal of the foreign object or closure of the tracheal opening) and observation.

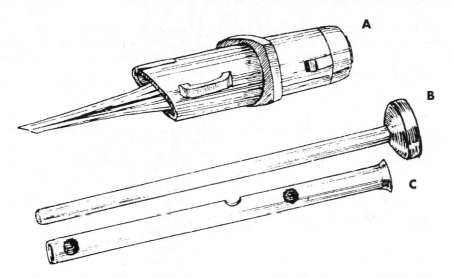

**Figure 11-34**  Components of the instrument used in cricothyrotomy. **A,** Needle and housing unit. **B,** Oburator. **C,** Airway.

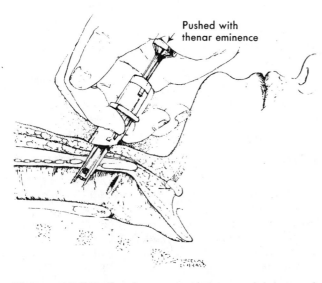

Pushed with thenar eminence

**Figure 11-35**  An obturator and airway unit is inserted into the needle or housing unit to open the airway. Next, the obturator is removed and the airway secured.

### Contraindications to cricothyrotomy

Although a useful and life-saving technique, cricothyrotomy is not recommended in all cases of upper-airway obstruction. The following are examples of a few such exceptions:

- Cricothyrotomy should not be performed without significant trepidation in children under 10 years and probably should not be performed at all in children under 5 years.[38] Although tracheostomy is the preferred emergency airway procedure in young patients, needle cricothyrotomy is more desirable in younger patients.[63]

- Preexisting pathologic processes in the larynx (for example, in the epiglottitis), chronic inflammation, or cancer make cricothyrotomy more difficult.
- Lack of familiarity with the technique and its complications are a major contraindication to cricothyrotomy. Inexperience may be the single-largest factor involved in cricothyrotomy complications.[64]
- Anatomic barriers, such as trauma to the neck region, should warn against performance of this technique.
- When uncontrolled hemorrhage is a possibility, the benefits of cricothyrotomy should be weighed carefully against its risks.

Acute, total airway obstruction is a very rare occurrence in dental offices. However, when it does occur, signs and symptoms must be recognized instantly and proper management initiated immediately. Thus all office staff members should receive training in the proper use of the Heimlich maneuver, which all individuals can and should learn to perform successfully. Noninvasive procedures for the maintenance of emergency airways are preferred over surgical procedures in all situations, but surgical techniques serve as vital last resorts when all else has failed.

## REFERENCES

1. Cameron SM, Whitlock WL, Tabor MS: Foreign body aspiration in dentistry: a review, *J Am Dent Assoc* 127(8):1224-1229, 1996.
2. Worthington P: Ingested foreign body associated with oral implant treatment: report of a case, *Int J Oral Maxillofac Implants* 11(5):679-681, 1996.

3. Lambrianidis T, Beltes P: Accidental swallowing of endodontic instruments, *Endod Dent Traumatol* 12(6):301-304, 1996.

4. Brunello DL, Mandikos MN: A denture swallowed: case report, *Aust Dent J* 40(6):349-351, 1995.

5. National Safety Council: *Accident facts,* Chicago, 1984, The Council.

6. American Heart Association, Emergency Care Committee and Subcommittees: Guidelines for cardiopulmonary resuscitation and emergency cardiac care, *JAMA* 268(16): 2171-2302, 1992.

7. Fitzpatrick PC, Guarisco JL: Pediatric airway foreign bodies, *J La State Med Soc* 150(4):138-141, 1998.

8. Rimell FL and others: Characteristics of objects that cause choking in children, *JAMA* 274(22):1763-1766, 1995.

9. Abman SH, Fan LL, Cotton EK: Emergency treatment of foreign-body obstruction of the upper airway in children, *J Emerg Med* 2:7-12, 1984.

10. Netter FH: *Atlas of human anatomy,* ed 2, East Hanover, NJ, 1997, Novartis.

11. Odelowo EO, Komolafe OF: Diagnosis, management and complications of oesophageal and airway foreign bodies, *Int Surg* 75(3):148-154, 1990.

12. Storey PS: Obstruction of the GI tract, *Am J Hospice and Palliative Care* 8(3):5, 1991.

13. Weissberg D: Foreign bodies in the gastrointestinal tract, *South Afr J Surg* 29(4):150-153, 1991.

14. Mu L, He P, Sun D: The causes and complications of late diagnosis of foreign body aspiration in children: report of 210 cases, *Arch Otolaryngol Head Neck Surg* 117(8): 876-879, 1991.

15. Barkmeier WW, Cooley RL, Abrams H: Prevention of swallowing or aspiration of foreign objects, *Am J Dent Assoc* 97:473, 1978.

16. Muth D, Scafermeyer RW: All that wheezes, *Pediatr Emerg Care* 6(2):110-112, 1990.

17. Lumpkin J: Airway obstruction, *Top Emerg Med* 2:15, 1990.

18. Jacob B and others: Laryngologic aspects of bolus asphyxiation—bolus death, *Dysphagia* 7(1):31-35, 1992.

19. Craig TJ, Richardson MA: Cafe coronaries in psychiatric patients, *JAMA* 248:2114, 1982 (letter to the editors).

20. Landing BH, Dixon LG: Congenital malformations and genetic disorders of the respiratory tract, *Am Rev Respir Dis* 120:15, 1979.

21. Munoz A, Ballesteros AI, Brandariz Castelo JA: Primary lingual abscess presenting as acute swelling of the tongue obstructing the upper airway: diagnosis with MR, *Am J Neuroradiol* 19(3):496-498, 1998.

22. Mayo-Smith MF and others: Acute epiglottitis: an 18-year experience in Rhode Island, *Chest* 108(6):1640-1647, 1995.

23. Mavrinac JM, Dolan RW: Acute lingual tonsillitis, *Am J Emerg Med* 15(3):308-309, 1997.

24. Deeb ZE: Acute supraglottitis in adults: early indicators of airway obstruction, *Am J Otolaryngol* 18(2):112-115, 1997.

25. Sdralis T, Berkowitz RG: Early adenotonsillectomy for relief of acute upper airway obstruction due to acute tonsillitis in children, *Int J Pediatr Otorhinolaryngol* 35(1):25-29, 1996.

26. Hamer R: Retropharyngeal abscess, *Ann Emerg Med* 11:549,1982.

27. Spitalnic SJ, Sucov A: Ludwig's angina: case report and review, *J Emerg Med* 13(4):499-503, 1995.

28. Bavitz JB, Collicott PE: Bilateral mandibular subcondylar fractures contributing to airway obstruction, *Int J Oral Maxillofac Surg* 24(4):273-275, 1995.

29. Myatt HM: Acute airway obstruction due to primary thyroid lymphoma, *Rev Laryngol Otol Rhinol (Bord)* 117(3):237-239, 1996.

30. Mordenfeld A, Andersson L, Bergstrom B: Hemorrhage in the floor of the mouth during implant placement in the edentulous mandible: a case report, *Int J Oral Maxillofac Implants* 12(4):558-561, 1997.

31. Watts AM, McCallum MI: Acute airway obstruction following facial scalding: differential diagnosis between a thermal and infective cause, *Burns* 22(7):570-573, 1996.

32. Kristoffersen MB, Rattenborg CC, Holaday PA: Asphyxial death: the roles of acute anoxia, hypercarbia, and acidosis, *Anesthesiology* 28:488, 1967.

33. Dailey RH: Acute upper airway obstruction, *Emerg Med Clin North Am* 1:261, 1983.

34. Arnold DN: Airway review, *Am Acad Gnathologic Orthoped* 7(2):4-7, 11, 1990.

35. Powell DM, Price PD, Forrest LA: Review of percutaneous tracheostomy, *Laryngoscope* 108(2):170-177, 1998.

36. Wood DE: Tracheostomy, *Chest Surg Clin N Am* 6(4):749-764, 1996.

37. Hamilton PH, Kang JJ: Emergency airway management, *Mt Sinai J Med* 64(4-5):292-301, 1997.

38. Walls RM: Cricothroidotomy, *Emerg Med Clin North Am* 6:725, 1988.

39. Tobias JD: Airway management for pediatric emergencies, *Pediatr Ann* 25(6):317-20, 323-8, 1996.

40. Bennett JD: High tracheostomy and other errors-revisited, *J Laryngol Otol* 110(11):1003-1007, 1996.

41. Heimlich HJ: A life-saving maneuver to prevent food-choking, *JAMA* 234:398, 1975.

42. Committee on Emergency Medical Services, Assembly of Life Sciences, National Research Council: *Report of emergency airway management,* Washington, DC, 1976, National Academy of Sciences.

43. Day RL, Crelin ES, DuBois AB: Choking: the Heimlich abdominal thrust vs back blows-an approach to measurement of inertial and aerodynamic forces, *Pediatrics* 70:113, 1982.

44. Heimlich HJ, Hoffman KA, Canestri FR: Food-choking and drowning deaths prevented by external subdiaphragmatic compression: physiologic basis, *Ann Thorac Surg* 20:188, 1975.

45. Heimlich HJ, Uhtley MH: The Heimlich maneuver, *Clin Symp* 31:22, 1979.

46. Patrick EA: Choking: a questionnaire to find the most effective treatment, *Emergency* 12:59, 1980.

47. Heimlich HJ: Pop goes the cafe coronary, *Emerg Med* 6:154, 1979.

48. Visintine RE, Baick CH: Ruptured stomach after Heimlich maneuver, *JAMA* 234:415, 1975.

49. Palmer E: The Heimlich maneuver misused, *Curr Prescribing* 154:155, 1979.

50. American Heart Association and National Academy of Sciences, National Research Council: Standards and guidelines for cardiopulmonary resuscitation (CPR) and emergency cardiac care (ECC), *JAMA* 244:453, 1980.

51. Gordon AS, Belton MK, Ridolpho RF: Emergency management of foreign body airway obstruction. In Safar P, Elam J, editors: *Advances in cardiopulmonary resuscitation,* New York, 1977, Springer-Verlag.

52. Guildner CW, Williams D, Subitch T: Airway obstructed by foreign material: the Heimlich maneuver, *JACEP* 5:675, 1976.

53. Ward RF: Current trends in pediatric tracheotomy, *Pediatr Pulmonol Suppl* 16:290-291, 1997.

54. Boyd AD and others: A clinical evaluation of cricothyroidotomy, *Surg Gynecol Obstet* 149:365, 1979.

55. Kostendieck JF: Airway management. In Rosen P, editor: *Emergency medicine: concepts and clinical practice,* ed 4, St Louis, 1998, Mosby.

56. Morris IR: Functional anatomy of the upper airway, *Emerg Med Clin North Am* 6:639-670, 1988.

57. Gilmore BB, Mickelson SA: Pediatric tracheostomy, *Otolaryngol Clin North Am* 19(1):141, 1986.

58. Weiss S: A new instrument for emergency cricothyrotomy, *JACEP* 23:331, 1973.

59. Barkin RM: Pediatric emergency management, *Emer Med Clin North Am* 6(4):687, 1988.

60. Kress TD, Balasubramaniam S: Cricothyroidotomy, *Ann Emerg Med* 11:197, 1982.

61. Narrod JA, Moore EE, Rosen P: Emergency cricothyrostomy: technique and anatomical considerations, *J Emerg Med* 2:443, 1985.

62. Weiss S: A new emergency cricothyroidotomy instrument, *J Trauma* 23:155, 1983.

63. McLaughlin J, Iserson KV: Emergency pediatric tracheostomy: a usable technique and model for instruction, *Ann Emerg Med* 15:463, 1986.

64. McGill J, Clinton JE, Ruiz E: Cricothyroidotomy in the emergency department, *Ann Emerg Med* 11:361, 1982.

# 12

# *Hyperventilation*

**H**YPERVENTILATION is defined as ventilation in excess of that required to maintain normal blood $PaO_2$ (arterial oxygen [$O_2$] tension) and $PaCO_2$ (arterial carbon dioxide [$CO_2$] tension).[1] It is produced by an increase in either the frequency or the depth of respiration, or both. Although the term *hyperventilation* is of recent origin, evidence of the syndrome dates back throughout history.[2] The term *vapors* appeared in eighteenth- and nineteenth-century literature to refer to the symptomatic manifestations of anxiety.[3] In Osler's time (the late 1800s) the terms *neurasthenia* or *psychasthenia* described the condition. During World War I, the terms *effort syndrome* and *soldier's heart* were used to describe the symptoms of anxiety encountered in the trenches of Europe.

Hyperventilation, one of the more common emergency situations that occur in the dental office, almost always is a result of extreme anxiety. However, organic causes for hyperventilation do exist; these include pain, metabolic acidosis, drug intoxication, hypercapnea, cirrhosis, and organic central nervous system disorders.[4] In most instances the hyperventilating patient remains conscious throughout the episode. Indeed unconsciousness secondary to hyperventilation is an extremely rare occurrence. Hyperventilation more commonly produces an altered level of consciousness. The patient complains of feeling faint, lightheaded, or both but does not lose consciousness.

# Predisposing Factors

Acute anxiety is the most common predisposing factor for hyperventilation. In dentistry, hyperventilation most commonly occurs in apprehensive patients who seek to hide their fears from the doctors and to "grin and bear it." Hyperventilation rarely occurs in adult patients who freely admit their fears and allow their doctors to employ stress-reduction techniques. Hyperventilation is encountered rarely in children, primarily because children usually make no attempt to hide their fears. Instead, apprehensive children voice uncertainties in rather obvious ways—crying, biting, kicking. If the patient's anxieties are released, hyperventilation and vasodepressor syncope rarely occur.

Likewise, patients older than 40 years do not experience hyperventilation and vasodepressor syncope as often as other age-groups; these patients are usually able to adjust to the stress of dental treatment and to admit their fears to the doctor. In my own experience, hyperventilation most often occurs in patients between 15 and 40 years. In addition, it has been stated that hyperventilation occurs more frequently in women[5]; however, recent reports and my experience have demonstrated that the condition occurs almost equally across the sexes.[6]

# Prevention

## MEDICAL HISTORY QUESTIONNAIRE

Hyperventilation can be prevented most effectively through the prompt recognition and management of anxiety. An anxiety questionnaire (see Chapter 2) may be included as part of the medical history the patient completes before the doctor begins treatment. Treatment can then be modified to accommodate the patient's fears. The stress reduction protocol is an invaluable asset in this quest. There are no specific questions on the long- or short-form medical histories that relate to hyperventilation.

## PHYSICAL EVALUATION

Through careful examination it is usually possible to detect a patient's anxiety. Shaking hands with the patient provides valuable information. Cold, wet (clammy) hands usually indicate apprehension. In extreme instances a mild tremor of the hands may be obvious. The patient may appear either flushed or pale; in either case the forehead is usually bathed in perspiration, and the patient may remark that the office is unusually warm, regardless of its actual temperature. Fearful patients simply appear uncomfortable when they sit in dental chairs and are overly concerned with the goings-on around them.*

## VITAL SIGNS

The vital signs of apprehensive patients may deviate from the normal, or baseline, values for that individual. The blood pressure becomes elevated, with the systolic pressure rising more than the diastolic. The heart rate (pulse) is rapid, significantly higher than the baseline level for that patient. In addition, the patient's rate of respiration increases above the normal adult rate of 14 to 18 breaths per minute, whereas the depth of respiration is either deeper or more shallow than normal.

The vital signs that are recorded on the patient's first visit to the dental office serve as baseline levels for all future readings. Therefore every effort should be made to minimize any anxiety at this initial visit. Indeed these efforts at anxiety reduction should continue at all times during treatment. To obtain more realistic baseline vital signs through stress reduction, the patient should be allowed to rest for a few minutes before recording vital signs. An easy way to accomplish this is to start a review of the medical history questionnaire (dialogue history) and then, after 5 minutes, measure the vital signs.

Another important factor to consider is that the recording of baseline vital signs at a visit during which no dental treatment is to be performed is often the best chance to obtain normal values. The patient in this situation is better able to relax, and vital signs will be closer to their normal values, not altered by dental stress. During subsequent visits, the monitoring of vital signs may reflect the patient's increased apprehension toward impending treatment.

## DENTAL THERAPY CONSIDERATIONS

The stress-reduction protocol outlined in Chapter 2 is the primary means of preventing hyperventilation. Care taken by the dental office staff to make every dental visit a pleasant one leads to the reeducation of the fearful patient and to a decrease in dental anxieties. Stress reduction is one of the most important factors in proper patient management.

---

*This overconcern becomes obvious; the patient's eyes follow every movement that the doctor and assistants make. Such patients also may appear stiff in the chair and seem ready at times to jump from the seat. The hands of the apprehensive patient are firmly attached to the chair ("white-knuckle syndrome") or they may squeeze and tear at a handkerchief or tissue.

# Clinical Manifestations

## SIGNS AND SYMPTOMS

At the onset of hyperventilation, which is frequently precipitated by the fear associated with receiving a local anesthetic injection, the patient may complain of chest tightness and a feeling of suffocation but be entirely unaware of overbreathing. As hyperventilation continues, the chemical composition of the blood changes and the patient begins to feel lightheaded or giddy, which serves to increase the apprehension even more. Increased apprehension leads to an increase in the severity of the episode, and a vicious cycle begins. Hyperventilation caused by dental anxiety leads to even further increased anxiety when the patient becomes aware of their hyperventilation, and then to an even further increase in hyperventilation because of the increased anxiety. The goal in management of the situation is to break this cycle.

At the onset of hyperventilation symptoms related to the cardiovascular system and gastrointestinal tract often appear. These symptoms include palpitation (a subjective feeling of a pounding of the heart), precordial discomfort, epigastric discomfort, and globus hystericus (a subjective feeling of a lump in the throat).

Left untreated, hyperventilation may last for relatively long periods. Patients have hyperventilated for 30 minutes or longer and have suffered several episodes per day. In instances in which hyperventilation continues for prolonged periods, the patient may experience tingling or paresthesias of the hands, feet, and perioral regions. Patients often describe these feelings as sensations of numbness or coldness.

If hyperventilation continues, the patient may develop muscular twitching and carpopedal tetany, a syndrome manifested by flexion of the ankle joints, muscular twitching and cramps, and convulsions. If the hyperventilating patient is not managed promptly and precisely, syncope may result. Table 12-1 summarizes the signs and symptoms associated with hyperventilation.

## EFFECT ON VITAL SIGNS

The primary clinical manifestation of hyperventilation is the change in the rate and depth of the patient's breathing. Normal respiratory rate for the adult is 14 to 18 breaths per minute. During hyperventilation the respiratory rate may exceed 25 to 30 breaths per minute. Not only does the rate of breathing increase, but the patient also usually exhibits an increase in the depth of breathing. To the person who has never seen or experienced hyperventilation,

| table 12-1 | Clinical manifestations of hyperventilation |

| SYSTEM | SIGNS AND SYMPTOMS |
| --- | --- |
| Cardiovascular | Palpitations |
| | Tachycardia |
| | Precordial pain |
| Neurologic | Dizziness |
| | Lightheadedness |
| | Disturbance of consciousness or vision |
| | Numbness and tingling of the extremities |
| | Tetany (rare) |
| Respiratory | Shortness of breath |
| | Chest pain |
| | Dryness of the mouth |
| Gastrointestinal | Globus hystericus |
| | Epigastric pain |
| Musculoskeletal | Muscle pains and cramps |
| | Tremors |
| | Stiffness |
| | Carpopedal tetany |
| Psychologic | Tension |
| | Anxiety |
| | Nightmares |

the nature of the patient's breathing may appear similar to that of an individual who has just finished performing strenuous exercise (for example, when a runner stands bent over and panting).

In the case of the runner, both the rate and the depth of breathing increase; these increases are normal physiologic responses to the increased metabolic rate as the body works to eliminate excessive $CO_2$ (produced during the exercise). Although the nature of a hyperventilating patient's breathing is similar to that of the athlete, it represents an abnormal physiologic response to the presence of anxiety because there is no elevation of $CO_2$ levels in the blood.

As previously stated, episodes of hyperventilation are most common in overtly apprehensive patients; however, many other patients may appear calm and totally unaware that they are hyperventilating (Box 12-1).

# Pathophysiology

Several distinct conditions—anxiety, respiratory alkalosis, an increase in the blood catecholamine level, and a decrease in the level of ionized calcium in the blood—produce the clinical signs and symptoms associated with hyperventilation.

Anxiety is responsible for both the increase in respiratory rate and depth and the increase in the levels of

box **12-1**    *Case report*

A 27-year-old female was scheduled for extraction of two third molars (nonimpacted). She appeared apprehensive when staff members first saw her and stated to the dental assistant that she was quite concerned about the procedure, particularly the local anesthetic injections. She appeared flushed and was perspiring; her blood pressure reading was 130/90 (baseline, 110/70), her heart rate was 110 (baseline, 84), and her respiratory rate measured 20 (baseline, 18). No preoperative medications were prescribed. The surgeon elected to use nitrous oxide ($N_2O$) and $O_2$ inhalation sedation during the procedure and titrated to a concentration of 60% $N_2O$ and 40% $O_2$, at which point the patient appeared adequately sedated. As the topical anesthetic was applied, the patient became visibly more tense and her respiratory rate began to increase. During administration of the local anesthetic, she began to hyperventilate (28 breaths per minute and deep), and the procedure was terminated.

The patient was permitted to breathe room air, and was calmed by the oral surgeon. She reported feeling a slight tingling of the fingers, but the symptom lasted only briefly. Within 10 minutes the patient was relaxed, and her vital signs returned to approximately baseline levels. The treatment was rescheduled, to be managed under intravenous (IV) sedation and local anesthesia.

The next week the patient received 30 mg flurazepam orally the evening before the treatment and 10 mg diazepam orally 1 hour before the appointment. A friend drove the patient to the office. An IV infusion with a 21-gauge scalp vein needle was begun in the woman's right forearm, and IV diazepam titrated to a dose of 17 mg; local anesthesia was then administered without complication and the surgery completed in 25 minutes. The patient tolerated the procedure well, commenting, "With the IV (drug), I didn't even need that local injection." She was discharged into the care of an adult companion.

the catecholamines epinephrine and norepinephrine in the blood (a result of the "fight or flight" response). The body's primary response to these respiratory changes is an increased exchange of $O_2$ and $CO_2$ by the lungs, which results in an excessive "blowing off" of $CO_2$. The partial pressure of $CO_2$ decreases from a normal level of 35 to 45 torr to a $PaCO_2$ below 35 torr (hypocapnea, or hypocarbia); this decrease produces an increase in the blood's pH to 7.55 (normal being 7.35 to 7.45), a condition known as *respiratory alkalosis.*

However, the same situation—increased ventilation—at the end of strenuous exercise does not produce respiratory alkalosis because exercise increases the body's rate of metabolism, producing an increased blood $PaCO_2$. Increased breathing in this case leads to the restoration of normal $CO_2$ blood levels. In the patient who starts with normal levels of $CO_2$, hyperventilation reduces the $PaCO_2$ to an abnormally low level (hypocapnea).

Hypocapnea and respiratory alkalosis are the result of hyperventilation in an individual who has not exercised. Hypocapnea produces vasoconstriction in cerebral blood vessels leading to a degree of cerebral ischemia, helping to explain the lightheadedness, dizziness, and giddiness associated with hyperventilation.[7] The degree of cerebral ischemia is usually insufficient to produce the loss of consciousness, although this may occur on rare occasions.[8-10] Many hyperventilating patients describe a "feeling of tightness" in their chests. In certain situations differentiation of this chest "pain" from that of angina pectoris may be difficult.

Anxiety also produces increased blood levels of catecholamines, which may be responsible for the palpitations, precordial oppression, trembling, and sweating frequently associated with spontaneously hyperventilating patients. It is interesting to note that volunteers who were asked to hyperventilate did not exhibit these symptoms, which are thought to be produced by catecholamine release although the symptoms related to increased rates and depths of breathing (for example, lightheadedness and faintness) are still present.[11]

Respiratory alkalosis also acts on the level of calcium in the blood. As blood pH rises from a normal of about 7.4 to approximately 7.55 in hyperventilation, calcium metabolism is disturbed. Although the total serum level of calcium remains approximately normal, the level of ionized calcium in the blood decreases as the blood's pH increases. Decreases in ionized calcium in the blood result in increased neuromuscular irritability and excitability, which if permitted to progress can result in a variety of symptoms, including tingling and paresthesias of the hands, feet, and perioral regions; carpopedal tetany; cramps; and possible convulsions.

## Management

The management of hyperventilation is directed at correcting the respiratory problem and reducing the patient's anxiety level.

Hyperventilation in the dental environment is almost always produced by a fear of dentistry that has been kept well-hidden by the patient. The subsequent inability of the patient to control the breathing further increases those fears. The doctor and staff members must initially attempt to calm the patient; they themselves must remain calm throughout the episode so that they do not exacerbate the situation.

*Step 1: termination of the dental procedure.* The presumed cause of the episode (for example, a syringe, handpiece, or pair of forceps) should be removed from the patient's line of vision.

*Step 2:* **P** *(position).* The hyperventilating patient will remain conscious but will demonstrate varying degrees of difficulty in breathing. The preferred position for this patient is usually upright. The supine position is normally uncomfortable for such patients because of the diminished ventilatory volume caused by the impingement of the abdominal viscera on the diaphragm. Most hyperventilating patients are most comfortable sitting fully or partially upright.

*Step 3:* **A-B-C** *(airway-breathing-circulation), (basic life support), as needed.* Hyperventilating individuals rarely require basic life support. Such victims are conscious and breathing efficiently (indeed, they are overventilating), and the heart is quite functional.

*Step 4:* **D** *(definitive care):*
*Step 4a: removal of materials from the mouth.* All foreign objects, such as rubber dam, clamps, and partial dentures, should be removed from the patient's mouth and any tight bindings (for example, a tight collar, tie, or tight blouse), which also may restrict respiration, loosened.

*Step 4b: calming of the patient.* Reassure the patient that all is well in a calm and relaxed manner. Attempt to aid the patient to regain control of breathing by speaking calmly. Have the patient breathe slowly and regularly at a rate of about 4 to 6 breaths per minute. This will permit the $PaCO_2$ to increase, reducing the pH of the blood to near normal and eliminating any symptoms produced by respiratory alkalosis. In many cases of hyperventilation these are the only steps necessary to terminate the episode.

*Step 4c: correction of respiratory alkalosis.* When the preceding steps are ineffective, helping the patient to increase the blood's $PaCO_2$ level is the next major concern. The patient may be instructed to breathe a gaseous mixture of 7% $CO_2$ and 93% $O_2$, which is supplied in compressed gas cylinders but is unlikely to be available in the dental office. More realistically, the patient will be told to rebreathe exhaled air, which contains an increased concentration of $CO_2$.

The most practical method of increasing $PaCO_2$ levels in the blood is to instruct the hyperventilating victim to cup the hands in front of the mouth and nose and to breathe in and out of this reservoir of $CO_2$-enriched exhaled air (Figure 12-1). In addition to elevating $PaCO_2$ levels, the warmth of the exhaled

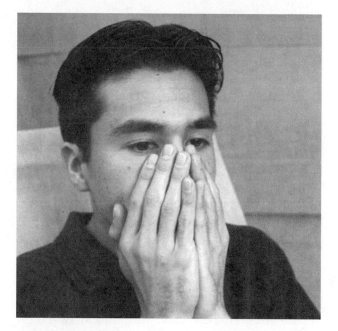

**Figure 12-1** The hyperventilating victim cups the hands together in front of the mouth and nose as a means of increasing the $PaCO_2$ level. *$PaCO_2$,* Arterial carbon dioxide tension.

air against the cold hands will warm the patient, alleviating one of the more frightening symptoms of hyperventilation. A full-face mask from an $O_2$ delivery unit may also be used. However, care must be taken not to administer $O_2$ to the hyperventilating patient. The patient should breathe into the full-face mask, which is held gently but firmly over the face. The use of a paper bag, into which the victim breathes while it is held over the mouth and nose, is no longer recommended.

$O_2$ is not indicated in the management of hyperventilation because its symptoms are produced in part by a decrease in the normal blood level of $CO_2$ and not by a decrease in $O_2$ levels. The blood's pH rises (respiratory alkalosis), and symptoms previously discussed may be observed. For this reason a major goal of management is to produce an increase, actually a return to normal, in the blood level of $CO_2$. The administration of 100% $O_2$ or of any enriched $O_2$ mixture further decreases the $PaCO_2$ level, delaying a return to normal. The administration of $O_2$, though not indicated, will not harm the hyperventilating patient. The administration of 100% $O_2$ will not resolve the clinical problem but might lead to a further progression of the clinical manifestations. A basic rule of thumb in the administration of $O_2$ is the following: If ever a patient's condition deteriorates when 100% $O_2$ is administered, the $O_2$ flow should be terminated and the patient instructed to breathe ambient air.

*Step 4d: drug management, if necessary.* If the previously discussed steps fail to terminate an episode of hyperventilation—an exceedingly unlikely situation—parenteral drugs may have to be administered to reduce the patient's anxiety and to slow the rate of breathing. The drugs of choice in this situation are diazepam or midazolam. If possible, the drug should be administered intravenously, in which case it is titrated until the patient's anxiety is visibly reduced and the patient is able to control breathing. This dose is approximately 10 to 15 mg diazepam, or 3 to 5 mg midazolam, for the average adult.

When the IV route is not available, 10 mg diazepam or 3 to 5 mg midazolam may be administered intramuscularly. Midazolam is preferred because diazepam is not water soluble and burns when injected intramuscularly. If diazepam is used, however, the drug should be injected deep into the muscle mass and the area massaged. Oral administration of diazepam may also be considered because the latent period for diazepam is actually longer after intramuscular administration than after oral administration.[12] An oral dose of 10 to 15 mg diazepam usually terminates hyperventilation within 30 minutes. It must be emphasized that drug therapy for the termination of hyperventilation is rarely required.

*Step 5: subsequent dental treatment.* Once the episode of hyperventilation is ended and all clinical signs and symptoms have resolved, the dentist must determine the cause of the hyperventilation. Like vasodepressor syncope, hyperventilation is often the first clinical manifestation of a deep-seated dental fear. Dental treatment may continue at this time if both the doctor and the patient are comfortable in doing so. However, subsequent dental treatment should be modified and the stress-reduction protocol consulted to prevent a recurrence of hyperventilation.

*Step 6: discharge.* After the episode has ended and all signs and symptoms are resolved, the patient may be discharged from the office as usual. If the doctor has any uncertainty about the patient's recovery, a friend or relative of the patient should drive the patient home. An entry about the episode and its management should be placed in the dental progress notes.

Box 12-2 summarizes the management of hyperventilation.

- **Drugs used in management:** No drugs are usually required in the management of hyperventilation. However, the rare patient who does not respond

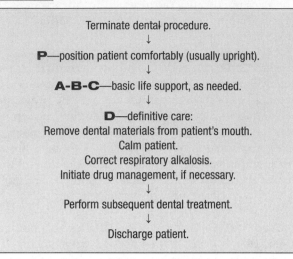

**box 12-2**    *Management of hyperventilation*

Terminate dental procedure.
↓
**P**—position patient comfortably (usually upright).
↓
**A-B-C**—basic life support, as needed.
↓
**D**—definitive care:
Remove dental materials from patient's mouth.
Calm patient.
Correct respiratory alkalosis.
Initiate drug management, if necessary.
↓
Perform subsequent dental treatment.
↓
Discharge patient.

**P,** Position; **A,** airway; **B,** breathing; **C,** circulation; **D,** definitive care.

to conservative management may require the administration of either diazepam or midazolam.
- **Medical assistance required:** None.

Like vasodepressor syncope, hyperventilation should not occur a second time in the same patient. Proper management of the fearful patient through the use of psychosedation can eliminate the recurrence of these two anxiety-produced, potentially life-threatening situations.

## REFERENCES

1. Anderson KN: *Mosby's medical, nursing, & allied health dictionary,* ed 5, St Louis, 1998, Mosby.
2. Paulley JW: Hyperventilation, *Recenti Prog Med* 81(9):594-600, 1990.
3. Dalessio DJ: Hyperventilation: the vapors, effort syndrome, neurasthenia-anxiety by any other name is just as disturbing, *JAMA* 239:1401, 1978.
4. Dailey RH: Difficulty in breathing. In Schwartz GR, editor: *Principles and practice of emergency medicine,* ed 3, Philadelphia, 1992, Lea & Febiger.
5. Sama A, Meikle JC, Jones NS: Hyperventilation and dizziness: case reports and management, *Br J Clin Pract* 49(2):79-82, 1995.
6. Lum LC: Hyperventilation: the tip and the iceberg, *J Psychosom Res* 19:375, 1975.
7. Gardner WN: The pathophysiology of hyperventilation disorders, *Chest* 109(2):516-534, 1996.
8. Edmeads J: Understanding dizziness: how to decipher this nonspecific symptom, *Postgrad Med* 88(5):255-258, 263-268, 1990.

9. Neill WA, Hattenhauer M: Impairment of myocardial O$_2$ supply due to hyperventilation, *Circulation* 52:854, 1975.

10. Wheatley CE: Hyperventilation syndrome: a frequent cause of chest pain, *Chest* 68:195, 1975.

11. Beck JG, Berisford MA, Taegtmeyer H: The effects of voluntary hyperventilation on patients with chest pain without coronary artery disease, *Behav Res Ther* 29(6):611-621, 1991.

12. Divoll M and others: Absolute bioavailability of oral and intramuscular diazepam: effect of age and sex, *Anesth Analg* 62:1, 1983.

# 13

## *Asthma*

**A**STHMA was defined in 1830 by Eberle, a Philadelphia physician, as "paroxysmal affection of the respiratory organs, characterized by great difficulty of breathing, tightness across the breast, and a sense of impending suffocation, without fever or local inflammation."[1] Today, *asthma* is defined by the American Thoracic Society as "a disease characterized by an increased responsiveness of the trachea and bronchi to various stimuli and manifested by widespread narrowing of the airways that changes in severity either spontaneously or as a result of therapy."[2]

Asthma affects an estimated 5% of adults and between 7% and 10% of children in the United States.[3] Approximately 15 million Americans suffer from asthma. A typical asthmatic patient is usually free of symptoms between acute episodes but exhibits varying degrees of respiratory distress during the acute episode. Although the degree of respiratory distress (dyspnea) is usually moderate, an estimated 1 in 100,000 individuals dies each year from complications associated with asthma.[4,5] It is estimated that asthma is responsible for 5000 to 6000 deaths in the United states annually.[6]

Asthma is primarily a disease of young people; one half of all cases develop before the individual reaches 10 years, and another third before 40 years.[5] Asthma is also the most chronic disease of childhood. Asthmatic children account for a significant number children who visit emergency rooms and up to 8% of all admissions at one large children's hospital.[7] Acute

box **13-1**  *Causative factors for acute asthma*

Allergy (antigen-antibody reaction)
Respiratory infection
Physical exertion
Environmental and air pollution
Occupational stimuli
Pharmacologic stimuli
Psychologic factors

asthmatic episodes are usually self-limiting; however, a clinical entity termed *status asthmaticus* is characterized by a persistent exacerbation of asthma.[8] This condition is potentially life threatening and is initially unresponsive to usually successful therapy, such as the administration of the adrenergic bronchodilators epinephrine and theophylline.

## Predisposing Factors

Asthma usually is classified according to causative factors into two major categories: extrinsic and intrinsic (Box 13-1). Individuals with extrinsic asthma have histories of allergy, whereas those with the intrinsic asthma do not. One factor, however, is common in all asthmatics—extreme sensitivity of the airways. This sensitivity is characterized not only by an increased contractile response of airway smooth muscle but also by an abnormal generation and clearance of secretions and an abnormally sensitive cough reflex.

### EXTRINSIC ASTHMA

Extrinsic asthma, also known as *allergic asthma,* accounts for 50% of asthmatics and occurs more often in children and younger adults. Most patients with this form of asthma demonstrate an inherited allergic predisposition. The inhalation of specific allergens may precipitate acute asthmatic episodes. The allergens may be airborne, such as house dust, feathers, animal dander, furniture stuffing, fungal spores, or a wide variety of plant pollens.[9] Foods and drugs also may precipitate the allergic form of asthmatic attacks. Highly allergenic foods include cow's milk, eggs, fish, chocolate, shellfish, and tomatoes. Penicillin,[10] vaccines, aspirin,[11] and sulfites[12,13] are examples of drugs and chemicals that often induce asthmatic episodes. Bronchospasm usually develops within minutes after exposure to the allergen (antigen). This response is called a *type I hypersensitivity reaction* in which im-

munoglobulin E (IgE) antibodies are produced in response to the allergen (see Chapter 24).

Acute episodes of extrinsic asthma usually occur with diminishing frequency and severity during middle and late adolescence and may disappear entirely later in life. Approximately 50% of asthmatic children become asymptomatic before reaching adulthood.[14] It is possible, however, for extrinsic asthma to become chronic in some individuals. This appears to be more common when asthma originally develops in early childhood and is associated with eczema.

### INTRINSIC ASTHMA

The second major category, which accounts for the other half of asthmatics, is intrinsic asthma. Intrinsic asthma usually develops in adults older than 35 years. Nonallergic factors—respiratory infection,[15] physical exertion,[16] environmental and air pollution,[17] and occupational stimuli[18]—precipitate these episodes. Intrinsic asthma also is referred to as *nonallergic asthma idiopathic asthma,* and *infective asthma.* Individuals who suffer this condition usually have negative histories to allergy, and the results of allergy testing (for example, skin tests) usually are negative.

Viral infection of the respiratory tract is the most common causative factor. Viral infections are known to enhance airway reactivity in both asthmatics[19] and nonasthmatics.[20] Individuals with exercise-induced asthma experience symptoms within 6 to 10 minutes after the start of the exercise, followed by a more severe delayed phase of bronchospasm that develops after the individual has completed the activity. The entire episode, which individuals in all age-groups and both sexes experience, classically lasts 30 to 60 minutes.[16]

Psychologic and physiologic stress can also contribute to asthmatic episodes in susceptible individuals.[21] Acute asthmatic episodes occur frequently in children during or after a disciplinary session with a parent.[22] The dental office is another common site for asthmatic attacks.[23] Simply walking into the treatment room may induce an acute episode in an asthmatic child. A dramatic resolution of acute signs and symptoms usually occurs by simply removing the child from the treatment room.[24] Psychologic factors may also be important in adult asthma. Stressful situations, such as dental appointments, produce symptoms in many adult asthmatics. For example, I have observed dental students with well-controlled asthma experience periods of chronic bronchospasm during final examination week.

Figure 13-1 illustrates a simplified view of the mechanisms involved in asthma. Acute episodes of intrinsic asthma usually are more fulminant and severe than

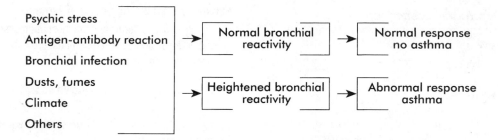

**Figure 13-1**  Predisposing factors for asthma. (From Pain MCE: The treatment of asthma, *Drugs* 6:118, 1973.)

those of allergic (extrinsic) asthma. The long-term prognosis of intrinsic asthma is also less optimistic because the disease usually becomes chronic and the patient eventually exhibits clinical signs and symptoms (for example, cough and sputum production) in the intervals between acute episodes.[25]

## MIXED ASTHMA

*Mixed asthma* refers to a combination of extrinsic and intrinsic asthma. The major precipitating factor in this form of asthma is the presence of infection, especially of the respiratory tract.

## STATUS ASTHMATICUS

Status asthmaticus is the most severe clinical form of asthma. Individuals who suffer from status asthmaticus experience wheezing, dyspnea, hypoxia, and others symptoms that are refractory to two to three doses of β-adrenergic agents.[26]

Status asthmaticus is a true medical emergency. If this condition is not managed adequately or promptly, the patient may die as a result of the respiratory changes that develop secondary to respiratory distress. These changes may include hypotension and respiratory acidosis secondary to hypoxemia and hypercapnea.

## Prevention

The primary-care physician's goal in the long-term management of asthma is to maintain the patient's pulmonary status as close to normal as possible for as long as possible. With the advent of newer and longer-acting medications, this goal is more realistic. A second factor that has helped to further this goal is the recognition that the pulmonary status of most asthmatic patients is far from normal in the period between acute episodes. Thus the goal in dental management of the asthmatic patient is the prevention of acute episodes, an end best accomplished through use of the information obtained from the patient's medical history and the dialogue history between the doctor and patient.

## Medical History Questionnaire

The University of Southern California medical history questionnaire contains several questions that relate to a prior history of asthma, hay fever, and allergy.

### Question 6: Have you taken any medicine or drugs during the past 2 years?

*Comment:* Many patients with asthma, especially children, take oral drugs in the period between acute episodes to prevent or reduce the frequency of recurrence. The five categories of such drugs include β-adrenergic agonists, methylxanthines, chromones, corticosteroids, and anticholinergics (Table 13-1). These drugs usually have little impact on the planned dental treatment.

Long-term glucocorticosteroid therapy may be used for patients who experience acute episodes frequently in spite of the previously mentioned forms of therapy. Glucocorticosteroids have been used to manage asthma since 1950; the beneficial effects of these drugs most likely are related to their antiinflammatory actions because they have little or no direct bronchodilating activity.[27] Patients receiving long-term glucocorticosteroid therapy should be evaluated carefully for possible adrenocortical insufficiency.

A recent addition to the preventive management of acute asthmatic episodes is cromolyn sodium (Intal), which is used primarily for patients with allergic (extrinsic) asthma. The drug is effective only during periods of remission to prevent recurrences and decrease the patient's corticosteroid requirement. Cromolyn sodium is available as an inhalant in a micronized powder. In addition, most asthmatic patients regularly carry a drug used to terminate the acute asthmatic episodes, most commonly nebulized epinephrine, isoproterenol, or albuterol. These drugs are discussed near the end of the chapter.

table **13-1**   *Commonly prescribed drugs for the management of obstructive airway disease*

| CATEGORY | GENERIC | PROPRIETARY |
| --- | --- | --- |
| **Bronchodilator** | | |
| Sympathomimetic | Albuterol | Proventil, Ventolin |
| | Salmeterol | Serevent |
| | Metaproterenol | Alupent, Metaprel |
| | Bitolterol | Tornalate |
| | Pirbuterol | Maxair |
| | Terbutaline | Brethaire, Bricanyl |
| | Isoetharine | Bronkometer, Bronkosol |
| | Isoproterenol | Isuprel and others |
| | Epinephrine | Many brands |
| Anticholinergic | Ipratropium bromide | Atrovent |
| Theophylline | Theophylline | Many brands |
| | Aminophylline | Aminophylline |
| **Corticosteroid** | | |
| | Beclomethasone Dipropionate | Beclovent, Vanceril |
| | Triamcinolone acetonide | Azmacort |
| | Prednisone | Several brands |
| | Methylprednisolone Sodium succinate | Several brands |
| | Hydrocortisone sodium succinate | Several brands |
| **Antimediator** | | |
| | Cromolyn sodium | Intal |
| | Nedocromil sodium | Tilade |

**Question 9: Circle any of the following that you have had or have at present:**

Asthma
Hay fever
Allergy

*Comment:* An affirmative response to any part of this question should prompt the doctor to conduct a more in-depth dialogue history to find out how severe the patient's condition is.

## DIALOGUE HISTORY

**Do you have asthma?**

*Comment:* A positive response prompts further questioning.

**What type of asthma do you have—allergic (extrinsic) or nonallergic (intrinsic)?**

*Comment:* Patients are usually aware of they type of asthma from which they suffer.

**At what age did you first develop asthma?**

*Comment:* Allergic asthma most often develops in children and younger adults, whereas nonallergic asthma more commonly develops in individuals older than 35 years.

**How often do you develop acute episodes?**

*Comment:* The more frequently these episodes occur, the greater the likelihood that an episode will develop during dental treatment.

**What precipitates your acute asthmatic attacks?**

*Comment:* Awareness of the factors involved in a patient's acute episodes helps in their prevention during treatment. Stress is a particularly important factor in the precipitation of attacks in both extrinsic and intrinsic asthma. Therefore the patient's attitude toward dentistry must be determined and appropriate steps taken to ensure as stress-free an appointment as possible. The stress-reduction protocol is an invaluable tool (see Chapter 2).

**How do you manage your acute asthmatic attacks?**

*Comment:* Determine which drugs are used by the patient to terminate acute episodes. Most patients keep their medications with them at all times. The doctor should ask to see the medications, note them in the patient's chart, and request that the patient have them available at each visit (with frequent reminders). These medications, usually nebulized β-adrenergic agonists, should be kept within reach throughout the appointment.

**Have you ever required emergency care or hospitalization for your acute asthmatic episodes?**

*Comment:* This question seeks to determine the severity of the acute episodes. Although bronchodilator administration readily terminates most episodes, status asthmaticus is refractory to the usual β-adrenergic therapy. Hospitalization of the patient is normally required in such instances. With a history of prior need for emergency medical assistance or hospitalization, the dentist would be more likely to seek out such assistance earlier in an acute asthmatic episode than in a situation in which an asthmatic patient has never required emergency care.

## DENTAL THERAPY CONSIDERATIONS

Modifications in dental treatment depend on the severity of the asthma. Acute episodes precipitated by emotional stress in a patient with many fears of dentistry require judicious handling by the doctor to prevent an acute asthmatic attack. Use of the stress-reduction protocol minimizes the likelihood of acute episodes.

No contraindications exist to the use of any conscious sedation technique in fearful asthmatic patients; some drug groups, barbiturates or opioids (especially meperidine) should not be administered. Barbiturates

table **13-2** *ASA classification for asthma*

| ASA CLASS | DESCRIPTION | TREATMENT MODIFICATIONS |
|---|---|---|
| II | Typical asthmatic—extrinsic or intrinsic<br>Infrequent episodes<br>Easily managed<br>No need for emergency care of hospitalization | Reduce stress, as needed.<br>Determine triggering factors.<br>Avoid triggering factors.<br>Keep bronchodilator available during treatment. |
| III | Patient with exercise-induced asthma<br>Fearful patient<br>Patient with prior need for emergency care or hospitalization | Follow ASA II modifications.<br>Administer sedation—inhalation with nitrous oxide and $O_2$ or oral benzodiazepines, if indicated. |
| IV | Patient with chronic sign and symptoms of asthma present at rest | Obtain medical consultation before beginning treatment.<br>Provide emergency care only, in office.<br>Defer elective care until respiratory status improves or until patient can be treated in controlled environment. |

*ASA*, American Society of Anesthesiologists (Physical Status Classification System); $O_2$, oxygen.

and opioids may increase the risk of bronchospasm in susceptible patients. Opioids, especially meperidine, may provoke histamine release, which can lead to bronchospasm.[28] Barbiturates may sensitize the respiratory reflexes, increasing the risk of bronchospasm.[29] Both drug groups therefore are relatively contraindicated in asthmatics. Inhalation sedation with nitrous oxide and oxygen, oral sedation with benzodiazepines, and parenteral sedation via intravenous or intramuscular routes are not contraindicated in apprehensive asthmatics.

On rare occasion the patient's primary-care physician may advise the dentist that nitrous oxide administration is contraindicated. This statement is unfounded. Inhalation anesthetic agents, such as ether, that irritate the respiratory mucosa are capable of inducing bronchospasm in these patients.[30] Nitrous oxide does not irritate the respiratory mucosa, is an excellent antianxiety agent, does not provoke bronchospasm, and is absolutely indicated for the management of dental fears in asthmatic patients.[31] An asthmatic who also happens to be claustrophobic, may be at increased risk for asthmatic episodes if the nasal hood is used for delivery of anesthetic gases. Although it is no longer a recommended means of nitrous oxide and $O_2$ delivery, a nasal cannula may be used instead.[11,32]

Between 3% and 19% of asthmatics are sensitive to aspirin administration.[11,32] However, the incidence rises to 30% to 40% in patients who have nasal polyps and pansinusitus.[33] Substitutes for these drugs may be prescribed, but because there is considerable cross-sensitivity between aspirin and other nonsteroidal antiinflammatory compounds, special care must be exercised when analgesics are prescribed. (Nonsteroidal antiinflammatory drugs include indomethacin, fenoprofen, naproxen, ibuprofen, mefenamic acid, sulindac, meclofenamate, tolmetin, piroxicam, oxyphenbutazone, and phenylbutazone.)[34]

The food industry has used sulfur dioxide and other sulfiting agents for years in the preservation of foods from oxidation (the sliced apple being an example of a food that oxidizes rapidly when exposd to air). Reports have documented numerous cases of death and other severe reactions predominantly among individuals with asthma or a sensitivity to sulfites after eating such foods at restaurants. Reactions included urticaria, gastrointestinal upset, bronchospasm, and anaphylactic shock.[12]

Sulfiting agents, such as sodium metabisulfite, are added to certain drugs and chemicals as antioxidants. Individuals have experienced asthmatic reactions (bronchospasm) when they inhaled the bronchodilators isoetharine (Bronkosol)[35] and isoproterenol (Isuprel).[36] Local anesthetic cartridges with vasopressors (for example, epinephrine and levonordefrin) also contain bisulfites to prevent oxidation of the vasopressor.[37] Although the volume of bisulfite in the local anesthetic cartridge is minimal, bisulfite-sensitive patients have suffered acute asthmatic attacks after administration of these drugs.[38] The use of local anesthetics containing bisulfites (that is, all local anesthetics that contain vasopressors) is absolutely contraindicated in these patients. (In some situations, the contraindication may be only relative.) Local anesthetics that do not contain vasopressors (for example, lidocaine plain, mepivacaine plain, and prilocaine plain) should be used instead in these patients.

Table 13-2 classifies asthma according to the American Society of Anesthesiologists' (ASA) Physical Status Classification System. The typical, well-controlled, easily managed asthmatic represents an ASA II risk during dental treatment. Asthmatics who experience acute episodes precipitated by stress or exercise or who previously required emergency medical care or hospitalization to terminate an acute episode are ASA III risks; the very few asthmatics exhibiting clinical symptomatology while at rest are ASA IV risks.

## Clinical Manifestations

Signs and symptoms of an acute asthmatic attack range in severity from episodes consisting of shortness of breath, wheezing, and cough and followed by complete remission (ASA II or III) to more chronic states in which clinical signs and symptoms, which vary in intensity, are present almost continuously (ASA IV). Because the inability to breathe normally may terrify the individual, a large psychologic component is present in most episodes of asthma. Symptoms of acute asthma classically consist of a triad–cough, dyspnea, and wheezing.

### USUAL CLINICAL PROGRESSION

Signs and symptoms of acute asthma may develop gradually or suddenly (Box 13-2). In the typical episode the patient becomes aware of a sensation of thickness or congestion in the chest. This sensation is usually followed by a coughing spell, which may or may not be associated with sputum production,[39] and wheezing, which is audible during both inspiration and expiration. These signs and symptoms tend to increase in intensity as the episode continues. The patient experiences a variable degree of dyspnea, and in most episodes the asthmatic patient sits up as if fighting for air. Although the expiratory phase of the respiratory cycle is actually more difficult than the inspiratory phase for the majority of asthmatics, many asthmatics report that inspiration is more difficult and frequently state that they do not know where their next breath is coming from. Air-trapping within the lungs occurs during the acute episode, and asthmatics will sit up and use accessory muscles of respiration (that is, the sternocleidomastoid and scalenus muscles) to lift the entire rib cage cephalad and generate high negative intrapleural pressures, thus increasing the work involved in breathing.[40]

Wheezing does not by itself designate the presence, severity, or duration of asthma.[41] The degree of wheezing or its absence varies according to the radius of the bronchial tube. Mild wheezing is an audible,

box **13-2**    *Signs and symptoms of acute asthma*

Feeling of chest congestion
Cough, with or without sputum production
Wheezing
Dyspnea
Patient wants to sit or stand up
Use of accessory muscles of respiration
Increased anxiety and apprehension
Tachypnea (>20 to >40 breaths per minute in severe cases)
Rise in blood pressure
Increase in heart rate (>120 beat per minute in severe episodes)
Diaphoresis
Agitation
Somnolence
Confusion
Cyanosis
Supraclavicular and intercostal retraction
Nasal flaring

low-pitched, coarse, discontinuous noise, whereas increased airway obstruction produces a more high-pitched and musical wheeze, but it remains a low-intensity sound. Wheezing vanishes in individuals suffering severe airway obstruction because there is insufficient air movement velocity to produce sound.[42,43]

As the degree of dyspnea increases, so do the levels of anxiety and apprehension. Breathing during an acute asthmatic attack is labored, and the respiratory rate increases to more than 20 breaths per minute in most episodes, but to more than 40 breaths per minute during more severe episodes. This increase in rate may be the result of apprehension, airway obstruction, or a change in blood chemistry.

The blood pressure may remain at approximately baseline levels in milder episodes, but it usually rises during acute asthmatic attacks. The rise reflects the increased levels of catecholamines in the blood as a result of increased anxiety. In addition, the heart rate increases. A rate of more than 120 beats per minute is common in cases of severe asthma.

Other clinical signs and symptoms may be present during an acute episode that are not diagnostic of asthma but are noted with respiratory distress. Such symptoms include diaphoresis, agitation, somnolence or confusion, cyanosis, soft-tissue retraction in the intercostal and supraclavicular regions, and nasal flaring.[44]

If left untreated, the acute asthmatic episode previously described may last minutes or hours. Termination of the attack is usually heralded by a period of intense coughing with expectoration of a thick, tenacious mucus plug. This is followed immediately by a sensation of relief and a clearing of the air passages. Prompt management with an aerosol spray usually aborts the attack within seconds.

Regardless of its precipitating cause, acute asthma is characterized by respiratory smooth muscle spasm, airway inflammation with edema, and mucus hypersecretion. Respiratory smooth muscle spasm most likely accounts for the rapidly reversible types of airway obstruction, whereas inflammatory edema and mucus plugging in the airways account for the nonresponsive forms of asthma.[45]

## STATUS ASTHMATICUS

Status asthmaticus is a clinical state in which a patient with moderate to severe bronchial obstruction does not respond significantly to the rapid-acting β-agonist agents administered in the initial treatment protocol. In this situation, bronchospasm may continue for hours or even days without remission.

Patients in status asthmaticus most commonly exhibit signs of extreme fatigue, dehydration, severe hypoxia, cyanosis, peripheral vascular shock, and drug intoxication as a result of intensive pharmacologic therapy. The blood pressure may be at or below baseline levels, and the heart rate is quite rapid. The status asthmaticus patient requires hospitalization because the condition is life-threatening. Chronic partial airway obstruction may lead to patient death as a result of muscle fatigue of the muscles of respiration and respiratory acidosis. Status asthmaticus may develop in any asthmatic.

# Pathophysiology

Regardless of the type of asthma present, one finding common to all asthmatics is an extreme sensitivity of the airways characterized not only by increased contractile response of the airway smooth muscle but also by an abnormal generation and clearance of secretions and an abnormally sensitive cough reflex.[43]

## NEURAL CONTROL OF THE AIRWAYS

The autonomic nervous system significantly influences airway reactivity. Stimulation of the vagus nerve releases acetylcholine, which produces maximal constriction of the airways with an initial diameter of 3 to 5 mm.[46] Acetylcholine also increases glandular or goblet cell secretion and dilates pulmonary vessels.[47] This vagally mediated reflex bronchoconstriction may result from stimulation of the receptors in the larynx and lower airways, chemoreceptors, and subepithelial irritant receptors.[48]

In the adrenergic nervous system, stimulation of β-receptors results in dilation of the airway smooth muscle and bronchial and pulmonary vascular beds. Additionally, ion and water transport into the airway lumen is facilitated, and glandular secretion is likewise stimulated.[48,49] Stimulation of sympathetic nerves innervating the proximal airways has been shown to provide minimal bronchodilation.[47] Therefore the preponderance of the β₂-adrenergic airway receptor stimulation most likely occurs as a result of systemic catecholamine release from the adrenal medulla.[50] Stimulation of α-adrenergic receptors results in bronchial smooth muscle constriction; however, significant α-adrenergic contractile effects do not occur clinically except under conditions of β-blockade.[51]

The neural component in the pathogenesis of airway hyperreactivity may be summarized as follows.[43] Vagal sensory receptors in airways with increased bronchomotor responses (as a result of viral respiratory-tract infections and exposure to oxidant air pollutants) are stimulated and produce constriction. As a result the normal homeostatic dilator responses (for example, a β₂-blockade provoking bronchoconstriction in asthmatics but not in normal subjects) may fail; other possibilities currently are being investigated.[21]

## AIRWAY INFLAMMATION

Airway inflammation is another important factor in the production of increased airway responsiveness. Inflammation may occur as a result of either immunologic or nonimmunologic airway insults, which produce airway edema and the immigration of inflammatory cells into the lumen through the epithelium.[43] Inflammation is associated with an opening of tight cellular junctions and an increase in mucosal permeability, which provides access from the lumen to the airway smooth muscle, submucosal mast cells, and irritant subepithelial receptors.[52] This access may provide an environment that induces multiple methods of airway obstruction, including a direct effect on smooth muscle, a stimulation of mast cells, or vagal reflexes.[43]

## IMMUNOLOGIC RESPONSES

It is thought that allergic or presumed allergic factors are involved in the majority of asthma cases.[39] These factors may induce bronchial hyperreactivity, trigger acute asthmatic episodes, or both. Extrinsic asthma is classified as a type I immune reaction, an immediate allergic reaction in which an antigen combines with an immunoglobulin E antibody on the surface of pulmonary mast cells in the submucosa of small peripheral airways and in larger central areas at the luminal surface interdigitating with the epithelium.[53] The reaction causes mast cell degranulation and the release or formation of a number of chemical mediators, including histamine, prostaglandins, acetylcholine, bradykinin, eosinophilic chemotactic factors, and leukotrienes (LT).[54]

In addition, slow-reacting substance of anaphylaxis (SRS-A) has been shown to be composed of the leukotrienes LTC, LTD, and LTE. In humans, LTC and LTD are the most potent bronchoconstrictors—approximately 1000 times more potent than histamine[55]—with a duration of effect from 15 to 20 minutes.[56] (The physiologic actions of these mediators are presented in Chapter 24.)

Once the mast cells release the mediators, their pharmacologic activities develop rapidly so that clinical symptoms and signs of an acute asthmatic reaction manifest quickly. Type I allergic reactions are characterized by the rapidity of the reaction time (within 15 to 30 minutes after exposure to the allergen) and are associated with immunoglobulin E. Clinical examples of the type I immune response include asthma, anaphylaxis, and hay fever.

## BRONCHOSPASM

Smooth muscle is present throughout the entire tracheobronchial tree.[57] Bronchial smooth muscle tone is regulated by the vagus nerve, which, when stimulated, causes constriction (bronchospasm), and by the sympathetic nervous system, which produces dilation (bronchodilation).[43]

In nonasthmatic patients, bronchial smooth muscle protects the lungs from foreign stimuli; the airways narrow (bronchial smooth muscle constriction) in response to the foreign stimulus. In the asthmatic patient, however, this response is exaggerated (increased constriction), producing clinical signs and symptoms of respiratory distress. This constriction is most prominent in the small bronchi (0.4 to 0.1 cm in diameter) and bronchioles (0.15 to 0.1 cm in diameter); however, smooth muscle constriction may occur wherever smooth muscle is present.

The site of the asthmatic reaction can vary, depending on the anatomic location of the stimulated bronchial smooth muscle. Stimulation of irritant receptors by foreign particles (for example, gases, pollens, and chemical mediators) initiates an autonomic, or vagal, reflex. The stimulus is carried by the afferent fibers in the vagus nerve to the central nervous system and then by the efferent fibers, again in the vagus nerve, returning to the lungs; there the efferent fibers terminate on bronchial smooth muscle, producing muscle constriction.

## BRONCHIAL WALL EDEMA AND HYPERSECRETION OF MUCOUS GLANDS

In gross and microscopic sections of the lungs of patients who die during asthmatic episodes (usually status asthmaticus), many changes become evident, including mucosal and submucosal edema and thickening of the basement membrane, infiltration by leukocytes (primarily eosinophils), intraluminal mucous plugs, and bronchospasm (see Box 13-2).[9] In cross section the lungs appear overdistended, and mucus plugs occlude many of the smaller bronchi. In spite of the appearance of overinflation, the lungs of these patients exhibit areas of hyperinflation alternating with areas of atelectasis produced by mucus plugs.

All of these factors help decrease the size of the airway lumen, increase airway resistance, and produce the clinical signs and symptoms of bronchospasm (relative to the degree of airway narrowing). Airway resistance varies inversely to the fourth power of its radius. Therefore cutting the radius of an airway in half leads to a sixteenfold increase in airway resistance (according to Poiseuille's approximation).[58] The result of this increased resistance is increased difficulty in gas exchange and ultimately in alterations of blood chemistry and pH.

## BREATHING

Breathing is composed of two phases—inspiration and expiration. The inspiratory phase is an active process; thoracic volume increases as the diaphragm and other inspiratory muscles function. As volume increases the intrapleural pressure increases in negativity (from $-2$ to $-6$ torr), and the lungs expand to fill the increasing chest volume. The body then draws air into the lungs until these pressures are equalized.[59]

The expiratory phase normally is a passive process that does not require the individual to expend muscular energy. As the respiratory muscles relax, the elastic tissues of the lungs, which were stretched during inspiration, are able to return to their normal unstretched state in a process termed *elastic recoil*. This shortening of fibers forces air from the lungs, which permits the thorax to return to its normal resting state.

The asthmatic patient experiences varying degrees of airway obstruction that may produce large increases in airway resistance, which compromises airflow during inspiration and expiration. To accommodate the increased resistance during inspiration, the workload of the respiratory muscles increases in order to produce a greater degree of chest expansion to permit more air into the lungs.

The deleterious effects of increased airway resistance occur during the expiratory phase of respiration in the majority of asthmatics. The elastic recoil of the lungs during expiration is no longer adequate to expel air against the increased airway resistance, and air becomes trapped in the lungs, producing hyperinflation.[60] To minimize hyperinflation, the normally passive expiratory phase becomes active with both the respiratory and accessory muscles being used to expel air from the lungs.[61] In addition, the increased resistance impairs ventilation, or the quantity of air exchanged per unit of time, which results in an increase in the rate of breathing (tachypnea).

As the asthmatic episode progresses and airway obstruction worsens, the expiratory phase of respiration becomes longer and air increasingly is trapped in the lungs. The alveoli hyperinflate, producing both an increase in airway diameter from the increased tension and an increase in energy use. The increased use of energy is necessary during the inspiratory phase to overcome the tension of the already stretched elastic lung tissues and allow air into the lungs.

Therefore if an acute asthmatic episode progresses unresolved, much of the body's energy is expended on respiration. The muscles of respiration eventually become fatigued, further decreasing respiratory efficiency and leading to alveolar hypoventilation.[62] Clinical manifestations at this stage include increased dyspnea, tachypnea, and possible cyanosis. Severe alveolar hypoventilation produces carbon dioxide retention (hypercarbia), which is exhibited as an increase in the rate and depth of respiration (hyperventilation) and a further increase in the work of breathing. Sweating, or diaphoresis, is another clinical sign of hypercarbia.

The process is self-limiting. If airway obstruction worsens and the patient's efforts at breathing increase, the increased hypercarbia and hypoxemia lead to acute respiratory acidosis. Table 13-3 lists the signs and symptoms associated with hypoxemia and hypercarbia. Respiratory failure may occur with the patient requiring artificial ventilation. Mortality rates at this stage are high.

The following review of the pathophysiology of mild and severe acute asthmatic episodes may prove helpful (Table 13-4):

- During the mild asthmatic episode, produced primarily by bronchospasm, moderate airway obstruction leads to a decrease in blood oxygenation. The ensuing hypoxia and increased work of breathing result in a heightened level of anxiety, producing hyperventilation. Hyperventilation produces a decrease in the blood's level of carbon dioxide (hypocapnea) and subsequent respiratory alkalosis (see Chapter 12).

- In the more severe asthmatic episode (greater influence of airway inflammation) or in status asthmaticus the greater degree of bronchial obstruction results in a more profound decrease in blood oxygenation. The respiratory workload increases; however, the body's responses soon prove ineffective as the obstruction becomes greater, leading to inadequate ventilation and carbon dioxide retention, or hypercapnea. Hypercapnea causes respiratory acidosis and may lead to respiratory failure.

table **13-3**   *Clinical signs and symptoms of hypoxia and hypercarbia*

| HYPOXIA | HYPERCARBIA |
|---|---|
| Restlessness, confusion, anxiety | Diaphoresis |
| Cyanosis | Hypertension (converting to hypotension if progressive) |
| Diaphoresis (sweating) | Hyperventilation |
| Tachycardia, cardiac dysrhythmias | Headache |
| Hypertension or hypotension | Confusion, somnolence |
| Coma | Cardiac failure |
| Cardiac or renal failure | |

table **13-4**   *Physiologic changes that develop during moderate and severe asthma*

| SEVERITY OF AIRWAY OBSTRUCTION | PaO$_2$ | PaCO$_2$ | pH | BASE EXCESS |
|---|---|---|---|---|
| Mild | WNL | L | I | Respiratory alkalosis |
| Moderate | LL | WNL or L | WNL or I | Normal |
| Severe | LLL | I | L | Metabolic acidosis Respiratory acidosis |

From Barkin RM, Rosen P: *Emergency pediatrics*, ed 3, St Louis, 1990, Mosby.
*WNL,* Within normal limits; *L,* lowered; *I,* increased; *PaO$_2$,* arterial O$_2$, tension; *PaCO$_2$,* arterial carbon dioxide tension.

# Management

## ACUTE ASTHMATIC EPISODE (BRONCHOSPASM)

Management of an acute asthmatic episode requires prompt and specific drug therapy and symptomatic management.

*Step 1: termination of the dental procedure.* Treatment should cease immediately when the individual exhibits signs of an acute asthmatic attack.

*Step 2:* **P** *(position).* The patient should be placed in a comfortable position as soon as signs become evident. The position almost always involves sitting, with the arms thrown forward (Figure 13-2). Other positions are equally acceptable, based upon the comfort of the patient.

*Step 3: removal of materials.* All dental materials or instruments should be removed from the patient's mouth immediately.

*Step 4: calming of the patient.* Many asthmatics, especially those with histories of easily managed bronchospasm, remain calm throughout the episode.

Others, primarily those with acute episodes that have been more difficult to terminate, may exhibit varying degrees of apprehension. Dental personnel must always remain calm themselves and attempt to calm anxiety-ridden patients.

*Step 5:* **A-B-C** *(airway-breathing-circulation), (basic life support), as needed.* During the acute asthmatic episode the patient remains conscious, is breathing (with a partially obstructed airway), and usually has an increased blood pressure and heart rate.

*Step 6:* **D** *(definitive care): administration of bronchodilator.* Before treating an asthmatic patient the doctor should place the patient's bronchodilator aerosol spray within reach. This medication then should be used to manage an acute episode (Figure 13-3).

Bronchodilators are the drugs used to manage bronchospasm. The most potent and effective dilators of bronchial smooth muscle are the β-adrenergic agonists, such as epinephrine (Adrenalin), isoproterenol (Isuprel), and metaproterenol (Alupent) (Figure 13-4). These drugs are agonists of $\beta_2$-receptors in the bronchial smooth muscle and relax bronchial, vascular, and uterine smooth muscle. In addition, $\beta_2$-stimulation inhibits histamine release from mast

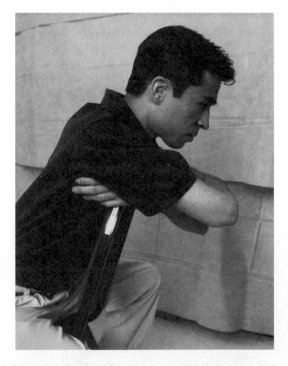

**Figure 13-2** Position for a patient suffering an acute asthmatic attack.

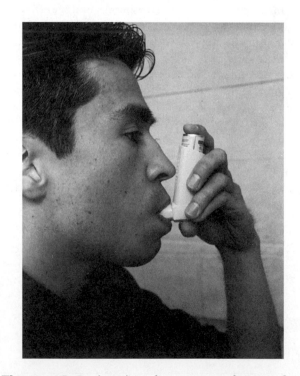

**Figure 13-3** A patient demonstrates the use of an aerosol inhaler.

cells, antibody production by lymphocytes, and enzyme release from polymorphonuclear leukocytes.[63]

These agents may be administered orally or sublingually, via aerosol inhalation or by injection. Although subcutaneous injection of epinephrine produces a rapid onset of relief, it is also associated with many other systemic actions, including dysrhythmias and hypertensive reactions; these reactions occur especially in patients receiving monoamine-oxidase inhibitors or tricyclic antidepressants.[64] Clinically, the best way to achieve bronchial smooth muscle relaxation is to administer β-adrenergic agonists via the inhalation of aerosolized sprays. This method provides an onset of action equal to injection but minimizes systemic absorption and side effects.[65] Aerosolized adrenergic bronchodilators are as effective as those administered via an IV route but have much less potential for serious side effects.[66]

The patient should be given the inhaler and instructed to take their usual dose to terminate the acute episode. Before ever needing to administer a bronchodilator, both the patient and the doctor should read the package insert to determine the maximum dose that may be administered safely in a given period.

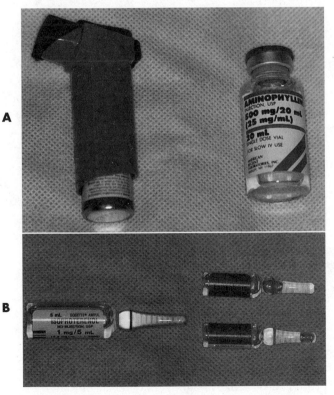

**Figure 13-4** **A,** Aerosol inhaler (left) and parenteral bronchilodator (aminophylline). **B,** A parenteral bronchodilator. Epinephrine (Adrenalin) may be administered via either an IV or intramuscular route.

Undesirable reactions associated with the use of these drugs relate primarily to the $\beta_1$- and $\alpha$–receptor-stimulating actions of epinephrine and isoproterenol. Metaproterenol is a partially selective $\beta_2$-agonist with little or no $\beta_1$- and $\alpha$-stimulating properties. The incidence of side effects (for example, tachycardia, 4%) is minimal.[67] Albuterol is a selective, fast-acting bronchodilator that lasts a long time and produces minimal side effects.[68] (I selected it as the bronchodilator of choice for inclusion in the office emergency kit.) Epinephrine and isoproterenol produce palpitations, tachycardia, and disturbances of cardiac rhythm and rate. In addition, epinephrine may produce headache and increased anxiety. Epinephrine is contraindicated in asthmatic patients with concomitant high blood pressure, diabetes mellitus (because epinephrine induces hyperglycemia), hyperthyroidism, and ischemic heart disease. Albuterol more frequently is recommended to treat acute asthma in patients with concomitant medical problems.

Another factor that should be considered is that prolonged use of these medications (months or years) may result in a state of refractoriness, which leads to prolonged episodes that are more difficult to terminate (status asthmaticus). Therefore these highly beneficial drugs must be used judiciously.

Aerosolized bronchodilators usually operate via a Freon-pressurized canister that dispenses a metered dose; only about 10% of the dose actually is inhaled.[69] The remaining amount becomes impacted in the oropharynx, but most is swallowed and biotransformed upon passage through the liver.

Proper use of the aerosol inhaler requires a very slow inhalation of the spray over approximately 5 to 6 seconds, as if the individual is sipping hot soup. The individual then should hold the breath at total lung capacity for 10 seconds and slowly exhale through pursed lips.[70] The onset of action of aerosolized bronchodilators is rapid, with improvement often noted within 15 seconds. To optimize inhalation of the aerosolized bronchodilator, the use of a spacer is recommended. The spacer serves as a reservoir into which the aerosolized bronchodilator is delivered and from which the drug is inhaled. Because the drug does not deliver to the patient rapidly, a greater percentage of the drug reaches the affected bronchi.

*Step 7: subsequent dental care.* Once the acute episode is terminated, the doctor should determine the cause of the attack. Appropriate steps in the stress-reduction protocol should be considered as a means to diminish the risk of future episodes. The planned dental treatment may continue at this visit if both the patient and the doctor feel that it is appropriate.

*Step 8: discharge.* After the acute asthmatic episode is resolved, the doctor may discharge the patient from the dental office without an escort if the doctor believes that the patient is in good condition. Such discharge is not usually a problem in cases of acute episodes that are terminated quickly with bronchodilator therapy.

## SEVERE BRONCHOSPASM

Management of the more severe acute asthmatic attack initially mimics the milder episode. However, more intensive treatment often must be used.

  *Step 1: termination of dental therapy.*
  *Step 2: P.* The patient should be placed in the most comfortable position.
  *Step 3: removal of materials from mouth.*
  *Step 4: calming of the patient.*
  *Step 5: A-B-C (basic life support), as needed.*
  *Step 6: D: definitive care.*
  *Step 6a: administration of bronchodilator.* In situations in which two doses of the aerosolized bronchodilator fail to resolve the acute episode, additional steps of management should be considered.
  *Step 6b: administration of $O_2$.* $O_2$ may be administered during any acute asthmatic episode, either through a full-face mask, nasal hood, or nasal cannula. (If a nasal cannula is used, a flow of 5 to 7 L per minute is adequate.) The presence of any clinical signs and symptoms of hypoxia and hypercarbia are indications for $O_2$ administration (see Table 13-3).
  *Step 6c: call for assistance.* When aerosolized bronchodilators fail to resolve bronchospasm, the appropriate team member should seek medical assistance (such as 9-1-1).
  *Step 6d: administration of parenteral bronchodilators.* In the management of more severe asthmatic episodes or in milder episodes that prove refractory to aerosol bronchodilators the injection of aqueous epinephrine is indicated. Epinephrine is available in a preloaded syringe containing 0.6 ml of a 1:1000 dilution in the basic emergency kit, whereas more advanced kits may contain epinephrine in a 1:10,000 concentration (in a 10-ml syringe). Both syringes contain 1 mg of epinephrine (see Figure 13-21). The usual subcutaneous or intramuscular dose of epinephrine (1:1000 dilution) in an adult patient is 0.3 ml, or 3 ml of a 1:10,000 solution administered via an IV route. This dose may be repeated as needed every 30 to 60 minutes.

Asthmatic children often cease exhibiting acute symptoms when they are removed from the treatment environment. If this simple measure proves ineffective, an aerosolized bronchodilator (for example, albuterol) should be administered. Only when this measure fails to resolve the bronchospasm should a 0.15- to 0.3-mg dose of epinephrine be considered.

  *Step 6e: administration of IV medications (optional).* Patients who prove refractory to the commonly used bronchodilators require additional drug therapy to terminate the acute episode. Drugs recommended for such patients include isoproterenol hydrochloride and corticosteroids (that is, hydrocortisone sodium succinate, 100 to 200 mg via an IV route). If the doctor possesses advanced training in emergency medicine and is able to start an IV infusion, these drugs should be considered for inclusion in the office emergency kit.

When respiratory failure appears imminent even after aggressive therapy with aerosols, isoproterenol should be administered. During and after isoproterenol administration the patient must be monitored closely because of the drug's propensity to provoke dysrhythmias.[71]

Glucocorticosteroids have been considered important in the management of severe acute asthma for more than 40 years. Although their direct bronchodilating activity is minimal, their antiinflammatory properties may make early administration of these drugs beneficial. After IV glucocorticosteroid administration, improvements in pulmonary function occur within 1 hour, usually peaking at 6 to 8 hours.[72] The general consensus is that "the early administration of steroids is perhaps the most important therapeutic measure to be taken in severe and resistant asthma, and they should be prescribed early in this situation and in higher doses."[73,74]

  *Step 6f: additional considerations.* Because asthmatic patients are usually quite anxious during acute attacks, the use of sedative drugs should be considered. However, the more severe the asthmatic attack, the more potentially dangerous the administration of any drugs that depress the central nervous or respiratory systems becomes. These drugs are absolutely contraindicated in cases of status asthmaticus or very severe asthma when any indication of carbon dioxide retention is present. Potential respiratory depression produced by sedative agents may be accentuated by concurrent hypoxia, and respiratory arrest may occur. In less severe episodes the judicious use of sedatives (for example 5 mg diazepam intramuscularly or via an IV route [preferred], titrated) may be indicated to decrease concomitant anxiety; however, their administration is rarely indicated. $O_2$ may be administered freely at any time during the asthmatic episode.

*Step 7: disposition of patient.* After the resolution of an acute episode of bronchospasm severe enough to require administration of parenteral drugs the patient frequently requires hospitalization so that physicians can reevaluate long-term asthma therapy. In other situations the emergency personnel may determine that the patient does not need hospitalization. In such cases a decision about how and when the patient may leave the office (that is, alone or escorted) should be made before the emergency personnel depart.

Box 13-3 summarizes the steps in the management of mild and severe asthmatic episodes. In addition, the following facts may prove helpful:

- **Drugs:** β-adrenergic agonists (epinephrine or albuterol) via aerosol, $O_2$, and isoproterenol and glucocorticosteroids (via an IV route) are used to manage severe acute attacks.
- **Medical assistance required:** No assistance is required if the attack is mild or easily terminated with aerosol therapy. However, if the attack is severe or refractory to aerosol therapy, the appropriate emergency team member should seek assistance.

---

**box 13-3**   *Management of acute asthma*

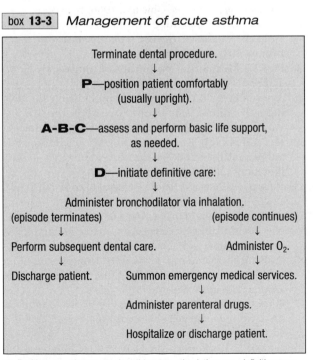

Terminate dental procedure.
↓
**P**—position patient comfortably
(usually upright).
↓
**A-B-C**—assess and perform basic life support,
as needed.
↓
**D**—initiate definitive care:
↓
Administer bronchodilator via inhalation.
(episode terminates)          (episode continues)
↓                                    ↓
Perform subsequent dental care.    Administer $O_2$.
↓                                    ↓
Discharge patient.          Summon emergency medical services.
↓
Administer parenteral drugs.
↓
Hospitalize or discharge patient.

**P,** Position; **A,** airway; **B,** breathing; **C,** circulation; **D,** definitive care; $O_2$, oxygen; *IV,* intravenous.

## REFERENCES

1. Eberle J: *A treatise on the practice of medicine,* vol 2, Philadelphia, 1830, John Grigg.
2. American Thoracic Society: Definitions and classifications of chronic bronchitis, asthma, and pulmonary emphysema, *Am Rev Respir Dis* 85:762, 1962.
3. Gregg I: Epidemiology of asthma. In Clark TJH, Godfrey S, editors: *Asthma,* London, 1977, Chapman & Hall.
4. Senior RM, Lefak SS: Status asthmaticus. In Fishman AP, editor: *Fishman's pulmonary diseases and disorders,* ed 3, New York, 1998, McGraw-Hill.
5. McFadden ER, Austin KF: Asthma. In Thorn GW and others, editors: *Harrison's principles of internal medicine,* ed 12, New York, 1991, McGraw-Hill.
6. Ford GT: Asthma—prognostic implications in the 1990s: morbidity-mortality evaluation, *Proc Annu Meeting of the Med Section of Am Council Life Insurance,* 1990.
7. Warner JO, Naspitz CK: Third International Pediatric Consensus statement on the management of childhood asthma, *Pediatr Pulmonol* 25(1):1-17, 1998.
8. Bone RC, Burch SG: Management of status asthmaticus, *Ann Allergy* 67(5):461-469, 1991.
9. Daniele RP: Pathophysiology of asthma. In Fishman AP, editor: *Pulmonary diseases,* New York, 1980, McGraw-Hill.
10. Kamada MM, Twang F, Leung DY: Multiple antibiotic sensitivity in a pediatric population, *Allergy Proc* 12(5):347-350, 1991.
11. Sonneville A: Asthma and aspirin, *Allerg Immunol* (Paris) 30(4):117-119, 1998.
12. Federal Drug Administration: Sulfite update, *FDA Drug Bull* 14:24, 1984.
13. Koepke JW and others: Inhaled metabisulfiite sensitivity, *J Allergy Clin Immunol* 75:135, 1984.
14. Levin RH: Advances in pediatric drug therapy of asthma, *Nurs Clin North Amer* 26(2):263-272, 1991.
15. Hudgel DW and others: Viral and bacterial infections in adults with chronic asthma, *Am Rev Respir Dis* 120:393, 1979.
16. Wilkerson LA: Exercise-induced asthma, *J Am Osteopath Assoc* 98(4):211-215, 1998.
17. Hijazi Z: Environmental pollution and asthma, *Pediatr Pulmonol Suppl* 16:205-207, 1997.
18. Murphy RH: Industrial disease with asthma. In Weiss E, Segal MS, editors: *Bronchial asthma: mechanisms and therapeutics,* Boston, 1976, Little, Brown.
19. Busse WW: The precipitation of asthma by upper respiratory infections, *Chest* 87:44(suppl), 1985.
20. Empey DW and others: Mechanisms of bronchial hyperreactivity in normal subjects after upper respiratory tract infection, *Am Rev Respir Dis* 113:131, 1976.
21. McFadden ER: Pathogenesis of asthma, *J Allergy Clin Immunol* 73:413, 1974.
22. Hamlett KW, Pellegrini DS, Katz KS: Childhood chronic illness as a family stressor, *J Pediatr Psychol* 17(1):33-47, 1992.

23. Fast TB, Martin MD, Ellis TM: Emergency preparedness: a survey of dental practitioners, *J Amer Dent Assoc* 112:499-501, 1986.

24. McCarthy FM: *Essentials of safe dentistry for the medically compromised patient,* Philadelphia, 1989, WB Saunders.

25. Ulrik CS, Backer V, Dirksen A: Mortality and decline in lung function in 213 adults with bronchial asthma: a ten-year follow-up, *J Asthma* 29(1):29-38, 1992.

26. Soler M, Imhof E, Perruchoud AP: Severe acute asthma: pathophysiology, clinical assessment, and treatment, *Respiration* 57(2):114-121, 1990.

27. Kussin PS: Pathophysiology and management of life-threatening asthma, *Respir Care Clin N Am* 1(2):177-192, 1995.

28. Ennis M and others: Histamine release induced by opioid analgesics: a comparative study using procine mast cells, *Agents Actions Suppl* 33(1-2):20-22, 1991.

29. Skidmore-Roth L: *Mosby's 1990 nursing drug reference,* St Louis, 1990, Mosby.

30. Tobias JD, Hirshman CA: Attenuation of histamine-induced airway constriction by albuterol during halothane anesthesia, *Anesthesiology* 72(1):105-110, 1990.

31. Little, Falace: *Dental management of the medically compromised patient,* ed 5, St Louis, 1997, Mosby.

32. McDonald JR, Mathison DA, Stevenson DD: Aspirin intolerance in asthma, *J Allergy Clin Immunol* 50:198, 1972.

33. Nagy GB: Acute severe asthma, *Acta Microbiol Immunol Hung* 45(1):147-152, 1998.

34. Mathison DA, Stevenson DD, Simon RA: Precipitating factors in asthma: aspirin, sulfites, and other drugs and chemicals, *Chest* 87:50s, 1985.

35. Twarog FJ, Laung DYM: Anaphylaxis to a component of isoetharine (sodium bisulfite), *JAMA* 249:2030, 1982.

36. Koepke JW and others: Inhaled metabisulfite sensitivity, *J Allergy Clin Immunol* 75:135, 1984.

37. Ciancio SG: Vasoconstrictors in local anesthetics, *Dent Management* 31(2):49-50, 1991.

38. Wright W and others: Effect of inhaled preservatives on asthmatic subjects: I. sodium metabisulfite, *Am Rev Respir Dis* 141(6):1400-1404, 1990.

39. Saunders NA, McFadden ER: Asthma: an update, *Dent Management* 24:1, 1978.

40. McFadden ER, Kiser R, DeGroot WJ: Acute bronchial asthma: relationships between clinical and physiologic manifestations, *N Engl J Med* 288:221, 1973.

41. McCombs RP, Lowell FC, Ohman JL: Myths, morbidity and mortality in asthma, *JAMA* 242:1521, 1979.

42. McFadden ER, Feldman NT: Asthma, pathophysiology and clinical correlates, *Med Clin North Am* 61:1229, 1977.

43. Nowak RM: Acute adult asthma. In Rosen P, editor: *Emergency medicine,* St Louis, 1988, Mosby.

44. Barkin RM, Rosen P: Pulmonary disorders. In Barkin RM, Rosen P: *Emergency pediatrics,* ed 3, St Louis, 1990, Mosby.

45. Hogg JC: The pathophysiology of asthma, *Chest* 82:8(suppl), 1982.

46. Olsen CR and others: Motor control of pulmonary airways studied by nerve stimulation, *J Appl Physiol Respir Environ Exercise Physiol* 20:202, 1965.

47. Cabezas GA, Graf PD, Nadel JA: Sympathetic versus parasympathetic nervous regulation of airways in dogs, *J Appl Physiol* 31:651, 1971.

48. Nadel JA: Airways: autonomic regulation and airway responsiveness. In Weiss EB, Segal MS, editors: *Bronchial asthma: mechanisms and therapeutics,* Boston, 1976, Little, Brown.

49. Richardson JB: Nerve supply to the lungs, *Am Rev Respir Dis* 119:785, 1979.

50. Leff A: Pathophysiology of asthmatic bronchoconstriction, *Chest* 83:13(suppl), 1982.

51. Leff AR, Munoz MN: Interrelationship between alpha- and beta-adrenergic agonists and histamine in canine airway, *J Allergy Clin Immunol* 68:300, 1981.

52. Nadel JA: Inflammation and asthma, *J Allergy Clin Immunol* 73:651, 1984.

53. Guerzon GM and others: The number and distribution of mast cells in monkey lungs, *Am Rev Respir Dis* 119:59, 1979.

54. Bisgaard H: Leukotrienes and prostaglandins in asthma, *Allergy* 39:413, 1984.

55. Dahlen SE and others: Leukotrienes are potent constrictors of human bronchi, *Nature* 288:484, 1980.

56. Weiss JW and others: Comparative bronchoconstriction effects of histamine and leukotrienes C and D (LTC and LTD) in normal human volunteers, *Clin Res* 30:571, 1982 (abstract).

57. Tortola GJ: The respiratory system. In *Principles of human anatomy,* ed 6, New York, 1992, Harper Collins.

58. Comroe JH: Mechanical factors in breathing. In *Physiology of respiration,* Chicago, 1966, Year Book.

59. Zamel N: Normal lung mechanics. In Baum GL, Wolinsky E, editors: *Textbook of pulmonary diseases,* ed 3, Boston, 1983, Little, Brown.

60. Mead J: Mechanical properties of lungs, *Physiol Rev* 41:281-330, 1961.

61. Agostini E: Action of respiratory muscles. In Fenn WO, Rahn H editors: *Handbook of physiology,* sec 3, vol I, Washington DC, 1964, American Physiological Society.

62. McFadden ER Jr, Kiser R, deGroot W: Acute bronchial asthma: relations between clinical and physiologic manifestations, *N Engl J Med* 228:221, 1973.

63. Nelson HS: Beta-adrenergic agonists, *Chest* 82:33(suppl), 1982.

64. Adverse reactions of drugs, *Med Lett Drugs Ther* 2:5, 1979.

65. Pliss LB, Gallaher EJ: Aerosol vs. injected epinephrine in acute asthma, *Ann Emerg Med* 10:353, 1981.

66. Williams SJ, Winner SJ, Clark TJH: Comparison of inhaled and intravenous terbutaline in acute severe asthma, *Thorax* 36:629, 1981.

67. Shim C, Williams MH: Bronchial response to oral versus aerosol metaproterenol in asthma, *Ann Intern Med* 93:428, 1980.

68. Godfrey S: Worldwide experience with albuterol (salbutamol), *Ann Allergy* 47:423, 1981.

69. Newman SP and others: Deposition of pressurized aerosols in the human respiratory tract, *Thorax* 36:52, 1981.

70. Dolovich M and others: Optimal delivery of aerosols from metered dose inhalers, *Chest* 80:911 (suppl), 1991.

71. Klaustermeyer WB, DiBernardo RL, Hale FC: Intravenous isoproterenol: rationale for bronchial asthma, *J Allergy Clin Immunol* 55:325, 1975.

72. Klaustermeyer WB, Hale FC: The physiologic effect of an intravenous glucocorticoid in bronchial asthma, *Ann Allergy* 37:80, 1976.

73. Fanta CH, Rossing TH, McFadden ER: Glucocorticoids in acute asthma: a critical controlled trial, *Am J Med* 74:845, 1983.

74. Leung FW, Santiago SM, Klaustermeyer WB: Corticosteroid therapy and death in cases of acute bronchial asthma, *West J Med* 138:565, 1988.

# 14

# Heart Failure and Acute Pulmonary Edema

**H**EART failure is generally described as the inability of the heart to supply sufficient oxygenated blood for the body's metabolic needs.[1] Congestion from fluid accumulates in the pulmonary circulation, systemic circulation, or both. When failure occurs solely in the left ventricle, the signs and symptoms are related to congestion of the pulmonary vasculature, whereas individuals with right ventricular failure commonly exhibit signs and symptoms of systemic venous and capillary congestion. Left and right ventricular failure may develop independently or occur simultaneously. The term *congestive heart failure (CHF)* refers to a combination of left and right ventricular failure in which evidence of both systemic and pulmonary congestion exists. *Acute pulmonary edema* is a life-threatening condition marked by an excess of serous fluid in the alveolar spaces or interstitial tissues of the lungs and is accompanied by extreme difficulty in breathing.

The human heart functions under normal conditions as a pump, supplying the tissues and organs of the body with a supply of blood that contains oxygen and nutrients sufficient to meet their metabolic needs both at rest and during activity. When viewed as a pump the heart is remarkable not only for its ability to adjust rapidly to the varying metabolic requirements of the body but also for its extreme durability. The heart lasts a lifetime—literally.

225

As durable as the heart is, it is also vulnerable to a large number of disorders—congenital, metabolic, inflammatory, and degenerative—that can affect its ability to function adequately as a pump. Cardiac dysfunction usually manifests itself clinically in one of two ways. In the first, signs and symptoms of the dysfunction occur directly at the site of the heart. These include chest pains and palpitations, represented clinically as angina pectoris (see Chapter 27), myocardial infarction (see Chapter 28), and cardiac dysrhythmias. The second type includes signs and symptoms that are extracardiac and originate in organs of the body that are either hyperperfused (congested) or hypoperfused (ischemic) with blood. Heart failure is a clinical expression of the former.

Under normal circumstances the right ventricle should outperform and outlast the left ventricle. In addition, the left ventricle is more vulnerable to heart disease and disorders in its blood supply than the right ventricle. Therefore the individual usually notes the first expression of heart failure in the left ventricle. Isolated right ventricular failure is extremely rare; usually the right ventricle fails shortly after left ventricular failure occurs. (Cardiac function, both normal and pathologic, will be discussed further in later sections of this chapter.)

Heart failure therefore represents a clinical diagnosis that is applied to a group of signs and symptoms that occur when the heart is unable to handle its load as a pump, thus depriving the various tissues and organs of an adequate supply of $O_2$ and nutrients. The degree of heart failure may vary dramatically; patients may exhibit only mild clinical signs and symptoms that arise solely on exertion, whereas patients with severe heart failure may demonstrate signs and symptoms in the resting state.

All patients with heart failure represent increased risk during dental treatment. The dental treatment plan may have to be modified to accommodate various degrees of cardiac dysfunction. Patients with more advanced heart failure or those with moderate degrees of heart failure who face physiologic or psychologic stress, or both, may experience exacerbation of their heart failure. This can lead to acute pulmonary edema, in which the patient exhibits extreme degrees of respiratory distress. Acute pulmonary edema is a life-threatening medical emergency that must be managed quickly and aggressively.

More than 2 million Americans suffer CHF.[1] In 1984 doctors discharged more than 450,000 patients from the hospital with a primary diagnosis of CHF.[2] Unfortunately, the prognosis for those with CHF is poor. One study found that after patients were initially diagnosed, 52% of males and 34% of females were dead within 4 years.[3] Another study reported an overall mortality of 75% 6 years after CHF diagnosis.[4]

Most individuals with progressive cardiovascular disease develop some degree of heart failure at some stage of their lives. (A discussion of the etiologic factors found in the majority of these cardiovascular diseases will be discussed in Chapter 26.) Thus the dentist must manage the dental needs of patients with varying degrees of heart failure. Most importantly, patients must be evaluated adequately before the actual treatment begins. In this way measures may be taken to prevent acute episodes of heart failure (acute pulmonary edema).

## Predisposing Factors

The tendency of heart failure to begin as left ventricular failure relates to the disproportionate workload of, and the prevalence of cardiac disease in, the left ventricle. Disease produces heart failure in one of the two basic ways:

1. Increasing the workload of the heart (for example, high blood pressure produces an increased resistance to the ejection of blood from the left ventricle, increasing the workload of the myocardium)
2. Damaging the muscular walls of the heart through coronary artery disease or myocardial infarction.

(Other causes of increased cardiac workload include cardiac valvular deficiencies [for example, stenosis or insufficiency of the aortic, mitral, tricuspid, or pulmonary valves], increases in the body's requirement for $O_2$ and nutrients [for example, pregnancy, hyperthyroidism, anemia, Paget's disease], and hypertension, which is responsible for more than 75% of all cases of congestive heart failure[5])

Left ventricular failure is the leading cause of right ventricular failure. Other causes of isolated right ventricular failure include mitral stenosis, pulmonary vascular or parenchymal disease, and pulmonary valvular stenosis, all of which significantly increase the workload of the right ventricle.

Any factor that increases the workload of the heart may precipitate an acute exacerbation of preexisting heart failure, which may result in acute pulmonary edema. Acute pulmonary edema may occur at any time, but occurs most often at night, after the individual has been asleep for a few hours. (This latter point will be discussed in more detail in later sections of this chapter.) Other factors that may increase cardiac workload include physical, psychologic, and climatic stress. Dental offices may easily precipitate such stress.

In pediatric patients heart failure may also be produced by an obstruction to the outflow of blood from the heart (for example, coarctation of the aorta or pulmonary stenosis). Of all children who develop CHF, 90% do so within the first year of life secondary to congenital heart lesions.[6] Older children may also develop CHF as a result of congenital heart lesions; however, much more common causes include disease acquired from cardiomyopathy, bacterial endocarditis, or rheumatic carditis.

## Prevention

The medical history questionnaire and the dialogue history are the best forms of prevention.

### Medical History Questionnaire

**Question 9: Circle any of the following that you have had or have at present:**

Heart failure
Heart murmur
Rheumatic fever
Congenital heart lesions
Scarlet fever

*Comment:* A positive response to any of the aforementioned conditions should prompt further questioning via dialogue history to determine the degree of severity and other relevant factors concerning the disease. All the conditions listed in Question 9 can lead to the development of varying degrees of heart failure.

**Question 10: When you walk up stairs or take a walk, do you ever have to stop because of pain in your chest, shortness of breath, or extreme fatigue?**

*Comment:* The ability to negotiate a normal flight of stairs or to walk two level city blocks is an excellent gauge of cardiorespiratory fitness. Shortness of breath that develops after mild exercise, termed *exertional dyspnea,* is an early sign of left ventricular failure.

**Question 11: Do your ankles swell during the day?**

*Comment:* In response to a positive answer, the time of night or day that the swelling develops should be determined. Dependent edema occurs late in the day after many hours of standing in most patients with right ventricular failure. This sign may also be seen in other clinical states, such as the later stages of pregnancy, varicose veins, or renal failure.

**Question 12: Do you use more than two pillows to sleep?**

*Comment:* Orthopnea is dyspnea that occurs while the patient is in the supine position; elevation of the trunk relieves

this condition.[7] Clinically, the patient cannot breathe comfortably while lying down and requires three or more pillows to do so, a condition termed three-pillow orthopnea. In severe cases the patient may rest or sleep only while maintaining an erect or upright position. Orthopnea is a sign of left ventricular failure. Modifications in the position of the patient or the dental chair may be required during treatment.

**Question 13: Have you lost or gained more than 10 pounds in the past year?**

*Comment:* An individual who reports having gained more than 10 pounds—especially if the gain occurred rapidly or without an apparent reason—may indicate the development of CHF. Retention of fluid is a significant factor in the development of CHF. An in-depth dialogue history must be performed to determine whether other reasons may explain the weight gain.

**Question 14: Do you ever awaken from sleep short of breath?**

*Comment:* Termed *paroxysmal nocturnal dyspnea,* this clinical sign usually indicates a more significant degree of left ventricular failure. Patients awaken from sleep short of breath and must sit up or stand, especially in front of an open window, to relieve their distress.

**Question 6: Have you taken any medicine or drugs during the past 2 years?**

*Comment:* Patients diagnosed with heart failure frequently take one or more of the following: diuretics, vasodilators, medications for high blood pressure, or inotropic agents such as digitalis.

Diuretics are often the first line of defense in the treatment of CHF. This class of drugs suppresses renal tubular reabsorption of sodium and helps in the management of diseases associated with excessive sodium and fluid retention. Several groups of diuretics are available, including thiazides, loop, and potassium-sparing diuretics (Box 14-1).

Inotropic agents, with the exception of digitalis, are reserved for the treatment of acute pulmonary edema and refractory CHF in hospitalized patients. These include dopamine,[8] dobutamine,[9] amrinone,[10] milrinone,[10,11] and aminophylline.

The fundamental action of digitalis glycosides is to increase the force and velocity of cardiac contraction, regardless of whether or not the heart is failing, through their positive inotropic actions. In CHF digitalis significantly increases cardiac output, decreases right atrial pressure, decreases venous pressure, and increases the excretion of sodium and water, thus correcting some of the hemodynamic and metabolic alterations that occur in heart failure. Digitalis decreases the heart rate, whereas it increases the demand of the myocardium for $O_2$.

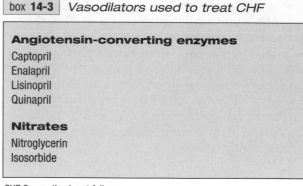

box **14-1**   *Diuretics used to manage CHF*

**Thiazides**
Hydrochlorothiazide
Chlorthalidone
Metazolone

**Loop diuretics**
Furosemide
Bumetanide
Ethacrynic acid

**Potassium-sparing diuretics**
Spironolactone
Triamterene
Amiloride

*CHF,* Congestive heart failure.

box **14-2**   *Inotropic agents used to treat CHF*

Digoxin
Dopamine
Dobutamine
Amrinone
Milrinone
Aminophylline

*CHF,* Congestive heart failure.

box **14-3**   *Vasodilators used to treat CHF*

**Angiotensin-converting enzymes**
Captopril
Enalapril
Lisinopril
Quinapril

**Nitrates**
Nitroglycerin
Isosorbide

*CHF,* Congestive heart failure.

## DIALOGUE HISTORY

After reviewing the medical history questionnaire, the dialogue history is used to gather additional information concerning the severity of the heart failure.

**Can you carry out your normal daily activities without becoming unduly fatigued?**

*Comment:* Related to question 10 on the medical history questionnaire, this question considers the presence of undue fatigue while the individual is at rest, not during exercise. Undue fatigue is a common symptom of left or right ventricular failure, or both. Fatigue and general weakness are usually the first clinical manifestations of heart failure.

**Can you climb a normal flight of stairs or walk two level city blocks without distress?**

*Comment:* As it relates to the preceding question, the inability to climb a normal flight of stairs or walk two level city blocks without distress signals an inefficient cardiorespiratory system. The following categories, based on the American Society of Anesthesiologists' (ASA) Physical Status Classification System, may indicate a patient's status in relation to this question (Figure 14-1):

- ASA I patients (that is, normal, healthy patients) can climb one flight of stairs or walk two level city blocks without having to pause because of shortness of breath, undue fatigue, or chest pain.
- ASA II patients can climb one flight of stairs or walk two level city blocks without distress but must stop once they complete either task because of distress. Patients with CHF most likely experience shortness of breath or undue fatigue.
- ASA III patients can climb one flight of stairs or walk two city blocks but must stop and rest before completing the task because of distress.
- ASA IV patients cannot negotiate a flight of stairs or walk two level city blocks because of shortness of breath or undue fatigue present at rest.

Although digitalis is still considered an important therapeutic modality for CHF, more and more frequently vasodilators, diuretics, and inotropic agents are replacing it (Box 14-2).

High blood pressure is one of the leading causes of left ventricular failure. Antihypertensive drugs are frequently prescribed for patients who suffer CHF. Knowledge of which drugs the patient takes helps the doctor to better understand the degree of cardiac dysfunction. This knowledge also enables the doctor to prevent the occurrence of certain side effects associated with many antihypertensive drugs.

Within the past 10 years, vasodilators have become significantly more popular in the management of CHF (Box 14-3). Depending on whether a drug is a venodilator, arteriodilator, or possesses mixed properties, CHF treatment can be tailored for the individual patient after a consideration of several factors, including blood pressure, degree of pulmonary congestion, degree of peripheral edema, concomitant presence of angina pectoris, renal hypoperfusion, heart rate, and likelihood of patient compliance.

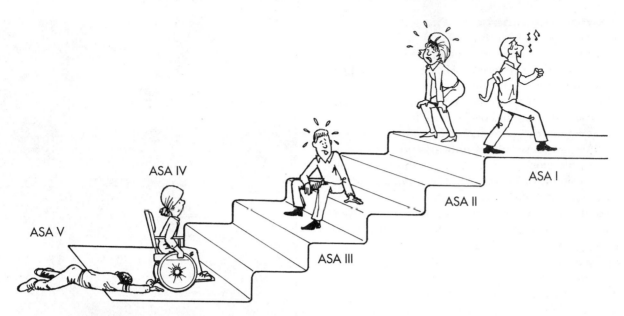

**Figure 14-1**  The ASA classification for CHF. *CHF,* Congestive heart failure. (Courtesy Dr. Lawrence Day.)

### Have you ever awakened at night short of breath?

*Comment: Paroxysmal nocturnal dyspnea,* awakening at night short of breath, usually occurs in more advanced left ventricular failure. Medical consultation should be considered seriously before any dental treatment is begun.

### What is the cause of your child's CHF?

*Comment:* Pediatric patients with CHF secondary to other diseases have a history of congenital or other heart problems. In such cases the parent or guardian should discuss the child's health status with the doctor. Consultation with the patient's primary-care physician is also warranted in cases of pediatric CHF. In the first year of life, 90% of children developing CHF do so because of congenital heart disease. Older children may also develop CHF as a result of congenital heart disease, but they more commonly suffer acquired CHF secondary to cardiomyopathy, bacterial endocarditis, or rheumatic carditis.[6]

In addition, the doctor may encounter patients who appear to have CHF but provide negative responses to the preceding questions. The doctor always must remember that many individuals accommodate their lifestyles to adapt to degrees of physical disability. For example, those persons who cannot climb a flight of stairs or walk two level city blocks may never try; they can use elevators or motor vehicles instead. The observant doctor always is on the lookout for clinical clues.

## PHYSICAL EVALUATION

Added to the steps outlined thus far, physical evaluation of the patient enables the doctor to determine the patient's current state of health more accurately than the medical history questionnaire or the dialogue history.

**Vital signs**    The patient's vital signs should be monitored and recorded. These include blood pressure, heart rate and rhythm (pulse), respiratory rate, and weight. Patients with CHF may demonstrate the following:

- The blood pressure may be elevated, with the increase in diastolic pressure greater than that in systolic pressure. The pulse pressure (the difference between the systolic and diastolic pressures) is narrowed. For example, a normal blood pressure of 130/80 yields a pulse pressure of 50; in contrast, a blood pressure of 130/100, as seen in cases of CHF, yields a pulse pressure of 30. In some situations the blood pressure may be decreased.

- The heart rate (pulse) and respiratory rate usually increase. Tachycardia is present because of the increased adrenergic activity, a principal compensatory mechanism for support of circulation in the presence of reduced cardiac output.[12] Tachypnea is evident early in the progression of CHF as the severity of dyspnea increases.

- Any recent, unexplained, large weight gain (more than 3 pounds in a 7-day period) may indicate the onset of acute heart failure. If such a gain occurs in conjunction with clinical signs of dependent edema (for example, ankle swelling), dental treatment should be postponed pending completion of a more extensive medical evaluation.

**Physical examination** The following areas should be inspected carefully:

- Skin and mucus membrane color: The skin color of a patient with more severe CHF may appear ashen-gray while the mucus membranes may be grayish-blue. Although skin color is important, perhaps more attention should be given to the patient's mucous membranes, particularly the nailbeds and lips. Cyanosis (a bluish tinge) indicates underoxygenation of the blood, and its presence should indicate the possibility of heart failure. Nail polish and lipstick may mask these areas, but the color of the intraoral mucous membranes can always be observed.

- Neck: Jugular vein distention develops in patients with right ventricular failure; when such patients are in the upright or semisupine position, their jugular veins may remain visible. In patients who do not suffer CHF, jugular vein pressure is negative when the patient is in the upright position and the veins are collapsed and invisible. However, in individuals with CHF whose central venous pressures are elevated, jugular veins remain visible.

Prominent jugular veins are normal when patients are in a supine position, but these veins gradually disappear as the patient slowly assumes a more upright position. At approximately a 30-degree angle or more upright, jugular veins should collapse and be undetectable (Figure 14-2). To determine increased jugular vein pressure, the distance that the jugular veins are distended is measured vertically above the sternal angle of Louis; to this distance is added 5 cm for the distance to the atrium. The patient should be situated in a 45-degree upright position and the right jugular vein evaluated.[13] Normally this distance is not less than 10 cm $H_2O$ (the unit of measurement). The causes of elevated jugular vein pressure include right ventricular failure, pulmonic and tricuspid valve stenosis, pulmonary hypertension, right ventricular hypertrophy, and constrictive pericarditis.

- Ankles: Ankle edema, also known as *pitting* or *dependent edema,* may occur in patients with right ventricular failure, pregnancy, varicose veins, and renal failure. It occurs in the more dependent parts of the body, where systemic venous pressures rise to their highest levels. If the patient follows a normal pattern of sleeping at night and staying awake during the day, ankle edema develops in the afternoon and disappears overnight.

Edematous tissue may be differentiated from adipose tissue by a simple test. Pressure placed on edematous tissue for 30 seconds results in a "pitting" effect as the pressure forces the edema fluid from the area (Figure 14-3). This pitting gradually disappears once the pressure is released and fluid returns. In

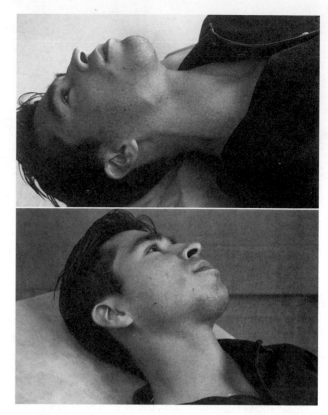

**Figure 14-2 A,** Prominent jugular veins. **B,** When the individual is positioned upright, the jugular vein disappears.

contrast, adipose or normal tissues return to their original shape immediately after the individual release of the pressure. As the severity of CHF intensifies, edema progresses, ascending to involve the legs, thighs, genitalia, and abdominal wall.[13]

## DENTAL THERAPY CONSIDERATIONS

The doctor now must examine all available information to determine the degree of risk that the CHF patient represents during dental treatment. The New York Heart Association[14] developed a functional classification of patients with heart disease based on the relationship between the symptoms and the amount of effort required to provoke them (Box 14-4).

The ASA physical status classification for CHF, which follows, is similar to the New York Heart Association's categorization:

- ASA I: The patient does not experience dyspnea or undue fatigue with normal exertion.
  *Comment:* If all items of the medical history are negative, this patient may be considered normal and healthy. No special modifications in dental

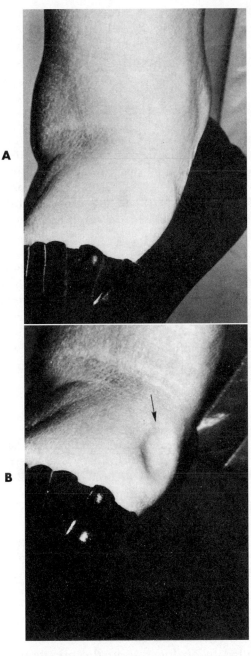

**Figure 14-3**  Ankle with dependent edema. **A,** The clinical appearance of an ankle before pressure is applied with a finger. **B,** Pressure on the right side of the ankle produces "pitting" *(arrow).*

treatment are indicated. Patients with heart failure are not ASA I risks.

- ASA II: The patient experiences mild dyspnea or fatigue during exertion.
  *Comment:* As with the ASA I patient, this patient may be managed normally if the rest of the medical history and physical examination prove to be non-

---

box **14-4**  *Functional classification for patients with heart disease*

**Class I: no limitation**
Ordinary physical activity does not cause undue fatigue, dyspnea, or palpitation.

**Class II: slight limitation of physical activity**
The patient is comfortable at rest. Ordinary physical activity results in fatigue, palpitation, dyspnea, or angina.

**Class III: marked limitation of physical activity**
Although the patient is comfortable at rest, less-than-ordinary activity produces symptoms.

**Class IV: Inability to carry on any physical activity without discomfort**
The patient experiences symptoms of CHF even while resting. Any physical activity produces increased discomfort.

*CHF,* Congestive heart failure.

contributory. In addition, use of the stress-reduction protocol should be considered if any physical or psychologic stress is evident or anticipated.

- ASA III: The patient experiences dyspnea or undue fatigue with normal activities.
  *Comment:* This patient is comfortable at rest in any position but may demonstrate a tendency toward orthopnea and have a history of paroxysmal nocturnal dyspnea. The ASA III CHF patient is an increased risk during dental treatment. Before beginning any treatment, medical consultation and use of the stress-reduction protocol and other specific treatment modifications should be seriously considered.

- ASA IV: The patient experiences dyspnea, orthopnea, and undue fatigue at all times.
  *Comment:* The ASA IV patient represents a definite risk. The heart cannot meet the body's metabolic requirements even at rest. Any degree of stress, which further increases metabolic demand, may exacerbate the condition and possibly provoke acute pulmonary edema. Dental treatment should be withheld for all elective procedures until the patient's cardiovascular disorder is corrected or controlled. Dental emergencies (for example, pain or infection) should be managed with medication; if physical intervention becomes necessary, the patient should be hospitalized under a physician's care before, during, and immediately after the dental procedure.

The stress-reduction protocol indicates the following general treatment modifications for CHF patients:

- Supplemental $O_2$: In patients with any degree of heart failure—indeed with any cardiovascular disorder (for example, angina pectoris or myocardial infarction)—no contraindication exists to the administration of $O_2$ during treatment. A nasal cannula or nasal hood from an inhalation sedation unit may also be used. A flow rate of 3 to 5 L per minute usually is adequate, but the flow rate should be adjusted in accordance with individual patient comfort (Figure 14-4).

- Positioning of the patient: Positioning of the CHF patient in the dental chair may require modification. If the patient finds it difficult to breathe while in the supine position, the doctor must modify the chair position until the patient is comfortable. As noted earlier, this condition is known as *orthopnea* and usually indicates a class III risk, which requires medical consultation before dental treatment. The

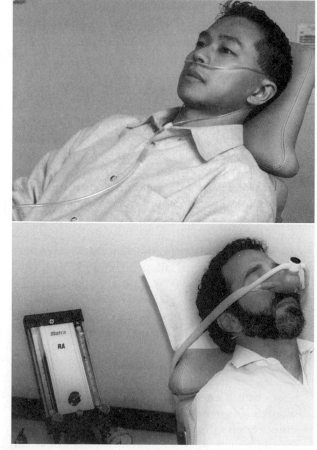

**Figure 14-4** The CHF patient may receive supplemental $O_2$ via nasal oxygen (**A**) or the face mask of an inhalation sedation unit (**B**). *CHF,* Congestive heart failure; $O_2$, oxygen.

use of rubber dam in this patient may be contraindicated as it may severely restrict the patient's already limited ability to obtain an adequate volume of air.

# Clinical Manifestations

Clinical manifestations of heart failure relate to the specific portion of the heart that is failing. Different individuals have varying degrees of heart failure so that not all patients exhibit all the symptoms and signs described in this chapter. In addition, most patients exhibit CHF, which is the combined failure of the left and right ventricles.

Clinical signs and symptoms are presented individually for each ventricle, followed by a description of acute pulmonary edema. Left ventricular failure is manifested clinically primarily by symptoms associated with pulmonary congestion, whereas right ventricular failure is dominated by signs of systemic venous congestion and peripheral edema. Undue fatigue and weakness are prominent symptoms present in both types of heart failure.

## LEFT VENTRICULAR FAILURE

Manifestations of left ventricular failure are associated primarily with respiratory distress; the severity of the distress is related to the degree of heart failure.

Weakness and undue fatigue are usually the first symptoms that the patient with left ventricular failure notices. The patient becomes aware of these symptoms when feeling fatigued during a level of exertion that previously caused no fatigue. As the degree of heart failure progresses, the patient becomes fatigued with less and less exertion until fatigue exists even at rest.

Dyspnea, or difficulty in breathing, is usually evident on exertion. This condition is commonly accompanied by an increase in the breathing rate (tachypnea). Cough and expectoration are present, related to reflexes produced by the congested lungs and bronchi. The patient with early left ventricular failure may report an increased frequency of urination at night (nocturia), a symptom produced by the rediffusion of edema fluid in the extremities from extracellular sites back into the general circulation.

Orthopnea and paroxysmal nocturnal dyspnea are later, more ominous signs related to more severe left ventricular failure. Orthopnea is dyspnea that occurs soon after the patient lies flat and disappears soon after the patient sits up. The patient with orthopnea can alleviate the breathing difficulty by elevating the head and thorax with more than two pillows. As the degree of heart failure progresses, this patient may have to remain in the upright position (for example, sitting in a chair) even during sleep. Positioning of this patient for dental treatment may be difficult. If present, orthopnea and paroxysmal nocturnal dyspnea confer upon the patient an ASA III medical risk and require specific modifications in treatment.

When orthopnea and paroxysmal nocturnal dyspnea are severe, the patient may require the use of supplemental $O_2$ 24 hours a day (ASA IV risk); such patients carry portable $O_2$ cylinders with a nasal cannula. They cannot lie down while sleeping but must sleep in an upright position. Paroxysmal nocturnal dyspnea is an exaggerated form of orthopnea. The patient with PND awakens from sleep acutely short of breath and gasping for air, with a degree of respiratory difficulty that verges on suffocation. The patient desperately seeks relief from this distress and usually sits up or rushes to an open window to breathe fresh air. For unknown reasons such patients may exhibit inspiratory and expiratory wheezing ("cardiac asthma"). These episodes usually resolve within a few minutes but may progress to acute pulmonary edema.

The patient with moderate to severe left ventricular failure appears pale and is usually diaphoretic (that is, sweating). The skin is cool to the touch, and the observer has no difficulty noticing that dyspnea, or difficulty in breathing is present. Monitoring of vital signs almost always demonstrates an increase in the blood pressure, with diastolic pressure elevated more than systolic pressure. The pulse pressure (systolic pressure minus diastolic pressure) therefore narrows. Heart rate most often is increased. *Pulsus alternans,* the appearance of alternating strong and weak heart beats, may be detected, even though the basic rhythm of the heart remains normal; this condition occurs frequently during the later stages of heart failure. Tachypnea, or an increased rate of breathing, and hyperventilation, an increased depth of breathing, are common signs of left ventricular failure as a consequence of pulmonary congestion.

## RIGHT VENTRICULAR FAILURE

Right ventricular failure usually develops after left ventricular failure has been present for a variable length of time. Signs indicative of systemic venous congestion primarily characterize this condition. The patient first notices signs of peripheral edema. Swelling of the feet and ankles develops during the day and subsides overnight in patients with right heart failure. This condition is referred to as *dependent,* or *pitting, edema.* If the patient is bedridden for extended periods, the edema fluid relocates in the sacral region. Dependent edema is a characteristic feature of right ventricular failure. *Pitting* refers to the depression, or pit, that remains in the tissue after pressure is applied to and removed from the area and is comparable to the impression that the foot leaves in wet sand when an individual walks on the beach. Within seconds the fluid returns, and the pit disappears.

Like left ventricular failure, individuals with right ventricular failure experience weakness and undue fatigue, which are produced by the deficient supply of $O_2$ and nutrients to the tissues of the body. In addition, this lack of $O_2$ produces cyanosis, which is prominent especially in mucous membranes (for example, nailbeds and lips). Cyanosis is produced by the removal by the tissues of a greater-than-normal amount of $O_2$ from the arterial blood in an effort to compensate for the decreased volume of circulating blood. This decreased blood supply is also the cause of the coolness often noted in the extremities.

Another sign of right ventricular failure is the presence of prominent jugular veins in the neck. In normal individuals the jugular veins are not visible in an upright position, except during moments of emotional or physical stress or exertion; however, as the right ventricle fails, systemic venous blood cannot be delivered to the heart normally and the jugular veins become engorged.

Engorgement of the liver (hepatomegaly) and spleen (splenomegaly) also occur. On examination, an enlarged liver may be palpated.[13] In normal situations the lower border of the liver is not palpable beneath the right lower costal margin. With hepatomegaly the liver may become palpable from one to four fingerbreadths below the right costal margin. This procedure evokes a degree of tenderness in the area of palpation. As right ventricular failure progresses, the edematous areas enlarge so that the legs, thighs, and eventually the abdomen (ascites) demonstrate clinical edema. Congestion of the gastrointestinal tract also occurs and is associated with clinical signs of anorexia, nausea, and vomiting. Signs of edema in the central nervous system include headache, insomnia, and irritability.

In left and right ventricular failure the patient will frequently be quite anxious. Once the patient first experiences difficulty in breathing, hyperventilation often follows. Indeed patients with heart failure may hyperventilate to the point of inducing respiratory alkalosis, with clinical symptoms of lightheadedness, coldness in the hands, and tingling in the fingers (see Chapter 12). In response to anxiety the workload of the heart increases even further, increasing the degree of heart failure.

## ACUTE PULMONARY EDEMA

Acute pulmonary edema is a life-threatening medical emergency in which a sudden and rapid transudation of fluid occurs from the pulmonary capillary bed into the alveolar spaces of the lungs.[15] Often, stressful situations—either physical or psychologic—precipitate this condition, but a salty meal, noncompliance with medications, or infection may also induce acute pulmonary edema.

The onset of symptoms is usually acute. A slight, dry cough is often the initial symptom; acute pulmonary edema may represent a direct extension of paroxysmal nocturnal dyspnea. Asthmatic-type wheezing (that is, cardiac asthma) may also be present. Dyspnea and orthopnea are commonly present. As the episode progresses, the patient experiences a feeling of suffocation and an acute sense of anxiety that further increases the rate and difficulty of breathing. Patients also may experience a sense of oppression in the chest. Physical signs that are evident at this time include tachypnea, dyspnea, and cough. If auscultated, the lungs demonstrate moist rales at their bases that progressively extend upward as the episode worsens.

In more severe episodes, patients exhibit pallor, sweating, cyanosis, and a frothy, pink (blood-tinged) sputum. Acute pulmonary edema is common during the period immediately after myocardial infarction if the degree of left ventricular myocardial damage is significant. Most individuals resist attempts at recumbency, may panic, and often remain uncooperative (Table 14-1).

## Pathophysiology

To view heart failure in its proper perspective, it is necessary to first review the function of the healthy human heart both at rest and during physical activity. The mechanisms of cardiac dysfunction then become more obvious.

The heart is designed to propel unoxygenated blood to the lungs and oxygenated blood to the peripheral tissues in accordance with their metabolic needs.[16] The human heart is composed of two individual pumps that work together (Figure 14-5). The right side of the heart receives venous (unoxygenated) blood from the body's systemic circulation and pumps this blood through the pulmonary arteries to the lungs, where it undergoes oxygenation. From the lungs, oxygenated (arterial) blood is delivered to the left atrium and then to the left ventricle, where it is pumped into the systemic circulation.

The amount of work that each ventricle requires to perform its task is considerably different. The right side of the heart may be considered as a low-pressure system. An average right ventricular pressure of $24/4-10$ mmHg is required to pump blood into the pulmonary artery, the only artery that normally contains unoxygenated blood. In contrast, the left side of the heart is a high-pressure system; left intraventricular pressure is approximately 120/80 mmHg during systole (contraction). Thus the left ventricle performs the lion's share

| table **14-1** | Clinical manifestations of heart failure and acute pulmonary edema |
| --- | --- |

| SIGNS | SYMPTOMS |
| --- | --- |
| **Heart failure** | |
| Pallor, cool skin | Weakness and undue fatigue |
| Sweating | Dyspnea during exertion |
| Left ventricular hypertrophy | Hyperventilation |
| Dependent edema | Nocturia |
| Hepatomegaly and splenomegaly | Paroxysmal nocturnal dyspnea |
| Narrow pulse pressure | Wheezing (cardiac asthma) |
| Pulsus alternans | |
| Ascites | |
| **Acute pulmonary edema** | |
| All the signs of heart failure | All the symptoms of heart failure |
| Moist rales at the base of the lungs | Increased anxiety |
| Tachypnea | Dyspnea at rest |
| Cyanosis | |
| Frothy pink sputum | |

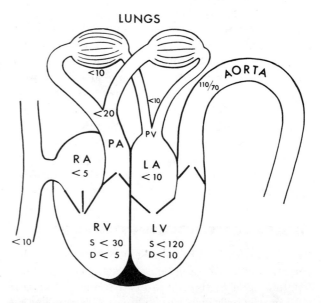

**Figure 14-5** Average blood pressures in various components of the circulatory system. *LA,* Left atrium; *LV,* left ventricle; *PA,* pulmonary arteries. (From Wylie WD, Churchill-Davidson HC: *A practice of anaesthesia,* ed 3, London, 1972, Lloyd-Luke.)

of the actual work of the heart. Before birth, both ventricles work equally because they bear the same pressure loads. After birth, pulmonary arterial pressure falls, the workload of the right ventricle decreases, and its walls become thin; conversely, the left ventricle's workload increases, and its walls enlarge.

The primary function of the heart is to serve as a pump, supplying oxygenated blood and nutrients to the body's tissues and cells. Table 14-2 lists minimal $O_2$ requirements per minute for the average adult performing various activities. If the heart for some reason cannot provide the body with its required $O_2$ supply, shortness of breath (dyspnea) and undue fatigue result. These signs normally appear when $O_2$ transport per minute falls below 1000 to 1250 ml per minute. At this level an individual can usually perform a light job and enjoy light recreation and sport without discomfort; the same individual cannot, however, perform more strenuous activities.

## NORMAL LEFT VENTRICULAR FUNCTION

The left ventricle is a thick muscular organ. At rest (diastole), left intraventricular pressure is approximately 6 to 8 mmHg, whereas the diastolic pressure in the aorta is approximately 80 mmHg. For blood to be expelled from the left ventricle into the aorta, intraventricular pressure must exceed aortic blood pressure so that the aortic valves can open. The following description outlines the normal sequence of left ventricular function when an individual is at rest.

Maximal left ventricular filling, termed *end diastolic volume,* occurs at the instant just before the start of systole. At this moment the muscles of the ventricle begin to contract, but blood is not yet ejected from the ventricle. Instead, the size of the ventricular cavity is rapidly decreasing, producing a sharp increase in intraventricular pressure. This interval, termed the *isovolemic period of systole,* normally lasts 50 milliseconds (ms), or about 0.050 seconds.

| table **14-2** | *Minimum adult $O_2$ requirements* |

| ACTIVITY | $O_2$ UTILIZATION (ML/MIN) |
| --- | --- |
| At rest | 250 |
| Standing | 375 |
| Walking | 400-1000 |
| Light work and exercise | 750-1250 |
| Intense exercise | 4000 and above |

*$O_2$,* Oxygen.

In a short time when intraventricular pressure exceeds diastolic aortic blood pressure (80 mmHg), the aortic valves are forced open and the ejection of blood into systemic circulation occurs. The ventricle continues to contract for a period of time (systole), after which relaxation occurs. The blood pressure within the left ventricle drops rapidly as the ventricle relaxes. Once the blood pressure in the left ventricle drops below that of the aorta, the aortic valve closes, signaling the end of systole and the beginning of diastole. During diastole, intraaortic blood pressure exceeds that in the ventricle, which permits the filling of the ventricle with blood.

When the aortic valves close, the volume of blood in the left ventricle is at its lowest level. The difference in volume between end-diastolic volume (maximum volume) and end-systolic volume (minimum volume) is termed the *ejection fraction.* In a normally functioning heart at rest, this fraction is 0.56 to 0.78; in other words, from 56% to 78% of the blood present in the left ventricle at the end of diastole is ejected into the aorta during systole. As left ventricular failure develops, the ejection fraction decreases and may reach levels as low as 0.1 to 0.2 in severe heart failure. Although this mechanism functions in normal situations, the demands on the heart change from second to second. The heart therefore must be able to respond rapidly to these ever-changing demands by increasing or decreasing the volume of blood it ejects per stroke (stroke volume).

Three factors—preload, afterload, and contractility—help to enable the heart to meet its obligations to the body's tissues. Preload is the end-diastolic volume. The greater the preload, the more the myocardial muscle fibers stretch. According to the Frank-Starling principle,[17] the greater the myocardial muscle stretches in diastole, the greater it will contract in systole; this is similar to the stretching of a rubber band. For example, with a preload of 100 ml of blood and an ejection fraction of 0.6 (60%), the stroke volume is 60 ml. If the preload increases to 140 ml and the ejection fraction remains 0.6, the stroke volume increases to 84 ml. In the same manner, decreased preload results in diminished stroke volume.

Afterload may be defined as the pressure that resists left ventricular ejection (aortic blood pressure). Increased afterload therefore makes more difficult the heart's attempt to eject a normal stroke volume. For example, if aortic blood pressure rises rapidly (as it may under extreme stress) from 120/80 to 200/120 mmHg, intraventricular pressure must rise to 120 mmHg (the aortic diastolic pressure) before the aortic valve can open. This valve will remain open for only a brief period before the aortic pressure once again exceeds that of the ventricle and closes the aortic valve. The ejection fraction in this instance is very low (0.1 to 0.2).

Such a stroke volume, if it continues indefinitely, is inadequate to support the body's requirements. Fortunately, the normal heart can compensate for this inadequate stroke volume. The end-systolic volume is larger than normal (because of the nonejected fraction of blood). To this is added the normal blood volume from the left atrium. This increase in preload (normal volume plus large end-systolic volume) causes increased stretch of the myocardial fibers, which results in a more forceful contraction with the next beat (the Frank-Starling principle). Within several beats the left ventricle can adjust the stroke volume to compensate for the increased aortic diastolic blood pressure, from 120/80 to 200/120 mmHg.

Limits to the Frank-Starling principle do exist, however, in that excessive stretch or a sudden increase in afterload is not met by an ever-increasing contraction of the myocardium. If the preload and afterload of the heart are permitted to remain the same, it is still possible for stroke volume to increase. Contractility is a basic property of cardiac muscle. The sympathetic nervous system can increase the heart's contraction through the release of epinephrine and norepinephrine. These catecholamines, which are released in increasing amounts under stress, increase the degree of myocardial fiber contraction, thus increasing the ejection fraction (from 0.6 to 0.8), resulting in an increase of stroke volume.

## HEART FAILURE

Heart failure may develop whenever the heart labors for extended periods of time against increased peripheral resistance (increased afterload), such as occurs in patients with high blood pressure or in patients with valvular defects (stenosis or insufficiency), or prolonged, continuous demands for increased cardiac output (as occurs in hyperthyroidism). These conditions, which demand a chronic increase in cardiac workload, all lead to structural changes in the heart muscle that eventually progress to muscular weakness and produce the clinical signs and symptoms of heart failure.

Another major cause of myocardial weakness is the presence of a disease state that directly attacks the myocardium (for example, coronary artery disease and myocarditis). In these conditions, cardiac muscle cannot respond normally to increases in afterload. The increase in fiber length that occurs as a result of increased ventricular filling is not met with the usual increase in stroke volume, and clinical heart failure results.

The chronic progression of heart failure is best illustrated by following the cardiac changes that develop in patients with high blood pressure, which is one of the primary causes of heart failure. In response to a sustained blood pressure elevation (afterload), the myocardium must contract more forcefully for an extended period to maintain an acceptable stroke volume. As with any muscle doing increased work for extended periods, the myocardial fibers hypertrophy, or increase in diameter and length. This response occurs primarily in the left ventricle and leads to the development of the first sign of heart failure, left ventricular hypertrophy.

A normal heart weighs approximately 250 to 350 g. In patients with mild heart failure the heart may weigh up to 500 g; in more severe cases of heart failure, the heart may weigh up to 1000 g. Left ventricular hypertrophy may be present for many years before being discovered, generally during a routine electrocardiogram or chest x-ray. Another important feature of hypertrophy is that along with the increased size of left ventricular muscle fibers there is not a corresponding increase in the number of capillaries to deliver blood to them; thus, myocardial blood supply becomes increasingly compromised as hypertrophy regresses. Because of the compromised blood supply seen in LVH a point is reached at which hypertrophy alone can no longer maintain an adequate stroke volume during a sustained increase in blood pressure.

At this point a second mechanism, called *dilation*, helps to maintain normal stroke volume. Dilation is an increase in the capacity of the left ventricle and is brought about by an elongation of the myocardial fibers. The force of ventricular contraction of these elongated myocardial fibers increases through the Frank-Starling principle, thus maintaining a normal stroke volume. However, both the end-diastolic (increased total blood volume in the ventricle) and end-systolic (increased residual blood after contraction) volumes are increased, and the ejection fraction of the left ventricle is decreased (<0.56). As the end-diastolic volume increases, the heart's workload increases, thereby increasing the myocardial $O_2$ requirement. In the presence of coronary artery disease or left ventricular hypertrophy this demand for $O_2$ may not be met, resulting in increasingly severe heart failure, angina pectoris, or myocardial infarction. As with left ventricular hypertrophy, dilation is evident on an electrocardiogram or chest x-ray.

If the blood pressure continues to rise or if the myocardium weakens, hypertrophy and dilation cannot maintain a stroke volume adequate to supply peripheral tissues with their required amounts of $O_2$ and nutrients. As this situation develops, the patient first begins to experience undue fatigue and dyspnea during exertion as the left ventricle becomes unable to increase its output in response to exercise. As left ventricular failure intensifies, dyspnea develops with less and less exertion (progressing from ASA II to III to IV risk levels).

Left ventricular failure also occurs at night when the individual lies down. At this time total blood volume increases as venous return from the lower extremities improves because of the decreased effect of gravity on the legs. To breathe comfortably, the individual must elevate the head and thorax at night with extra pillows. The elevation is necessary because the now-increased fluid volume begins to produce respiratory distress (for example, orthopnea) as fluid from the cardiovascular bed diffuses into alveolar sacs in the lungs, preventing the normal exchange of $O_2$ and carbon dioxide.

Blood volume increases in a second and perhaps more important manner that involves the kidneys. Decreased stroke volume leads to a decrease in renal blood flow and glomerular filtration rate, thereby decreasing the excretion of sodium. In fact, tubular reabsorption of sodium is actually stimulated through the increased secretion of renin and its attendant chemical reactions (secondary to a decreased GFR). Increased sodium retention prompts the pituitary gland to secrete decreased amounts of antidiuretic hormone, which is responsible for further water retention. These mechanisms result in a further increase in total blood volume (hypervolemia).

Hypervolemia produces increased hydrostatic pressure within the capillaries, leading at first to interstitial edema and then to an actual transudation of fluid into tissues with decreased tissue pressure. Edema of the ankles and lower extremities develops during the day when the individual is upright because of the downward effect of gravity; it develops in the sacral region when the individual is recumbent, either at night or for long periods during illness or convalescence. Clinical signs and symptoms of left ventricular failure become more prominent at night, when most individuals assume recumbent positions for sleep. During the day, when an individual is in an erect position, the force of gravity causes the excessive fluid volume to be deposited into the subcutaneous tissues in the most dependent portions of the body (for example, the ankles), producing signs of right ventricular failure.

When an individual assumes the supine position, the edematous fluid in the dependent portions of the body is reabsorbed into the cardiovascular system, leading to an increase in blood volume and venous return to the heart. This increase may result in overdistention of an already-weakened left ventricle, producing an acute reduction in cardiac output and a large increase in the end-diastolic and end-systolic volumes. As a result the end-diastolic pressure may also rise. A normal end-diastolic pressure of 6 to 8 mmHg may rise to 30 to 40 mmHg or greater. The increased left ventricular pressure leads to increased pressure in the left atrium. The Frank-Starling principle enables the left atrium to accommodate this increasing pressure, and after a few heartbeats the pressure in the left atrium increases to 30 to 40 mmHg or above, remaining elevated for as long as the left ventricle is failing. This increased left atrial pressure is next transmitted backward to the pulmonary veins and capillaries so that the pulmonary capillary pressure also increases to 30 to 40 mmHg. When this occurs, water and solutes diffuse from the capillaries into the alveolar air sacs, producing paroxysmal nocturnal dyspnea, acute pulmonary edema, or both.

When the alveolar air sacs contain fluid, $O_2$ and carbon dioxide cannot be exchanged and dyspnea results. Bronchospasm (cardiac asthma) is a common complicating factor of paroxysmal nocturnal dyspnea. Positional changes (for example, from the supine to upright position) commonly produce dramatic relief from symptoms of left ventricular failure by causing fluid to move from the alveolar sacs and concentrate in the base of the lungs.

Right ventricular and atrial failure occur shortly after left ventricular failure as the increased pressure in the left side of the heart continues to back up, resulting in signs and symptoms of systemic venous and capillary congestion. As this increase in pressure develops, fluid leaves the blood vessels in the most dependent portions of the body (for example, the ankles and feet). In addition, venous return from the head and upper extremities is impaired because of the elevated right atrial pressure, and the jugular veins become engorged. Impaired venous return from the lower portions of the body is evident through engorgement of the liver (hepatomegaly) and spleen (splenomegaly) with blood.

*Nocturia,* or increased frequency of urination at night, is yet another sign of heart failure. During the day, when the individual is awake, renal function is poor because the individual's activities increase the degree of heart failure. Therefore less urine is produced during the day. At night cardiac and renal functions improve. Increased glomerular filtration produces more urine, and nocturia results.

One final sign of heart failure is cyanosis, which is most evident in mucous membranes and is produced by the heart's failure to provide an adequate stroke volume. To secure an adequate $O_2$ supply, the body's tissues extract more $O_2$ than normal from the capillary blood. Therefore the red blood cells within the capillaries and veins are poorly oxygenated and appear darker in color, which is clinically manifested as cyanosis.

# Management

The patient suffering acute pulmonary edema represents a true medical emergency requiring immediate management. The protocol outlined below should be followed to treat the dental patient who has a history of heart failure—either left or right ventricular failure—or combined failure (CHF):

Step 1: termination of the dental procedure. As soon as the patient begins to exhibit signs and symptoms of heart failure, all dental treatment should cease.

Step 2: removal of dental materials. All dental materials and instruments should be removed from the patient's mouth.

Step 3: P (position). As with patients suffering other forms of acute respiratory distress, the patient suffering acute pulmonary edema usually remains conscious. This patient may appear panicky and uncooperative.[1] The patient should be positioned comfortably, which in most cases will be the upright position. The upright position allows excess fluid within the alveolar sacs to concentrate at the bases of the lungs, permitting a greater exchange of $O_2$. If at any time the patient loses consciousness, that individual should be placed in the supine position.

Step 4: summoning of emergency medical services. At the onset of acute respiratory distress in a patient with preexisting CHF, the appropriate office team member should summon emergency medical personnel immediately. The patient usually requires hospitalization. Further medical management in the hospital may include phlebotomy, $O_2$, and drugs, such as digitalis and diuretics.

Step 5: calming of the patient. Dental personnel must reassure the patient that they are making every effort to manage the problem and that they have summoned emergency personnel.

Step 6: A-B-C (airway-breathing-circulation), (basic life support), as needed. In acute pulmonary edema the airway, breathing, and circulation are (usually) adequately maintained by the patient.

Step 7: D definitive care:
Step 7a: administration of $O_2$. $O_2$ should be administered to all patients who demonstrate signs of acute pulmonary edema or severe CHF. Such patients require high concentrations at high flows to prevent or alleviate hypoxia. Face masks should be used with a flow rate of 10 L or more of $O_2$ per minute.

Step 7b: monitoring of vital signs. Vital signs, including blood pressure, heart rate and rhythm, and respiratory rate, should be monitored and recorded every 5 minutes. The blood pressure, heart rate, and respiratory rate increase in those suffering heart failure; these changes demonstrate the presence of extreme apprehension and cardiac and pulmonary congestion.

Step 7c: alleviation of symptoms. The immediate goal in the management of acute pulmonary edema is to alleviate the patient's breathing difficulties. Proper positioning (per patient wishes, but usually upright) is extremely important. If respiratory distress is still evident, however, additional steps may be required. In cases of acute pulmonary edema the heart cannot adequately handle the quantity of blood being delivered to it.

Step 7d: bloodless phlebotomy. Phlebotomy is a procedure that may be performed in the hospital. Approximately 350 to 500 ml of blood is removed from the patient. Phlebotomy is sometimes rapidly effective in the reduction of respiratory symptoms because venous return to the right side of the heart is reduced while the left side drains some excess fluid from the lungs.

Phlebotomy in the dental office is not often indicated. However, a bloodless phlebotomy may achieve a similar effect. Bloodless phlebotomy temporarily removes approximately 12% of circulating blood volume, or 700 of 6000 ml in the average adult male, permitting the heart to function more effectively and dyspnea to be alleviated.[18] Tourniquets or blood pressure cuffs are applied to three extremities, using wide, soft, rubber tubing for the tourniquets. The tourniquets are placed approximately 6 inches below the groin and approximately 4 inches below the shoulders. Tourniquets are applied to only three extremities at a time. Every 5 to 10 minutes, one of the tourniquets is released and applied to the free extremity. The tourniquets (or blood pressure cuffs) should be applied at a pressure less than the systolic blood pressure but greater than the diastolic pressure. An arterial pulse should be palpable distal to each tourniquet or cuff.

Bloodless phlebotomy actually leads to a total

reduction in the circulating blood volume. While trapped in the extremities, a protein-poor filtrate is forced out of the capillaries into the tissues, where it remains for a period even after the tourniquet is removed.

*Step 7e: administration of a vasodilator.* Within the past few years the administration of vasodilators in the management of CHF and acute pulmonary edema has gained popularity. Venodilators, such as nitroglycerin, reduce the preload (the filling pressure) but not the systemic pressure (afterload). Nitrates are predominantly venodilators. Side effects associated with their administration include headache, dizziness, hypotension, and flushing. Between 0.8 to 1.2 mg (two to three tablets or sprays) every 5 to 10 minutes may be administered in the rapid treatment of acute pulmonary edema.[19] Onset of action is within 2 minutes, and the duration is about 15 to 30 minutes. When sublingual nitroglycerin tablets are used, the patient should be asked whether the tablet tingles as it dissolves to ensure the potency of the preparation. The use of nitroglycerin should be considered only when the systolic blood pressure is above 100 mmHg.

In the past, calcium channel blockers were used sublingually in lieu of nitroglycerin in the management of acute pulmonary edema. However, recent clinical trials have shown that they may accelerate the progression of CHF.[20] In general, calcium-channel blockers should be avoided unless they are being used in a patient to treat associated angina pectoris or high blood pressure.

The angiotensin-converting enzyme inhibitors are now standard therapy for the treatment of heart failure.[21] Their beneficial effects include both vasodilation and inhibition of increased neurohormonal activity. The United States' Food and Drug Administration has approved captopril and enalapril for the treatment of heart failure, both to prolong survival and to alleviate symptoms.

*Step 7f: alleviation of apprehension.* Most patients suffering acute pulmonary edema are extremely apprehensive, bordering on panic. Increased apprehension leads to increases in cardiac and respiratory workloads, both of which are absolutely contraindicated in these patients. For this reason the dental personnel must take special care to eliminate patient anxiety.

If the preceding steps diminished the degree of respiratory distress, the patient may no longer be apprehensive. However, in the presence of continued respiratory distress and anxiety, drug therapy should be considered. Administration of an opioid agonist,

such as meperidine (25 to 50 mg via an intramuscular or IV route, titrated slowly) or morphine (2 to 10 mg IV in 2-mg increments), is a possibility. (These suggested doses are for adult patients only. Pediatric doses of morphine in the treatment of pulmonary edema are 0.1 to 0.2 mg IV per kilogram of body weight.) These drugs act to reduce anxiety and agitation and also produce vasodilation, thereby decreasing cardiac and pulmonary workloads.[22] Absolute contraindications to these drugs in the management of heart failure include the clinical presence of hypoxia (see Table 13-1) with cyanosis or of mental confusion or delirium. Opioids further depress respiration in these individuals, who already suffer severely compromised respiratory function. Naloxone, an opioid antagonist, must be available whenever opioid agonists are administered. Nalbuphine, a opioid agonist-antagonist, has also been used with considerable success.

*Step 8: discharge.* The patient suffering acute pulmonary edema requires hospitalization for additional management. Once medical assistance becomes available, subsequent emergency treatment of pulmonary edema consists of the following steps:

- Continuous cardiac monitoring
- Establishment of an IV line
- Administration of furosemide, 40 mg IV
- Dopamine infusion, administered at 10 mg/kg/min, to increase renal perfusion and elevate blood pressure
- Tracheal intubation if the patient is in extremely poor condition
- Emergency transport

*Step 9: subsequent dental treatment.* Even after the patient has been stabilized in the hospital and returns home, the episode must be considered in all future dental treatments to prevent a repeat occurrence. The stress-reduction protocol can help minimize future risk. Consultation with the patient's primary-care physician is essential in the development of a reasonable plan for dental treatment.

Box 14-5 summarizes the management of CHF and acute pulmonary edema.

- **Drugs used in management:** O₂, at high flow; nitroglycerin, sublingual, or nifedipine; and morphine or meperidine (optional) are used in the management of CHF and acute pulmonary edema.
- **Medical assistance required: Yes.** Emergency assistance is required in the treatment of patients suffering heart failure.

box **14-5**  *Management of heart failure and acute pulmonary edema*

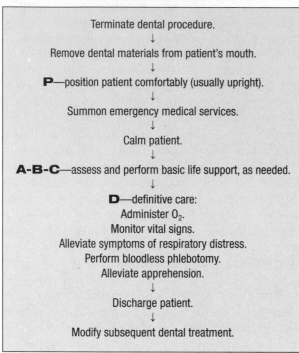

Terminate dental procedure.

↓

Remove dental materials from patient's mouth.

↓

**P**—position patient comfortably (usually upright).

↓

Summon emergency medical services.

↓

Calm patient.

↓

**A-B-C**—assess and perform basic life support, as needed.

↓

**D**—definitive care:

Administer $O_2$.

Monitor vital signs.

Alleviate symptoms of respiratory distress.

Perform bloodless phlebotomy.

Alleviate apprehension.

↓

Discharge patient.

↓

Modify subsequent dental treatment.

**P,** Position; $O_2$, oxygen; **A,** airway; **B,** breathing; **C,** circulation; **D,** definitive care.

## REFERENCES

1. Stirling EL: Congestive heart failure. In Rosen P, editor: *Emergency medicine,* ed 2, St Louis, 1988, Mosby.
2. Kannel WB, Thom TJ: Incidence, prevalence, and mortality of cardiovascular disease. In Alexander RW, Schlant RC, Fuster V, editors: *Hurst's the heart, arteries and veins,* ed 9, New York, 1998, McGraw-Hill.
3. McKee PA and others: The natural history of congestive heart failure: the Framingham study, *N Engl J Med* 285:1441, 1971.
4. Gibson TC, White KR, Klaimer LM: The prevalence of congestive heart failure in two rural communities, *J Chronic Dis* 19:141, 1966.
5. Hutter AM: Congestive heart failure. In Rubinstein E, Federman D, editors: *Scientific American medicine,* New York, 1985, Scientific American Illustrated Library.
6. Barkin RM, Rosen P: Congestive heart failure. In Barkin RM, Rosen P, editors: *Emergency pediatrics,* ed 3, St Louis, 1990, Mosby.
7. Franciosa JA, Dunkman WB: Congestive heart failure. In Rose LF, Kaye D, editors: *Internal medicine for dentistry,* ed 2, St Louis, 1990, Mosby.
8. Schulz H: Inotropic drugs and their mechanism of action, *J Am Coll Cardiol* 4:389, 1984.
9. Sonnenblick EH and others: Dobutamine: a new synthetic cardioactive sympathetic amine, *N Engl J Med* 300:17, 1979.
10. Maskin CS and others: Long-term amrinone therapy in patients with severe heart failure, *Am J Med* 72:113, 1982.
11. Zelcer AA, LeJemtel TH, Sonnenblick EH: Inotropic therapy in heart failure, *Heart Failure* 1:7, 1985.
12. Chidsey CA, Braunwald E, Morrow AG: Catecholamine excretion and cardiac stores of norepinephrine in congestive heart failure, *Am J Med* 39:442, 1962.
13. Braunwald E: The physical examination. In Braunwald E, editor: *Heart disease,* Philadelphia, 1980, WB Saunders.
14. Criteria Committee, New York Heart Association: *Diseases of the heart and blood vessels: nomenclature and criteria for diagnosis,* ed 6, Boston, 1964, Little, Brown.
15. Visscher MB, Haddy FJ, Stephens G: The physiology and pharmacology of lung edema, *Pharmacol Rev* 8:389, 1956.
16. Braunwald E, Sonnenblick EH, Ross J Jr: Contraction of the normal heart. In Braunwald E, editor: *Heart disease,* Philadelphia, 1980, WB Saunders.
17. Starling EH: *Lecture on the law of the heart* (1915), London, 1918, Longmans, Green.
18. McCarthy FM: Cardiovascular disease. In McCarthy FM: *Essentials of safe dentistry for the medically compromised patient,* Philadelphia, 1989, WB Saunders.
19. Cohn JN, Franciosa MD: Vasodilator therapy of cardiac failure, *N Engl J Med* 297:254, 1977.
20. Pieper JA: Evolving role of calcium channel blockers in heart failure. *Pharmacotherapy* 16(2 Pt 2):43S-49S, 1996.
21. Michael KA, Parnell KJ: Innovations in the pharmacologic management of heart failure, *AACN Clin Issues* 9(2):172-191, 1998.
22. Vismara LA, Leaman DM, Zelis R: The effects of morphine on venous tone in patients with acute pulmonary edema, *Circulation* 54:335, 1976.

# 15

# Respiratory Distress

## Differential Diagnosis

*N* most clinical situations the cause of respiratory distress is readily evident, thereby expediting definitive management of the patient. However, situations do exist in which the cause of respiratory distress is less than obvious. In these cases consideration of the following factors may assist the doctor in determining the cause of the clinical problem, thereby permitting definitive therapy to proceed.

## Medical History

Patients suffering respiratory distress almost always remain conscious throughout the episode. The doctor may take advantage of this by asking the patient about any previous similar episodes. In addition, the medical history questionnaire usually includes questions about respiratory problems, such as asthma, heart failure, or a history of hyperventilation; this helps facilitate a differential diagnosis. If the patient loses consciousness at any time, management must follow the protocol for management of unconsciousness (see Section II).

## Age

Respiratory distress in younger patients (under the age of 10) most commonly is related to asthma (usually allergic asthma); hyperventilation and heart failure are significantly less common in this age-group.

241

Hyperventilation is more likely to be the cause of respiratory distress for individuals between 12 and 40 years. Asthma may also occur in this age-group, but in most instances patients already know whether they suffer from this condition. Clinically significant heart failure is rarely seen before the age of 40 years. The peak incidence of heart failure in men is between 50 and 60 years; in women, this peak is between 60 and 70 years.

## Sex

The incidence of hyperventilation, asthma, and heart failure does not differ markedly between males and females, although the incidence of heart failure is slightly greater among males in that age-group, compared with females under the age of 70 years.

## Related Circumstances

Stress, whether physiologic or psychologic, is present in most instances of respiratory distress and increases in severity as the episode progresses. Hyperventilation is precipitated almost exclusively by extreme apprehension. Stressful situations may acutely exacerbate asthma, especially in children, regardless of the type of asthma (intrinsic or extrinsic). In addition, stress causes the physical conditions of patients with heart failure to progressively deteriorate.

## Clinical Symptoms between Acute Episodes

The patient with heart failure may exhibit clinical signs and symptoms at all times, either during physical activity or at rest. Orthopnea, dependent edema, peripheral cyanosis, dyspnea, and undue fatigue may be evident in the patient during dental appointments, depending on the degree of pump failure. Asthmatics are usually asymptomatic between acute episodes; however, noisy breathing and chronic coughs may be present while these patients are at rest. No clinical signs and symptoms of hyperventilation are present between episodes.

## Position

The position of the patient at the onset of clinical symptoms is most relevant in patients with heart failure. Respiratory distress becomes progressively more severe as the dental chair is reclined toward the supine position. Dramatic relief of symptoms can often be achieved by simply allowing the patient to sit upright. Signs and symptoms of asthma and hyperventilation do not respond to repositioning although most patients in respiratory distress can breathe more easily in an upright position.

## Accompanying Sounds

*Wheezing* is usually present in patients with asthma. Wheezing may also be present in paroxysmal nocturnal dyspnea and pulmonary edema (cardiac asthma), although in these circumstances it is associated with other signs and symptoms of heart failure. Partial obstruction of the trachea or bronchi by a foreign object may also produce wheezing. Individuals with heart failure may also exhibit moist, wet respirations, especially those suffering acute pulmonary edema, which is often associated with a frothy, pink-tinged sputum and cough. Hyperventilating individuals breathe deeper and more rapidly than normal, but produce no accompanying abnormal sounds.

## Symptoms Associated with Respiratory Distress

Most individuals in respiratory distress experience shortness of breath (SOB). In cases of heart failure SOB progressively worsens as the patient reclines (orthopnea) and increases as the patient with exertion. Shortness of breath during episodes of hyperventilation is related to anxiety and a feeling of suffocation; it is not related to exertion. In addition, hyperventilation is not associated with cough. Asthmatics exhibit shortness of breath associated with episodic wheezing during acute periods. Most asthmatics are asymptomatic between acute episodes.

## Peripheral Edema and Cyanosis

Patients with heart failure may exhibit peripheral edema and cyanosis. Other possible causes of peripheral edema include renal disease, varicose veins, and pregnancy, whereas cardiorespiratory disease and polycythemia vera are possible causes of cyanosis. In cases of severe asthma with hypoxia or hypercarbia, cyanosis may be present; however, peripheral edema is not noted. Neither peripheral edema nor cyanosis usually accompany hyperventilation.

# Paresthesia of the Extremities

Tingling and numbness of the fingers, toes, and perioral regions, are experienced during hyperventilation. These symptoms may also be present in milder episodes of asthma and heart failure, produced by hyperventilation secondary to acute anxiety.

# Use of Accessory Respiratory Muscles

The patient with acute asthma uses accessory muscles of respiration (abdominal and neck muscles) in an effort to breathe adequately. This may also be noted with acute pulmonary edema.

# Chest Pain

Hyperventilating patients often experience chest pain, describing it as a "weight," a "pressing" sensation, or as a "shooting" or "stabbing" feeling. However, these patients rarely exhibit other clinical manifestations of cardiac disease. The age of the hyperventilating patient (under 35 years) is usually below that at which cardiovascular disease normally occurs. Patients suffering asthma and heart failure usually do not experience chest pain along with their other clinical symptoms.

# Heart Rate and Blood Pressure

Both heart rate and blood pressure usually increase during periods of respiratory distress. This elevation occurs in hyperventilation and during acute asthmatic episodes as a result of anxiety. In these cases the blood pressure (both systolic and diastolic) and heart rate are elevated.

Although both the systolic and the diastolic pressures increase in during heart failure, diastolic blood pressure is usually elevated to a greater degree; therefore the pulse pressure (systolic − diastolic) narrows (to <40). The heart rate increases with heart failure.

# Duration of Respiratory Distress

Respiratory distress associated with heart failure often improves dramatically with repositioning (when the patient sits upright). However, when pulmonary edema is present, respiratory distress does not improve until definitive management is initiated.

Most asthma attacks will not resolve for a considerable period without drug management. Therefore bronchodilator therapy is employed as soon as it becomes available. Status asthmaticus requires more definitive management—possibly even hospitalization.

Hyperventilation is usually manageable without drug intervention and rarely, if ever, necessitates the help of additional personnel or hospitalization.

(An algorithm for the diagnosis and management of respiratory difficulty appears on page 214.)

# ALTERED CONSCIOUSNESS

# 16

# Altered Consciousness

## General Considerations

**A** *STATE* of altered consciousness may be a clinical manifestation of any number of systemic medical conditions. Almost every one of the situations that most commonly produce altered consciousness may also result in the loss of consciousness, which is another clinical expression of altered consciousness (Table 16-1). However, in most cases the prompt recognition of clinical signs and symptoms and the equally prompt institution of corrective measures permit the victim to retain consciousness until definitive management becomes available. Box 16-1 lists some of the terms and definitions frequently associated with altered consciousness.

Altered consciousness may be the first clinical sign of a serious medical problem requiring immediate and intensive therapy. Therefore the doctor must be aware of the patient's medical history before beginning any treatment so that prompt recognition and treatment are possible. Such knowledge will also help in the modification of future dental treatment to prevent episodes.

## Predisposing Factors

The most common cause of altered consciousness in a dental setting is the ingestion or administration of drugs. With increasing use of pharmacosedation in dentistry, dentists are likely to encounter greater numbers of reports of inadvertent overadministration

table **16-1**    *Causes of altered consciousness*

| CAUSE | FREQUENCY | TEXT DISCUSSION |
|---|---|---|
| Drug overdose (alcohol, barbiturates, insulin) | Most common | Drug-related emergencies (Section Six) |
| Hyperventilation | Common | Respiratory distress (Section Three) |
| Hypoglycemia | Common | Altered consciousness (Section Four) |
| Hyperglycemia | Less common | Altered consciousness (Section Four) |
| CVA, transient ischemic attack | Less common | Altered consciousness (Section Four) |
| Hyperthyroidism | Rare | Altered consciousness (Section Four) |
| Hypothyroidism | Rare | Altered consciousness (Section Four) |

*CVA,* Cerebrovascular accident.

box **16-1**

**confusion**  A mental state marked by the mingling of ideas with consequent disturbances in comprehension and understanding, which eventually leads to bewilderment

**delirium**  A mental disturbance marked by illusions, delusions, cerebral excitement, physical restlessness, and incoherence

**dizziness**  A disturbed sense of relationship to space; a sensation of unsteadiness accompanied by a feeling of movement within the head

of these drugs. Knowledge of drug pharmacology and proper use of such drugs, however, can help minimize these incidents.

One particular psychosedative, which doctors rarely prescribe, may be the drug that dental patients most commonly use—alcohol. Most practicing dentists, at one time or another, have had to manage the needs of a patient who has accidentally (or in some instances, intentionally) ingested an overdose of alcohol; in other words, the patient is intoxicated. In such instances dental treatment should be postponed and the patient strictly admonished against self-administration of drugs. In addition, the doctor may need to discover the patient's reasons for overdosing on alcohol (or other psychoactive drugs) and, if appropriate, take steps to alleviate the patient's dental anxiety. The administration of additional drugs (for example, local anesthetics or sedatives) that further depress the central nervous system of a patient who has ingested an unknown quantity of an unknown drug that also possesses CNS-depressant properties invites serious and often dire consequences.

Hyperventilation is the most common nondrug cause of altered consciousness in dentistry. Although hyperventilation rarely causes an individual to lose consciousness, this can occur with delays in recognition and management. Fear and anxiety are the pri-

mary precipitating factors in almost all cases of hyperventilation in the dental setting, which occurs predominantly in adolescents and young adults; patients under 40 years comprise the majority of cases (see Chapter 12).

This section discusses three additional systemic problems that manifest clinically as altered consciousness—diabetes mellitus, cerebrovascular ischemia and infarction, and thyroid gland dysfunction. Diabetes mellitus and its acute clinical complication, hypoglycemia, are not encountered frequently in dental patients. However, inadequate medical management of diabetes and the presence of additional stress rapidly may result in an altered state of consciousness and possibly in the loss of consciousness. In addition, a nondiabetic individual may develop hypoglycemia under certain circumstances. Cerebrovascular ischemia and infarction (also known as *stroke* or *brain attack*) are less common but potentially more serious causes of altered consciousness. Proper management of the post-cerebrovascular accident (CVA) patient greatly reduces the risk that dental treatment may precipitate a second attack. A prodromal form of cerebrovascular ischemia, known as *transient ischemic attack,* is also discussed.

Thyroid gland dysfunction is another situation in which alterations in consciousness may be observed. Although acute clinical complications resulting from thyroid gland hypofunction or hyperfunction are extremely rare in dental settings, the doctor must be aware of a patient's thyroid gland dysfunction and be able to recognize the signs and symptoms associated with them. Even more importantly, the doctor must also monitor the increased incidence of cardiovascular disease that often accompanies patients with thyroid dysfunction.

In all of these situations, an increase in physiologic or psychologic stress during dental treatment increases the potential for an acute exacerbation of the patient's underlying medical condition.

# Prevention

Recognition of unusually high levels of apprehension in a prospective patient can help in treatment modification and minimize the occurrence of vasodepressor syncope and hyperventilation; the proper use of pharmacosedative techniques can help prevent treatment-related drug overdose. In addition, a patient's medical history permits the doctor to modify the treatment plan to minimize any risk to the patient. The questionnaire, physical examination, and monitoring of vital signs are invaluable in the proper pretreatment assessment of a patient; specific questions and examinations should be used as references before treatment begins.

# Clinical Manifestations

A spectrum of signs and symptoms may be present in patients with altered consciousness: the cold, wet appearance, mental confusion, and bizarre behavior of the hypoglycemic patient contrasts markedly with the hot, dry, florid appearance of the hyperglycemic diabetic patient. The presence of acetone on the breath further aids in the clinical recognition of hyperglycemia (ketoacidosis).

CVAs may develop with a sudden loss of consciousness (presenting an extremely grave prognosis) or with a more gradual onset of symptoms that are related to central nervous system dysfunction. These may include a variable degree of derangement in speech, thought, motion, sensation or vision. The state of consciousness may remain unimpaired, or the patient may demonstrate varying degrees of altered consciousness, ranging from headache, dizziness, and drowsiness to mental confusion.

If left untreated, hypothyroidism may produce weakness, fatigue, lethargy, and slow speech, among other signs and symptoms. In contrast, untreated hyperthyroidism causes restlessness, nervousness, irritability, and degrees of motor incoordination that range from fine, mild tremulousness to gross tremors. Thyroid storm, or thyroid crisis, is an example of one serious consequence of unmanaged hyperthyroidism. This condition may arise spontaneously but more commonly follows periods of sudden stress in patients who are clinically hyperthyroid. The death rate associated with thyroid storm is significant.

# Pathophysiology

In all three situations discussed in this section the clinical manifestations are evident systemically even though a specific factor causes the onset of symptoms and signs. A blood-glucose level that is either too high or too low causes most clinical signs and symptoms of diabetes mellitus. Although it is considered a disease of impaired carbohydrate utilization, diabetes mellitus is also a blood-vessel disease; for this reason, diabetic patients exhibit a greater incidence of cardiovascular disease than nondiabetic patients. A change in the quality of circulating blood is responsible for most of the acute clinical problems associated with diabetes.

Signs and symptoms of thyroid gland dysfunction are related clinically to the circulating blood level of thyroid hormone (thyroxine) and its pharmacologic actions on other parts of the body. Inadequate blood flow to the brain also produces signs and symptoms of impaired consciousness. Temporary insufficiency leads to transient ischemic attack; more prolonged insufficiency results in permanent neurologic changes, termed cerebrovascular infarctions (strokes).

# Management

When altered consciousness is recognized, several basic steps must be performed immediately (Box 16-2). (Each of the subsequent chapters in this section will discuss definitive management of those specific emergencies.)

*Step 1: recognition of altered consciousness.* Changes in the level of consciousness occurring during dental treatment should be a warning to the doctor to terminate treatment. (The following chapters will describe specific signs and symptoms.) In most cases changes in levels of consciousness are gradual (occurring over hours [hypoglycemia] to weeks or longer [thyroid dysfunction]), so the change in level of consciousness may be visible prior to the start of dental treatment.

*Step 2: termination of dental treatment.*

*Step 3: **P** (position).* Proper positioning for patients with altered levels of consciousness varies according to the causative factor. In most instances the patient remains conscious; therefore the supine, semi-supine, or erect positions all are acceptable; patient comfort and vital signs (particularly blood pressure) will also influence positioning. The conscious diabetic or thyroid dysfunction patient may be most comfortable sitting up. However, if a patient ever loses consciousness, initial management must follow the protocol for the treatment of unconsciousness.

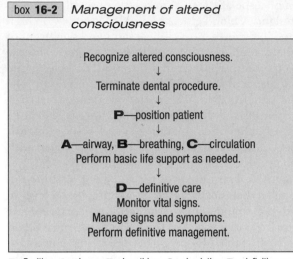

| box 16-2 | *Management of altered consciousness* |

Recognize altered consciousness.
↓
Terminate dental procedure.
↓
**P**—position patient
↓
**A**—airway, **B**—breathing, **C**—circulation
Perform basic life support as needed.
↓
**D**—definitive care
Monitor vital signs.
Manage signs and symptoms.
Perform definitive management.

**P,** Position; **A,** airway; **B,** breathing; **C,** circulation; **D,** definitive care.

CVAs are often associated with extreme elevations of blood pressure. In such situations a nonrecumbent (nonsupine) position is important; in an upright position, cerebral blood pressure is somewhat reduced through the actions of gravity. If a CVA leads to a rapid loss of consciousness is associated with high blood pressure, the patient's positioning is altered slightly. Because the supine position causes an increase in cerebral blood pressure that may not prove beneficial at this time, the patient should be placed in the supine position, with the head elevated slightly.

*Step 4:* **A-B-C** *airway-breathing-circulation, (basic life support), as needed.* The steps of basic life support should be initiated as soon as possible:
- Assessment of airway patency and airway maintenance, if needed
- Assessment of spontaneous breathing and artificial ventilation, if needed
- Assessment of circulatory adequacy and artificial circulation, if needed

*Step 5:* **D** *(definitive care):*

*Step 5a: monitoring of vital signs.* The blood pressure, heart rate and rhythm, and respiratory rate should be monitored and recorded approximately every 5 minutes throughout the episode. A permanent record should also be retained.

*Step 5b: management of signs and symptoms.* Clinical signs and symptoms should be treated in an effort to increase patient comfort. Blankets should be available if the patient is shivering, and tight garments should be loosened or removed to allow the patient easier breathing.

*Step 5c: definitive management.* At this point a decision must be made as to the definitive management of the problem. In-office management ranges from basic life support (CVA) to the administration of drugs to terminate the episode (hypoglycemia). (The following chapters will describe in detail the management recommended for each situation.)

# 17

# Diabetes Mellitus

## Hyperglycemia and Hypoglycemia

**D**IABETES mellitus represents a syndrome of disordered glucose metabolism and inappropriate hyperglycemia that results from an absolute deficiency in insulin secretion, a reduction in the biologic effectiveness of insulin, or both. Approximately 200 million individuals worldwide and 15.7 million Americans (5.9% of the U.S. population) suffer from diabetes mellitus,[1] representing a 50% increase in the incidence of diabetes within the past two decades.[2-5] Although 10.3 million of these Americans have been diagnosed with diabetes, 5.4 million individuals are unaware that they have the disease. Approximately 798,000 Americans are diagnosed with diabetes annually.

In addition, diabetes is prevalent in children, with about 1 in 600 school-age children diagnosed with the disease.[6] Statistics also indicate that one half of all children who currently have diabetes die of renal disease an average of 25 years after the initial diagnosis.[2] Diabetes is the seventh leading cause of death in the United States.[7] Morbidity and mortality from diabetes most often relates to its vascular complications.[8] A study of mortality in diabetics reported 36.8% of deaths related to cardiovascular causes, 17.5% to cerebrovascular disorders, 15.5% to diabetic coma, and 12.5% to renal failure.[9]

The incidence of diabetes increases with age.[10] Table 17-1 illustrates the incidence of diabetes and its relationship to age-group; approximately 80% of diabetics are older than 45 years. Nearly 18.4% of the

251

| table 17-1 | Incidence of diabetes by age in the United States |

| AGE-GROUP (IN YEARS) | INCIDENCE (PER 1000 INDIVIDUALS) |
|---|---|
| 0-17 | 1.3 |
| 25-40 | 17 |
| 45-65 | 45 |
| 65 or older | 79 |

Data from Little JW, Falace DA: *Dental management of the medically compromised patient,* ed 4, St Louis, 1993, Mosby.

U.S. population between 65 and 74 years has diabetes. Little and Falace[11] estimate that a dental practice serving an adult population of 2000 people may expect to encounter about 40 to 70 individuals with diabetes, about a third of whom are unaware of their condition.

## Acute Complications

Hyperglycemia, or high blood sugar, and its sequelae represent one of two clinically significant complications for the doctor who is called upon to treat the diabetic patient. The second and more acutely life-threatening complication is hypoglycemia, or low blood sugar. Hypoglycemia may be present in diabetic and nondiabetic individuals. Blood glucose levels below 50 mg per 100 ml (venous blood) usually indicate hypoglycemia in adults, whereas blood glucose values of less than 40 mg per 100 ml indicate hypoglycemia in children.[12]

Signs and symptoms of hypoglycemia may become evident within minutes, leading rapidly to the loss of consciousness, or as is more common, develop gradually, leading to alterations in consciousness. Hyperglycemia may also result ultimately in the loss of consciousness (diabetic coma), but this usually represents the end of a much longer process. (The time elapsed from the onset of symptoms to the loss of consciousness is usually at least 48 hours.) Loss of consciousness due to hyperglycemia is an extremely unlikely occurrence in the dental office. Conversely, low blood sugar is significantly more likely to lead to profound changes in levels of consciousness or to the loss of consciousness. Regardless of cause the doctor must be able to recognize the clinical problem and initiate the proper management protocol. To aid in the differential diagnosis of diabetic complications, this chapter stresses the differences between hyperglycemia and hypoglycemia.

## Chronic Complications

In addition to hyperglycemia and hypoglycemia, the diabetic is subject to other, more chronic complications. It is important to note that most cases of morbidity and mortality in diabetics results from these complications (Table 17-2).

Three major categories of diabetic complications exist—large blood vessel disease, small blood vessel disease (microangiopathy), and increased susceptibility to infection. Large blood vessel disease, such as arteriosclerosis, frequently occurs in nondiabetic individuals; however, it is more common in diabetics and develops at an earlier age (diabetics being two to four times more likely to have heart disease than nondiabetics).[13] Clinical manifestations are related to an inadequate blood supply to the heart (angina pectoris, myocardial infarction, sudden death), the brain (cerebrovascular ischemia or infarction [again, diabetics being two to four times more likely to suffer cerebrovascular disease]), the kidneys (glomerulosclerosis), and the lower extremities (gangrene). High blood pressure also occurs more frequently and at an earlier age in the diabetic patient.[14,15] Death rates from heart disease are two to four times as high in diabetics than in nondiabetics.

Diabetic microangiopathy, or small blood vessel disease, is related to disorders affecting the arterioles, venules, and capillaries. It is thought that the disease is specific, occurring only in patients with diabetes mellitus. Clinical manifestations of microangiopathy most often appear in the eye (diabetic retinopathy),[16] kidney (arteriolar nephrosclerosis),[17] and lower extremities (gangrene).[18] The cause of diabetic microangiopathy is not yet entirely clear, but two interpretations are most often accepted. In the first the cause is related to the carbohydrate intolerance associated with diabetes mellitus; however, documented instances do exist in which microangiopathy develops in the absence of carbohydrate intolerance. A second theory links microangiopathy to a genetic factor that also manifests as diabetes.

Regardless of the cause, diabetic microangiopathy may represent a more serious disease than carbohydrate intolerance itself. Studies have not yet demonstrated that careful control of blood-glucose levels decreases or retards small vessel disease. The extent of diabetic microangiopathy is such that approximately 11% to 18% of all diabetics have treatable diabetic retinopathy.[19] Diabetic retinopathy is the leading cause of new blindness in individuals between 20 and 74 years.[20]

| table 17-2 | Chronic complications of diabetes mellitus |
|---|---|

| AFFECTED BODY PART OR CONDITION | COMPLICATIONS |
|---|---|
| Vascular system | Atherosclerosis<br>   Large vessel disease<br>   Microangiopathy |
| Kidneys | Diabetic glomerulosclerosis<br>Arteriolar nephrosclerosis<br>Pyelonephritis |
| Nervous system | Motor, sensory, and autonomic<br>   neuorpathy |
| Eyes | Retinopathy<br>Cataract formation<br>Glaucoma<br>Extraocular muscle palsies |
| Skin | Diabetic xanthoma<br>Necrobiosis lipoidica diabeticorum<br>Pruritus<br>Furunculosis<br>Mycosis |
| Mouth | Gingivitis<br>Increased incidence of dental<br>   caries and periodontal disease<br>Alveolar bone loss |
| Pregnancy | Increased incidence of large babies,<br>   stillbirths, miscarriages, newborn<br>   deaths, and congenital defects |

Approximately 60% to 70% of diabetics suffer mild to severe forms of diabetic nerve damage (neuropathy), which in severe forms can lead to lower limb amputation. Diabetes is the most frequent cause of nontraumatic lower-limb amputation. The risk of a leg amputation is 15 to 40 times greater for an individual with diabetes. Each year, 56,200 Americans lose their feet and legs to diabetes.[18,20]

In addition, diabetics are more prone to infections than nondiabetics. Although the precise cause is yet undetermined, the propensity for infection is most likely related to the combination of vascular lesions and infections.[21] Uncontrolled diabetics also suffer inflammatory periodontal diseases with increased frequencies, but the extent of such diseases is no greater than in well-controlled diabetics.[22] To prevent severe infection, diabetics must practice scrupulous personal hygiene.

About 10% to 21% of diabetics will develop renal disease (diabetic nephropathy), a major cause of illness and death, particularly in female diabetics. Diabetic nephropathy may be related to high glucose levels in the urine, which serves as an excellent growth medium for microorganisms. Microangiopathy of diabetic renal disease occurs in two thirds of diabetics 20 years after the onset of the disease; microangiopathy generally causes proteinuria.[1] Within 5 years of the onset of proteinuria, uremia may ensue. Diabetic nephropathy is the most common cause of end-stage renal disease, a condition in which the individual requires dialysis or a kidney transplant to survive.[20] As many as 4000 cases of end-stage renal disease occur annually among diabetics in the United States.[23]

Impotence, secondary to diabetic neuropathy or blood vessel blockage, afflicts approximately 13% of men with type I diabetes and 8% of men with type II diabetes. Reports have documented that diabetic men older than 50 years may experience impotence rates as high as 50% to 60%.[20]

The doctor called upon to treat the dental needs of a diabetic patient must be aware of the acute complications of diabetes (that is, hypoglycemia and hyperglycemia) and take measures to avoid their occurrence. That doctor must also seek out any chronic complications associated with diabetes that may increase the patient's medical risk during dental treatment. In such cases modifications in the planned treatment are likely to be required.

## Predisposing Factors

Major factors leading to the development of diabetes mellitus include the following:
- Genetic disorder
- Primary destruction of the islets of Langerhans in the pancreas caused by inflammation, cancer, or surgery
- An endocrine condition, such as hyperpituitarism or hyperthyroidism
- The administration of steroids, resulting in iatrogenic diabetes

The most important factor in the development of diabetes mellitus is heredity. If one identical twin has diabetes, the other twin will also be a diabetic if that individual lives long enough. In addition, the offspring of two diabetic parents have almost a 100% chance of developing the disease. Table 17-3 demonstrates the prediction of risk factors for the development of diabetes mellitus based on family history.

## Classification of Diabetes

Until recently, classifications of diabetes were based upon (1) the age of onset of the disease and (2) whether

table **17-3** *Prediction of diabetic risk*

| RELATIVES WITH DIABETES | DIABETIC RELATIVE ON OTHER SIDE OF FAMILY | MAXIMUM RISK (%) |
|---|---|---|
| Parent + | Grandparent and aunt or uncle | 85 |
| Parent + | Grandparent, aunt, or uncle | 60 |
| Parent + | First cousin | 40 |
| Parent | | 22 |
| Grandparent | | 14 |
| First cousin | | 9 |

From Steinberg AG: *Ann NY Acad Sci* 82:197, 1959.

box **17-1** *Prior classification of diabetes by the American Diabetes Association, 1975*

### Hereditary, primary, or idiopathic diabetes

Prediabetes
Subclinical, latent, or stress diabetes
Chemical diabetes
Overt, or clinical, diabetes
Juvenile, or early-onset, diabetes
Maturity-, adult-, or late-onset diabetes

### Nonhereditary, secondary diabetes

Damage to or removal of pancreatic islet tissue
Disorders of other endocrine glands
Drugs or chemicals

Modified from National Diabetes Data Group: Classification and diagnosis of diabetes mellitus and other categories of glucose intolerance, *Diabetes* 28:1039-1057, 1979.

box **17-2** *Classification of diabetes mellitus and other categories of glucose intolerance*

### Diabetes mellitus

Insulin-dependent diabetes mellitus (IDDM)—type I
Non–insulin-dependent diabetes mellitus (NIDDM)—type II
  Nonobese
  Obese
Other types (including diabetes mellitus associated with other conditions and syndromes)
  Pancreatic diseases
  Diseases of hormonal etiology
  Drug- or chemical-induced conditions
  Insulin-receptor abnormalities
  Certain genetic syndromes
  Miscellaneous pathologic processes

### Imparied glucose tolerance (IGT)

Nonobese
Obese
Impaired glucose tolerance associated with certain conditions and syndromes
  Pancreatic diseases
  Diseases of hormonal etiology
  Drug- or chemical-induced conditions
  Insulin-receptor abnormalities
  Certain genetic syndromes
  Miscellaneous pathologic processes
Gestational diabetes
Statistical risk classes (subjects with normal glucose tolerance but statistically increased risks for diabetes)
Previous abnormality of glucose tolerance
Potential abnormality of glucose tolerance

Modified from Bennett PH: The diagnosis of diabetes: new international classification and diagnostic criteria, *Ann Rev Med* 34:295, 1983.
*IGT,* Impaired glucose tolerance.

the condition required an injection of insulin in its management. In other words the classifications were adult-onset versus juvenile-onset diabetes (Box 17-1) and insulin-dependent diabetes mellitus (IDDM) versus non–insulin-dependent diabetes mellitus (NIDDM).

However, the age of onset no longer is considered a criterion for classification of the disease. Instead, in 1979 the National Diabetes Data Group recommended a therapeutic classification, which the American Diabetes Association subsequently endorsed. Box 17-2 outlines this classification, and Table 17-4 presents a comparison and contrast of the types of diabetes. More recently, reports have described diabetes as either type I or type II, without mention of the insulin requirement.

Yet another category—impaired glucose homeostasis—is relatively new. The name refers to a condition in which blood sugar levels are higher than normal but not high enough to meet the classification for diabetes. In addition, two subcategories—impaired glucose tolerance (IGT) and impaired fasting glucose (IFG)—are considered risk factors for the future development of diabetes and cardiovascular disease. The IGT test is positive when results of a 2-hour oral glucose tolerance test are between 140 and 199 mg/dl. IGT is a major risk factor for type II diabetes and is present in about 11% of adults. Approximately 40% to 45% of individuals 65 years and older have either IGT or type II diabetes. The IFG test is positive when results of an 8-hour fasting plasma glucose test are greater than 110 but less than 126 mg/dl.

IGT and IFG are significant in that they are not associated with the complications, either chronic or acute, of diabetes mellitus.[23] Many individuals who fall within the IGT group spontaneously develop normal glucose tolerance. However, between 1% to 5% of the IGT group will progress to become diabetics.[24]

table **17-4** *Clinical classification of idiopathic diabetes mellitus syndromes*

| TYPE | KETOSIS | ISLET CELL ANTIBODIES | HUMAN LYMPHOCYTE ANTIGEN ASSOCIATION | TREATMENT |
|---|---|---|---|---|
| Insulin-dependent (Type I) | Present | Present at onset | Positive | Insulin (mixtures of rapid-acting and intermediate-acting insulin at least twice daily) and diet |
| Non–insulin-dependent (Type II) Nonobese | Absent | Absent | Negative | Eucaloric diet alone *or* Diet plus insulin or sulfonylureas |
| Obese | Absent | Absent | Negative | Weight reduction *and* Hypocaloric diet plus sulfonylureas or insulin for symptomatic control only |

Modified from Karam JH: Diabetes mellitus and hypoglycemia. In Tierney LM Jr, McPhee SJ, Papadakis MA, editors: *Current medical diagnosis and treatment,* ed 35, 1996, Stamford, Conn, Appleton & Lange.

Still another type of the disease—gestational diabetes—develops in 2% to 5% of all pregnant women but disappears when the pregnancy ends. Women who have had gestational diabetes are increased risks for developing type II diabetes as they age. Other types of diabetes result from specific genetic syndromes, surgery, drugs, malnutrition, infections, and other illnesses.

## TYPE I*

The primary form of diabetes is genetic, or hereditary. Approximately 8% of diabetic patients in the United States have type I diabetes. This is a more severe form of diabetes, characterized in its untreated state by ketoacidosis (DKA, diabetic ketoacidosis). More common in adolescents, type I diabetes may also develop in adults, usually in the nonobese, and in those who are elderly when hyperglycemia appears. The prevalence of type I diabetes varies significantly worldwide. Prevalence is highest in Scandinavia, where as many as 20% of diabetics are type I. In Southern Europe this incidence falls to 13%, whereas in Japan and China fewer than 1% of diabetics are type I.

In type I diabetes, circulating insulin is essentially absent (thus the term *insulinopenic*), plasma glucagon levels are elevated, and pancreatic β–cells do not respond to all insulinogenic stimuli. These individuals require exogenous insulin to reverse their catabolic state, prevent diabetic ketoacidosis, reduce hyperglucagonemia, and reduce elevated blood glucose levels. Studies have

demonstrated that the incidence of type I diabetes is linked to the presence or absence of certain genetically determined cell surface antigens found on lymphocytes. Human lymphocyte antigens (HLA), which are located on the sixth human chromosome adjacent to the immune response genes, are closely associated with the development of type I diabetes.[25]

Research also suggests that type I diabetes may be an autoimmune response because of the discovery of autoantibodies to pancreatic β–cells and other endocrine organs.[26] Because of the immune factors associated with the development of type I diabetes, it is felt that this type of diabetes is the result of an infectious or environmental insult to pancreatic β–cells in genetically predisposed individuals. These extrinsic factors include damage produced by viruses, such as mumps or coxsackie-virus B; toxic chemicals; or destructive cytotoxins and antibodies released from sensitized immunocytes.[27,28]

## TYPE II*

Type II diabetes describes a heterogeneous group composed of milder forms of diabetes that occur most frequently in adults and only occasionally in children. More than 90% of all U.S. diabetics are type II. Circulating endogenous insulin blood levels are adequate to prevent ketoacidosis (insulinoplethoric), but are either subnormal or inadequate to meet the individual's increased needs, which are caused by insensitivity of the tissues.

Type II diabetes mellitus is a nonketotic form of diabetes that is not linked to human lymphocyte anti-

*Formerly known as *juvenile-onset diabetes* and *insulin-dependent diabetes mellitus (IDDM)*.

*Formerly known as *adult-onset diabetes* and *non–insulin-dependent diabetes mellitus*.

gen markers on the sixth chromosome; it has no islet cell antibodies. Most type II diabetics do not require exogenous insulin therapy to sustain life. Regardless of body weight, the tissues of type II diabetics demonstrate a degree of insensitivity to insulin, which is produced by either a lack of insulin receptors in peripheral tissues or an insensitivity of the existing receptors.

Two subcategories exist for type II diabetes mellitus, based on the presence or absence of obesity. The degree and prevalence of obesity in diabetics varies among racial groups. For example, fewer than 30% of type II diabetics in Japan and China are obese; however, among Africans, Europeans, and North Americans with type II diabetes, 75% to 80% are obese. This statistic approaches 100% among Pacific Islanders from Nauru or Samoa and among the Pima Indians of Arizona.

### Nonobese type II diabetes

The nonobese type II diabetic demonstrates either an absent or significantly blunted early phase of insulin release in response to a glucose challenge. The same poor insulin release may also be demonstrated in response to other insulinogenic stimuli, such as acute intravenous (IV) administration of glucagon or sulfonylureas. Hyperglycemia in these diabetics often responds to oral hypoglycemic agents or occasionally to dietary therapy alone. In rare instances such individuals may require insulin therapy to achieve satisfactory control of blood sugar levels, although it is not required to prevent ketosis.

### Obese type II diabetes

Obese type II diabetes occurs secondary to extrapancreatic factors that produce an insensitivity to endogenous insulin. The condition is characterized by a nonketotic mild form of diabetes that occurs primarily in adults and occasionally in children. The primary problem is a target organ disorder, which results in a lack of sensitivity to insulin. Hyperplasia of pancreatic β-cells often appears and most likely accounts for the fasting hyperinsulinism and exaggerated insulin responses to glucose and other stimuli that occur in patients with milder forms of this disorder.

Obsesity is commonly seen in this disorder because of excess caloric intake, perhaps resulting from hunger caused by mild postprandial hypoglycemia after excess insulin release. In this form of diabetes insulin insensitivity correlates with the presence of distended adipocytes. Liver and muscle cells also resist the deposition of additional glycogen and triglycerides in their storage depots.

Two mechanisms may explain the insensitivity of tissues to insulin in the obese form of type II diabetes. Chronic overfeeding may lead to either (1) sustained pancreatic β-cell stimulation and hyperinsulinism,

which by itself may induce receptor insensitivity to insulin, or (2) a postreceptor defect associated with overdistended storage depots and a reduced ability to clear nutrients from circulation. Consequent hyperinsulinism induces receptor insensitivity to insulin.[24] A reduction in food intake may interrupt either cycle, regardless of the mechanism. In the first case a restricted diet reduces islet cell stimulation of insulin release, thereby restoring insulin receptor sites and improving tissue sensitivity to insulin. In the second situation normal tissue sensitivity returns as storage depots become less saturated.

Other possible causes of carbohydrate intolerance and hyperinsulinism in response to glucose include chronic muscle inactivity or disease and liver disease. Secondary causes of carbohydrate intolerance include endocrine disorders (for example, tumors) associated with excessive production of growth hormone, glucocorticoids, catecholamines (for example, epinephrine), or glucagon; in such cases the peripheral response to insulin is decreased.

The prognosis for both forms of diabetes mellitus, even in individuals who maintain scrupulous control over blood sugar levels, remains uncertain. The belief that tight glycemic control limits or reverses diabetic complications has led to more aggressive diabetic therapy and monitoring.[29] Recent research with pancreatic islet transplants[30,31] and improved insulin delivery systems, such as the insulin pump,[32] may make possible the ability to determine whether adequate control can minimize the severity of the disease or delay the onset of complications.

In one series of 164 juvenile-onset type I diabetics (median age of onset being 9 years), data were collected after 25 years. In the study one of five diabetics who received standard dietary and insulin control died and one became incapacitated with severe proliferative retinopathy and renal failure. Two other members of the group were active, contributing members of society despite mild background retinopathy, mild nephropathy, neuropathy, and some degree of ischemia of the feet. The fifth diabetic was completely free of complications.[33]

It appears that the period between 10 and 20 years after the onset of diabetes is a critical one. If the patient does not experience significant complications during this period, a strong possibility exists that that individual may remain in reasonably good health. Knowledge of the type of diabetes enables the doctor to estimate the risk factor in each case. However, other factors over which the individual has no control, such as infection and pregnancy, may lead to the exacerbation of a diabetic patient's condition. Table 17-5 compares type I and type II diabetes.

table **17-5**   *Comparison of type I and type II diabetes mellitus*

| FACTOR | TYPE I | TYPE II |
|---|---|---|
| Frequency (% of total diabetic population) | 5 | 85 |
| Age at onset (years) | 15 | 40 and older |
| Body build | Normal to thin | Obese |
| Severity | Severe | Mild |
| Use of insulin | Almost all | 25%-30% |
| Response to oral hypoglycemic agents | Very few respond | 50% respond |
| Ketoacidosis | Common | Uncommon |
| Complications | 90% in 20 years | Less common than with type I |
| Rate of clinical onset | Rapid | Slow |
| Stability | Unstable | Stable |
| Family history of diabetes | Common | Less common than with type I |
| Human lymphocyte antigen and abnormal autoimmune reactions | Present | Not present |
| Insulin receptor defects | Usually not found | — |

From Little JW, Falace DA: Dental management of the medically compromised patient, ed 4, St Louis, 1993, Mosby.

# Hyperglycemia

Any of the following factors, all of which increase the body's demand for insulin, may precipitate hyperglycemia:

- Weight gain
- Cessation of exercise
- Pregnancy
- Hyperthyroidism or thyroid medication
- Epinephrine therapy
- Corticosteroid therapy
- Acute infection
- Fever

Although hyperglycemia usually by itself does not lead to an acute, life-threatening emergency, it may if left untreated progress to diabetic ketoacidosis and subsequent diabetic coma, both of which are life threatening. Diabetic ketoacidosis most often occurs in type I diabetics and is associated with infection or inadequate administration of insulin. However, DKA can occur in type II diabetics and may be associated with any kind of medication, epinephrine therapy, or stress.[34] Infection and a secondary disease state also are common causes of hyperglycemia in diabetics. Diabetic ketoacidosis is slow in onset, producing 1 day to 2 weeks of malaise, nausea, polydipsa, polyuria, and polyphagia in younger individuals.[35] In such situations, it is not uncommon for the patient to experience vomiting and shortness of breath.

# Hypoglycemia

Unlike hyperglycemia, hypoglycemia may develop rapidly, especially in patients receiving injectable insulin therapy who may lose consciousness within minutes after insulin administration. In patients receiving oral hypoglycemic agents, the onset of symptoms is slower, usually developing over several hours.

The following factors decrease the body's requirement for insulin:

- Weight loss
- Increased physical exercise
- Termination of pregnancy
- Termination of other drug therapies (for example, epinephrine, thyroid, or corticosteroid)
- Recovery from infection and fever

Administration of the usual dose of insulin at this time is associated with an increased risk of hypoglycemia. Common causes of hypoglycemia include the omission or delay of meals, excessive exercise before meals, and insulin overdose. Table 17-6 lists some frequently observed causes of hypoglycemia in known diabetic patients.

Dental treatment is a potential threat to the diabetic and to control of the disease state. Stress—physiologic and psychologic—increases the body's requirement for insulin, which increases the diabetic dental patient's chance of developing hyperglycemia. (Both the doctor and the patient must be aware of this possibility so that modifications may be made in management and, if necessary, the patient's insulin dose to preclude a progression into diabetic coma.) In addition, dental treatment may necessitate that the patient alter their normal eating habits for variable lengths of time. Some patients purposefully avoid eating before dental appointments so that their teeth are "clean." The doctor, out of necessity, may need to schedule a treatment appointment during a normal lunch or dinner

**table 17-6** *Causes of 240 consecutive cases of hypoglycemia in diabetic patients**

| CAUSE | % |
|---|---|
| Inadequate food (carbohydrate) intake | 66 |
| Excessive insulin dose | 12 |
| Sulfonylurea therapy | 12 |
| Strenuous exercise | 4 |
| Ethanol intake | 4 |
| Other (kidney failure, liver failure, decrease in corticosteroid dose) | 2 |

Modified from Davidson JK: Hypoglycemia. In Schwartz GR and others, editors: *Principles and practice of emergency medicine*, Philadelphia, 1978, WB Saunders.
*Patients were observed at Grady Memorial Hospital Emergency Clinic from 1973 to 1975.

hour, forcing the patient to delay or miss a meal. The dental procedure may also delay the patient's ingestion of food. Prolonged anesthesia after treatment and extensive dental procedures (for example, periodontal or oral surgery or endodontics), using drugs such as bupivacaine and etidocaine, may delay the patient's next meal, increasing the risk of hypoglycemia.

## Control of Diabetes

Diabetes is a fascinating disease in that it produces a myriad of clinical signs and symptoms. In addition, there are many factors that affect control of the disease on a daily basis. For these reasons diabetics must be able to monitor the status of their disease and initiate modifications in its management. To manage diabetes, the patient must learn to control the disease. Treatment cannot cure diabetes; therefore the patient must continue to monitor and manage the disease for life. Long-term compliance with management regimens is a major problem that diabetics and individuals with other controllable, but not curable, conditions such as high blood pressure often find difficult to maintain.

Diabetes mellitus is a chronic disease requiring ongoing medical care and patient and family education to prevent acute illness and reduce the risk of long-term complications. These goals should not unduly restrict the individual's quality of life. However, the dramatic results of the Diabetes Control and Complications Trial indicate that the therapeutic objective of diabetes control is the restoration of known metabolic derangements to as close to normal as possible to prevent and delay the progression of diabetic complications (Box 17-3). This objective should be approached while every effort is made to avoid severe hypoglycemia.[36]

**box 17-3** *Results of the diabetes control and complications trial*

In the study, 1441 type I diabetics in 29 U.S. centers reported that near normalization of blood glucose resulted in a delay in the onset and a major slowing of the progression of established microvascular and neuropathic complications during a follow-up of up to 10 years. In addition, the following facts characterized smaller groups of patients who received differing treatments:

- The intensively treated group received multiple insulin injections (66%) or insulin pumps (34%). Conventionally treated groups received no more than two insulin injections. The goal was clinical well-being.
- About 50% of intensive therapy subjects achieved a mean blood glucose level of 155 mg/dl. Conventionally treated groups averaged a blood glucose level of 225 mg/dl.
- Over a study period that lasted 7 years, there was an approximately 60% reduction in risk between the two groups in regard to diabetic retinopathy, nephropathy, and neuropathy.
- Intensively treated patients experienced greater tendencies toward weight gain and threefold greater risks for serious hypoglycemia.

Data from DTTC Research Group: The effect of intensive treatment of diabetes on the development and progression of long-term complications in insulin-dependent diabetes mellitus, *N Engl J Med* 329:977, 1993.

When compared to the older method of testing urinary glucose levels, at-home monitoring of capillary blood glucose has permitted greater flexibility in the management of diabetes while achieving improved glycemic control. The improved control is especially important for type I diabetics, who try to achieve "tight" metabolic control. More accurate electronic blood glucose monitoring devices, such as the portable, battery-operated Glucometer II (Ames), have helped reduce the risk of hypoglycemic episodes in individuals with tight control of blood sugar levels.[37,38] Glucose meters are relatively inexpensive, costing between $50 and $100 each, a one-time expense. Test strips, used with every blood test, cost a hefty 50 cents to 75 cents apiece.

The diabetic must be able to perform the following three essential steps when using a glucometer (Figures 17-1 and 17-2):

1. Obtain a drop of capillary blood from a finger prick. (Newer lancets are 28 gauge, compared with the original [and more painful] 21-gauge lancets.)
2. Apply the blood sample to a test strip and remove the sample at the proper time (usually 60 seconds). Newer glucose meters, One-Touch II [Lifescan] and ExacTech [Baxter], automatically time the reaction as soon as blood is applied to the test strip. In this way the patient need not wipe the strip at a precise time.
3. Accurately evaluate the color that develops, a skill that requires careful education and training.

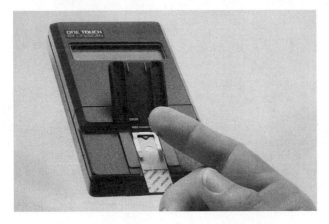

**Figure 17-1**   The One Touch is used to prick the finger to obtain a drop of capillary blood for glucose testing.

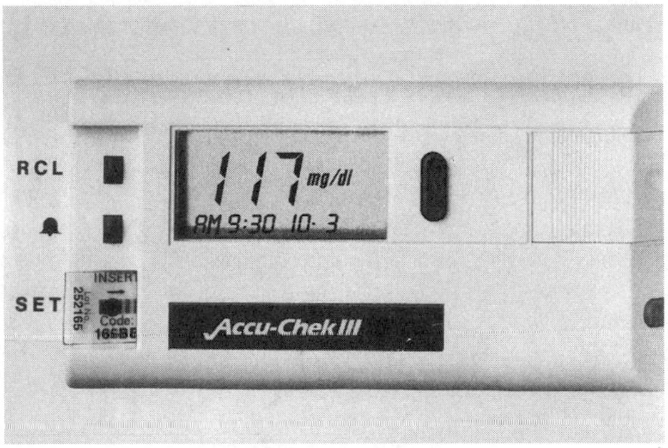

**Figure 17-2**   The blood sample then is applied to test strip and removed at the proper time.

table **17-7**   *Diagnosis of diabetes mellitus*

| | NORMAL GLUCOSE TOLERANCE | IMPAIRED GLUCOSE TOLERANCE | DIABETES MELLITUS |
|---|---|---|---|
| Fasting plasma glucose (mg/dl) | <115 | 116-139 | >140 |

Self-monitoring of blood glucose is especially important for brittle diabetics (that is, those who are unable to maintain a stable blood sugar level and exhibit extremes of both hyperglycemia and hypoglycemia despite therapy), women trying to maintain ideal glycemic control during pregnancy, and individuals with little or no warning of impending hypoglycemic episodes. This type of self-monitoring has proved a safe and reliable clinical tool in compliant diabetics. Diagnostic strips, such as Chemstrip-bG (Bio-Dynamics), permit visual estimation of glucose concentrations with a series of color standards.

Capillary blood glucose levels are closer to arterial levels than are those obtained from venous blood. Normal fasting blood glucose levels for venous blood range from 60 to 100 mg/100 ml (60 to 100 mg%). In 1979 the National Diabetes Data Group[39] stated that a fasting blood glucose level of 140 mg/100 ml on two or more occasions is adequate for the diagnosis of diabetes mellitus. Fasting hyperglycemia is replacing oral glucose tolerance tests in the diagnosis of diabetes mellitus (Table 17-7).[40]

Diabetics can be managed by maintaining control over diet and physical activity and administering oral antidiabetic drugs and insulin, as needed. Many type II diabetics use the combination of weight loss, exercise, and diet control. However, when this regimen fails, they must add oral antidiabetic drugs (Table 17-8). Sulfonylurea agents, such as tolbutamide, tolazamide, chlorpropamide, acetohexamide, and the newer second-generation sulfonylurea drugs, glyburide and glipizide, remain the most widely prescribed oral drugs for the treatment of hyperglycemia.[40-43] Glyburide and glipizide,[44] newer oral antidiabetic drugs, are 100-fold more potent than the earlier oral antidiabetics such as tolbutamide. For this reason, they are used in significantly lower doses. The incidence of adverse side effects, which occur commonly with first-generation sulfonylurea drugs, is remarkably diminished with these newer drugs.

In December 1994 the FDA approved the use of metformin, a biguanide drug, for clinical use as an oral antidiabetic. Unlike the sulfonylureas, which work by stimulating the pancreas to secrete more insulin, metformin decreases hyperglycemia via other mechanisms. The drug is an "insulin-sparing" drug that does not causes weight gain in treated diabetics. Its tendency to produce lactic acidosis is only one-tenth that of phenformin, another biguanide, which the FDA removed from the market in the U.S. and in many other countries in 1977. Exactly how metformin works is unclear. It reduces both the fasting level of blood glucose and the degree of postprandial hyperglycemia in type II diabetics; however, the drug does not affect fasting blood glucose in normal subjects.

table **17-8** *Currently available oral antidiabetic drugs*

| GENERIC NAME | PROPRIETARY NAME | DAILY DOSE | DURATION (HR) |
|---|---|---|---|
| Tolbutamide | Orinase | 0.5-2 g in 2-3 divided doses | 6-12 |
| Tolazamide | Tolinase | 01.-1 g as single dose or in two divided doses | up to 24 |
| Acetohexamide | Dymelor | 0.25-1.5 g as single dose or in two divided doses | 8-24 |
| Chlorpropamide | Diabinese | 0.1-0.5 g as single dose | 24-72 |
| Glyburide | DiaBeta, Micronase | 1.25-20 mg as single dose or in two divided doses | Up to 24 |
| | Glynase | 1.5-18 mg in single dose or in two divided doses | Up to 24 |
| Glipizide | Glucotrol | 2.5-40 mg as single dose or in two or three divided doses on an empty stomach | 6-12 |
| Metformin | Glucophage | 1-2.55 g in one tablet with meals 2 or 3 times daily | 7-12 |

Some question does remain regarding the safety of oral antidiabetic agents. The University Group Diabetes Program reported that the number of deaths due to cardiovascular disease in diabetics treated with tolbutamide or the no-longer-used phenformin was excessive, compared with either insulin-treated patients or those receiving placebos. At present, each package of sulfonylureas or metformin contains a warning label concerning potential cardiac death. However, there is no restriction upon recommending their use by the American Diabetes Association.

The type I diabetic requires insulin to control blood glucose levels. In addition, the nonobese type II diabetic with insulinopenia whose hyperglycemia does not respond to diet therapy either alone or in combination with oral antidiabetic drugs requires insulin. Until recently, diabetics received insulin extracted from the pancreas of the cow and pig. A risk of adverse reactions accompanied administration of this bovine or porcine insulin, including both localized allergy and systemic allergy, immune insulin resistance, and localized lipoatrophy at the injection site. Improvements in the purification of beef and pork insulin have minimized the occurrence of serious adverse reactions in most type I diabetics. In 1983 genetically designed human insulin became available.[45] This insulin is synthesized in a non–disease-producing special laboratory strain of *Escherichia coli* bacteria that has been genetically altered by the addition of the human gene for insulin production. Although the risk of serious adverse reaction is diminished, reports of such responses still appear.[46]

Insulin is available in several preparations that differ in their onset and duration of action (Table 17-9). They are characterized as rapid-acting, intermediate-acting, and long-acting insulin. Regular insulin is absorbed rapidly and administered before meals, whereas NPH and Lente preparations are intermediate acting and administered once a day. Long-acting

table **17-9** *Currently available insulin preparations in the United States*

| ACTION | TYPE OF INSULIN | ONSET | DURATION (HR) |
|---|---|---|---|
| Short | Regular | 15 min | 5-7 |
| Intermediate | Lente | 2 hr | 18-24 |
| | NPH | 2 hr | 18-24 |
| Long | Ultralente | | 24-36 |

insulin (protamine) preparations are available, but are rarely required.

Patients requiring insulin therapy are initially regulated under conditions of optimal diet and normal daily activities. If "tight" control (near-normalization of blood glucose levels) is the goal, at least three measurements of capillary blood glucose are required daily to prevent frequent hypoglycemic reactions. Insulin is administered via either a conventional split-dose mixture or intensive insulin therapy.

A typical initial dose schedule for a 70-kg patient taking 2200 kcal divided into six or seven feedings may be 10 units of regular and 15 units of NPH insulin in the morning, followed by 5 units each of regular and NPH insulin in the evening. Diabetics are taught to adjust insulin intake by observing their pattern of glycemia and correlating it with the approximate duration of action and the time of peak effect after injection of the various insulin preparations.

When intensive insulin therapy is deemed necessary (when conventional split doses of insulin mixtures fail to maintain near normalization of blood glucose without hypoglycemia), multiple insulin injections may be required. A popular regimen consists of decreasing the evening dose of intermediate insulin and adding a portion of it at bedtime. The administration of three smaller doses of regular insulin (before meals) and one injection of long-acting insulin at bedtime is yet another possible regimen.[47] Other options available today include the use of continuous subcutaneous infusions with portable open-loop insulin pumps, which require subcutaneous needle insertion only every 48 hours.

# Prevention

An adequate preliminary patient evaluation can help avert acute complications of diabetes. In addition, the dental health professional is in a position to aid in the detection of previously undiagnosed diabetes (the United States having approximately 10 million undiagnosed diabetics). Relevant questions from the medical history questionnaire and the ensuing dialogue history may lend some insight.

## Medical History Questionnaire

**Question: Circle any of the following that you have had or have at present:**

Diabetes

Cortisone medicine

*Comment:* If the patient is aware that he or she is diabetic, a definitive dialogue history should be obtained. In addition, the prolonged use of corticosteroid medications may lead to the onset of diabetes. The dialogue history is used to determine the presence of signs and symptoms.

**Question 13: Have you lost or gained more than 10 pounds in the past year?**

*Comment:* An affirmative response to unexplained weight loss may indicate the presence of previously undetected diabetes mellitus.

**Question 15: Are you on a special diet?**

*Comment:* An affirmative response may indicate the presence of type II diabetes. Dietary restrictions in type II diabetics vary, ranging from a strict balance between carbohydrate, protein, and fat intake to a more liberal diet in which only total caloric intake is controlled.[48]

**Question 6: Have you taken any medicine or drugs during the past 2 years?**

*Comment:* Table 17-8 lists the oral drugs currently prescribed for the management of type II diabetes. In addition, the doctor should know that other drugs are capable of producing alterations in blood sugar levels (Box 17-4).

| box **17-4** | *Commonly used medications that lower blood sugar levels* |

**Potentiate action of sulfonylureas**

Barbiturates*
Dicumarol
Monoamine-oxidase inhibitors
Salicylates*
Thiazides

**Increase insulin production**

α-Adrenergic blockers
β-Adrenergic stimulators
Monoamine-oxidase inhibitors

**Decrease hepatic glycogenolysis**

Propranolol

**Perform unknown mechanisms**

Antihistamines
    Tripelennamine HCl
Morphine*
Propylthiouracil
Tuberculostatic drugs
    Isoniazid
    Aminosalicylic acid

*These agents are administered or prescribed frequently in the practice of dentistry.

## DIALOGUE HISTORY

If the patient responds negatively to question 9 but positively to any or all of questions 6, 13, or 15, the following dialogue history should be considered:

**Questions: Are you frequently thirsty?**
**Are you hungry much of the time?**
**Do you wake up at night to void (urinate) frequently?**
**Have you gained or lost weight recently without dieting; if so, how many pounds?**

*Comment:* Although these symptoms are not specific for diabetes mellitus, they can lead to a presumptive diagnosis of the disease. The classical triad of diabetic symptoms—the three *p*'s: polydipsia (increased thirst), polyphagia (increased appetite), and polyuria (increased frequency of urination)—when accompanied by unexpected weight loss should alert the doctor to the possible presence of diabetes. If the response to question 9 in the medical history questionnaire is negative and the responses to the dialogue questions are positive, the doctor should continue with the preliminary medical and dental examination and consult the patient's primary-care physician before initiating dental treatment.

If the response to question 9 is positive, the doctor should conduct the following dialogue history:

**Question: How long have you had diabetes, and what type of treatment do you use to control it?**

*Comment:* The severity of the diabetes and the potential for the development of its acute complications are greatest in insulin-dependent and brittle non–insulin-dependent diabetics who manage the disease through injectable insulin and diet control. Patients who successfully control their blood glucose levels through diet alone or through diet and oral hypoglycemic agents (type II diabetics) usually retain some pancreatic function; these patients are more resistant to diabetic ketoacidosis (see Table 17-8).

**Question: How often do you monitor your urine or blood glucose levels? What have your results shown over the past few days?**

*Comment:* For nearly five decades diabetics tested their urine samples for the presence of glucose. Urine tests for glucose and ketones are still important in the management of some cases; however, monitoring urinary glucose levels is significantly less reliable than direct monitoring of capillary blood glucose levels. Indeed some patients may "spill" sugar into the urine at blood glucose values that are significantly below those for hyperglycemia, whereas others do not demonstrate glucose in the urine with blood glucose levels of 300 to 400 mg/100 ml.

Recently, however, most diabetics have begun to self-monitor blood glucose levels at home, a procedure that has rapidly gained acceptance, especially because many necessary products are available over the counter.[49] Although a significant departure in appearance from traditional diabetic testing procedures, capillary blood glucose testing is a more sophisticated and logical extension of tests usually performed by physicians and laboratories. Proprietary names for home blood glucose testing kits include Chemstrip bG (Bio-Dynamics), Dextrostix (Miles Labs), and Glucostix (Miles Labs). Portable, battery-operated devices, such as the Glucometer II (Ames) or Glucosan II, provide a digital readout of the patient's blood glucose level within 60 seconds. Newer devices, such as the One Touch II (Lifescan) and ExacTech (Baxter), automatically time the reaction, eliminating timing errors by the patient. Studies have demonstrated that 8 of 10 diabetics would rather prick their fingers than obtain urine samples.[50]

In addition to their convenience, such tests are accurate, producing results similar to those obtained in professional laboratories. Sonkson[51] demonstrated that patients can maintain normal blood glucose levels more easily through self-assessment of blood, not urine, samples. Levels are recorded in milligrams of glucose per deciliter (100 ml) of whole blood (also read as mg %). In children and adults, values below 50 mg/dl indicate hypoglycemia. The upper range of values (Chemstrip bG) is 240 mg/dl for a 2-minute reading or 800 mg/dl for a 3-minute reading.

For diabetics who still monitor urine, the levels of blood glucose obtained are less reliable. Readings are 0, trace, 1+, 2+, 3+, and 4+. Patients who can keep their glucose levels in the trace or 1+ ranges have relatively well-controlled blood sugar and may be managed normally during dental treatment. Patients with consistently negative (0) readings are more likely to become hypoglycemic. The diabetic with 2+ readings should be evaluated carefully before treatment. Some primary-care physicians prefer that their patients remain in the 1+ to 2+ ranges, in which case they are less likely to become hypoglycemic. If no clinical signs and symptoms associated with hyperglycemia or hypoglycemia are present, dental treatment may proceed without modifications. In contrast, urinary glucose readings of 3+ and 4+ indicate that the diabetic is not in control of the disease. The stress frequently associated with dental treatment further elevates blood sugar and may help precipitate ketoacidosis and potentially, although rarely, diabetic coma. Medical consultation should be performed before treatment so that appropriate adjustments in insulin doses and overall diabetic management may be made.

Table 17-10 summarizes the optimal ASA physical classification for type I and type II diabetics, whereas Table 17-11 presents modifications in these optimal classifications based on urinary or blood glucose levels.

**Question: How frequently (if ever) do you experience hypoglycemic episodes?**

*Comment:* Some diabetics have a greater tendency to become hypoglycemic. Awareness of this tendency better prepares the doctor to manage it. Patients who frequently test negative for urinary glucose or low for blood glucose are more likely to become hypoglycemic.

## PHYSICAL EXAMINATION

After completing the medical history questionnaire and dialogue history, the diabetic patient should be evaluated carefully for signs and symptoms of secondary disease, particularly of the cardiovascular system. Vital signs should be recorded before and after all dental treatment.

The skin of a diabetic patient may indicate the possible presence of acute complications associated with overly high or low blood sugar levels. Hyperglycemic patients appear flushed and their skin dry (absence of sweating because of dehydration), whereas hypoglycemic patients appear cold and wet (clammy). Patients with diabetic ketoacidosis exhibit the characteristic smell of acetone (a sweet, fruity odor) on the breath. The blood pressure of the hyperglycemic, ketoacidotic patient is decreased due to hypovolemia, with a compensatory tachycardia. Hypoglycemic patients exhibit increased blood pressures as well as tachycardia (increased sympathetic response).

## DENTAL THERAPY CONSIDERATIONS

After the medical and dental evaluations are completed, proper patient management must be considered. If any doubt exists about the patient's medical status, contable **17-10**  *Optimal physical status classifications for diabetic patients*

| TYPES OF DIABETES | TREATMENT | SEVERITY | OPTIMAL ASA PHYSICAL STATUS |
|---|---|---|---|
| Type I (IDDM) | Insulin plus diet control | Severe | III |
| Type II (NIDDM) | | | |
| Nonobese | Insulin plus diet control | Moderate to severe | II-III |
| | Oral medication plus diet control | Mild to moderate | II |
| Obese | Oral medication plus diet control | Mild to moderate | II |

*ASA*, American Society of Anesthesiologists; *IDDM*, insulin-dependent diabetes mellitus; *NIDDM*, non–insulin-dependent diabetes mellitus.

table **17-11**  *Physical status classification for diabetes mellitus*

| GLUCOSE MEASUREMENT | | CHANGE IN PHYSICAL STATUS‡ | COMMENT |
|---|---|---|---|
| URINARY* | BLOOD† | | |
| 0 | <50 mg/dl | +1 | May accept for treatment but more likely to be or become hypoglycemic |
| Trace, 1+, 2+ | 80, 120, 180 mg/dl | 0 | May accept for treatment |
| 3+ | 240 mg/dl | +1 | Evaluate carefully before treatment |
| 4+ | >400 mg/dl | +2 | If consistently in this range, obtain medical consultation before treatment |

*Tes-Tape.
†Chemstrip bG.
‡This table lists the change in physical status from the optimal presented in Table 17-10.
Thus an individual with an ASA (American Society of Anesthesiologists) II classification who has a 3+ urinary glucose or 240 mg/dl blood glucose becomes an ASA III.

sultation with the patient's primary-care physician is warranted.

The type II diabetic is less prone to acute fluctuations in blood glucose levels and more apt to tolerate any and all forms of dental treatment, including general anesthesia, parenteral sedation, and local anesthesia, without increased concern. Basic dental treatment modifications may be considered with type I (ketosis-prone) diabetics through use of the stress-reduction protocol. The individual should also be advised to maintain normal dietary habits by taking the usual insulin dose and eating a normal breakfast before a dental appointment. Scheduling dental appointments earlier in the day also helps minimize episodes of hypoglycemia. The use of appropriate local anesthetics (for example, shorter-acting [mepivacaine plain] versus longer-acting [bupivacaine with epinephrine]) minimize posttreatment eating impairment. If the nature of the dental procedure is likely to hamper the patient's normal eating habits either preoperatively (IV sedation) or postoperatively (surgery), the insulin dose should be adjusted accordingly. In addition, medical consultation should be considered for the type I diabetic who requires large doses of insulin to maintain blood glucose levels (>40 units daily) or in any case in which doubt remains concerning adjustment of the patient's insulin dose.

Diabetics are better able to tolerate transient periods of hyperglycemia than periods of hypoglycemia. After extensive dental procedures (for example, oral or periodontal surgery), reconstruction, or endodontics, type I patients should be instructed to check their blood glucose levels more frequently for the next few days. If glucose or ketone levels become elevated, the patient should initiate changes in the insulin dose and contact the primary-care physician. Antibiotic coverage is recommended to minimize the risk of postoperative infections in ASA III or IV diabetics undergoing extensive surgical procedures (Table 17-12).

## Clinical Manifestations

### HYPERGLYCEMIA

Hyperglycemia, or high blood sugar, may manifest itself in different ways depending on the severity of the diabetes. It may be evident in previously undiagnosed diabetics or in known diabetics who neglect their therapeutic regimens. The type II diabetic may not exhibit any clinical signs or symptoms of hyperglycemia. Quite commonly, this form of diabetes is detected during a routine physical examination through evidence of elevated blood glucose levels.

table **17-12**  *Diabetes mellitus—dental therapy considerations*

| ASA PHYSICAL STATUS | TREATMENT CONSIDERATIONS |
|---|---|
| II | Follow usual ASA II considerations, plus the following:<br>Eat a normal breakfast and take usual insulin dose in morning, if possible.<br>Avoid missing meals before and after surgery.<br>If missing meal is unavoidable, consult physician or decrease insulin dose by half. |
| III | Follow usual ASA III considerations, plus the following:<br>Monitor blood glucose levels more frequently for several days after surgery or extensive procedure and modify insulin doses accordingly.<br>Consider medical consultation. |
| IV | Follow usual ASA IV considerations, plus the following:<br>Consult a physician before beginning dental treatment. |

*ASA,* American Society of Anesthesiologists.

Generally, diabetes mellitus is first diagnosed after a clinical episode brought about by an advanced degree of atherosclerosis associated with the disease. Myocardial infarction in a younger man or woman or development of peripheral vascular insufficiency at an early age may also prompt the doctor to suspect diabetes. Other indicators for further evaluation for the presence of diabetes include individuals who are obese, are older than 40 years, have delivered babies larger than 10 pounds, have suffered spontaneous abortion or stillbirth, or have diabetic relatives.[52]

The type I diabetic presents a more severe clinical picture of hyperglycemia. The classic diabetic triad of *p*'s, or *poly's*—polydipsia, polyphagia, and polyuria—is evident for a day or more and is associated with a marked loss of weight, fatigue, headache, blurred vision, abdominal pain, nausea and vomiting, constipation, dyspnea, and mental stupor, which can progress into a state of unconsciousness known as *diabetic coma.*[53]

Clinical signs of hyperglycemia include a florid appearance of the face (bright red color) associated with hot and dry skin, both of which indicate dehydration. Respirations are commonly deep and rapid (signs of Kussmaul's respiration), with a fruity, sweet smell of acetone evident if diabetic ketoacidosis is present. The heart rate is rapid, whereas the blood pressure is lower than normal. This combination of tachycardia and hypotension is yet another indication of dehydration and salt depletion (Table 17-13).

table **17-13**  *Clinical manifestations of hyperglycemia*

|  | TYPE I DIABETES (IDDM) | TYPE II DIABETES (NIDDM) |
|---|:---:|:---:|
| Polyuria | ++ | + |
| Polydipsia | ++ | + |
| Polyphagia with weight loss | ++ | − |
| Recurrent blurred vision | + | ++ |
| Vulvovaginitis or pruritus | + | ++ |
| Loss of strength | ++ | + |
| Nocturnal enuresis | ++ | − |
| Absence of symptoms | − | ++ |

| Other symptoms—type I | Other symptoms—type II |
|---|---|
| Repeated skin infections | Decreased vision |
| Marked irritability | Paresthesias |
| Headache | Loss of sensation |
| Drowsiness | Impotence |
| Malaise | Postural hypotension |
| Dry mouth | |

Modified from Karan JH: Diabetes mellitus and hypoglycemia. In Tierney LM Jr, McPhee SJ, Papadakis MA, editors: *Current medical diagnosis and treatment,* ed 35, Stamford, Conn, 1996, Appleton & Lange; and Little JW, Falace DA: *Dental management of the medically compromised patient,* ed 2, St Louis, 1984, Mosby.
*IDDM,* Insulin-dependent diabetes mellitus; *NIDDM,* non–insulin-dependent diabetes mellitus; −, not usually present; +, occasionally present; ++, usually present.

# HYPOGLYCEMIA

Hypoglycemia, the second and much more common acute complication of diabetes, may rapidly progress to the loss of consciousness, or it may take a relatively mild form, representing a less ominous clinical picture. Episodes of hypoglycemia usually develop when the patient has not eaten for several hours. Initially, hypoglycemia usually manifests as diminished cerebral function, such as the inability to perform simple calculations, decreased spontaneity of conversation, and change in mood (for example, lethargy). Throughout this text I have categorized these symptoms as altered consciousness.

Signs and symptoms of central nervous system involvement include hunger, nausea, and an increase in gastric motility. This is followed by a phase of sympathetic hyperactivity, marked clinically by signs of increased epinephrine activity that include sweating, tachycardia, piloerection, and increased anxiety. The skin is cold and wet, in marked distinction to the hot, dry skin of hyperglycemia. The individual is conscious but may exhibit bizarre behavioral patterns that often lead onlookers to suspect alcohol or drug intoxication. If the condition progresses, the hypoglycemic patient may lose consciousness, and seizures may develop (Box 17-5).

Because hypoglycemia is a more acute problem than hyperglycemia, diabetic patients always carry with them a source of carbohydrate, such as a packet of sugar or hard candy. Tablets containing 3 g of glucose (Dextrosol) are available. It is also recommended that every diabetic receiving insulin therapy be given an ampule of glucagon (1 mg), and the primary-care physician should instruct family and friends on intramuscular (IM) administration technique in case the patient loses consciousness or refuses food. In addition, the state of altered consciousness produced by hypoglycemia may mimic drug intoxication; thus diabetics may not be able to respond rationally to questioning. For this reason, diabetic individuals wear either a MedicAlert bracelet* or necklace or carry a card stating the individual's condition and primary-care physician's number and asking the reader to call in an emergency (Figure 17-3).

# Pathophysiology

## INSULIN AND BLOOD GLUCOSE

Glucose is a major fuel and energy source for all the body's cells. In fact glucose is the only fuel that the brain can use to replenish its continuous need. Blood sugar

---

*MedicAlert Foundation International, Turlock, Calif., 1-800-ID-ALERT.

---

box **17-5** | *Clinical manifestations of hypoglycemia*

**Early stage—mild reaction**
Diminished cerebral function
    Changes in mood
    Decreased spontanteity
Hunger
Nausea

**More severe stage**
Sweating
Tachycardia
Piloerection
Increased anxiety
Bizarre behavioral patterns
    Belligerence
    Poor judgment
    Uncooperativeness

*Later severe stage*
Unconsciousness
Seizure activity
Hypotension
Hypothermia

---

**I Am a Diabetic and Take Insulin**

If I am behaving peculiarly but am conscious and able to swallow, give me sugar or hard candy or orange juice slowly. If I am unconscious, call an ambulance immediately, take me to a physician or a hospital, and notify my physician. *I am not intoxicated.*

My name _____

Address _____

Telephone _____

Physician's name _____

Physician's address _____

Telephone _____

**Figure 17-3** Example of an identification card carried by many diabetics.

that is too high (hyperglycemia) or too low (hypoglycemia) produces varying degrees of central nervous system dysfunction (altered consciousness). The body's homeostatic mechanisms are targeted at maintaining the blood glucose level within a range of 50 to 150 mg/100 ml of blood (mg %). The mean blood glucose level in normal individuals who fast overnight is 92 mg/100 ml, with a range of from 78 to 115 mg/100 ml. The minimal blood glucose level that the brain requires to maintain normal cerebral function is 50 mg/100 ml. When blood glucose levels exceed the saturation point of renal reabsorption (approximately 180 mg/100 ml), glucose "spills" into the urine, resulting in loss of energy (glucose is fuel) and water.

Insulin is the most important factor in the regulation of the blood glucose level. It is synthesized in β-cells of the pancreas and rapidly secreted into the blood in response to elevations in blood sugar levels (for example, after a meal). The half-life of insulin in the blood is 3 to 10 minutes, with biotransformation occurring in the liver and kidneys. Insulin promotes the uptake of glucose into the body's cells and its storage in the liver as glycogen; it also promotes the uptake of fatty acids and amino acids into cells and their subsequent conversion into storage forms (triglycerides and proteins). In this way, insulin produces a decrease in the blood glucose level, preventing its loss through urinary excretion.

Without insulin, the cell membranes of many cells are impermeable to glucose. Muscle and adipose cells are insulin dependent; they require its presence to enable glucose to cross the cell membrane, even in hyperglycemic states.[54] In the absence of insulin these cells break down triglycerides into fatty acids, which the body can use as an alternative energy source. This process gives rise to the hyperglycemic state known as *diabetic ketoacidosis* (DKA). Other tissues and organs, such as nerve tissue (including the brain), the kidneys, and hepatic tissue, are not insulin dependent. These tissues can transfer glucose across cell membranes without insulin.

In the fasting stage, decreased blood sugar levels (hypoglycemia) inhibit insulin secretion. The body's cells still require glucose, however, and several mechanisms exist through which it is made available. The goal of these mechanisms is to provide the central nervous system with the minimal glucose level required to maintain normal function. The body breaks down glycogen stores in the liver into glucose through a process called *glycogenolysis* while amino acids are converted into glucose through a process known as *gluconeogenesis*. This newly formed glucose is available principally to the central nervous system; in fact, insulin-dependent cells actually suffer a decreased uptake of glucose. Fuel for these cells (e.g., muscle and adipose) is provided through the breakdown of triglycerides, the storage form of fat, into free fatty acids.

Thus insulin is a signal to the body that it has been fed and a means for the maintenance of glucose homeostasis. After a meal the high blood level of insulin tells the body's cells to absorb and store any fuel that is not immediately required for metabolic needs. In the fasting state, low insulin levels tell the body that no food is entering and that storage forms of nutrients should be utilized for fuel.

## HYPERGLYCEMIA, KETOSIS, AND ACIDOSIS

After the diabetic or nondiabetic individual eats a meal, hyperglycemia occurs. However, the diabetic's blood glucose level remains elevated for a prolonged period because of a lack of insulin (type I) or because of a lack of response by tissues to circulating insulin (type II). Other factors that help increase blood glucose levels include an increase in the hepatic production of glucose from glycogenolysis and a decreased uptake of glucose by the peripheral insulin-dependent tissues (muscle and adipose).

Glucose appears in the urine when the blood glucose level exceeds the renal reabsorption threshold of approximately 180 mg/100 ml. The presence of glucose in the urine is called *glycosuria*. Because of its large molecular size, glucose in the urine, through osmosis, carries with it large volumes of water as well as the electrolytes sodium and potassium. This, in addition to the presence of ketones, which also increase the secretion of sodium and potassium in the urine, helps produce the clinical symptoms of polyuria (an increased frequency of urination) and the dehydrated state of the hyperglycemic patient, which is characterized by a florid appearance, dry skin, and polydipsia (increased thirst).

Weight loss accompanying a normal or increased appetite is a common feature of type I diabetes. Weight loss initially is due to depletion of water, glycogen, and triglyceride stores. In addition, the body loses muscle mass as it converts amino acids into glucose and ketone bodies. Without insulin, most of the body's cells cannot use the large quantities of glucose in the blood. The fasting state mechanisms previously described respond to the call for required energy. Glycogen in the liver and muscle is converted to glucose via glycogenolysis, and proteins are broken into their component amino acids, which are subsequently converted into glucose through gluconeogenesis in the liver. The body also converts triglycerides into free fatty acids in the liver. In the absence of glucose the body's muscles use these free fatty acids, primarily acetoacetate and β-hydroxybutyrate (ketone bodies), as fuel. The metabolism of acetoacetate creates as a by-product—acetone, which is responsible for the characteristic fruity, sweet breath odor noted in this stage, called *diabetic ketoacidosis.*

If the insulin deficiency is severe, gluconeogenesis and ketogenesis continue to increase, regardless of the blood glucose level. However, the tissues decrease their use of ketones over time so that blood levels of acetoacetate and β-hydroxybutyrate increase. This leads to a decrease in the blood's pH, a condition known as *metabolic acidosis (ketoacidosis).* As blood levels of ketones increase, the renal threshold quickly becomes exceeded and ketones become detectable in the urine. Ketoacidosis depresses cardiac contractility and decreases the response of arterioles to the catecholamines epinephrine and norepinephrine.

More significant perhaps is the effect of metabolic acidosis on blood pH and respiration. As the blood level of ketoacids rises, the blood's pH drops below 7.3. This level induces hyperventilation, the body's attempt to raise the pH by means of respiratory alkalosis (see Chapter 12). When severe, this type of breathing is called *Kussmaul's respirations,* which describes deep respirations that may be either slow or rapid. When severe, this type of breathing may cause the individual to lose consciousness, as in a hyperglycemic or diabetic coma. Hyperglycemic coma is associated with either severe insulin deficiency (diabetic ketoacidosis) or mild-to-moderate insulin deficiency (hyperglycemic nonketotic hyperosmolar coma). Poor patient compliance is one of the most common causes of ketoacidosis, particularly when episodes are recurrent.

## HYPOGLYCEMIA

Hypoglycemia is the most commonly encountered acute complication of diabetes; nondiabetics also may develop this condition. Approximately 70% of cases of nondiabetic hypoglycemia are caused by functional hyperinsulinism, a condition related to an oversecretion of insulin by β-cells in the pancreas because of an exaggerated response to glucose absorption, muscular exertion, pregnancy, or anorexia nervosa, all of which increase insulin requirements.

Whatever its cause, diabetic or nondiabetic, the clinical manifestations of hypoglycemia are the same. By arbitrary definition, hypoglycemia in adults is equated with blood glucose values below 50 mg/100 ml, whereas a blood sugar of <40 mg/100 ml defines the condition in children.[12] Hypoglycemia is characterized by varying degrees of neurologic dysfunction, may occur with or without signs of epinephrine overactivity, and is responsive to the administration of glucose. Although the definition of hypoglycemia indicates a blood glucose level of less than 50 mg/100 ml, hypoglycemic reactions may occur in individuals with normal or higher-than-normal blood glucose levels. Indeed, published reports of hypoglycemic reactions in diabetic patients document blood sugar levels ranging from 82 to 472 mg/100 ml, with reactions developing within 40 minutes of IV insulin administration.[55] On the other hand, blood glucose levels of 25 to 30 mg/100 ml have been reported in patients who exhibit no clinical evidence of hypoglycemia.[56]

One of the most important factors in the precipitation of clinical hypoglycemia is the rate at which the blood glucose level drops. After the administration of insulin, the signs and symptoms of hypoglycemia may develop within a few minutes and progress rapidly to the loss of consciousness. In diabetics receiving oral hypoglycemics, the onset of signs and symptoms is normally more gradual, developing over a period of hours. Clinical signs and symptoms of hypoglycemia are similar to those exhibited by individuals during acute anxiety states or after the administration of excessive doses of epinephrine ("epinephrine reaction").

The lack of adequate blood glucose levels alters the normal functioning of the cerebral cortex and manifests clinically as mental confusion and lethargy. This lack of glucose further manifests itself in the increased activities of the parasympathetic and sympathetic nervous systems. Part of this response is mediated by increased epinephrine secretion, which produces increases in the systolic and mean blood pressures, increases sweating, and produces tachycardia. When the blood sugar level drops even further, the individual may lose consciousness and enter a state of hypoglycemic coma, or insulin shock. During this stage, the diabetic frequently experiences tonic-clonic convulsions, which may lead to permanent cerebral dysfunction if they are not treated promptly.

## Management

Prompt recognition of diabetes-related complications is vital. Equally important is the doctor's ability to differentiate between hyperglycemia and hypoglycemia. Because of the differing rates of onset of these acute complications, diabetic patients who behave bizarrely or lose consciousness should be managed as if they were hypoglycemic until proved otherwise.

Hyperglycemia and ketoacidosis usually develop over a period of many hours or days, and the diabetic appears and behaves chronically ill. Another important factor in differential diagnosis is the hot, dry appearance seen in hyperglycemia, which contrasts to the cold, wet look of hypoglycemia. The odor of acetone on the breath further confirms a diagnosis of hyperglycemia. When doubt remains as to the cause of the condition, supportive therapy (**P-A-B-C** [position-airway-breathing-circulation]) is indicated until additional medical assistance becomes available.

## HYPERGLYCEMIA

Definitive management of hyperglycemia, ketosis, and acidosis consists of the administration of insulin to normalize the body's metabolism, restoration of fluid and electrolyte deficiencies, determination of the precipitating cause, and avoidance of complications. Diabetic ketoacidosis is a life-threatening medical emergency with a mortality rate just under 5%. It is most common in type I diabetics; cases of severe stress, such as sepsis, may result in ketoacidosis in type II diabetics. Usually, dental office management of patients who are hyperglycemic or ketoacidotic is supportive.

The following signs serve as diagnostic clues to the presence of hyperglycemia and its emergency manifestations, diabetic ketoacidosis and diabetic coma:

- Hyperglycemia (>250 mg/dl)
- Acidosis with blood pH <7.3
- Dry, warm skin
- Kussmaul's respirations
- Fruity, sweet breath odor
- Rapid, weak pulse
- Normal to low blood pressure
- Altered level of consciousness

**Hyperglycemia—conscious patient**  The dental patient with clinical signs and symptoms of hyperglycemia represents an ASA IV risk and should not receive any dental treatment until a physician is consulted. In most cases, medical consultation results in the scheduling of an immediate appointment between patient and physician or hospitalization.

> NOTE: Emergency medical technicians are trained to regard any unknown diabetic emergency as hypoglycemia until shown otherwise. If the patient is awake and alert, the EMT may administer oral glucose; if the patient's level of consciousness is altered, glucose paste may be used while monitoring airway management.[57] The reason for this is that if hypoglycemia is not treated rapidly, the patient is likely to die or suffer serious neurologic damage. In contrast, death or permanent disability usually takes longer to develop in hyperglycemic patients.[58]

**Hyperglycemia—unconscious patient**
*Step 1: termination of the dental procedure.*

*Step 2:* **P** *(position).* The unconscious patient should be placed into the supine position with the legs elevated slightly.

*Step 3:* **A-B-C** *(BLS, as indicated).* If the diabetic patient loses consciousness in the dental office, the doctor should implement the steps of BLS quickly (check airway, check breathing, and check the pulse). These steps ensure adequate oxygenation and cerebral blood flow. However, this patient will remain unconscious until the doctor can correct the underlying metabolic cause (for example, hyperglycemia, metabolic acidosis). Usually the only steps of BLS required in diabetic coma are positioning and airway management. Breathing is usually spontaneous, deep, and either rapid or slow. It may be possible to detect the sweet, fruity odor of acetone. Adequate circulation will usually be present.

*Step 4:* **D** *(definitive care):*
*Step 4a: summoning of medical assistance.* Medical assistance should be sought if any unconscious person does not demonstrate improvement after the steps of BLS are initiated.
*Step 4b: IV infusion (if available).* An IV infusion of 5% dextrose and water or of normal saline may be started before emergency personnel arrive. Access to a patent vein facilitates subsequent patient management. Insulin has no place in the office emergency kit (unless the doctor or staff member is an insulin-dependent diabetic). Insulin must be administered carefully and blood tests performed to monitor its effect on blood glucose. The patient requires hospitalization to correct the hyperglycemia and other deficits that occur.
*Step 4c: administration of oxygen.* Oxygen may be administered at any time during this emergency. Although oxygen will not help this patient recover, no harm can result from its administration.
*Step 4d: transportation of the patient to the hospital.* As soon as emergency personnel arrive and stabilize the patient, they will transport the patient to the emergency department of a local hospital for definitive diagnosis (if in doubt) and treatment (Box 17-6).

## HYPOGLYCEMIA

Management of hypoglycemia presents more dramatic results than management of hyperglycemia; most individuals experience a rapid relief from symptoms in a short period of time. The method of management depends on the patient's level of consciousness.

The following signs provide diagnostic clues to the presence of hypoglycemia, also known as *insulin shock:*

- Weakness, dizziness
- Pale, moist skin
- Normal or depressed respirations

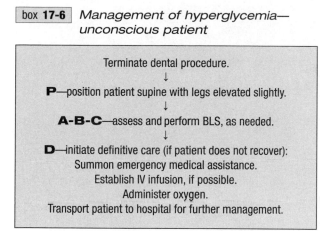

box **17-6**    *Management of hyperglycemia—unconscious patient*

Terminate dental procedure.
↓
**P**—position patient supine with legs elevated slightly.
↓
**A-B-C**—assess and perform BLS, as needed.
↓
**D**—initiate definitive care (if patient does not recover):
Summon emergency medical assistance.
Establish IV infusion, if possible.
Administer oxygen.
Transport patient to hospital for further management.

*BLS,* Basic life support; **P,** position; **A,** airway; **B,** breathing; **C,** circulation; **D,** definitive care; *IV,* intravenous.

- Headache
- Altered level of consciousness

## Hypoglycemia—conscious and responsive patient

*Step 1: recognition of hypoglycemia.* Bizarre behavior or changes in personality (if the patient's breath does not smell of alcohol) and other clinical signs of possible glucose insufficiency should prompt the doctor to suspect hypoglycemia. The condition may develop in both diabetic and nondiabetic individuals. If the patient is diabetic, the doctor should determine how long ago the patient ate or injected a dose of insulin.

NOTE: Hypoglycemics may be unable to respond rationally to such questions (concerning diet and insulin) even though they may appear to be functioning normally.

*Step 2: termination of the dental procedure.*

*Step 3:* **P** *(position).* As with any conscious individual in an emergency situation, positioning is dictated by the individual's comfort. In most situations the hypoglycemic patient prefers to sit upright. Depending on the patient's wishes, the doctor may vary the position.

*Step 4:* **A-B-C** *(BLS, as indicated).* The conscious patient should be capable of maintaining adequate control over airway, breathing, and circulation.

*Step 5:* **D** *(definitive care).*
*Step 5a: administration of oral carbohydrates.* If the patient is conscious and cooperative but still demonstrates clinical symptoms of hypoglycemia, an oral carbohydrate is the treatment of choice. The emergency kit should contain sugar, which can be dissolved and ingested by the patient. Other available items might include orange juice, soft drinks, and candy bars. A 6- to 12-oz portion of soft drink contains 20 to 40 g of glucose. The carbohydrate should be administered in 3- or 4-oz doses every 5 to 10 minutes until the symptoms disappear.

*Step 6: recovery.* The patient should be observed for approximately 1 hour before being permitted to leave the office. The patient may leave the office unescorted if the dentist believes the patient has recovered completely from the episode. If the doctor retains any doubts about the recovery, either the patient should remain in the office longer or arrangements should be made for an adult relative or friend to escort the patient home. In addition, the doctor should determine whether the patient ate before the appointment and reaffirm the importance of eating before each dental visit.

## Hypoglycemia—unresponsive conscious patient

If the patient does not respond to oral glucose or cooperate in ingesting the glucose, the doctor continues with the management.

*Step 1: recognition of hypoglycemia.*
*Step 2: termination of the dental procedure.*
*Step 3:* **P** *(position).*
*Step 4:* **A-B-C** *(BLS, as needed).*
*Step 5:* **D** *(definitive care).*
*Step 5a: administration of oral carbohydrates.*
*Step 5b: summoning of medical assistance.* When oral carbohydrates prove ineffective, outside medical assistance should be summoned immediately.
*Step 5c: administration of parenteral carbohydrates.* If oral carbohydrates do not reverse the signs and symptoms of hypoglycemia or if the individual refuses to ingest the oral carbohydrate, parenteral drug administration must be considered. Glucagon, 1 mg, may be administered IM or IV, or if available, 50 ml of a 50% dextrose solution may be administered IV over 2 to 3 minutes (Figure 17-4). The patient usually responds within 10 to 15 minutes after IM injection of glucagon and within 5 minutes following 50% dextrose IV. Oral carbohydrates should be started as soon as they are tolerated by the patient.
*Step 5d: monitoring of the patient.* Vital signs should be monitored and recorded at least every 5 minutes during the episode until medical assistance becomes available.

*Step 6: discharge and subsequent dental treatment.* Emergency medical personnel will provide the patient with definitive care either in the dental

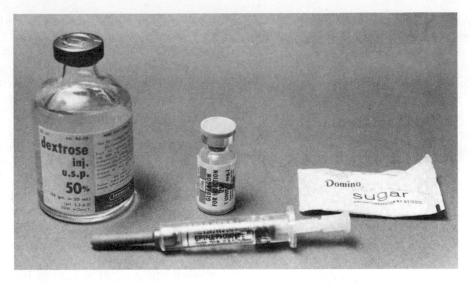

**Figure 17-4**  Antihypoglycemic agents. The 50% dextrose solution must be administered via an IV route, but glucagon and epinephrine may be administered either IM or IV. Sugar is administered orally to the conscious patient.

office or after transport to a hospital. In most instances the patient will be hospitalized, at least until blood sugar levels return to normal. Before scheduling subsequent dental appointments, the doctor should discuss with the patient possible reasons that the episode may have occurred and seek ways in which its recurrence can be prevented.

### Hypoglycemia—unconscious patient

*Step 1: termination of the dental procedure.*

*Step 2:* **P** *(position).* The unconscious patient should be placed in the supine position with the legs elevated slightly.

*Step 3:* **A-B-C** *(BLS, as needed).* If a diabetic patient loses consciousness in the dental office, the doctor should implement quickly the steps of BLS. These steps ensure the maintenance of adequate oxygenation and cerebral blood flow. However, the hypoglycemic patient remains unconscious until the underlying metabolic problem (low blood sugar) is corrected. Usually the only step of BLS that such patients require is airway management. Breathing will be spontaneous, and circulation is adequate.

*Step 4:* **D** *(definitive care):*
*Step 4a: summoning of medical assistance.* If the unconscious patient fails to respond to the steps of BLS, medical assistance should be sought.
*Step 4b: administration of carbohydrates.* An unconscious patient with a history of diabetes should be

presumed to be hypoglycemic unless other obvious causes of unconsciousness exist. Definitive management of the unconscious diabetic requires the administration of carbohydrates via the most effective route available. In most instances this is the IV injection of a 50% dextrose solution or the IM injection of glucagon or epinephrine. (All insulin-dependent diabetics should carry glucagon.) The unconscious patient must never receive via mouth any liquid or other substance that can run into the throat because this increases the possibility of airway obstruction, pulmonary aspiration, or both.

Administration of glucagon (1 mg IM or IV) leads to an elevation of blood glucose via the breakdown of glycogen stores in the liver. The response to glucagon is variable,[59] with an onset of action in approximately 10 to 20 minutes and a peak response in 30 to 60 minutes.[60] If neither glucagon nor a 50% dextrose solution are available, 0.5 mg of a 1:1000 epinephrine concentration may be administered via the subcutaneous or IM route and repeated every 15 minutes, as needed. Epinephrine increases blood glucose levels but should be used with extreme caution in patients with known cardiovascular disease. Once consciousness is restored, the patient should receive fruit juice or soft drinks orally.

In the absence of the parenteral route or of parenteral drugs, the doctor should maintain BLS until medical assistance arrives. Although liquids should never be placed in the mouth of an unconscious or stuporous patient—the risk of aspiration or airway obstruction being too great—a thick paste of concentrated glucose may be used with a high degree of safety. A small amount of honey or syrup may be placed into the patient's buccal fold.[61] Perhaps even more effective for use in a dental office is a small tube of decorative icing designed for bakers; its consistency is similar to or thicker than that of toothpaste. A small, thin strip of this icing may be placed in the patient's maxillary and mandibular buccal folds. Onset is not rapid (usually 30 to 40 minutes), but the blood sugar level will slowly rise; during this wait BLS should continue, and the oral cavity should be evaluated and suctioned every 5 minutes, if necessary.

> NOTE: Previous editions of this text have recommended the transmucosal application of sugar in certain clinical situations. Because of its slow onset of action and the ready access to emergency medical care available to most individuals in the United States and Canada, transmucosal application of sugar is now recommended for use only when access to assistance is considerably delayed (for example, more than 30 minutes).

Although not applicable in many dental settings, the rectal administration of honey or syrup (30 ml per 500 ml of warm water), the so-called honey bear enema, is another effective method in the management of hypoglycemia.[61]

*Step 5: recovery and discharge.* The unconscious hypoglycemic recovers consciousness when blood glucose levels elevate, as long as no additional damage occurred (for example, from hypoxia). Once the individual is conscious, oral carbohydrates, such as fruit juice or soft drinks, may be administered. On arrival, emergency personnel ensure BLS, establish an IV line, and administer any necessary drugs. Once stabilized, the patient then is transported to a hospital for definitive care and observation.

Another important point to remember is that severe hypoglycemia may be associated with the development of generalized tonic-clonic seizures. Management of hypoglycemia-induced seizures follows the guidelines discussed in the section on seizure disorders (see Chapter 21). However, such seizures may persist until the blood sugar level increases.

Box 17-7 outlines the management of hypoglycemia. In addition, the following facts may prove helpful in its treatment:

- **Drugs:** The conscious patient may receive oral forms of sugar. For the unconscious patient, administration of a 50% dextrose solution IV, glucagon IM or IV, sugar paste transmucosally, or syrup or honey rectally is recommended.
- **Medical assistance:** If the individual suffers only a mild alteration of consciousness, no assistance is re-

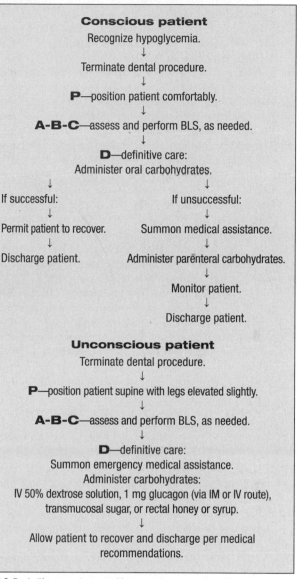

box **17-7**    *Management of hypoglycemia*

**Conscious patient**

Recognize hypoglycemia.
↓
Terminate dental procedure.
↓
**P**—position patient comfortably.
↓
**A-B-C**—assess and perform BLS, as needed.
↓
**D**—definitive care:
Administer oral carbohydrates.

If successful:          If unsuccessful:
↓                  ↓
Permit patient to recover.     Summon medical assistance.
↓                  ↓
Discharge patient.      Administer parenteral carbohydrates.
                       ↓
                       Monitor patient.
                       ↓
                       Discharge patient.

**Unconscious patient**

Terminate dental procedure.
↓
**P**—position patient supine with legs elevated slightly.
↓
**A-B-C**—assess and perform BLS, as needed.
↓
**D**—definitive care:
Summon emergency medical assistance.
Administer carbohydrates:
IV 50% dextrose solution, 1 mg glucagon (via IM or IV route),
transmucosal sugar, or rectal honey or syrup.
↓
Allow patient to recover and discharge per medical recommendations.

*BLS,* Basic life support; **P,** position; **A,** airway; **B,** breathing; **C,** circulation; **D,** definitive care; *IV,* intravenous.

quired. However, if the diabetic loses consciousness or does not respond to the administration of sugar, emergency assistance should be summoned at once.

## REFERENCES

1. Graber TW: Diabetes. In Rosen P, editor: *Emergency medicine: concepts and clinical practice,* ed 4, St Louis, 1998, Mosby.
2. Winter RJ: Recent developments in diabetes research, *Compr Ther* 4:6, 1978.
3. Bingley PJ, Gale EA: Rising incidence of IDDM in Europe, *Diabetes Care* 12(4):289, 1988.

4. Olefsky JM: Diabetes mellitus. In Bennett JC, Plum F, editors: *Cecil textbook of medicine,* ed 20, Philadelphia, 1996, WB Saunders.

5. Skillman TG: Diabetes mellitus. In Massaferri EL, editor: *Endocrinology case studies,* ed 3, Flushing, N.Y., 1986, Medical Examination.

6. Cahill GF: Diabetes mellitus. In Beeson PB, McDermott W, Wyngaarden JB, editors: *Cecil textbook of medicine,* Philadelphia, 1979, WB Saunders.

7. American Heart Association: *1992 Heart and stroke facts,* Dallas, 1991, The Association.

8. Skyler JS: Complications of diabetes mellitus: relationship to metabolic dysfunction, *Diabetes Care* 2:499, 1979.

9. Patel JC, Deshpande PS: Diabetes mellitus the cause of death: its ranking, *Indian J Med Sci* 31:150, 1977.

10. Owen OE and others: Pathogenesis and diagnosis of diabetes mellitus. In Rose LF, Kaye D, editors: *Internal medicine for dentistry,* ed 2, St Louis, 1992, Mosby.

11. Little JW, Falace DA: Diabetes. In Little JW, Falace DA, editors: *Dental management of the medically compromised patient,* ed 4, St Louis, 1993, Mosby.

12. Barkin RM, Rosen P: Hypoglycemia. In Barkin RM, Rosen P, editors: *Emergency pediatrics: a guide to ambulatory care,* ed 4, St Louis, 1994, Mosby.

13. Pyoeralae K: Diabetes and coronary heart disease: what a coincidence, *J Cardiovasc Pharmacol* 16(suppl 9):S8, 1990.

14. Douglas JG: Hypertension and diabetes in blacks, *Diabetes Care* 13(11):1191, 1990.

15. Hamilton BP: Diabetes mellitus and hypertension, *Am J Kidney Dis* 16(suppl 4)1:20, 1990.

16. Davis MD: Diabetic retinopathy, *Diabetes Care* 15:1884, 1992.

17. Humphrey LL, Ballard DJ: Renal complications in non–insulin-dependent diabetes mellitus, *Clin Geriatr Med* 6(4):807, 1990.

18. Fylling CP, Knighton DR: Amputation in the diabetic population: incidence, causes, cost, treatment, and prevention, *J Enterostomal Ther* 16(6):247, 1989.

19. Turner GS, Kohner EM: Diabetic retinopathy, *Practitioner* 228:161, 1984.

20. Frank N: On the pathogenesis of diabetic retinopathy, *Ophthalmology* 91:626, 1984.

21. Rosenberg CS: Wound healing in the patient with diabetes mellitus, *Nurs Clin North Am* 25(1):247, 1990.

22. Wilson TG Jr: Periodontal diseases and diabetes, *Diabetes Educ* 15(4):342, 1989.

23. Al Sayegh H, Jarrett RJ: Oral glucose-tolerance tests and the diagnosis of diabetes: results of a prospective study based on the Whitehall Survey, *Lancet* 2:432, 1979.

24. Keen H, Jarrett RJ, McCartney P: The ten-year follow-up of the Bedford Survey (1962-1972): glucose tolerance and diabetes, *Diabetologia* 22:73, 1982.

25. Goldstein S: Cellular and molecular biological studies on diabetes mellitus, *Pathol Biol* (Paris) 32:99, 1984.

26. MacDonald MJ: Etiology and classification of diabetes in children: practical genetics and prognosis counseling, *Prim Care* 10:531, 1983.

27. Rayfield EJ, Mento SJ: Viruses may be etiologic agents for non-insulin-dependent (type II) diabetes, *Rev Infect Dis* 5:341, 1983.

28. Bodansky HJ and others: Which virus causes the initial islet lesion in type 1 diabetes? *Lancet* 1:401, 1984.

29. Hollander P: The case for tight control in diabetes, *Postgrad Med* 75:80, 1984.

30. Sutherland DE: Pancreas and islet transplant registry statistics, *Transplant Proc* 16:593, 1984.

31. McMaster P: What to expect from pancreas transplantation, *Transplant Proc* 16:587, 1984.

32. Raskin P: Treatment of insulin-dependent diabetes mellitus with portable insulin infusion devices, *Med Clin North Am* 66:1269, 1982.

33. Knowles HC Jr: Long-term juvenile diabetes treated with unmeasured diet, *Trans Assoc Am Physicians* 84:95, 1971.

34. Kitabchi AE, Wall BM: Diabetic ketoacidosis, *Med Clin North Am* 79:9, 1995.

35. Fleckman AM: Diabetic ketoacidosis, *Endocrinol Metab Clin North Am* 22:181, 1993.

36. DTTC Research Group: The effect of intensive treatment of diabetes on the development and progression of long-term complications in insulin-dependent diabetes mellitus, *N Engl J Med* 329:977, 1993.

37. Bell PM, Walshe K: Home blood glucose monitoring: impact on lifestyle and diabetes control, *Practitioner* 228:197, 1984.

38. Aziz S, Hsiang Y: Comparative study of home blood glucose monitoring devices: Visidex, Chemstrip bG, Glucometer, and Accu-Chek bG, *Diabetes Care* 6:529, 1983.

39. National Diabetes Data Group: Classification and diagnosis of diabetes mellitus and other categories of glucose intolerance, *Diabetes* 28:1039, 1979.

40. University Group Diabetes Program: Effects of hypoglycemic agents on vascular complications in patients with adult-onset diabetes. II. Mortality results, *Diabetes* 19(suppl 2):785, 1970.

41. University Group Diabetes Program: Effects of hypoglycemic agents on vascular complications in patients with adult-onset diabetes. V. Evaluation of phenformin therapy, *Diabetes* 24(suppl 1):65, 1975.

42. University Group Diabetes Program: Effects of hypoglycemic agents on vascular complications in patients with adult-onset diabetes. VI. Supplementary report on nonfatal events in patients treated with tolbutamide, *Diabetes* 25:1129, 1976.

43. University Group Diabetes Program: Effects of hypoglycemic agents on vascular complications in patients with adult-onset diabetes. VIII. Mortality and selected nonfatal events with insulin treatment, *JAMA* 240:37, 1978.

44. Glyburide and glipizide: *Med Lett Drugs Ther* 26:79, 1984.

45. Human insulin: *Med Lett Drugs Ther* 25:63, 1983.

46. Grammer LC, Metzger BE, Patterson R: Cutaneous allergy to human (recombinant DNA) insulin, *JAMA* 251:1459, 1984.

47. Stephenson JM, Schernthaner G: Dawn phenomenon and Smogyi effect in IDDM, *Diabetes Care* 12:245, 1989.

48. Williams G: Management of non–insulin-dependent diabetes mellitus, *Lancet* 343:95, 1994.

49. Tomky DM, Clarke DH: A comparison of user accuracy, techniques, and learning time of various systems for self blood glucose monitoring, *Diabetes Educator* 16(6):483-486, 1990.

50. Sonkson PH, Judd S, Lowy C: Home monitoring of blood glucose: new approach to management of insulin-dependent diabetic patients in Great Britain, *Diabetes Care* 3:100, 1980.

51. Sonkson PH, Judd S, Lowy C: Home monitoring of blood glucose, *Lancet* 1:729, 1978.

52. Andreani D, DiMario U, Pozzilli P: Prediction, prevention, and early intervention in insulin-dependent diabetes, *Diabetes Metab Rev* 7(1):61-77, 1991.

53. Nabarro JD: Diabetes in the United Kingdom: a personal series, *Diabetic Med* 8(1):59-68, 1991.

54. Garland PB, Newsholm EA, Randle PJ: Regulation of glucose uptake by muscle, *Biochem K* 93:665, 1964.

55. Hepburn DA and others: Symptoms of acute insulin-induced hypoglycemia in humans with and without IDDM: factor-analysis approach, *Diabetes Care* 14(11):949-957, 1991.

56. Arogyasami J and others: Effects of exercise on insulin-induced hypoglycemia, *J Appl Physiol* 69(2):686-693, 1990.

57. Pollakoff J, Pollakoff K: *EMT's guide to treatment,* Los Angeles, 1991, Jeff Gould.

58. Pollakoff J: Diabetes. In *EMT news update,* Pacoima, Calif, 1989, Poicoma Skills Center.

59. Bobzien WF: Suicidal overdoses with hypoglycemic agents, *JACEP* 11:467, 1979.

60. Lorber D: Nonketotic hypertonicity in diabetes mellitus, *Med Clin North Am* 79:39, 1995.

61. Karam JH: Diabetes mellitus & hypoglycemia. In Tierney LM Jr, McPhee SJ, Papadakis MA, editors: *Current medical diagnosis & treatment,* ed 35, 1996, Stamford, Conn, Appleton & Lange.

# 18

# *Thyroid Gland Dysfunction*

*HE* thyroid gland is composed of two elongated lobes on either side of the trachea that are joined by a thin isthmus of thyroid tissue located at or below the level of the thyroid cartilage.[1]

The thyroid gland produces and secretes three hormones that are vital in the regulation of the level of biochemical activity of most of the body's tissues. These hormones are thyroxine ($T_4$), triiodothyronine ($T_3$), and calcitonin. Proper functioning of the thyroid gland from the time of birth is vital for normal growth and metabolism.

Thyroid gland dysfunction may occur either through overproduction (hyperthyroidism) or underproduction (hypothyroidism) of thyroid hormone. In both instances the observed clinical manifestations may encompass a broad spectrum, ranging from subclinical dysfunction to acute life-threatening situations. Fortunately, most patients with thyroid dysfunction suffer the milder forms of the disease.

Like adrenal insufficiency, thyroid gland dysfunction presents initially as a slow, insidious process in which nonspecific signs and symptoms develop over months or years and then are acutely precipitated by intercurrent stress. Thyroid dysfunction is relatively uncommon, and the characteristic symptoms are not easy to recognize. All three thyroid conditions are potentially lethal if untreated and constitute medical emergencies in their extreme stages.[2]

This chapter focuses primarily on the detection of clinical signs and symptoms of thyroid gland dysfunction. In addition, parts of the discussion consider the life-threatening situations myxedema coma and thyroid "storm", or crisis—both of which are extremely rare.

Hypothyroidism is a clinical state in which the body's tissues do not receive an adequate supply of thyroid hormones. Clinical signs and symptoms of hypothyroidism are related to the age of the patient at the time of onset and to the degree and duration of the hormonal deficiency. A deficiency of thyroid hormone during fetal or early life can produce a clinical syndrome known as *cretinism* in infants and children.[3] Severe hypothyroidism that develops in an adult is called *myxedema* and refers to the appearance of nonpitting, gelatinous, mucinous infiltrates beneath the skin.[4] Severe, unmanaged hypothyroidism ultimately may induce the loss of consciousness, a condition known as *myxedema coma.* The mortality rate in myxedema coma is high (up to 50%) even with optimal treatment.[5,6]

Hyperthyroidism is also known by several other names, including *thyrotoxicosis, toxic goiter (diffuse or nodular), Basedow's disease,*[7] *Graves' disease,*[8] *Parry's disease,* and *Plummer's disease.* It is a state of heightened thyroid gland activity associated with the production of excessive quantities of the thyroid hormones L-thyroxine ($T_4$) and L-triiodothyronine ($T_3$). Because the thyroid hormones affect the cellular metabolism of virtually all organ systems, signs and symptoms of hyperthyroidism may be noted in any part of the body. Left untreated, hyperthyroidism may lead to an acute life-threatening situation known as *thyroid storm,* or *thyroid crisis,* which manifests as severe hypermetabolism, including high fever, and cardiovascular, neurologic, and gastrointestinal dysfunction.[9] Although uncommon today, thyroid storm still has a high mortality rate.

# Predisposing Factors

Dysfunction of the thyroid gland is a relatively common medical disorder. Excluding diabetes mellitus, the most common endocrine disorder, thyroid gland dysfunction accounts for 80% of all such disorders.

## HYPOTHYROIDISM

Thyroid failure usually occurs as a result of diseases of the thyroid gland (primary hypothyroidism), pituitary gland (secondary), or hypothalamus (tertiary).[2] Secondary failure accounts for less than 4% of cases,[10] whereas tertiary failure is even less common. Primary thyroid disease causes the remaining cases. Adult hypothyroidism usually develops as a result of idiopathic atrophy of the thyroid gland, which many researchers

currently believe occurs via an autoimmune mechanism.[11] Other causes of hypothyroidism include total thyroidectomy or ablation after radioactive iodine therapy, both of which are used commonly to manage thyroid gland hyperfunction, and chronic thyroiditis. Thyroid hypofunction occurs 3 to 10 times more frequently in females than males,[12] with the greatest incidence in the seventh decade of life.[13] Myxedema coma, the end stage of untreated hypothyroidism, carries a mortality rate of up to 50% but is seen infrequently clinically.[5,6] Myxedema coma is associated with severe hypothermia,[10] hypoventilation, hypoxia, hypercapnea, and hypotension.[14] Box 18-1 lists possible causes of hypothyroidism.

The dentist should be aware of possible hypothyroid patients because if medically untreated or inadequately managed, they represent increased risks during dental treatment. The clinically hypothyroid patient is unusually sensitive to most central nervous system (CNS) depressant drugs, including sedatives, opioids, and antianxiety drugs, which are commonly used in dentistry. Usual therapeutic doses of these drugs may result in extreme overreactions in clinically hypothyroid individuals.

## HYPERTHYROIDISM

Like hypothyroidism, hyperthyroidism, also called *thyrotoxicosis,* usually begins insidiously and may progress, resulting in the more severe form of the disorder, thyroid storm, or thyroid crisis, if left untreated.

Approximately 3 out of 10,000 adults develop thyroid gland hyperfunction each year; eight females are diagnosed for every male.[15] Hyperthyroidism occurs

| box **18-1** | *Causes of hypothyroidism* |

**Primary**
Autoimmune hypothyroidism
Idiopathic causes
Postsurgical thyroidectomy
External radiation therapy
Radioiodine therapy
Inherited enzymatic defect
Iodine deficiency
Antithyroid drugs
Lithium, phenylbutazone

**Secondary**
Pituitary tumor
Infiltrative disease (sarcoid) of pituitary

Modified from Wogan JM: Endocrine disorders. In Rosen P, editor: *Emergency medicine: concepts and clinical practice,* ed 4, St Louis, 1998, Mosby.

most often in patients between 20 and 40 years.[16] By far the most common form of thyrotoxicosis is that associated with diffuse enlargement of the thyroid gland and the presence of antibodies against different fractions of the thyroid gland. This autoimmune thyroid disorder, called *Graves' disease* (*Basedow's disease* in Europe and Latin America), has a familial tendency. Box 18-2 lists other causes of hyperthyroidism.

Although rare, thyroid storm, or crisis, occurs in patients with untreated or incompletely treated thyrotoxicosis. Only about 1% to 2% of patients with hyperthyroidism will progress to thyroid storm.[17] On rare occasions thyroid storm may occur suddenly in a patient who has not previously been diagnosed with hyperthyroidism. More commonly, thyroid storm follows a long history of uncomplicated hyperthyroidism. The patient usually experiences 6 to 8 months of milder symptoms and may have developed hyperthyroidism as long as 2½ to 5 years before.[17,18] Thyroid storm represents a sudden and severe exacerbation of the signs and symptoms of hyperthyroidism. It is usually accompanied by hyperpyrexia (elevated body temperature) and precipitated by some form of stress, intercurrent disease, infection, trauma, thyroid surgery, or radioactive iodine administration.

Clinically hyperthyroid patients are unusually sensitive to catecholamines, such as epinephrine, and may respond to their administration with hypertensive episodes, tachycardia, or significant dysrhythmias. In addition, hyperthyroid patients may appear apprehensive, which may suggest the need for sedation during dental treatment. However, sedatives may prove futile in such patients, whose "anxiety" is not psychologic, but hormonally-induced. Both hyperthyroidism and hypothyroidism are associated with an increased incidence of cardiovascular disease.[19,20]

Milder forms of both types of dysfunction may go easily unnoticed. Although both hyperthyroidism and hypothyroidism can potentially create increased risks during dental treatment, the more severe, undiagnosed, or untreated patient presents the greatest risk. The doctor must be able to recognize each form of thyroid dysfunction and take the steps necessary to decrease potential risks.

## Prevention

Two goals are essential in the management of patients with thyroid dysfunction:

1. Prevention of the occurrence of the life-threatening situations myxedema coma and thyroid storm
2. Prevention of the exacerbation of complications associated with thyroid dysfunction, notably cardiovascular disease

Only Question 9 on the University of Southern California medical history questionnaire relates to thyroid disease. However, several other questions may provide important information about potential thyroid gland dysfunction. Most other medical history questionnaires do not specifically mention thyroid disease.

### Medical History Questionnaire

**Question 4: Have you been a patient in the hospital during the past 2 years?**
**Question 5: Have you been under the care of a medical doctor during the past 2 years?**
**Question 9: Circle any of the following that you have had or have at present:**

Thyroid disease

*Comment:* Patients with a known history of thyroid gland dysfunction most often mention the problem in one or more of these three questions.

**Question 6: Have you taken any medicine or drugs during the past 2 years?**

*Comment:* Patients with thyroid gland hypofunction receive thyroid extract or a synthetic preparation.[21] The most frequently used drug, which is also the drug of choice, is L-thyroxine sodium (Synthroid). Other drugs commonly used in management of thyroid hypofunction include liotrix (Euthroid, Thyrolar) and dextrothyroxine sodium (Choloxin). The goal in thyroid dysfunction management is to achieve a normal level of glandular functioning, known as the *euthyroid state.*

---

box **18-2**    *Causes of hyperthyroidism*

Toxic diffuse goiter (Graves' disease)
Toxic multinodular goiter
Toxic uninodular goiter
Factitious thyrotoxicosis
$T_3$ thyrotoxicosis
Thyrotoxicosis associated with thyroiditis
    Hashimoto's thyroiditis
    Subacute (de Quervain's) thyroiditis
Jod-Basedow
Metastatic follicular carcinoma
Malignancies with circulating thyroid stimulators
TSH-producing pituitary tumors
Struma ovarii with hyperthyroidism
Hypothalamic hyperthyroidism

From Wogan JM: Endocrine disorders. In Rosen P, editor: *Emergency medicine: concepts and clinical practice,* ed 4, St Louis, 1998, Mosby.
*T₃,* Triiodothyronine; *TSH,* thyroid-stimulating hormone.

Patients with a hyperfunctioning thyroid gland undergo treatment aimed at halting the excessive secretion of thyroid hormone. Three methods—medical therapy, subtotal thyroidectomy, and radioactive iodine ablation of the gland—help to achieve this goal.[22] Frequently prescribed antithyroid drugs include propylthiouracil (Propyl-Thyracil) and methimazole (Tapazole).[23] Propranolol (Inderal), dexamethasone, and lithium also are used to manage thyrotoxicosis (Table 18-1).[23]

### Question 13:  Have you lost or gained more than 10 pounds in the past year?

*Comment:* Unexplained weight loss in a patient with a ravenous appetite should alert the doctor to the possible presence of hyperthyroidism. Conversely, an unexplained increase in weight accompanied by other clinical signs and symptoms may indicate hypothyroidism.

### Question 16:  Has your medical doctor ever said you have a cancer or a tumor?

*Comment:* Thyroid dysfunction is frequently discovered during a routine examination of the patient's neck; the condition often manifests itself as a lump or bump. Question 16 prompts the individual to explain the type of thyroid dysfunction and mode of treatment. Subtotal thyroidectomy is a common mode of treatment for thyroid hyperfunction. Surgical intervention is especially common in patients whose glands develop benign or malignant thyroid nodules. Irradiation with radioactive iodine (iodine-131) is another common technique in the destruction of hyperactive thyroid tissue.

### Question 7:  Are you allergic to (that is, experience itching, rash, swelling of hands, feet, or eyes) or made sick by penicillin, aspirin, codeine, or any drugs or medications?

*Comment:* Clinically hypothyroid patients are unusually sensitive to the pharmacologic actions of opioids and other CNS depressants. Any adverse response to a strong analgesic, such as codeine, or other CNS depressant should prompt a careful patient evaluation for a precise description of the response. Individuals who overreact (see Chapter 23) to usual doses of these drugs may be hypothyroid.

## DIALOGUE HISTORY

If the patient indicates on Question 9 of the medical history questionnaire a positive history of thyroid disease, an in-depth dialogue history is indicated.

### Question: What is the nature of the thyroid dysfunction—either hypofunction or hyperfunction?
### Question: How do you manage the disorder?

*Comment:* These questions prompt the individual to disclose general information about the thyroid problem.

A physical examination should be performed next to uncover any clinical evidence of thyroid dysfunction. In most instances the patient is euthyroid and represents only a normal  risk during dental treatment. According to the American Society of Anesthesiologists' (ASA) Physical Classification System, this patient represents an ASA II-risk.

However, when the patient has no history of thyroid dysfunction but clinical evidence leads to a suspicion of its presence, the following dialogue history is warranted.

### Question:  Have you unexpectedly gained or lost weight recently?

*Comment:* Recent weight gain (10 or more pounds) is noted commonly in clinically hypothyroid individuals, whereas those with hyperthyroidism often lose weight despite an increased appetite. Note, however, that a number of other medical conditions, including diabetes, congestive heart failure (CHF), and malignancy, may also induce weight gain or loss.

### Question:  Are you unusually sensitive to cold temperatures or pain-relieving medications?

*Comment:* Individuals with a hypofunctioning thyroid often exhibit these symptoms.

### Question:  Are you unusually sensitive to heat?
### Question:  Have you become increasingly irritable or tense?

*Comment:* Patients with a hyperfunctioning thyroid gland frequently exhibit the previous two symptoms. The patient may become more aware of changes in temperature and less aware

table **18-1**  *Medications used to manage hypothyroidism and hyperthyroidism*

| HYPOTHYROIDISM | | HYPERTHYROIDISM | |
| --- | --- | --- | --- |
| GENERIC | PROPRIETARY | GENERIC | PROPRIETARY |
| Thyroid USP (dessicated) | Armour Thyroid, Thyrar, Throid Strong, Westhroid | Prophylthiouracil | |
| Levothyroxine ($T_4$) | Leo-T, Levoxine, Synthroid, Eltroxin | Methimazole | Tapazole |
| Liothryronine ($T_3$) | Cytomel | Carbimazole | |
| Liotrix | Euthroid, Thyrolar | Propanolol | Inderal |

of changes in temperament, whereas a close acquaintance (for example, a spouse) is more likely to notice subtle changes in temperament.

## PHYSICAL EXAMINATION

In most cases the patient who reports a history of thyroid gland dysfunction has received or is currently undergoing treatment. These individuals are usually in an euthyroid state (a condition of normal thyroid hormone levels) and do not represent increased risks during dental treatment.

On the other hand the patient with undetected thyroid dysfunction represents a possibly significant elevation in risk during dental treatment. Fortunately, clinical signs and symptoms enable the doctor to recognize these thyroid dysfunctions and to modify treatment accordingly. The clinically hypothyroid patient may have a large, thick tongue with atrophic papillae and thick edematous skin with puffy hands and face. The skin is dry, and the patient does not sweat. The blood pressure is approximately normal, with the diastolic pressure slightly elevated, and the heart rate is slow (bradycardia). The patient appears lethargic and speaks slowly.

Hyperthyroid patients often appear nervous and have warm, sweaty hands that may mildly tremble. The blood pressure is elevated (systolic more than diastolic), and the heart rate is increased markedly (tachycardia). It is very difficult to make a differential diagnosis between hyperthyroidism and acute anxiety. One possible clue is that the patient with hyperthyroidism has warm, sweaty palms, whereas acutely anxious individuals' palms are cold and clammy.

## DENTAL THERAPY CONSIDERATIONS

**Euthyroid**     Patients with thyroid gland dysfunction who are receiving or have received therapy to treat the condition (for example, surgery, medication, or irradiation), who have normal levels of circulating thyroid hormone, and are asymptomatic are considered euthyroid. These patients are ASA II risks and may be managed normally during dental treatment. In addition, if mild clinical manifestations of either hyperthyroidism or hypothyroidism are present, elective treatment may proceed although certain possible modifications should be considered. These patients are ASA III risks.

**Hypothyroid**     If hypothyroidism is suspected, certain precautions are recommended. Medical consultation with the patient's primary-care physician should be considered before any dental treatment begins. In ad-

dition, caution must be exercised when prescribing any CNS-depressant drugs. Of particular concern are the sedative-hypnotics (barbiturates), opioid analgesics, and antianxiety drugs. Because hypothyroid patients are overly sensitive to the CNS-depressant actions of these drugs, administration of a "normal" dose may prove to be an overdose (known as a *relative* overdose) leading to respiratory or cardiovascular depression, or both.[24]

Furthermore, an increased incidence of cardiovascular disease is associated with the hypothyroid state. Barnes and Barnes[25] theorized that hypofunction of the thyroid gland produces most instances of cardiovascular disease and that correction of thyroid deficiency leads to the elimination of cardiovascular disease. Although controversial, this theory is intriguing. A history of thyroid gland hypofunction should direct the doctor to seek other possible signs and symptoms of cardiovascular disease. In an individual with more intense signs and symptoms of thyroid hypofunction (for example, mental apathy, drowsiness, or slow speech), dental treatment should be postponed until consultation with the patient's primary-care physician or definitive management of the clinical disorder is achieved.

**Hyperthyroid**     Mild degrees of thyroid hyperfunction may pass for acute anxiety, with little increase in clinical risk. However, various cardiovascular disorders, primarily angina pectoris, are exaggerated in cases of hyperthyroidism. If the individual develops one or more of these cardiovascular disorders, the management protocol for the specific situation should be followed (see Section Seven).

Patients who exhibit severe hyperfunction should receive immediate medical consultation. Dental treatment should be postponed until the underlying metabolic disturbance is corrected. A point worth remembering is that psychologic or physiologic stress may precipitate thyroid crisis in untreated or incompletely treated hyperthyroid individuals.

Furthermore, the use of atropine, a vagolytic agent (that is, inhibiting the vagus nerve, which decelerates the heart) should be avoided. Atropine increases the heart rate and may be a factor in precipitating thyroid storm. In addition, epinephrine and other vasopressors should be used with caution in clinically hyperthyroid patients. Vasopressors stimulate the cardiovascular system and may precipitate cardiac dysrhythmias, tachycardia, and thyroid storm in hyperthyroid patients, whose cardiovascular systems already are stimulated. However, local anesthetics with vasoconstrictors may be used when the following precautions are taken:

- Using the least-concentrated effective solution

- Injecting the smallest effective volume of anesthetic/vasopressor
- Aspirating before each injection (see Chapter 23)

Of greater potential risk, however, is the use of racemic epinephrine for gingival retraction. This form of epinephrine is more likely to precipitate unwanted side effects, especially in the presence of clinical hyperthyroidism. The use of racemic epinephrine is absolutely contraindicated in the clinically hyperthyroid patient.

Patients who are mildly hyperthyroid easily may be mistaken for those who are apprehensive. The use of conscious sedation techniques in these individuals is not contraindicated. However, because the apparent nervousness of the hyperthyroid individual is induced by hormones, not fear, sedative drugs may be less than effective (the patient requiring larger-than-normal doses to achieve sedation).

Hypothyroid or hyperthyroid patients who have been treated and are currently euthyroid are ASA II risks, whereas patients who exhibit clinical manifestations of thyroid dysfunction are ASA III risks (Table 18-2).

## Clinical Manifestations

### HYPOTHYROIDISM

Hypothyroidism is a state in which all bodily functions progressively slow down, a process caused by an insufficient supply of the thyroid hormones. When this deficiency occurs during childhood, the child exhibits alterations in growth and development and the syndrome is termed *cretinism*. Children who suffer cretinism lack the necessary thyroid hormone in utero or shortly after birth, which retards the child's entire physical and mental development. Ossification of bone is delayed, tooth development is poor, tooth

eruption is delayed, and permanent neurologic damage is evident. Clinically, the infant is dull and apathetic, and the body temperature is usually subnormal. Physically, the tongue is enlarged, the skin and lips are thick, the face is broad and puffy, and the nose is flat (Figure 18-1).

When hypothyroidism occurs in the adult, the onset is usually insidious. A friend or spouse often persuades the individual to seek medical assistance because of noticeably increased weakness and fatigue, sudden weight gain (usually about 7 or 8 pounds) not associated with an increased appetite,[26] or cold intolerance, present in half the cases.[27] The patient is frequently unaware of these changes.

As the disease progresses, the individual may exhibit slowing of the speech, hoarseness, absence of sweating, moderate weight gain, constipation (in 25% of cases), decreased sense of taste and smell, peripheral nonpitting edema, dyspnea, and anginal pain. Clinical signs include puffiness of the face and eyelids,[28] carotenemic (orange-red) skin color and rosy cheeks,

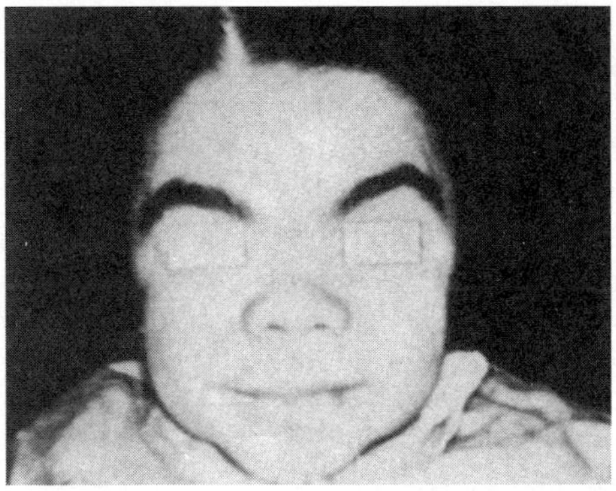

**Figure 18-1** A clinical picture of an individual with cretinism demonstrates the characteristic flat nose and broad, puffy face.

| table **18-2** | *Physical status classifications of thyroid gland dysfunction* |

| DEGREES OF DYSFUNCTION | PHYSICAL STATUS (ASA) | CONSIDERATIONS |
|---|---|---|
| Hypofunctioning or hyperfunctioning patient receiving medical therapy; no signs or symptoms of dysfunction evident | II | Usual ASA considerations |
| Hypofunction or hyperfunction; signs and symptoms of dysfunction evident | III | Usual ASA III considerations, including avoidance of vasopressors (hyperfunction) or CNS depressants (hypofunction)<br>Evaluation for cardiovascular disease |

*ASA,* American Society of Anesthesiologists; *CNS,* central nervous system.

thickened tongue, and thickened edematous skin (non-pitting). The blood pressure measurement remains approximately normal, with the potential for slight elevation of diastolic pressure[13]; however, the heart rate decreases (sinus bradycardia being the most common dysrhythmia in individuals who have hypofunctioning thyroids). Patients with severe, untreated hypothyroidism may develop CHF with pulmonary congestion.

Pseudomyotonic deep tendon reflexes and paresthesias are extremely common (almost 100% occurrence) in hypothyroid patients. Pseudomyotonic deep tendon reflexes are characterized by a prolonged relaxation phase, which is confirmed through testing of the Achilles tendon reflex while the patient kneels on a chair. The relaxation phase is at least twice as long as the contraction phase in these patients.[29] About 80% of cases include paresthesias,[30] in which the median nerve in carpal tunnel syndrome is the most common. Indeed 5% of patients with carpal tunnel syndrome suffer hypothyroidism.[31]

The most severe complication of hypothyroidism, however, is myxedema coma. This condition has a high mortality rate and is marked by hypothermia (29.5 degrees Celsius to 30 degrees Celsius), bradycardia, hypotension, and intense cerebral obtundation (loss of consciousness). Myxedema coma is rare, occurring in only 0.1% of all cases of hypothyroidism, and extremely rare in patients younger than 50 years; the condition is most common in elderly women.[28] About 80% of patients with myxedema experience hypothermia, some with recorded temperatures as low as 24 degrees Celsius.[10]

Symptoms that are essential to a diagnosis of hypothyroidism include weakness, fatigue, cold intolerance, constipation, menorrhagia, and hoarseness. Signs necessary for diagnosis include dry, cold, yellow, puffy skin; scant eyebrows; thick tongue; bradycardia; and the delayed return of deep tendon reflexes (Table 18-3).[32]

## HYPERTHYROIDISM

Like hypothyroidism, hyperthyroidism is rarely severe at the time of onset. In most cases, questioning of the patient reveals clinical evidence of the dysfunction over a period of months before its "discovery." As with hypofunction, the individual who actually discovers the disease frequently is a spouse or friend, someone who notices changes in the habits and personality of the patient. Nervousness, increased irritability, and insomnia are usually the first evident clinical signs and symptoms. Other clinical manifestations include increased intolerance to

heat; hyperhidrosis, or a marked increase in sweating; overactivity, including quick, uncoordinated movements that range from mild to gross tremors; and rapid speech. Unexplained weight loss accompanied by an increased appetite is another important signal. Up to half of all emergency room patients with thyroid storm have lost more than 40 pounds.[18] Hyperthyroid patients become fatigued easily and may notice heart palpitations.

Clinical signs include excessive sweating; the skin of a hyperthyroid individual feels warm and moist to the touch. The extremities, especially the hands, exhibit varying degrees of tremulousness. When hyperthyroidism results from Graves' disease, ophthalmopathy may be noted, the severity of which does

| table **18-3** | Clinical manifestations of hypothyroidisim |
|---|---|

| SYMPTOMS (10% OR GREATER INCIDENCE) | % MANIFESTATION |
|---|---|
| Paresthesias | 92 |
| Loss of energy | 79 |
| Intolerance to cold | 51 |
| Muscular weakness | 34 |
| Pain in muscles and joints | 31 |
| Inability to concentrate | 31 |
| Drowsiness | 30 |
| Constipation | 27 |
| Forgetfulness | 23 |
| Depressed auditory acuity | 15 |
| Emotional instability | 15 |
| Headaches | 14 |
| Dysarthria | 14 |
| **SIGNS** | **% MANIFESTATION** |
| "Pseudomyotonic" reflexes | 95 |
| Change in menstrual pattern | 86 |
| Hypothermia | 80 |
| Dry, scaly skin | 79 |
| Puffy eyelids | 70 |
| Hoarse voice | 56 |
| Weight gain | 41 |
| Dependent edema | 30 |
| Sparse axillary and pubic hair | 30 |
| Pallor | 24 |
| Thinning eyebrows | 24 |
| Yellow skin | 23 |
| Loss of scalp hair | 18 |
| Abdominal distension | 18 |
| Goiter | 16 |
| Decreased sweating | 10 |

Modified from Wogan JM: Endocrine disorders. In Rosen P, editor: *Emergency medicine: concepts and clinical practice*, ed 4, St Louis, 1998, Mosby.

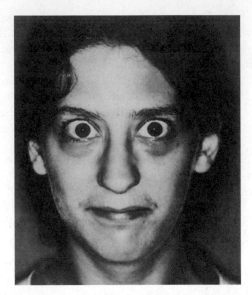

**Figure 18-2**   Hyperthyroid patient exhibiting exophthalmos.

not parallel the intensity of the thyroid gland dysfunction. Werner[33,34] classified the clinical manifestations of ophthalmopathy in hyperthyroid patients, including upper-lid retraction, staring, lid lag, proptosis, exophthalmos (Figure 18-2), and extraocular muscle palsies. Cardiovascular manifestations of hyperthyroidism vary, from an increase in blood pressure (systolic pressure increasing more than diastolic pressure), widening of the pulse pressure, sinus tachycardia (more common during sleep), and on occasion paroxysmal atrial fibrillation and CHF. In addition, hyperthyroid individuals experience mitral valve prolapse significantly more than the general population.[16]

Untreated hyperthyroidism may eventually result in thyroid storm, an acutely life-threatening emergency. Although extremely rare today, thyroid storm is essentially an acute exacerbation of the signs and symptoms of hyperthyroidism manifested by signs of severe hypermetabolism. Clinical manifestations include hyperpyrexia (highly elevated body temperature); excessive sweating; nausea, vomiting, and abdominal pain; cardiovascular disturbances, such as tachycardia and atrial fibrillation; and CHF with possible pulmonary edema. CNS manifestations usually begin as mild tremulousness; the patient then becomes severely agitated and disorientated, which turns into psychotic behavior, stupor (partial unconsciousness), and eventual coma. Thyroid storm has a high mortality rate, often even with proper management.

**table 18-4**   *Clinical manifestations of hyperthyroidism*

| SYMPTOMS | % MANIFESTATION |
|---|---|
| Weight loss | 72-100 |
| <20 lb | Up to 14 |
| 20-40 lb | 27-36 |
| >40 lb | 23-45 |
| Palpitations | |
| Dyspnea | |
| Edema | |
| Chest pain | |
| Nervousness | |
| Weakness | |
| Tremor | |
| Psychosis | |
| Diarrhea | |
| Hyperdefacation | |
| Abdominal pain | |
| Myalgias | |
| Disorientation | |

| SIGNS | % MANIFESTATION |
|---|---|
| Fever | 100 |
| <103° F | 57-70 |
| >103° F | 30-43 |
| Tachycardia | 100 |
| 100-139 | 24 |
| 140-169 | 62 |
| 170-200 | 14 |
| Sinus tachycardia | 67 |
| Dysrhythmias | 37 |
| Wide pulse pressure | 86-100 |
| 40-59 mm Hg | 38 |
| 60-100 mm Hg | 62 |
| Tremor | 73 |
| Thyrotoxic stare or lid retraction | 60 |
| Hyperkinesis | 55 |
| CHF | 50 |
| Weakness | 23 |
| Coma | 18-23 |
| Tender liver | 17 |
| Infiltrative ophthalmopathy | 17 |
| Somnolence or obtundence | 14-46 |
| Psychosis | 9-29 |
| Jaundice | 9-24 |

Modified from Wogan JM: Endocrine disorders. In Rosen P, editor: *Emergency medicine: concepts and clinical practice*, ed 4, St Louis, 1998, Mosby. *CHF,* Congestive heart failure.

Symptoms necessary for the diagnosis of hyperthyroidism include weakness, sweating, weight loss, nervousness, loose stools, and heat intolerance. Signs include warm, thin, soft, moist skin; exophthalmos; staring; and tremors (Table 18-4).[32]

# Pathophysiology

## HYPOTHYROIDISM

Insufficient levels of circulating thyroid hormone produce the signs and symptoms of hypothyroidism. All the body's functions in effect slow down. In addition, mucopolysaccharides and mucoproteins progressively infiltrate the skin of individuals with chronic hypofunction, lending the skin its characteristic puffy appearance. This hard, nonpitting, mucinous edema, called *myxedema,* is characteristic of hypothyroidism. Initially, the edema does not appear in dependent areas.[28]

Myxedema may also cause significant cardiac enlargement, which leads to pericardial and pleural effusions and to the cardiovascular and respiratory difficulties associated with hypothyroidism.[25,36] Research has demonstrated that coronary artery disease is often accelerated in clinically hypothyroid patients.[19]

Myxedema coma is the end point of the progression of severe hypothyroidism. The loss of consciousness may be produced by hypothermia, hypoglycemia, or carbon dioxide retention, all of which are present in this clinical condition.

## HYPERTHYROIDISM

Hyperthyroidism is the result of excessive production of endogenous thyroid hormone by the thyroid gland or excessive administration of exogenous thyroid hormone (as in treatment of hypothyroid states). Clinically observed signs and symptoms relate to the level of these hormones in the blood. Thyroid hormones produce an increase in the body's energy consumption and an elevation of the basal metabolic rate. The increased use of energy results in fatigue and weight loss.

Cardiovascular findings in hyperthyroid patients are related to the direct actions of thyroid hormones on the myocardium. They are characterized by a hyperdynamic, electrically excitable state. These findings include an increased heart rate and increased cardiac irritability. The increased incidence of cardiac problems (for example, angina pectoris and CHF) and cardiac symptoms (for example, palpitations, dyspnea, chest pain) in hyperthyroid individuals most likely relates to the increased cardiac workload.[18,20] Subclinical cardiac disease may have been present before the onset of the hyperthyroid state or in the hypothyroid state before therapy; however, clinically significant cardiac disease becomes evident with the addition of thyroid hormone, which creates the increase in the heart's workload and myocardial oxygen requirement.

In addition, hyperthyroidism decreases liver function. Jaundice may appear but is readily eliminated through treatment of thyrotoxicosis.[37] Because of the variable degree of liver dysfunction associated with thyrotoxicosis, all drugs and medications metabolized primarily in the liver should be administered judiciously and in smaller-than-normal doses. Because of the effects of atropine and epinephrine on the heart and cardiovascular systems, their use is contraindicated in severely hyperthyroid individuals.

Thyroid storm, or crisis, is the end point of untreated hyperthyroidism. The primary difference between thyroid storm and severe hyperthyroidism is the presence of hyperpyrexia; if this condition is left untreated, the body's temperature may reach a lethal level (105 degrees Fahrenheit or higher) within 24 to 48 hours. In this severe hypermetabolic state the body's demand for energy overtaxes the cardiovascular system, which helps produce the clinical signs and symptoms of cardiac dysrhythmia, CHF, and acute pulmonary edema. The thyroid storm patient also exhibits profound delirium, vomiting, diarrhea, and dehydration.

# Management

Acute thyroid-related emergencies are unlikely to develop during dental treatment of patients with thyroid disease. When loss of consciousness does occur, management is supportive in nature.

## HYPOTHYROIDISM

No special management is necessary for most patients who exhibit clinical evidence of thyroid hypofunction. If the doctor has doubts or concerns after a complete medical and dental evaluation, medical consultation is warranted before treatment begins.

It is worth remembering that hypothyroid patients may be unusually sensitive to the following categories of drugs:

- Sedatives (for example, barbiturates)
- Opioids (for example, meperidine and codeine)
- Antianxiety drugs (for example, diazepam)
- Most other CNS depressants, such as histamine-blockers (antihistamines).

Moderate to severe overdose reactions may develop following administration of "normal" doses of these drugs.

Effective management of the hypothyroid individual is usually easily achieved through oral administration of desiccated thyroid hormone. In almost all cases, therapy must continue for the rest of the patient's life. Within 30 days of the start of therapy the patient usually returns to a normal body weight, and all clinical signs and symptoms disappear. On the whole the prognosis for treated hypothyroidism is a return to normal health.

Diagnostic clues to the presence of hypothyroidism include:
- Cold intolerance
- Weakness
- Fatigue
- Dry, cold, yellow, puffy skin
- Thick tongue

**Unconscious patient with history of hypothyroidism**  The possibility that the undiagnosed, untreated, clinically hypothyroid patient may lose consciousness and not respond to resuscitative measures is extremely unlikely. More likely is the possibility that a patient may lose consciousness because of a fear of dental treatment. In this situation the individual usually regains consciousness after the steps in the management protocol for any unconscious patient are performed.

*Step 1: termination of the dental procedure.*

*Step 2:* **P** *(position).*  The unconscious patient should be placed in the supine position with the legs elevated slightly.

*Step 3:* **A-B-C** *(airway-breathing-circulation), basic life support (BLS), as needed.*  If a hypothyroid patient loses consciousness, the possibility of myxedema coma must be considered. Management of this situation includes establishment of a patent airway, assessment of breathing, administration of $O_2$, and assessment of the adequacy of circulation.

*Step 4:* **D** *(definitive care):*
*Step 4a: summoning of medical assistance.*  Because the underlying cause of unconsciousness is not a lack of cerebral blood flow or $O_2$, this patient does not regain consciousness after BLS is initiated. Medical assistance should be summoned immediately whenever a patient does not regain consciousness after implementation of BLS.

*Step 4b: establishment of an intravenous (IV) line (if available).*  If available, an IV infusion of 5% dextrose and water or normal saline may be started before the arrival of emergency personnel. Availability of a patent vein facilitates subsequent medical management of this patient.

*Step 4c: administration of $O_2$.*  $O_2$ may be administered at any time during this emergency. Although

$O_2$ administration will not lead to the recovery of consciousness, no harm can result.

*Step 4d: definitive management.*  Definitive management of myxedema coma includes the transport of the individual to a hospital emergency department, the administration of massive IV doses of thyroid hormones (for example, triiodothyronine or levothyroxine) for several days, and the reversal of hypothermia. Additional therapy may vary according to the patient's clinical state. The mortality rate associated with myxedema coma is high (40%), even with proper, rigorous management (Box 18-3).

## HYPERTHYROIDISM

Clinically, hyperthyroid individuals most often appear nervous and apprehensive. If clinical symptoms are so intense that the doctor remains doubtful as to the nature of the patient's problem, medical consultation is indicated before dental treatment begins. Although the risk of thyroid storm is minimal, undue stress can induce this acute life-threatening situation. In addition, the use of certain drugs, particularly atropine and epinephrine, may precipitate thyroid crisis; therefore these drugs should not be administered to clinically hyperthyroid individuals.

The following are diagnostic clues that may prompt a suspicion of hyperthyroidism:
- Sweating
- Heat intolerance
- Tachycardia
- Warm, thin, soft, moist skin
- Exophthalmos
- Tremor

box **18-3**  *Management of the unconscious patient with thyroid disease*

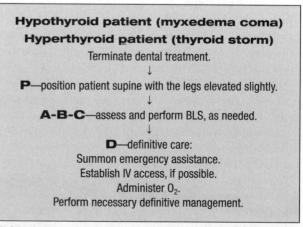

**Hypothyroid patient (myxedema coma)**
**Hyperthyroid patient (thyroid storm)**
Terminate dental treatment.
↓
**P**—position patient supine with the legs elevated slightly.
↓
**A-B-C**—assess and perform BLS, as needed.
↓
**D**—definitive care:
Summon emergency assistance.
Establish IV access, if possible.
Administer $O_2$.
Perform necessary definitive management.

*BLS,* Basic life support; *$O_2$,* oxygen; *IV,* intravenous; **P,** position; **A,** airway; **B,** breathing; **C,** circulation; **D,** definitive care.

**Unconscious patient with history of hyperthyroidism**    As with the hypothyroid patient, the undiagnosed, untreated, clinically hyperthyroid patient is unlikely to lose consciousness to the point at which resuscitation is impossible. Vasodepressor syncope is a much more likely cause of unconsciousness. In this situation the patient should regain consciousness rapidly after implementation of the basic steps in the management of an unconscious patient.

*Step 1: termination of the dental procedure.*

*Step 2:* **P** *(position). The patient should be placed in the supine position with the legs elevated slightly.*

*Step 3:* **A-B-C,** *or BLS, as indicated.* If a hyperthyroid patient loses consciousness, the possibility of thyroid storm must be seriously considered, especially if the temperature is elevated. Management of this situation includes implementing the steps of BLS, including establishment of a patent airway, assessment of breathing and circulation, and administration of $O_2$, as needed.

*Step 4:* **D** *(definitive care):*
*Step 4a: summoning of medical assistance.* Because the underlying cause of unconsciousness is not a lack of cerebral blood flow or $O_2$, the hypothyroid patient will not regain consciousness after these basic procedures are implemented. Medical assistance should be sought immediately whenever the patient does not regain consciousness after the steps of BLS have been performed.

*Step 4b: establishment of an IV line (if available).* An IV infusion of a 5% solution of dextrose and water or normal saline may be begun before emergency personnel arrive. Availability of a patent vein facilitates subsequent medical management of this patient.

*Step 4c: administration of $O_2$.* $O_2$ may be administered at any time during the emergency. Although its administration does not lead to recovery, $O_2$ cannot harm the individual.

*Step 4d: definitive management.* Definitive management of thyroid storm includes transport of the patient to a hospital emergency department and administration of large doses of antithyroid drugs (for example, propylthiouracil). Additional therapy includes administration of propranolol to block the adrenergic-mediated effects of thyroid hormones and large doses of glucocorticosteroids to prevent the occurrence of acute adrenal insufficiency. Other measures may include $O_2$, cold packs, sedation, and careful monitoring of hydration and electrolyte balance. The prognosis is poor for individuals with thyroid storm.

Box 18-3 outlines the management of an unconscious patient who suffers thyroid disease. In addition, the following information may prove useful:

- **Drugs used in management:** No drugs are used to manage thyroid disease in the dental office.
- **Medical assistance required:** If the hyperthyroid or hypothyroid individual loses consciousness, medical assistance is required.

## REFERENCES

1. Nikolai TF: The thyroid gland. In Rose LF, Kaye D, editors: *Internal medicine for dentistry,* ed 2, St Louis, 1992, Mosby.
2. Wogan JM: Endocrine disorders. In Rosen P, editor: *Emergency medicine: concepts and clinical practice,* ed 4, St Louis, 1998, Mosby.
3. LaFranchi S: Diagnosis and treatment of hypothyroidism in children, *Compr Ther* 13:20, 1987.
4. Ord WM: On myxedema, a term proposed to be applied to an essential condition in the cretinoid affection occasionally observed in middle-aged women, *Med Chir Trans London* 61:57, 1877.
5. Jordan RM: Myxedema coma: pathophysiology, therapy and factors affecting prognosis, *Med Clin North Am* 79:185, 1995.
6. Nichols AB, Hunt WB: Is myxedema coma respiratory failure? *South Med J* 69:945, 1976.
7. von Basedow CA: *Exophthalmos durch Hypertrophie des Zellgewbes in der Augenhohle, Wochenschrift fur die gesammte Heilkunde,* Berlin, 1840. Reprinted in Major RH: *Classic descriptions of disease,* Springfield, Ill, 1978, Charles C Thomas.
8. Graves RJ: Newly observed affection of the thyroid gland in females, *London Med Surg J* 7(2):516. Reprinted in Major RH: *Classic descriptions of disease,* Springfield, Ill, 1978, Charles C Thomas.
9. Tietgens ST, Leinung MC: Thyroid storm, *Med Clin North Am* 79:169, 1995.
10. Senior RM and others: The recognition and management of myxedema coma, *JAMA* 217:61, 1971.
11. Amino N: Autoimmunity and hypothyroidism, *Clin Endocrinol Metab* 2:591, 1988.
12. Swanson JW, Kelly JJ, McConahey WM: Neurologic aspects of thyroid dysfunction, *Mayo Clin Proc* 56:504, 1981.
13. Nickerson JF and others: Fatal myxedema, with and without coma, *Ann Intern Med* 53:475, 1960.
14. Wartofsky L: Myxedema coma. In Ingbar SH, Braverman LE, editors: *The thyroid: a fundamental and clinical text,* ed 5, Philadelphia, 1986, Lippincott.
15. Gittoes NJ, Franklyn JA: Hyperthyroidism: current treatment guidelines, *Drugs* 55(4):543-553, 1998.
16. Toft AD, editor: Hyperthyroidism (symposium), *Clin Endocrinol Metab* 14(2): entire issue, 1985.

17. Wartofsky L: Thyrotoxic storm. In Ingbar SH, Braverman LE, editors: *The thyroid: a fundamental and clinical text,* ed 5, Philadelphia, 1986, Lippincott.

18. Dillmann WH: Thyroid storm, *Curr Ther Endocrinol Metab* 6:81-85, 1997.

19. Becker C: Hypothyroidism and atherosclerotic heart disease: pathogenesis, medical management, and the role of coronary artery bypass surgery, *Endocr Rev* 6:432, 1985.

20. Waldstein SS and others: A clinical study of thyroid storm, *Ann Intern Med* 52(3):626, 1960.

21. Fish LH and others: Replacement dose, metabolism, and bioavailability of levothyroxine in the treatment of hypothyroidism: role of triiodothyronine in pituitary feedback in humans, *N Engl J Med* 316:764, 1987.

22. Becker DV: Choice of therapy for Graves' hyperthyroidism, N Engl J Med 311:464, 1984 (editorial).

23. Dunn JT: Choice of therapy in young adults with hyperthyroidism of Graves' disease, *Ann Intern Med* 100:891, 1984.

24. Urbanic RC, Mazzaferri EL: Thyrotoxic crisis and myxedema coma, *Heart Lung* 7:435, 1978.

25. Barnes BO, Barnes CW: *Solved: the riddle of heart attacks,* Fort Collins, Colo, 1976, Robinson.

26. Gaitan E, Cooper DS: Primary hypothyroidism, *Curr Ther Endocrinol Metab* 6:94-98, 1997.

27. Hierholzer K, Finke R: Myxedema, *Kidney Int Suppl* 9:S82-S89, 1997.

28. Pittman CS, Zayed AA: Myxedema coma, *Curr Ther Endocrinol Metab* 6:98-101, 1997.

29. Maclean D, Taig DR, Emslie-Smith D: Achilles tendon reflex in accidental hypothermia and hypothermic myxedema, *Br Med J* 2:87, 1973.

30. Tsitouras PD: Myxedema coma, *Clin Geriatr Med* 11(2):251-258, 1995.

31. Doyle JR, Carroll RE: The carpal tunnel syndrome: a review of 100 patients treated surgically, *Calif Med* 108:263, 1968.

32. Endocrine disorders. In Schroeder SA and others, editors: *Current medical diagnosis & treatment 1990,* Norwalk, Conn, 1990, Appleton & Lange.

33. Werner SC: Classification of the eye changes in Graves' disease, *Am J Ophthalmol* 68(4):646, 1969.

34. Werner SC: Modification of the classification of eye changes in Graves' disease, *Am J Ophthalmol* 83(5):725, 1977.

35. Bartalena L, Marcocci C, Pinchera A: Treating severe Graves' ophthalmopathy, *Baillieres Clin Endocrinol Metab* 11(3):521-536, 1997.

36. Gomberg-Maitland M, Frishman WH: Thyroid hormone and cardiovascular disease, *Am Heart J* 135(2 Pt 1):187-196, 1998.

37. Greenberger NJ and others: Jaundice and thyrotoxicosis in the absence of congestive heart failure, *Am J Med* 38:840, 1964.

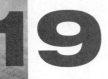

# 19

# *Cerebrovascular Accident*

**C**EREBROVASCULAR accident (CVA) is a focal neurologic disorder caused by destruction of brain substance as a result of intracerebral hemorrhage, thrombosis, embolism, or vascular insufficiency. CVA is also known as *stroke, cerebral apoplexy,* and "brain attack".[1,2] The latter term, *brain attack,* has gained popularity in recent years in order to stress the need of these patients for immediate emergency medical care; the parallel to the term *heart attack* is intentional.

A CVA is a fairly common occurrence in the adult population. In the United States approximately 600,000 new instances of acute CVA are reported annually. Although mortality rates for the different forms of CVA vary considerably, the overall death rate is relatively high. In 1995, 157,991 individuals in the United States died as a result of CVA, making it the third-leading cause of death in the country, behind only cancer (second) and heart disease (first).[3,4] Most stroke victims survive but often with significant disability. The frequency with which CVAs occur is emphasized by the fact that approximately 25% of routine autopsies demonstrate evidence of CVA, even though the patient may never have exhibited evidence of stroke.

CVA is the most common form of brain disease. The average age of an individual at the time of the first CVA is approximately 64 years. In addition, 28% of all CVAs occur in individuals under 65 years. Recent evidence indicates that the incidence of CVA is decreasing; in the last decade it declined 17.3%, but the actual number of CVA deaths rose by 3.2%.[3] For every 100 first cases of CVA that occurred in a unit of population between 1945 and 1949, only 55 first episodes occurred between 1970 and 1974. This decline encompasses both sexes and all age-groups but is most notable in the elderly.[5-7]

The incidence of stroke in children is 2.5 per 100,000 per year. Although stroke can occur at any age between infancy and childhood, such episodes occur most frequently between 1 and 5 years.[8,9] Cyanotic heart disease is the most common underlying systemic disorder that predisposes children to stroke.

The incidence of death from stroke also varies by race and sex. In 1995, death rates from CVA were 26.5% for white males and 52.2% for black males, and 23.1% for white females and 39.6% for black females.[3] In addition, a transient ischemic attack (TIA), or mini-stroke, shows a prevalence of 2.7% in males between 65 and 69 years and 3.6% for those 75 to 79 years.[2] For women the prevalence for mini-stroke is 1.6% for those 65 to 69 years and 4.1% for those 75 to 79 years.[3]

## Classification

CVA is usually classified by cause. Two major classes of stroke are hemorrhagic and occlusive; in addition, a lacunar infarction is a type of occlusive stroke. Table 19-1 presents the various forms of CVA and their relative incidence. In addition to the forms of CVA presented in the table, a syndrome variously known *TIA, transient cerebral ischemia, incipient stroke,* or *mini-stroke* also exists. It consists of brief episodes of cerebral ischemia that result in no permanent neurologic damage, whereas CVA victims almost always suffer some degree of permanent neurologic damage.

### Lacunar Infarction

Lacunar infarcts are among the most common cerebrovascular lesions. Small in size (<5 mm in diameter), lacunar infarcts often are associated with poorly controlled hypertension or diabetes. They involve penetration of cerebral arterial branches that lie deep in the cerebrum or brain stem.[10,11] Prognosis for recovery from the deficits produced by lacunar infarction is usually good, with many individuals experiencing partial or complete resolution over the subsequent 4 to 6 weeks.[11]

## CEREBRAL INFARCTION

The most prevalent form of CVA is the occlusive stroke, accounting for more than 85% of all CVAs. Occlusive stroke most commonly results from atherosclerotic disease and cardiac abnormalities. Thrombosis of intracranial and extracranial arteries and cerebral embolization from various origins throughout the body are the primary causes of cerebral infarction. *Cerebral infarction* may be defined as the death of neural (brain) tissue as a result of ischemia. The primary cause of ischemia is a prolonged decrease in blood flow to the brain. Cerebral infarction is most common in individuals 60 to 69 years and occurs more frequently in males (a 2:1 ratio).

Cerebral infarction is usually accompanied by abnormalities in the arterial blood supply from the heart to the brain. In most instances atherosclerosis, which is found commonly in certain anatomic areas, produces this alteration in arterial blood supply. Emboli most often originate in a heart in atrial fibrillation and after myocardial infarction,[12] and in neck veins, specifically in the internal carotid artery at the carotid bifurcation in the neck and the junction of the vertebral and basilar arteries (Figure 19-1). By the third decade of a normal adult's life, there is usually significant atherosclerotic plaque in arteries. However, in most cases, clinical evidence, in form of acute myocardial infarction or cerebral infarction, does not develop until the individual reaches the fifth or sixth decade of life.

Narrowing of atherosclerotic vessels must be significant (a lumenal reduction of approximately 80%)

table **19-1**  *Classification of cerebrovascular disease*

| CAUSE | APPROXIMATE % OF ALL CVAs | INITIAL MORTALITY RATE (%) | RECURRENCE RATE (%) |
|---|---|---|---|
| **Cerebral ischemia and infarction** | 88 | 30 | * |
| Atherosclerosis and thrombosis | 81 | * | 20 |
| Cerebral embolism | 7 | * | * |
| **Intracranial hemorrhage** | 12 | 80 | * |
| Arterial aneurysms | * | 45 | 33 |
| Hypertensive vascular disease | * | 50 | Rare |

*CVA,* Cerebrovascular accident; *, unknown.

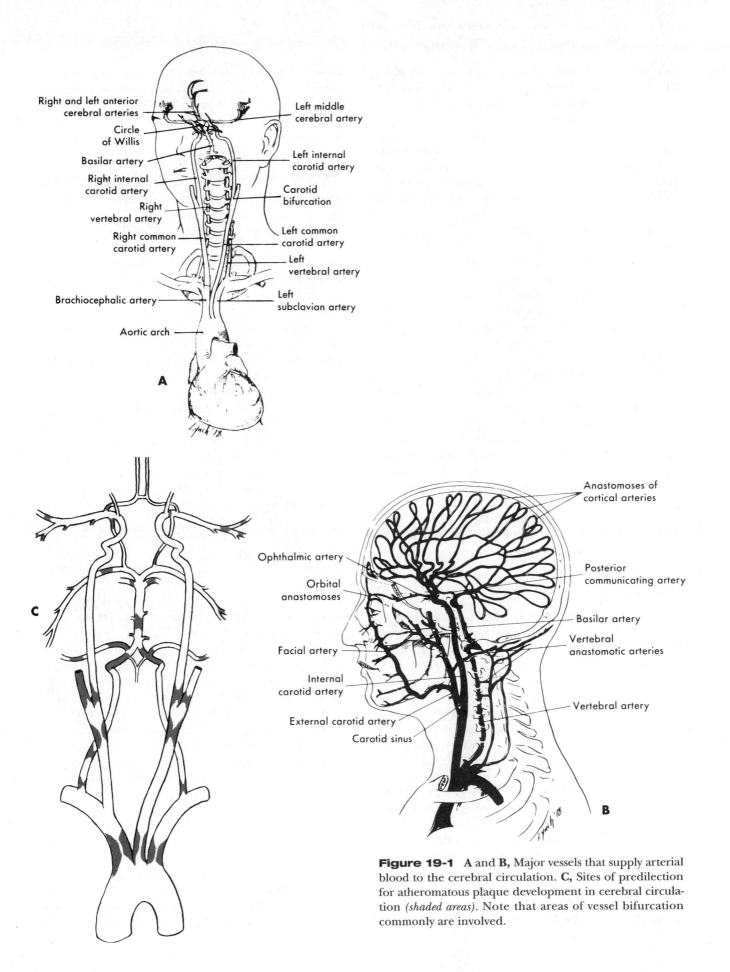

**Figure 19-1** **A** and **B**, Major vessels that supply arterial blood to the cerebral circulation. **C**, Sites of predilection for atheromatous plaque development in cerebral circulation (*shaded areas*). Note that areas of vessel bifurcation commonly are involved.

before blood flow drops to clinically significant levels. A second factor of importance in atherosclerotic vessels is the formation of thrombi (blood clots). Thrombus formation is more likely to occur in atherosclerotic than in nonatherosclerotic vessels. In either atherosclerosis or thrombosis, the blood supply to the area of the brain distal to the vessel narrowing, or occlusion, is severely reduced so that a portion of brain tissue becomes ischemic, and its cells become necrotic and shrunken or infarcted, producing signs and symptoms of neurologic deficit. Patients with certain diseases have been shown to be more likely to develop atherosclerosis, especially at relatively early ages, and to experience more severe forms of the condition. Foremost among these diseases are high blood pressure and diabetes mellitus.[13,14] Acute episodes of cerebral ischemia and infarction may develop at any time; however, approximately 20% occur during sleep.

Cerebral embolization is a causative factor in approximately 7% of CVAs. A major source of emboli is in the hearts of individuals with impaired flow or damaged valves. Rheumatic heart disease with mitral stenosis and atrial fibrillation is the most common cause of cerebral embolization in individuals under 50 years. Other causes include prosthetic valves, acute myocardial infarction, atrial fibrillation, bacterial endocarditis, mitral valve prolapse, and thyrotoxicosis with atrial fibrillation.[15] Cerebral embolization occurs throughout the age spectrum of 20 to 70 years; however, it is most frequent in individuals older than 40 years.

## TRANSIENT ISCHEMIC ATTACK (TIA)

The TIA, also termed *incipient stroke, transient cerebral ischemia,* or *mini-stroke,* is considered a "temporary stroke" in much the same manner that angina pectoris is considered a "temporary heart attack." TIAs are characterized by focal ischemic cerebral neurologic deficits that last for less than 24 hours. These attacks rarely last more than 8 hours and often resolve within 15 to 60 minutes. Attacks may occur many times a day or at weekly or monthly intervals. In the periods between episodes the patient is asymptomatic. Platelet, fibrin, or other atherosclerotic embolic material from the neck or heart may lodge in a cerebral vessel and interfere transiently with blood flow, causing the TIA.[16]

Clinically, TIAs signal the existence of a significant degree of cerebrovascular disease and clearly demonstrate a potential danger of cerebral infarction.[17] Patients with TIAs that last more than 1 to 2 hours are greater risks for suffering stroke.[18] In an older population, 3.6% of males between 75 and 79 years experience TIAs; the incidence for females in the same age category is 4.6%.[3] Older individuals have 4 to 10 times greater risks of suffering CVAs than a control population. This incidence may reach 35% within a 4-year period.[19]

## INTRACEREBRAL HEMORRHAGE

The second major category of CVA is intracerebral hemorrhage, also called *apoplexy.* This category is responsible for approximately 10% of all acute cases of cerebrovascular disease and, regardless of the specific cause, represents a serious problem with a high mortality rate. It occurs most commonly in individuals older than 50 years. Intracerebral hemorrhage may develop in any blood vessel, but the usual source of bleeding is from arteries. Hemorrhagic stroke is categorized by the location of the bleeding. Subarachnoid hemorrhage occurs on the surface of the brain within the subarachnoid space, whereas intracerebral hemorrhage occurs within the parenchyma of the brain.

The two major sources of intracerebral hemorrhages are ruptured arterial aneurysms and hypertensive vascular disease. In both cases the walls of the blood vessels involved are defective—congenital defects in the former and acquired defects in the latter—producing weakened areas. The cause of the actual vessel wall rupture is most likely an acute change or elevation in the systolic blood pressure. Subarachnoid hemorrhage most commonly occurs when an aneurysm ruptures as a result of weakened vessel walls at arterial bifurcations.[20] Rupture occurs with a sudden increase in local pressure within a critically stretched aneurysm sac. Intracerebral hemorrhage occurs when weakened arterioles rupture as a result of chronic, systemic hypertension.[16]

Clinically, most cases of intracerebral hemorrhage occur while patients are engaged in normal activities, such as heavy lifting or straining while passing a stool, factors categorized as physical stress and that are associated with elevations in blood pressure. Although intracerebral hemorrhage is responsible for only 10% of all CVAs, it represents more of a potential risk to the dental practitioner, who must manage acutely anxious patients during potentially painful procedures. Both anxiety and pain are associated with potentially significant increases in the heart rate and blood pressure of the patient, making the development of a hemorrhagic CVA more likely.

Survivors of episodes of cerebrovascular disease have a high risk of recurrence (Table 19-1). Within 12 to 24 months, 20% of individuals who have suffered CVAs as a result of atherosclerotic vascular disease experience repeat attacks; more than 33% of patients with ruptured aneurysms develop recurrent episodes.[21] However, the risk of recurrent CVA is not the major threat to survival of these patients. Cardiovascular disease is *the* major limiting factor for the status post-CVA patient.

More than 50% of post-CVA victims die as a result of acute myocardial infarction or heart failure.[22] A status post-CVA patient therefore represents a definite increased risk during dental treatment. Thorough evaluation of this patient before dental treatment begins and special considerations during treatment can minimize potential risk.

## Predisposing Factors

A number of factors have been shown to significantly increase the risk that an individual may suffer a CVA (Table 19-2). These factors include high blood pressure (hypertension), diabetes mellitus, cardiac enlargement (as determined with electrocardiology), hypercholesterolemia, the use of oral contraceptives, and cigarette smoking. Some reports have associated the use of birth control pills with a ninefold increased risk of thrombotic stroke,[23] but recent analyses suggest that this risk is confined to those women who also smoke cigarettes.[24]

| table 19-2 | Types of stroke and associated risk factors |

| STROKE SYNDROME | RISK FACTORS |
| --- | --- |
| **Occlusive** | |
| Emboli | Atrial fibrillation |
| | Acute myocardial infarction |
| | Abnormal valves |
| Thrombi | |
|   TIA | Hypertension |
|   Reversible ischemic neurologic deficit | Smoking |
|   Progressive | Lipids |
|   Completed | Age |
| | Diabetes |
| | Prior TIA |
|   Lacunar | Hypertension (90%) |
| **Hemorrhagic** | |
| Subarachnoid | None |
| Intracerebral | Hypertension (50%) |
| Cerebellar | Hypertension (50%) |

*TIA,* Transient ischemic attack.

Other reports indicate that consistently elevated blood pressure is a major risk factor in the development of both occlusive and hemorrhagic stroke. Evidence from the National Heart, Lung and Brain Institute's Framingham Heart study has led many professionals to believe that high blood pressure may be the major predisposing factor in the development of a hemorrhagic CVA.[25] The risk that an individual may develop a hemorrhagic CVA increases an estimated 30% for every 10 mm Hg elevation of the systolic blood pressure above 160 mm Hg.[26] Prolonged periods of elevated blood pressure also produce thickening and fibrinoid degeneration of cerebral arteries. Atherosclerosis develops at earlier ages and to more severe degrees in patients with elevated blood pressure.

The normal response of cerebral arteries to elevations in blood pressure is yet another mechanism by which high blood pressure promotes an increased incidence of CVA. Cerebral arteries, primarily smaller ones, constrict in response to blood pressure elevations. This constriction reduces the local cerebral blood flow and leads to ischemia of certain areas of brain tissue, which may produce infarction if it occurs over prolonged periods of time.

It is worth repeating that high blood pressure is the single greatest risk factor in the development of all forms of cerebrovascular disease. Fortunately, however, high blood pressure is also the only major risk factor that, if reversed, is associated with a decreased incidence of CVA. This fact is of particular importance to the dental profession because so many dental treatments are associated with pain, either real or imagined, which leads to increased apprehension. Therefore a significant percentage of dental patients exhibit signs of increased cardiovascular activity. Clinical manifestations of such increases include elevated blood pressure and increased heart rate. In patients with evidence of other CVA risk factors, such as diabetes and atherosclerosis, the increases in cardiovascular activity may precipitate an acute CVA, most likely of the more ominous hemorrhagic type.

The status post-CVA patient represents an even greater risk in the dental office. Chances are good that CVA survivors may recover some degrees of function. According to 1998 National Heart, Lung and Brain Institute statistics, 31% of CVA survivors need help caring for themselves, 20% need help walking, and 71% suffer impaired vocational capacity, as determined upon physical examination an average of 7 years later; in addition, 16% require institutionalization.[25] Only 10% of the individuals escaped functional deficits completely.

CVA is the leading cause of serious, long-term disability in the United States, and survivors may be correctly termed "the walking wounded." As McCarthy[27] stated, CVA survivors are "accidents waiting to happen." An independently mobile post-CVA patient expects to receive dental treatment; however, a point worth stressing is that the recurrence rate for CVA is high (see Table 19-1) and that factors such as pain and anxiety only add to the risk such a patient presents. Therefore proper management of pain and anxiety are of the utmost importance in the treatment of a post-CVA patient.

# Prevention

Prevention of the occurrence or recurrence of CVA is based on the recognition of the risk factors discussed and possible modifications in dental treatment that accommodate the diminished ability of the status post-CVA patient to effectively handle stress. The medical history questionnaire contains a number of questions that may prompt the patient to discuss problems that may indicate cerebrovascular complications. In addition, the dialogue history may help in the determination of what modifications if any are needed.

## Medical History Questionnaire

### Question 6: Have you taken any medicine or drugs during the past 2 years?

*Comment:* In the past, all CVA patients received anticoagulant therapy. In contrast, these drugs are used more cautiously today in light of information in a number of studies demonstrating that there is little benefit to be gained from their administration in most forms of stroke and that they may increase the risk of hemorrhage.[28,29] Anticoagulant therapy is valuable, however, in the treatment of embolic stroke victims when there is a cardiac source for the embolization, such as atrial fibrillation or valvular disease.[30,31] Antiplatelet therapy using dipyridamole (Persantine) or aspirin has been successful in the reduction of recurrent TIAs, but such treatment has not yet demonstrated a convincing decrease in the risk of long-term stroke.[32] This reduction in risk is limited to males in some studies but not all. Aspirin doses range from 100 mg/day to more than 1 g/day, without a notable change in efficacy, but lower doses have demonstrated fewer associated side effects.[33] The currently recommended dose is 325 mg/day.[34]

Antihypertensive drugs are prescribed for the 66% of post-CVA patients whose blood pressures are elevated. Diuretics (see Chapter 14, Table 14-1), methyldopa (Aldomet), and propranolol (Inderal) are examples of some commonly used drugs in the management of high blood pressure. The doctor must be aware of the potential side effects associated with each drug and possible interactions with commonly used dental drugs (for example, propranolol and epinephrine).[35] Postural hypotension is one common side effect of many antihypertensive drugs. In addition, the doctor should have available a variety of drug references, including the *Physicians' Desk Reference.*[36-39]

### Question 9: Circle any of the following that you have had or have at present:

High blood pressure
Stroke
Fainting or dizzy spells

*Comment:* High blood pressure is the single most important risk factor in causing CVA and the only risk factor that, if altered, results in a decreased risk of CVA. High blood pressure is present in more than two thirds of status post-CVA patients. Routine blood pressure screening of all prospective dental patients and all medically compromised individuals has significantly helped to minimize the development of CVA and other acute high blood pressure sequelae, such as acute myocardial infarction and renal dysfunction, in dental patients.

Fainting or dizzy spells may indicate the presence of TIAs. In such cases further patient evaluation is warranted through dialogue history. A positive response to a history of stroke requires that a dialogue history be conducted to determine the degree to which that individual is at risk during dental treatment.

## DIALOGUE HISTORY

**Question: When did you have your stroke (CVA)?**
**Question: What type of stroke did you suffer?**
**Question: Were you hospitalized? If so, for how long?**

*Comment:* These questions seek basic information about the nature and severity of the CVA. Following a CVA a degree of recovery from neurologic deficit occurs. Although the length of time varies from patient to patient, maximal improvement usually occurs within 6 months. All but emergency dental treatment should be withheld during this period. The status post-CVA patient is classified routinely according to the American Society of Anesthesiologists (ASA) as a type ASA IV for 6 months, at which time the risk is reevaluated.[40]

**Question: What degree of neurologic deficit (paralysis) did you suffer after the CVA, and what degree of function have you recovered?**

*Comment:* Although motor deficit (hemiplegia) may be fairly evident in a CVA survivor, minor degrees of neurologic deficit may be less obvious. Patients are normally willing to discuss these problems with their doctor.

**Question: What medications are you currently taking?**

*Comment:* Question 6 of the medical history questionnaire should be referred to for discussion. Many post-CVA patients receive antihypertensive and antiplatelet drugs in their long term management.

**Question: If you experienced high blood pressure at the time of the CVA, how high or low was your blood pressure when you suffered the CVA?**

**Question: How often do you measure your blood pressure, and what is the normal reading?**

*Comment:* A large percentage of CVA patients have high blood pressure. In many cases the elevation remains undetected until the CVA occurs. Patients who are aware of their high blood pressure and seek to lower it monitor their blood pressures regularly. These recordings may serve as reference points to compare with the recordings obtained in the dental office. In general, the blood pressure of a status post-CVA patient should not be elevated significantly.

**Question: Have you ever experienced episodes of unexplained dizziness, numbness of the extremities, or speech defects?**

*Comment:* Transient episodes of cerebral ischemia may produce fainting or dizzy spells. These episodes may occur daily or at more infrequent intervals. In many instances the patient is aware of the TIA and is receiving drug therapy (for example, anticoagulant, antihypertensive, or antiplatelet drugs) to reduce the risk of CVA. Such patients should be managed as though they have suffered a CVA (ASA II or III). If a patient with no history of CVA experiences signs and symptoms of unexplained dizziness, numbness of the extremities, or speech defects, medical consultation with the patient's primary-care physician is warranted before dental treatment is begun.

## PHYSICAL EXAMINATION

Physical evaluation of the status post-CVA patient should include a thorough visual examination to determine the extent of any residual neurologic deficit. The exam should include the recording of vital signs, including blood pressure, heart rate and rhythm, and respiratory rate.

## VITAL SIGNS

Proper technique is essential for the accurate measurement of blood pressure (see Chapter 2). The medical risk associated with elevated blood pressure increases steadily with each millimeter of mercury that the blood pressure rises; no blood pressure exists below which risk is absent and above which risk increases. Therefore guidelines for clinical use must be provided (see Table 2-4).

The doctor must be aware at the beginning of each dental appointment of the blood pressure of the post-CVA patient. Because marked elevations in blood pressure increase the risk of recurrent CVAs, such elevations may be life threatening. Guidelines indicate that any adult patient with a blood pressure of 200 mmHg systolic and/or 115 mmHg diastolic or above should not receive elective dental treatment until the blood pressure is brought under better control (for example, an ASA IV patient becoming an ASA III or II). This usually necessitates immediate medical consultation and a delay in dental treatment while antihypertensive therapy is begun or corrected. Physical status (ASA) III blood pressure (between 160 and 199 mmHg systolic and between 95 and 114 mmHg diastolic) in a post-CVA patient warrants immediate medical consultation before dental treatment is begun.

## APPREHENSION

In addition, the presence of unusual apprehension should be determined. Increased anxiety increases circulating blood levels of the catecholamines epinephrine and norepinephrine, which increase the heart rate and blood pressure.

## DENTAL THERAPY CONSIDERATIONS

The post-CVA patient represents an increased risk during dental treatment. Several basic factors must be considered in the management of such patients.

### Length of time elapsed since the CVA

Post-CVA patients should not undergo elective dental care within 6 months of the episode. The risk of recurrence is presumably greater during this time. Noninvasive emergency care for pain or infection should be managed, if at all possible, noninvasively with medication. All invasive dental treatment should be delayed, if possible, or carried out in a controlled environment, if necessary. The clinic of a hospital or teaching institution (for example, a dental school or hospital training program) might prove to be more appropriate sites for invasive dental treatment of post-CVA patients.

### Minimization of stress

The stress-reduction protocol is ideal for use on the post-CVA patient. Of importance are the following:

- Short, morning appointments that do not exceed the patient's limit of tolerance
- Effective pain control (for example, local anesthetics with epinephrine in 1:200,000 or 1:100,000 concentrations used in judicious volumes)

- Psychosedation during treatment (for example, with nitrous oxide and oxygen inhalation sedation or light oral sedation)

NOTE: All central nervous system depressants are relatively contraindicated in the post-CVA patient. Any such depressant may produce hypoxia, leading to aggravated confusion, aphasia, and other complications associated with CVA. In my experience, light levels of sedation, such as those produced with nitrous oxide and $O_2$ or the oral benzodiazepines, have proved safe and highly effective in the reduction of stress in post-CVA patients. However, these techniques should be used only if a particular condition warrants them.

- Avoidance of the epinephrine-impregnated gingival retraction cord

### Assessment of when the post-CVA patient is too great a risk for treatment

Blood pressure and heart rate are indicators of the patient's cardiovascular status at the time of dental treatment. Marked elevations in blood pressure should be viewed with great concern and dental treatment withheld until medical consultation is obtained or corrective therapy achieved. Recommended patient management for ASA adult blood pressure categorizations is modified in the post-CVA patient. I recommend medical consultation with the patient's primary-care physician when the blood pressure increases significantly, compared with previous measurements, or exceeds 160 mmHg in the post-CVA patient if no previous values are available. In addition, post-CVA patients should not receive elective dental treatment for 6 months after the episode.

NOTE: Routine preoperative monitoring of blood pressure in all post-CVA patients is of utmost importance in the prevention of recurrent episodes.

### Assessment of bleeding

Most CVA survivors and those who suffer TIAs receive antiplatelet (aspirin) or anticoagulant therapy to reduce the morbidity and mortality associated with recurrent episodes. If a patient is receiving such drugs, medical consultation is indicated before any dental procedures are begun that may produce significant bleeding. Although excessive hemorrhage in the post-CVA patient rarely presents a clinical problem in dentistry, both the dentist and the physician must consider the possibility and take safeguards against it:

- Proceed with dental treatment without altering the anticoagulant blood level, which may increase postoperative bleeding.

- Lower the prothrombin time (that is, decrease anticoagulant levels) before the procedure to decrease the risk of excessive bleeding with a possible increased risk of CVA.
- Alter the treatment plan to avoid excessive bleeding in instances in which the risk of reducing the prothrombin time is too great.

In most instances, dental treatment may proceed without alterations in the patient's anticoagulant drug therapy or difficulty with excessive bleeding.

Prothrombin time can be obtained from the patient or primary-care physician. Considering a prothrombin time of 11 to 14 seconds to be normal, a level up to two and a half times that amount is considered acceptable for surgical procedures. Prothrombin times greater than 35 seconds demand a delay in dental treatment, medical consultation, and possible modifications in anticoagulant doses. In addition, bleeding time should be determined for those patients receiving antiplatelet therapy with aspirin or dipyridamole.

When a patient with an elevated prothrombin time undergoes treatment, the doctor should consider several of the following precautionary steps to minimize the risk of significant postoperative bleeding:

- Advice to the patient and primary-care physician on the possible need for vitamin K if excessive bleeding occurs
- Use of hemostatic agents, such as oxidized cellulose in extraction sockets
- Use of multiple sutures in surgical extraction sites and periodontal surgery areas
- Use of pressure packs for 6 to 12 hours postoperatively (longer if necessary)
- Availability of the doctor via telephone for 24 hours after treatment

The doctor called on to manage a patient who has previously experienced a CVA should not proceed with the contemplated dental care until there is no doubt about the physical ability of this patient to safely tolerate the planned treatment. Whenever doubt or concern persists, discussion of the contemplated dental procedures and the physical status of the patient with the physician is strongly recommended (Table 19-3).

NOTE: Patients with a history of TIAs should be managed the same as those with a history of CVA.

## Clinical Manifestations

Signs and symptoms of cerebrovascular disease vary, depending on the area of the brain and type of CVA (Box 19-1). The onset may be violent; the patient may fall to the ground, unmoving, exhibiting a flushed face and bounding pulse. Respiratory efforts may be

| table **19-3** | *Physical status classifications for CVA and TIA* |
|---|---|

| HISTORY | PHYSICAL STATUS (ASA) | DENTAL THERAPY CONSIDERATIONS |
|---|---|---|
| One documented CVA at least 6 months before treatment; no residual neurologic deficit or history of TIA | II | ASA II considerations include the following:<br>• Light levels of sedation only<br>• Routine postoperative follow-up via telephone |
| One or more documented CVAs at least 6 months before treatment; some degree of neurologic deficit evident | III | ASA III considerations include the following:<br>• Light levels of sedation only<br>• Routine follow-up via telephone |
| Documented CVA within 6 months of treatment with or without residual neurologic deficit | IV | ASA IV considerations |

*CVA,* Cerebrovascular accident; *TIA,* transient ischemic attack; *ASA,* American Society of Anesthesiologists.

| box **19-1** | *Clinical manifestations of CVAs* |
|---|---|

**Infarction**

Gradual onset of signs and symptoms (minutes to hours to days)
TIA frequently preceding
Headache, usually mild
Neurologic signs and symptoms*
Transient monocular blindness—TIA

**Embolism**

Abrupt onset of signs and symptoms (seconds)
Mild headache preceding neurologic signs and symptoms* by several hours

**Hemorrhage**

Abrupt onset of signs and symptoms (seconds)
Sudden, violent headache
Nausea and vomiting
Chills and sweating
Dizziness and vertigo
Neurologic signs and symptoms*
Loss of consciousness

*CVA,* Cerebrovascular accident; *TIA,* transient ischemic attack.
*Neurologic signs and symptoms include the following:
• Paralysis on one side of the body
• Difficulty in breathing and swallowing
• Inability to speak or slurring of speech
• Loss of bladder and bowel control
• Pupils that are unequal in size

slow, and one arm and leg may become flaccid. In some cases the onset may be more gradual, with no alteration in consciousness and only minimal impairments in speech, thought, motor, and sensory functions.

Commonly observed signs and symptoms of CVAs include headaches, dizziness and vertigo, drowsiness, sweating and chills, nausea, and vomiting. Loss of consciousness, a particularly ominous sign, and convulsive movements are much less common. Weakness

or paralysis occurs in the extremities contralateral to the CVA. Speech defects also may be noted.

## TRANSIENT ISCHEMIC ATTACK

Like all CVAs, clinical manifestations of TIAs vary according to the area of the brain affected; however, the symptoms in any given individual tend to be constant. The onset is abrupt and without warning, and recovery usually is rapid, often within a few minutes. Most TIAs cause transient numbness or weakness of the contralateral extremities (legs, arms, hands), which many patients describe as a feeling of "pins and needles." Transient monocular blindness is a distinctive, common sign of TIA. A gray-black shade progressively obscures all or part of the vision in the involved eye. The shade later recedes painlessly as the tiny embolus dislodges from the retinal artery.[16] During a TIA, consciousness is usually unimpaired although the thought process may be dulled.

Transient ischemic episodes normally last about 2 to 10 minutes, although some documented cases have lasted as long as 1 hour and as briefly as 10 seconds. The rate of frequency varies from patient to patient.

## CEREBRAL INFARCTION

Patients who suffer cerebral infarction as a result of atherosclerotic changes in cerebral blood vessels or thrombosis normally experience a more gradual onset of symptoms (neurologic signs and symptoms appearing over a period of hours to days), which are usually preceded by TIAs. Headaches, if present, are usually mild and generally limited to the side of the infarction. Vomiting is rare, and significant obtundation is unusual unless the infarction involves a massive area of the brain or the brain stem or occurs in a previously diseased brain.

## CEREBRAL EMBOLISM

A CVA that occurs as a result of embolism differs clinically from other CVAs in that the onset of symptoms is usually abrupt. A mild headache is the first symptom, and it normally precedes by several hours the onset of neurologic symptoms, which occur on the contralateral side of the body only. Seizures usually herald the onset of a thrombotic stroke but are not specific indicators for this condition.[41]

Lacunar strokes, a subtype of thrombotic stroke, occur almost exclusively in patients with high blood pressure. They are small, well-localized infarcts with resultant characteristic neurologic abnormalities. Lacunar strokes are abrupt in onset, stabilize over a period of a few days, and do not affect higher-language function or consciousness.[10]

## CEREBRAL HEMORRHAGE

Because of the stressful nature of dental treatment and its possible effects on cardiovascular function, intracerebral hemorrhage is the most likely form of CVA to develop in a dental setting. The onset of clinical signs and symptoms usually is abrupt, the first manifestation being a sudden, violent headache of maximal intensity at onset, often accompanied by vomiting. Different victims have described the headache as "excruciating," "intense," and "the worst I have ever experienced." The headache is at first localized but gradually becomes generalized. Other clinical signs and symptoms include nausea and vomiting, chills and sweating, dizziness, and vertigo. Signs of neurologic deficit may occur at any time but usually occur several hours after the onset. Severe cases are characterized by confusion, coma, or death.[10]

Hemorrhagic CVAs most commonly occur during periods of exertion—sexual intercourse, Valsalva's maneuver, and labor and delivery—or physical and psychologic stress, which may occur during dental treatment. Consciousness is lost or impaired in about half of all patients. This is an ominous sign that usually indicates the occurrence of a large hemorrhage.[42] Of conscious patients, 50% demonstrate marked deterioration in consciousness and lose consciousness at a later time. The initial mortality rate from all hemorrhagic CVAs is approximately 50%, but the rate for comatose patients rises to between 70% and 100%.[43]

## Pathophysiology

The following two important factors work together to produce a CVA:
1. The brain's continual requirement for large amounts of $O_2$ and energy substrate

2. The inability of the brain to expand within its confining bony space, the cranium

The brain cannot store $O_2$ or glucose in reserve for use in times of increased need or deprivation. Acute disruption of the $O_2$ supply to the brain (for example, via embolism or hemorrhage) produces alterations in brain activity that can be detected by an electroencephalogram within 10 to 20 seconds and irreversible neurologic death after 5 minutes.[44] Gradual deprivation (atherosclerotic change) produces the same result over a longer period of time.

## CEREBROVASCULAR ISCHEMIA AND INFARCTION

As ischemia develops, changes occur in the affected neural tissues. The ischemic tissue becomes soft, and the normally well-demarcated border between white and gray matter becomes less distinct. When viewed under a microscope, neurons in the ischemic area appear necrotic and shrunken. A second factor now emerges.

Edema is a normal occurrence following cerebral infarction. On a cellular level, ischemia results in anaerobic glycolysis with the production of lactate. Mitochondrial dysfunction develops, resulting in disruption of the membrane and vascular endothelium. Thus the blood-brain barrier breaks down, and edema forms.[45]

The degree of edema is related to the size of the infarcted area. Edema increases the mass of the tissue within the cranium and causes the mild headache characteristic of atherosclerotic CVAs. In more severe CVAs the degree of edema may be so great as to force portions of the cerebral hemisphere into the tentorium cerebelli, further reducing blood and cerebrospinal fluid flow to the brain (Figure 19-2). The degree of ischemia and neurologic deficit therefore increases, potentially leading to ischemia and infarction of the upper brain stem (medulla), which produces a loss of consciousness and is invariably fatal.

The clinical significance of edema and of its management is that during the first 72 hours after a nonhemorrhagic CVA, a gradual increase in neurologic deficit and decrease in consciousness commonly occur. Cerebral edema in and around the infarcted area is the usual cause of these changes. A gradual return of some neurologic function normally follows as collateral circulation to the infarcted region improves. Maximal recovery normally occurs within 6 months.

## HEMORRHAGIC CVA

Hemorrhagic CVAs differ clinically from nonhemorrhagic CVAs in that their onset is generally more rapid,

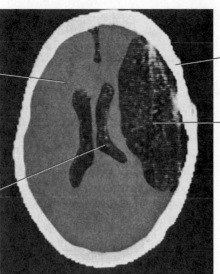

Compressed
left hemisphere

Compressed,
displaced
lateral ventricle

Skull

Zone of
infarcted
edematous
brain

**Figure 19-2** CAT scan of the cranium during cerebral vascular infarction *(top)*. Explanation of the CAT scan *(bottom)*. *CAT,* Computerized axial tomography.

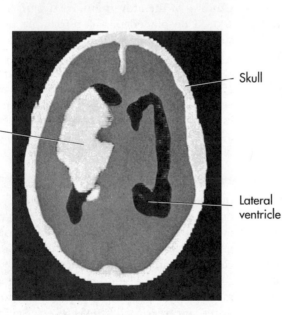

Intracerebral
hemorrhage

Skull

Lateral
ventricle

**Figure 19-3** CAT scan of a hemorrhagic CVA *(top)*. Explanation of the CAT scan *(bottom)*. *CAT,* Computerized axial tomography; CVA, cerebrovascular accident.

the symptoms more intense, and the risk of death much greater. The most common source of blood in hemorrhagic CVAs is arterial. Two primary causes exist for this form of CVA—subarachnoid hemorrhage resulting from ruptured aneurysms and intracranial hemorrhage resulting from hypertensive vascular disease. Aneurysms, which are dilations in blood vessels, muscular walls have weakened, which can rupture under increased pressure. In contrast, hypertensive vascular disease produces degenerative changes in blood vessel walls—usually smaller arterioles—over a greater period, which weakens them and makes them more susceptible to rupture. In addition, intracranial hemorrhage may result from an idiopathic vascular disease, known as *amyloid angiopathy,* that occurs in older individuals.[46] Rupture of these vessels invari-

ably occurs during periods of activity that produce blood pressure elevations.

Once vessels rupture, arterial blood rapidly fills the cranium, increasing intracerebral pressure, which may cause rapid displacement of the brain into the tentorium cerebelli and ultimately death. Cerebral edema, which always develops, only serves to increase the already high mortality rate for this type of CVA (Figure 19-3).

The intense headache noted in cases of hemorrhagic CVA is related to the irritating effects of blood and its breakdown products on blood vessels, meninges, and neural tissues of the brain. The headache is localized at first but becomes more generalized as meningeal irritation increases because of the spread of blood. The rapid increase in intracranial pressure brought on by hemorrhage and edema is responsible for the significant clinical differences noted between hemorrhagic and nonhemorrhagic CVAs. The area of neural tissue that loses its blood supply and becomes infarcted determines the neurologic deficits that the individual suffers.

# Management

Management of the patient suffering an acute CVA depends on the rapidity of the onset of symptoms and the severity of the episode. In almost all cases supportive therapy and basic life support (BLS) are indicated.

The American Heart Association attached the term "brain attack" to the CVA to alert individuals to the immediate need for emergency management. Until recently it was generally believed that little or nothing could be done to help the CVA victim or to minimize the degree of neurologic damage. With the advent of the neurointensive care unit (NICU) and thrombolytic drugs, this is no longer true. The neurointensive care unit provides the monitoring and treatment for a progressing CVA and its complications. Patients who may be suitable for neurointensive care include the following:
- Patients with severe CVAs
- Patients receiving thrombolytic therapy
- Patients receiving hypervolemia-hypertensive-hemodilution therapy
- Patients at risk for and medical complications
- Patients experiencing in-hospital CVAs after medical and surgical procedures

In addition, thrombolysis has been demonstrated to be an effective treatment for ischemic stroke. Lack of awareness about this treatment, coupled with a short therapeutic window (<6 hours) are major obstacles to its use. Indiscriminate use of thrombolytic therapy can lead to an unacceptably high rate of hemorrhage. Early recognition of the onset of CVA, immediate transfer of the individual to a properly equipped facility, and careful screening of a computed tomographic scan of the head for signs of early infarction all are necessary for the safe administration of intravenous thrombolysis.[2,47-49]

## CEREBROVASCULAR ACCIDENT AND TRANSIENT ISCHEMIC ATTACK

In most cases of CVA and TIA the victim remains conscious. Indeed differentiating between a TIA and a CVA may initially be difficult. In such instances the duration of the episode becomes most important. Most TIAs last approximately 2 to 10 minutes, whereas the signs and symptoms of a CVA do not regress.

The following conditions provide diagnostic clues to the presence of CVA or TIA[50]:
- Hypertension (blood pressure above 140/90 mmHg)
- Altered consciousness
- Hemiparesis, hemiparalysis
- Headache and blurred vision
- Asymmetry of face and pupils of eyes
- Incontinence
- Aphasia

Because of the uncertainty of diagnosis, initial management of any patient with signs and symptoms indicating cerebrovascular disease should be identical, regardless of the ultimate cause.

*Step 1: termination of the dental procedure.*

*Step 2:* **P** *(position).* A conscious patient complaining of the aforementioned signs and symptoms should be placed in a comfortable position; most such patients prefer sitting upright or semiupright.

*Step 3:* **A-B-C** *(airway-breathing-circulation), (BLS), as indicated.* The victim's airway, breathing, and circulation are assessed and the necessary steps implemented. When the victim is conscious, a rapid assessment can determine the adequacy of airway, breathing, and circulation.

*Step 4: monitoring of vital signs.* The blood pressure is usually elevated markedly during the episode, whereas the heart rate may be normal or elevated. In most cases either the radial or brachial arterial pulses, or both, are bounding. Comparison of vital signs with baseline values almost always demonstrates significant blood pressure elevation. The heart rate and rhythm and blood pressure should be monitored and recorded at least every 5 minutes during the acute episode.

*Step 5:* **D** *(definitive care):*
*Step 5a: summoning of medical assistance.* When signs and symptoms indicating possible cerebrovascular disease and an elevation in blood pressure appear, medical assistance should be sought immediately, regardless of whether the individual has a history of cerebrovascular disease. Because thrombolytic therapy may help minimize residual neurologic deficit if it is begun early after the onset of a CVA, the prompt summoning of emergency personnel is critical.
*Step 5b: management of signs and symptoms.* Most TIA and CVA victims remain conscious throughout the episode. The patient should be allowed to

remain seated upright (45 degrees, or semi-Fowler's position, being recommended[50]), and attempt to maintain the patient's comfort. The semi-Fowler's position decreases slightly the intracerebral blood pressure, whereas the supine position increases blood flow to the brain, a potentially dangerous situation during this time of significantly elevated blood pressure.

O$_2$ may be administered via a nasal cannula or nasal hood during this time. However, central nervous system depressants are not indicated for patients believed to be suffering a stroke or TIA. Any drug producing central nervous depression (for example, analgesics, antianxiety agents, opioids, or inhalation sedatives) may affect the patient's condition adversely, masking any neurologic signs that might be present and making definitive diagnosis more difficult.

**Transient ischemic attack**    If the clinical signs and symptoms resolve rapidly before emergency personnel arrive, the episode was likely a TIA. When the victim has no history of cerebrovascular disease, emergency personnel are likely to transport that individual to the hospital for further neurologic evaluation. However, when a history of TIA is present, the individual should either be hospitalized or immediately referred to the primary-care physician.

*Step 6: follow-up management.* After termination of the TIA for which the individual does not require hospitalization, the patient's primary-care physician should be contacted. In addition, medical examination and modifications in future dental treatment should be discussed. The patient should not operate a motor vehicle, and an adult friend or relative should escort that individual home.

**CVA**    If neurologic signs and symptoms do not resolve by the time emergency assistance arrives, the victim will be stabilized and transported to a hospital.

Loss of consciousness is associated with a poor clinical prognosis in CVA (70% to 100% initial mortality rate). The hemorrhagic CVA, that most likely to develop during dental treatment, is also the most likely to produce unconsciousness. An intense headache is likely to precede the loss of consciousness, an additional clue to the presence of this problem.

*Step 1:* **P** *(position).* The victim who loses consciousness should be placed in the supine position. Minor alterations in this position may be indicated later.

*Step 2:* **A-B-C,** *BLS, as needed.* The steps of BLS should be initiated immediately. Airway main-

tenance and respiratory support are particularly critical, and O$_2$ should be administered as soon as it becomes available. Although cardiac arrest is a possibility at this time, the victim is likely to require airway management only. Breathing is usually spontaneous, and the carotid pulse strong and bounding.

*Step 3: monitoring of vital signs.* Vital signs (blood pressure, heart rate, and respiration) should be monitored and recorded. In most instances the heart rate is normal or slow and the pulse full and bounding. If either heart rate, blood pressure, or both is absent, cardiopulmonary resuscitation should be initiated immediately. The blood pressure frequently is elevated significantly (systolic pressure >200 mmHg).

*Step 4: repositioning of the patient (if necessary).* When the unconscious patient's blood pressure is markedly elevated, the position should be altered slightly from the normally recommended supine position. Because of the increase in cerebral blood flow in the supine position and the markedly elevated blood pressure observed in what is likely a hemorrhagic CVA, the patient should be placed in an almost-supine position with the head and chest elevated slightly. This new position must still allow for the maintenance of a patent airway and ventilation, if necessary. If cardiac arrest ensues and cardiopulmonary resuscitation becomes necessary, the patient must be repositioned into the supine position with the feet elevated.

*Step 5:* **D** *(definitive care):*
*Step 5a: establishment of an intravenous (IV) line, if available.* An IV infusion of 5% dextrose and water or normal saline may be started before the emergency personnel arrive. The availability of a patent vein will facilitate subsequent medical management.
*Step 5b: definitive management.* Once the patient is stabilized at the scene and transported to the hospital, immediate management of the hemorrhagic CVA patient is predicated upon preventing an increase in intracranial pressure. This requires terminating intracranial bleeding, surgical evacuation of blood from the cranium, and preventing or minimizing edema of the brain.

Box 19-2 summarizes the management of CVAs and TIAs.

- **Drugs used in management:** O$_2$ is used to manage CVAs and TIAs.
- **Medical assistance required:** Those suffering CVAs or TIAs require emergency assistance.

box **19-2**    *Management of CVA and TIA*

**Conscious patient**
Terminate dental procedure.
↓
**P**—position patient comfortably.
↓
**A-B-C**—assess and perform BLS, as needed.
↓
Monitor vital signs.
↓
**D**—definitive care:
Summon emergency personnel.
Manage signs and symptoms.
If blood pressure is elevated, use semi-Fowler's position.
Administer $O_2$.
Do not administer central nervous system depressants.

| Symptoms resolve. | Symptoms persist. | Patient loses consciousness. |
|---|---|---|
| (TIA?) | (CVA or TIA) | (hemorrhagic CVA?) |
| ↓ | ↓ | ↓ |
| Perform follow-up management. | Hospitalize patient. | **P**—position patient supine with feet elevated slightly. |
| | | ↓ |
| | | **A-B-C**—perform BLS, as needed. Monitor vital signs. |
| | | ↓ |
| | | Reposition patient (slight head and chest elevation) if blood pressure is elevated. |
| | | ↓ |
| | | **D**—initiate definitive care: Establish intravenous line, if available. Perform definitive management (provide for transportation to hospital). |

*CVA,* Cerebrovascular accident; *TIA,* transient ischemic attack; **P,** position; **A,** airway; **B,** breathing; **C,** circulation; **D,** definitive care; *BLS,* basic life support; $O_2$, oxygen.

# REFERENCES

1. Whisnant JP: The decline of stroke, *Stroke* 15:160, 1984.
2. Heros RC, Camarata PJ, Latchaw RE: Brain attack: introduction, *Neurosurg Clin N Am* 8(2):135-44, 1997.
3. American Heart Association: Stroke (brain attack) statistics—1998, Dallas, 1998, The Association.
4. National Center for Health Statistics, Bethesda, Md, 1998.
5. Garraway WM and others: The declining incidence of stroke, *N Engl J Med* 300:449, 1979.
6. Levy RI: Stroke decline: implications and prospects, *N Engl J Med* 300:489, 1979.
7. Furlan AJ and others: Decreasing incidence of primary intracerebral hemorrhage: a population study, *Ann Neurol* 5:367, 1979.
8. Golden GS: Stroke syndromes in childhood, *Neurol Clin* 3:59, 1985.
9. Ferrera PC, Curran CB, Swanson H: Etiology of pediatric ischemic stroke, *Am J Emerg Med* 15(7):671-679, 1997.
10. Fischer CM: Lacunar strokes and infarcts: a review, *Neurology* 32:871, 1982.
11. Mohr MP: Lacunes, *Neurol Clin* 1:201, 1983.
12. Komrad MS and others: Myocardial infarction and stroke, *Neurology* 34:1403, 1984.
13. Walker AE, Robins M, Weinfeld FD: National survey of stroke: clinical findings, *Stroke* 12(suppl 1):13, 1981.
14. Khaw KT and others: Prediction of stroke-associated mortality in the elderly, *Stroke* 15:244, 1984.
15. Easton JD, Sherman DG: Management of cerebral embolism of cardiac origin, *Stroke* 11:433, 1980.
16. Frommer DA: Stroke. In Rosen P, editor: *Emergency medicine: concepts and clinical practice,* ed 4, St Louis, 1998, Mosby.
17. Earnest MP: Emergency diagnosis and management of brain infarctions and hemorrhages. In Earnest MP, editor: *Neurologic emergencies,* New York, 1983, Churchill Livingstone.
18. Harrison, MJG, Marshall J: Atrial fibrillation, TIAs and completed strokes, *Stroke* 15:441, 1984.
19. Stone WM: Ischemic stroke syndromes: classification, pathophysiology and clinical features, *Med Health R I* 81(6):197-203, 1998.
20. Wiebers DO, Whisnant JP, O'Fallon WM: The natural history of unruptured intracranial aneurysms, *N Engl J Med* 304:696, 1981.
21. Barrett HJM: Progress toward stroke prevention, *Neurology* 30:1212, 1980.
22. Hennekens CH: Lessons from hypertension trials, *Am J Med* 104(6A):50S-53S, 1998.
23. Collaborative Group for the Study of Stroke in Young Women: Oral contraceptives and stroke in young women, *JAMA* 231:718, 1975.
24. Bronner LL, Kanter DS, Manson JE: Primary prevention of stroke, *N Engl J Med* 333(21):1392-4000, 1995.
25. Gresham GE and others: Survival and functional status 20 or more years after first stroke: the Framingham Study, *Stroke* 29(4):793-797, 1998.
26. Kannel WB and others: Systolic blood pressure, arterial rigidity and risk of stroke, *JAMA* 245:1225, 1981.
27. McCarthy FM: Sudden, unexpected death in the dental office, *J Am Dent Assoc* 83:1091, 1971.
28. Duke RJ and others: Intravenous heparin for prevention of stroke progression in acute partial stable stroke: a randomized controlled trial, *Ann Intern Med* 105:825, 1986.

29. Wittkowsky AK: The stroke pharmacopeia: current medical therapies, *Pharmacotherapy* 18(3 Pt 2):94S-100S; discussion, 85S-86S, 1998.

30. Albers GW: Choice of antithrombotic therapy for stroke prevention in atrial fibrillation: warfarin, aspirin, or both? *Arch Intern Med* 158(14):1487-1491, 1998.

31. Calandre L, Ortega JF, Bermejo F: Anticoagulation and hemorrhagic infarction in cerebral embolism secondary to rheumatic heart disease, *Arch Neurol* 41:1152, 1984.

32. Diener HC: Antiplatelet drugs in secondary prevention of stroke, *Int J Clin Pract* 52(2):91-97, 1998.

33. Raskob GE: Oral anticoagulant therapy, *Curr Opin Hematol* 3(5):361-364, 1996.

34. Grotta JC: Current medical and surgical therapy for cerebrovascular disease, *N Engl J Med* 317:1505, 1987.

35. Merck S: Adverse effects of epinephrine when given to patients taking propranolol (Inderal), *J Emerg Nurs* 21(1):27-32, 1995.

36. Physicians' Desk Reference, ed 52, Oradell, NJ, 1998, Medical Economics.

37. Olin BR, editor: *Facts and Comparisons*, St Louis, 1992, Facts and Comparisons.

38. *USP Drug Information for the Health Care Professional*, ed 15, 1995, Rockville, Md, US Pharmacopeial Convention.

39. American Dental Association Council on Dental Therapeutics: *ADA Guide to Dental Therapeutics*, Chicago, 1998, The Association.

40. McCarthy FM: *Essentials of safe dentistry for the medically compromised patient*, Philadelphia, 1989, WB Saunders.

41. Cocito L, Favale E, Reni K: Epileptic seizures in cerebral arterial occlusive disease, *Stroke* 13:189, 1982.

42. Caplan L: Intracerebral hemorrhage revisited, *Neurology* 38:624, 1988 (editorial).

43. Sedzimir CB, Robinson J: Intracranial hemorrhage in children and adolescents, *J Neurosurg* 38:269, 1973.

44. White BC, Wiegenstein JG, Winegar CD: Brain ischemic anoxia: mechanisms of injury, *JAMA* 251:1586, 1984.

45. Rehncrona S, Rosen I, Siesjo BK: Brain lactic acidosis and ischemic cell damage: biochemistry and neurophysiology, *J Cereb Blood Flow Metab* 1:297, 1981.

46. Drury I, Whisnant JP, Garraway WM: Primary intracerebral hemorrhage: impact of CT on incidences, *Neurology* 34:653, 1984.

47. Torner JC, Davis P, Leira E: Epidemiology of stroke in requiring intensive care, *New Horiz* 5(4):422-432, 1997.

48. Testani-Dufour L, Morrison CA: Brain attack: correlative anatomy, *J Neurosci Nurs* 29(4):213-222, 1997.

49. Selman WR, Tarr R, Landis DM: Brain attack: emergency treatment of ischemic stroke, *Am Fam Physician* 55(8):2655-2662, 2665-2666, 1997.

50. Pollakoff J, Pollakoff K: *EMT's guide to treatment*, Los Angeles, 1991, Jeff Gould.

# 20

# Altered Consciousness:

## Differential Diagnosis

**A**number of clinical conditions may cause alterations in an individual's state of consciousness (see Table 16-1). In almost all such situations the doctor must maintain the life of a patient who remains conscious but is exhibiting unusual behavior. If not recognized and managed promptly, several of these conditions may worsen, leading to the loss of consciousness. Basic management of each of these situations is similar and is all that is required in some cases; however, others will require definitive management, which can be performed only if the precise cause of the problem is known. The following is provided to aid in the determination of this diagnosis.

## Medical History

Several of the clinical conditions discussed in this section normally become evident on review of the medical history questionnaire. The patient with diabetes mellitus or thyroid gland dysfunction or the post-cerebrovascular accident (CVA) patient is aware of the problem and indicates it on the questionnaire. A thorough dialogue history should then enable the doctor to further determine the degree of risk this patient presents during dental treatment. Unless a previous episode is reported, neither hyperventilation nor drug overdose can be diagnosed from data on the medical history.

303

## Age

The age of the patient with altered consciousness may assist in the diagnosis. Hyperventilation occurs only rarely in children or in older individuals (>50 years); its greatest incidence is in those between 15 and 40 years. Hyperthyroidism most often occurs between the ages of 20 and 40, and more than 80% of diabetics develop the disease after the age of 35 years. Cerebrovascular disease is extremely rare in individuals under 40 years; its incidence increasing with age. Drug overdose may occur at any age. In pediatric patients the most likely cause of altered consciousness is hypoglycemia secondary to insulin-dependent diabetes mellitus.

## Sex

Hyperthyroidism (thyrotoxicosis) occurs predominantly in females. However, hyperventilation and the other clinical conditions discussed in this section demonstrate little or no sex differentiation.

## Related Circumstances

Undue stress resulting from anxiety and pain may predispose an individual to hyperventilation. Indeed this syndrome is primarily a clinical expression of extreme fear. Stress may also be related to the onset of a hemorrhagic CVA. In addition, individuals with hyperthyroidism and hypoglycemia may appear acutely anxious, but specific clinical signs and symptoms associated with these problems usually permit an accurate differential diagnosis to be made.

## Onset of Signs and Symptoms

The onset of clinical manifestations of altered consciousness is gradual in individuals suffering hyperglycemia (many hours to several days), hyperthyroidism and hypothyroidism (days to months), and CVAs produced by atherosclerotic changes in blood vessels (days to weeks). A patient will arrive in the dental office already exhibiting signs and symptoms. When the office staff members know the patient well, the alteration in consciousness may be obvious.

In contrast, hyperventilation, hypoglycemia, and CVAs produced by thrombosis, embolisms, and especially intracerebral hemorrhages are accompanied by the more rapid onset of clinical manifestations (signs and symptoms developing more acutely within the dental office).

## Presence of Symptoms between Acute Episodes

The patient with undiagnosed thyroid dysfunction or inadequately managed thyroid dysfunction exhibits clinical evidence at all times. Post-CVA patients usually demonstrate some residual neurologic deficit, the severity of which ranges from flaccid paralysis to barely perceptible motor or sensory changes. In contrast, patients who experience transient ischemic attacks (TIAs) remain clinically free of symptoms between acute episodes. Brittle adult diabetics may manifest the signs and symptoms of hyperglycemia at all times.

## Loss of Consciousness

Although all the clinical conditions discussed in this section manifest primarily as alterations in consciousness, several may lead to the loss of consciousness. CVA, particularly the hemorrhagic type, may be associated with unconsciousness, a particularly ominous clinical sign.

Patients with clinical evidence of thyroid dysfunction may also lose consciousness if the condition is poorly controlled. Significant mortality rates accompany the two clinical situations in which unconsciousness occurs—myxedema coma (hypothyroid) and thyroid crisis, or storm (hyperthyroid). In addition, hyperglycemic and hypoglycemic individuals may ultimately lose consciousness; however, the hypoglycemic is more likely to lose consciousness rapidly. Hyperventilation only rarely leads to unconsciousness.

## Signs and Symptoms

### APPEARANCE OF SKIN (FACE)

The presence or absence of perspiration and the temperature of the skin may assist in the determination of a differential diagnosis. The skin of the clinically hyperglycemic diabetic is hot and dry to the touch (produced by dehydration), whereas that of the hypoglycemic is cold and wet (clammy). The skin of the clinically hyperthyroid individual is hot and wet, whereas the hypothyroid individual has dry skin and may demonstrate a subnormal body temperature.

## OBVIOUS ANXIETY

The clinical signs of agitation, perspiration, and possible fine tremor of the extremities (hands) give the appearance of nervousness and are apparent in patients who are hypoglycemic, hyperthyroid, or hyperventilating, as well as in patients who are simply quite nervous but otherwise healthy.

## PARESTHESIA

Paresthesia, the feeling of numbness or "pins and needles" in various portions of the body, occurs in several situations. If it accompanies a rapid respiratory rate, paresthesia of the perioral region, fingertips, and toes is diagnostic of hyperventilation. Patients with TIAs exhibit unilateral paresthesia or muscle weakness unaccompanied by a change in respiration, which often develops in the absence of anxiety. An acute CVA demonstrates the aforementioned signs of TIA but continues to progress, whereas signs and symptoms of TIA commonly subside within 10 minutes.

## HEADACHE

Individuals with hypothyroidism may suffer headaches, but those experiencing acute CVAs are more likely to have them. A severe, intense headache, the kind described by many individuals as "the worst headache I have ever experienced" is an important clinical finding in intracerebral hemorrhage, a form of CVA.

## "DRUNKEN" APPEARANCE

The clinical appearance of drunkenness is most commonly evident after a patient overindulges in alcohol or another drug that depresses the central nervous system. However, hypoglycemia may present a similar clinical picture. The patient demonstrates signs of mental confusion and bizarre behavioral patterns that may lead to a suspicion of alcohol or other drug use. A history of diabetes, especially type I, or of not eating before dental appointments may assist in differential diagnosis.

## BREATH ODOR

The telltale odor of alcohol on the breath aids in a diagnosis of patient-administered "predmedication." Severely hyperglycemic patients may have the characteristic fruity, sweet smell of acetone on their breath.

# Vital Signs

## RESPIRATION

The respiratory rate increases when hyperventilation, hyperthyroidism, or hyperglycemia is present. In hyperglycemic patients, this increase is frequently associated with the previously discussed odor of acetone. Patients suffering CVAs (unconscious patients with slow but deep respirations), those who have ingested an overdose of CNS-depressant drugs (alcohol, sedatives, antianxiety drugs, or opioids), and some hypoglycemics may demonstrate respiratory depression.

## BLOOD PRESSURE

Elevated blood pressure is found in hyperventilation, hyperthyroidism, and many kinds of CVA (intracerebral hemorrhage, subarachnoid hemorrhage, and cerebral thrombosis). In hyperglycemia there may be a slight decrease in blood pressure, whereas the blood pressure of the hypothyroid patient changes very little.

## HEART RATE

Rapid heart rates (tachycardia) accompany hyperventilation, hypoglycemia, hyperglycemia, and hyperthyroidism. Hypothyroid patients often demonstrate slower-than-normal heart rates.

# Summary

Each of the clinical conditions that produces altered consciousness possesses certain relevant clinical features. The following statements summarize the distinctive characteristics of each:

*Hyperventilation:* The respiratory rate is rapid, and the individual demonstrates deep breaths, acute anxiety, and elevations in blood pressure and heart rate; some patients may experience paresthesia of the extremities and circumoral region. The condition occurs primarily in those between 15 and 40 years and seldom results in unconsciousness.

*Hypoglycemia:* Most such individuals have histories of diabetes (usually type I) or lack of food ingestion. The patient may appear drunk, and the skin may feel cold and wet to the touch. The heart rate is rapid, and the patient may exhibit hand tremors. The onset of symptoms may appear rapidly and lead quickly to the loss of consciousness.

*Hyperglycemia:* These individuals often have histories of inadequately controlled diabetes. The skin of the hyperglycemic appears hot and dry; the breath may emit the odor of acetone, and breathing is rapid and deep, known as *Kussmaul's respirations*. Such patients experience more gradual onsets of symptoms and rarely lose consciousness.

*Hypothyroidism:* These patients are sensitive to cold, and their body temperatures are lowered (no sweating). Their speech and mental capabilities appear slower than normal. Peripheral edema (nonpitting) is present, particularly around the face and eyelids, and skin color is carotenemic. Hypothyroid patients are

overly sensitive to central nervous system-depressant drugs and often note a history of recent unexplained weight gain.

*Hyperthyroidism:* These individuals are nervous and hyperactive, with elevations in blood pressure, heart rate, and body temperature. Their skin feels wet and warm to the touch and is sensitive to heat. Most patients report recent unexplained weight loss accompanied by an increase in appetite.

*CVA:* Those individuals suffering hemorrhagic CVAs complain of unusually intense headaches. They experience unilateral neurologic deficits (for example, flaccid paralysis, speech defects). The level of consciousness is normally unchanged though unconsciousness may occur.

# SEIZURES

# 21

## Seizures

**W**ITNESSING a seizure is a traumatic experience for most individuals. The belief persists that a seizure is a life-threatening emergency requiring the prompt intervention of a trained individual to prevent death; this is not normally the case. Although they are in no sense benign, most convulsive episodes are simply transient alterations in brain function characterized clinically by an abrupt onset of motor, sensory, or psychic symptoms. In these instances the prevention of injury to the victim during the seizure and supportive therapy after the episode constitute the essentials of management. Proper management helps ensure that significant morbidity and mortality are rare. Only if seizures follow one another closely or if they become continuous do they create a life-threatening medical emergency. In these cases prompt action and specific therapy are required to prevent death or significant postseizure morbidity.

Box 21-1 lists some relevant terms and definitions introduced in this section.

## Types of Seizure Disorders

The clinical manifestations of paroxysmal excessive neuronal brain activity (seizures) span a wide range of sensory and motor activities that may involve any or all of the following:

- Altered visceral function
- Sensory, olfactory, auditory, visual, and gustatory phenomena

309

## box 21-1    *Terms related to seizures*

**convulsion, seizure** Defined in 1870 by Hughlings Jackson as "a symptom . . . an occasional, an excessive, and a disorderly discharge of nerve tissue;"[1] a more modern definition emphasized the same essentials, stating that a seizure is "a paroxysmal disorder of cerebral function characterized by an attack involving changes in the state of consciousness, motor activity, or sensory phenomena; a seizure is sudden in onset and usually of brief duration;" the terms *convulsion* and *seizure* are synonymous

**epilepsy** Derived from the Greek term *epilepsia,* meaning "to take hold of;" the World Health Organization[2] defines epilepsy as "a chronic brain disorder of various etiologies characterized by recurrent seizures due to excessive discharge of cerebral neurons;" Sutherland and Eadie[3] updating this definition to read: "Epilepsy should be regarded as a symptom due to excessive temporary neuronal discharging, which results from intracranial or extracranial causes; epilepsy is characterized by discrete episodes, which tend to be recurrent, in which there is a disturbance of movement, sensation, behavior, perception, and/or consciousness."

**status epilepticus** Condition in which seizures are so prolonged or so repeated that recovery does not occur between attacks; a life-threatening medical emergency

**tonic** A sustained muscular contraction; patient appearing rigid or stiff during the tonic phase of a seizure

**clonic** Intermittent muscular contractions and relaxation; the clonic phase being the actual convulsive portion of a seizure

**stertorous** Characterized by snoring; used to describe breathing

**ictus** A seizure

## box 21-2    *Clinical and electroencephalographic classification of epileptic seizures*

**Partial seizures (focal, local) ++***
Simple partial seizures
   Motor signs
   Somatosensory or special sensory symptoms
   Autonomic symptoms or signs
   Psychic symptoms
Complex partial seizures (psychomotor, temporal lobe)
   Simple partial onset followed by impairment of
      consciousness ++++†
   Impairment of consciousness at onset
Partial seizures evolving to generalized tonic-clonic convulsions
   (secondarily generalized) ++++‡
   Simple partial seizures evolving to generalized tonic-clonic
      convulsions
   Complex partial seizures evolving to generalized tonic-clonic
      convulsions (including simple partial seizure to complex
      partial seizure to generalized tonic-clonic convulsion)

**Generalized seizures (convulsive or nonconvulsive) +++++§**
Absence seizures (true petit mal)
Atypical absence seizures
Myoclonic seizures
Clonic seizures
Tonic seizures
Tonic-clonic seizures (grand mal)
Atonic seizures
Unclassified epileptic seizures

Modified from the Commission on Classification and Terminology of the International League Against Epilepsy: Proposal for revised clinical and electroencephalographic classification of epileptic seizures, *Epilepsia* 22:489, 1981.
*++ Partial seizures have behavioral or electroencephalographic evidence showing that the ictal discharge begins in one area of the brain. Seizures that do not alter consciousness are called *simple partial;* those that do are called *complex partial.*
†++ + Complex partial seizures are said to evolve from simple partial seizures when they begin without an alteration in consciousness (for example, an aura).
‡++++ Partial seizures can progress to generalized tonic-clonic convulsions and are called *secondarily generalized seizures.*
§+++++ Behavioral and electroencephalographic manifestations of true generalized seizures are generalized from the start. Several types of generalized seizures are recognized; some have no known structural or chemical causes (for example, true petit mal), whereas others are associated with diffuse brain damage.

- Abnormal motor movements
- Changes in mental acuity and behavior
- Alterations in consciousness

Box 21-2 presents a recent classification of the types of epilepsies by the Commission on Classification and Terminology of the International League Against Epilepsy.

Between 30 to 50 individuals per 100,000 (about 0.5% of the U.S. population) develop epilepsy (recurrent seizure activity) each year in general populations (all age-groups).[4] If isolated, nonrecurrent seizures and febrile convulsions are added to this group, the incidence rises considerably. One study reported the incidence of epilepsy at 48 per 100,000 individuals per year; however, when isolated, nonrecurrent seizures were added, the rate increased to 75 per 100,000, and to 115 per 100,000 with the addition of febrile convulsions.[5] United States estimates indicate that more than 10 million individuals report having suffered at least one convulsive episode (an isolated, nonrecurrent seizure) and more than 2 million admit suffering two or more such episodes. In addition, it is estimated that more than 200,000 U.S. individuals suffer seizures more than once a month despite medical treatment.[6]

When seizures are examined by age of onset, a specific pattern becomes evident. The highest rates of incidence occur in the first year of life, with a consistent and rapid decline toward adolescence and a gradual leveling off thereafter; however, when the individual reaches 50 years, a sharp upswing is noted.[5] More than three quarters of patients with epilepsy experienced their first seizure before reaching 20 years. In addition, the risk that an individual may suffer a second seizure after an initial, unprovoked episode is 30%. The chance for remission of seizures in childhood epilepsy is 50%,[7] whereas the recurrence rate in children after withdrawal from anticonvulsant drug therapy is 30%.[8,9]

The seizures that occur most frequently and possess the greatest potential for morbidity and mortality are known as *generalized seizures*. Included in this group are tonic-clonic convulsive episodes, known clinically as *grand mal epilepsy*, and petit mal epilepsy, also called *absence attacks*.

## PARTIAL SEIZURES

Partial, or focal, seizures are those involving a specific region of the brain. Clinical signs and symptoms of focal seizures relate to the affected area of the brain (the ictal focus). Signs and symptoms evident in individuals suffering partial seizures may include specific motor or sensory symptoms, or both; therefore they are called *simple partial seizures*. Such seizures may also appear as "spells" associated with more complex symptoms, including illusions, hallucinations, or déjà vu, known as *complex partial seizures*. Focal seizures may remain localized, in which case the individual's consciousness or awareness usually is somewhat disturbed, and variable degrees of amnesia may be evident. On the other hand, a focal seizure can turn into a generalized seizure, in which case the individual loses consciousness. Although all seizures are significant, generalized seizures are clinically more dangerous in the dental office due to their greater potential for injury and postseizure complications.

## GENERALIZED SEIZURES

The majority of patients with recurrent, generalized seizures develop one of three major forms—grand mal, petit mal, or psychomotor. Of all persons with epilepsy, 70% suffer only one type of seizure disorder, whereas the remaining 30% suffer two or more types.[10]

**Grand mal epilepsy**   More properly known as *generalized tonic-clonic seizure (GTCS)*, grand mal epilepsy is the most common form of seizure disorder, present in 90% of epileptics. GTCS is what most individuals characteristically think of as "epilepsy." Approximately 60% of epileptics suffer this form alone, whereas 30% experience additional seizure types. Grand mal epilepsy occurs equally in both sexes and in any age-group, although more than two thirds of cases occur by the time the individual reaches puberty.[10]

GTCS may be produced by neurologic disorders or may develop in a neurologically sound brain secondary to a systemic metabolic or toxic disturbance. Causes include drug withdrawal, photic stimulation, menstruation, fatigue, alcohol or other intoxications, and falling asleep or awakening.[11] Neurologically induced GTCSs usually last about 2 to 3 minutes and seldom more than 5 minutes (clonic phase). The entire seizure, including the immediate postictal period, lasts 5 to 15 minutes, but a complete return to normal, preictal cerebral function may take up to 2 hours.[12] The GTCS forms the basis for this section's discussion.

**Petit mal epilepsy**   Also known as *absence seizures*, petit mal epilepsy is found in 25% of epileptics. Only 4% of those individuals, however, report petit mal as their sole type of seizure disorder; the other 21% suffer petit mal in addition to other forms, most commonly grand mal.[10] The incidence of petit mal seizures among those with childhood epilepsy is less than 5%[13]; such seizures almost always occur in children and adolescents between 3 and 15 years.[14] The incidence of petit mal seizures decreases with age, and its persistence beyond 30 years is rare. However, 40% to 80% of individuals who suffer petit mal seizures go on to develop GTCS.[15]

Petit mal seizures may occur frequently, and individuals may experience multiple daily episodes. Petit mal seizures tend to occur shortly after awakening or during periods of inactivity. Conversely, exercise reduces the incidence of petit mal seizures.[16] Clinically, a petit mal seizure consists of a brief lapse of consciousness, normally lasting from 5 to 10 seconds and only rarely beyond 30 seconds. The individual exhibits no movement during the episode other than perhaps a cyclic blinking of the eyelids. The episode usually terminates just as abruptly as it began. If the individual is standing at the onset of the seizure, the posture usually remains erect throughout the episode. In addition, a petit mal triad is recognized, consisting of myoclonic jerks, akinetic seizures, and brief absences or blank spells without associated falling and body convulsions. Individuals also exhibit characteristic electroencephalographic patterns consisting of 3 cycles per second.

**Jacksonian epilepsy**  With jacksonian epilepsy (simple partial seizure), the individual often remains conscious despite an obvious impairment of consciousness. The focal convulsions of jacksonian epilepsy may be motor, sensory, or autonomic in nature. Commonly, this type of epilepsy begins in the limb as convulsive jerking or as paresthesias or on the face as a localized chronic spasm that spreads ("marches") in a more or less orderly manner. For example, it may start in the great toe and extend to the leg, thigh, trunk, and shoulder, possibly involving the upper limb. If the seizure crosses to the opposite side, the individual usually loses consciousness.[12]

**Psychomotor seizures**  Also known as *complex partial seizures* or *temporal lobe epilepsy,* psychomotor seizures are present in approximately 2% to 25% of children and 15% to 50% of adults[14,17,18] (6% experiencing this type only and 12% experiencing them in combination with other forms[10]). These seizures involve extensive cortical regions and produce a variety of symptoms. They last longer than simple partial seizures (usually 1 to 2 minutes), their onset and termination are more gradual, and they involve an associated impairment of consciousness.[12] Such episodes often progress into generalized seizures.[17] Common causes of psychomotor seizures include birth injury, tumors, and trauma.[19] The usual age of onset extends from late childhood to early adulthood.[14]

Psychomotor seizures includes most seizures that do not meet the criteria described previously for grand mal, petit mal, or jacksonian seizures. Individuals with psychomotor epilepsy often exhibit automatisms, apparently purposeful movements, incoherent speech, turning of the head, shifting of the eyes, smacking of the lips, twisting and writhing movements of the extremities, clouding of consciousness, and amnesia.

**Status epilepticus**  Status epilepticus is defined as a seizure that persists for more than 1 hour or repeated seizures that produce a fixed and enduring epileptic condition for more than 1 hour.[20,21] The definition of the Academy of Orthopedic Surgeons may be more clinically practical, defining status epilepticus as a seizure that continues for more than 5 minutes or a repeated seizure that begins before the individual recovers from the initial episode.[22]

The incidence of status epilepticus among epileptic patients is about 5%, although the reported range varies from 1.3% to 10%.[23,24] Although status epilepticus may occur with any type of seizure, it usually is categorized as convulsive status or nonconvulsive status. Convulsive (tonic-clonic) status is a true medical emergency and carries an acute mortality rate of 10%[25] and a long-term mortality rate of more than 20%.[26] Convulsive seizures typically are generalized tonic-clonic seizures.[27]

The most common factor precipitating status epilepticus is failure of the epileptic patient to take antiepileptic drugs.[28] Status epilepticus is also more common in patients whose epileptic causes are known.[29] Of 2588 patients with epilepsy, only 1.8% of the 1885 with epilepsy of unknown cause (idiopathic) experienced status epilepticus, whereas 9% of those with epilepsy of known cause suffered status epilepticus. The most common causes in the latter group were tumor or trauma.[29]

Prolonged petit mal and psychomotor seizures are examples of nonconvulsive status and include mild to severe alterations in the level of consciousness and confusion with or without automatisms.[23] Petit mal status may last hours or days and is usually precipitated by hyperventilation, photic stimulation, psychogenic stress, fatigue, or minor trauma, frequently terminating in a generalized seizure.[30] Nonconvulsive status does not constitute an acutely life-threatening medical emergency in the dental office.

## Causes

Many known causes exist to explain seizures. Classification by cause involves two major categories—primary and secondary.[31] More than 65% of individuals with recurrent seizures (that is, epileptics) may suffer from idiopathic or genetic epilepsy, in which no definitive causative factor for the seizures can be found or the seizures are attributed to a genetic predisposition. This condition is known as *primary epilepsy.* Relatives of individuals with primary epilepsy have a 3% to 5% incidence rate, which is 6 to 10 times the expected rate in a given population. Secondary epilepsy, or acquired (symptomatic) epilepsy, is present in the remaining nearly 35% of individuals who experience recurrent seizures. The word *secondary* implies that evaluation of the individual demonstrates a probable cause or causes for the seizures. Some possible causes of secondary epilepsy include the following:
- Congenital abnormalities
- Perinatal injuries
- Metabolic and toxic disorders
- Head trauma
- Tumors and other space-occupying lesions
- Vascular diseases
- Degenerative disorders
- Infectious diseases

Congenital and perinatal conditions include maternal infection (rubella), trauma, or hypoxia during delivery.

Metabolic disorders, such as hypocalcemia, hypoglycemia, phelylketonuria, and alcohol or drug withdrawal, may also produce seizures. Metabolic disorders account for between 10% and 15% of all cases of acute isolated seizures.[32,33] Drugs and toxic substances account for about 4% of acute seizures. Commonly used drugs associated with the ability to provoke seizures (epileptogenic) include penicillin, hypoglycemic agents, local anesthetics, physostigmine,[34] and phenothiazines.[35] Withdrawal from addictive drugs like cocaine also may provoke seizures.[36]

Head trauma is of great importance at any age, but especially in young adults. Posttraumatic epilepsy is more likely to develop when the dura mater is penetrated; seizures manifest within 2 years after the injury, with 75% occurring within the first year.[37] Epilepsy caused by craniocerebral injuries accounts for 5% to 15% of all cases of acquired epilepsy,[38] with a peak incidence between 20 and 40 years.[39]

Tumors and other space-occupying lesions may occur at any age but are especially common from middle age on, when the incidence of neoplastic disease increases. Tumors are relatively uncommon in children (accounting for 0.5% to 1% of childhood epilepsy[40]) but represent the most common acquired cause of seizures between 35 and 55 years, accounting for 10% of all cases of adult-onset secondary epilepsy.[41] Approximately 35% of cerebral tumors are associated with seizures, which are the initial symptom in 40% of this percentage group.[41,42]

The importance of vascular diseases in the production of seizures increases with age; such diseases are the most common causes of seizures that develop after 60 years. Any disease that impairs blood flow to the brain can provoke a seizure, the likelihood varying with the severity of cerebral ischemia. Arteriosclerotic cerebrovascular insufficiency and cerebral infarction, both of which present increased risks with increased age, are the most common vascular disorders provoking seizures.[43] In elderly patients such diseases account for 25% to 70% of acquired epilepsy[44] and 10% to 24% of acute isolated seizures.[45]

Infectious diseases, which are considered reversible causes of seizures, can occur at any age. Central nervous system (CNS) infections, such as bacterial meningitis or herpes encephalitis, frequently cause seizures. Infections account for 3% of acquired epilepsy[46] and 4% to 12% of acute isolated seizures.[45]

A phenomenon exists in which children and adults who are exposed to television interference and to the flickering lights and geometric patterns of video games develop seizures.[47] This phenomenon, called *photosensitive epilepsy,* was recently responsible for the occurrence of seizure and seizurelike activity in thousands of Japanese children watching one television show that featured flickering colored lights.[48]

The introduction of new, noninvasive neurodiagnostic techniques—most significantly, computerized axial tomography scans and nuclear magnetic resonance (also called *magnetic resonance imaging*)—has improved the detection of underlying lesions in individuals with epileptic disorders. Thus newly diagnosed cases of seizures will increasingly be diagnosed in the secondary category.

Febrile convulsions are usually associated with and precipitated by marked elevations in body temperature. They occur almost exclusively in infants and young children, particularly during the first year of life. Criteria for febrile seizures include the following:

- Age 3 months to 5 years (most occurring between 6 months and 3 years)
- Fever of 38.8 degrees Celsius (102 degrees Fahrenheit)
- Infection not associated with the CNS

Approximately 2% to 3% of children suffer febrile convulsions. Most such convulsions are short, lasting less than 5 minutes. Only 2% to 4% of children with febrile convulsions develop epilepsy in later childhood or as adults.[49] Febrile convulsions are not a significant issue in the dental setting.

Table 21-1 presents the most common causes of seizures according to the age of the patient. The most likely causes for any type of seizure in the dental office include the following:

- Seizure in an epileptic patient
- Hypoglycemia
- Hypoxia secondary to syncope
- Local anesthetic overdose

## Predisposing Factors

Management of most patients with a history of epilepsy is based on minimizing or preventing acute seizures. In almost all cases this goal is accomplished through the use of long-term anticonvulsant drug therapy. In spite of such therapy, acute seizure activity may still develop. In some cases no apparent predisposing factor can be determined; the seizure episode develops suddenly without warning. However, factors do exist that increase the frequency with which seizure activity develops. For instance, the immature brain is much more susceptible to biochemical alteration in cerebral blood flow than the adult brain. Therefore convulsions caused by hypoxia, hy-

table **21-1**  *Top causes of seizures by age*

| NEONATAL (FIRST MONTH) | INFANCY (1 TO 6 MONTHS) | EARLY CHILDHOOD (6 MONTHS TO 3 YRS) | CHILDHOOD AND ADOLESCENCE | EARLY ADULT LIFE | LATE ADULT LIFE |
|---|---|---|---|---|---|
| 1. Hypoxia<br>2. Metabolic disorder<br>3. Infection<br>4. Congenital deformity | Same causes as neonatal | 1. Febrile seizures<br>2. Birth injury<br>3. Infection<br>4. Toxin<br>5. Trauma<br>6. Metabolic disorder<br>7. Cerebral degenerative disease | 1. No known cause<br>2. Infection<br>3. Trauma<br>4. Cerebral degenerative disease | 1. Trauma<br>2. Tumor<br>3. No known cause<br>4. Birth injury<br>5. Infection<br>6. Cerebral degenerative disease | 1. Vascular disease<br>2. Trauma<br>3. Tumor<br>4. Cerebral degenerative disease |

Data modified from Tomlanovich MC, Yee AS: Seizure. In Rosen P, editor: Emergency medicine, ed 2, St Louis, 1988, Mosby.

poglycemia, or hypocalcemia are more likely to occur in younger age-groups.[50] In addition, a "breakthrough" of seizure activity in a well-managed adult patient may also occur. Many cases have demonstrated that such episodes are often correlated with sleep or menstrual cycles.[51]

In many instances of seizure activity an acute triggering disturbance is evident. Such triggering factors include flashing lights (especially prominent in precipitating petit mal seizures), fatigue or decreased physical health, a missed meal, alcohol ingestion, and physical or emotional stress. Seizures may, therefore, be said to be precipitated by a combination of several factors. The genetically determined predisposition to seizures (primary epilepsy) and the presence of a localized brain lesion are among these factors. One or more of the following factors also may induce acute seizure activity:

- A generalized metabolic or toxic disturbance that produces an increase in cerebral neuronal excitation
- A state of cerebrovascular insufficiency
- An acute triggering disturbance, such as sleep, menstrual cycle, fatigue, flickering lights, or physical or psychologic stress

Each of these factors also may produce seizure activity individually.

# Prevention

## NONEPILEPTIC CAUSES

The prevention of acute seizure activity in the dental office may be difficult due to the idiopathic nature of most seizures. However, physical evaluation of the patient before treatment may facilitate the prevention of seizures produced by metabolic or toxic disturbances. (See Chapter 17 for a discussion of the prevention of hypoglycemic reactions.)

A local anesthetic overdose (toxic reaction) is the most likely nonepileptic cause of a seizure in the dental office. Adequate patient evaluation and preparation, care in selection of local anesthetic agents, and use of the proper administration technique go far in preventing toxic reaction (see Chapter 23).

## EPILEPTIC CAUSES

The doctor's goal with most epileptic patients is to determine the probability that an acute seizure may develop during dental treatment and to take any of the steps necessary to minimize that possibility. In addition, the doctor and staff members should be prepared to manage any patient who has a seizure that may arise despite preventive techniques and should attempt to minimize any associated clinical complications (for example, soft tissue injury or fractures).

## Medical History Questionnaire

**Question 9: Circle any of the following that you have had or have at present:**

Epilepsy or seizures
Fainting or dizzy spells

*Comment:* An affirmative response to either question indicates that the patient is aware of such a disorder. Most epileptics are aware of their condition and respond appropriately to such questions.

**Question 6: Have you taken any medicine or drugs during the past 2 years?**

table **21-2**   *Drugs used in the long-term management of epilepsy*

| | USUAL DAILY ADULT DOSE (MG/KG/DAY)* | USUAL PEDIATRIC TOTAL DAILY DOSE (MG/KG/DAY)* | DIVIDED DOSES/ DAY | THERAPEUTIC BLOOD LEVEL (μG/ML)*,†, ‡ | SIDE EFFECTS*,†,‡ |
|---|---|---|---|---|---|
| **GTCS (grand mal) or partial (focal) seizures** | | | | | |
| Phenytoin (Dilantin) | 4-8 | 5-10 | 1 a<br>1-2 c | 10-20 | GI distress, ataxia, sedation, gingival hypertrophy, rash fever |
| Carbamazepine (Tegretol) | 5-25 | 15-25 | 2 a<br>2-4 c | 5-12 | Nystagmus, ataxia, drowsiness, nausea, rash |
| Phenobarbital | 2-5 | 3-8 | 1 a,c | 10-40 | Sedation, hyperactivity in children, ataxia, confusion, rash, possible learning difficulties |
| Primidone (Mysoline) | 5-20 | 10-25 | 3 a<br>3-4 c | 5-15 | Sedation, vertigo, GI distress, anorexia, rash, dizziness |
| Valproic acid (Depakene, Depakote) | 10-60 | 15-60 | 3 a<br>2-4 c | 50-100 | GI distress, sedation, ataxia, weight gain |
| Felbamate | 1200-1600 | | 3 | ? | Anorexia, nausea, vomiting, hepatotoxicity |
| Gabapentin | 900-1800 | | 3 | ? | Sedation, fatigue, ataxia, nystagmus |
| Lamotrigine | 100-500 | | 2 | ? | Sedation, skin rash, visual disturbances, dyspepsia, ataxia |
| **Absence (petit mal) seizures** | | | | | |
| Ethosuximide (Zarontin) | 20-35 | 10-40 | 2 a<br>1-2 c | 40-100 | GI distress, sedation, dizziness, headache |
| Valproic acid (Depakene, Depakote) | 10-60 | 15-60 | 3 a<br>2-4 c | 50-100 | GI distress, sedation, ataxia, weight gain |
| Clonazepam (Klonopin) | 0.05-0.2 | 0.1-0.2 | 2 a<br>2-3 c | 20-80 ng | Sedation, ataxia, behavioral changes, hypotension |
| **Myoclonic seizures** | | | | | |
| Valproic acid (Depakene, Depakote) | 10-60 | 15-60 | 3 a<br>2-4 c | 50-100 | GI distress, sedation, ataxia, weight gain |
| Clonazepam (Klonopin) | 0.05-0.2 | 0.1-0.2 | 2 a<br>2-3 c | 20-80 ng | Sedation, ataxia, behavioral changes, hypotension |

*Modified from Aminoff MF: Neurologic disorders. In Watts HD, editor: *Handbook of medical treatment,* ed 17, Greenbriar, Calif, 1983, Jones.
†Modified from Moe PG, Seay A: Seizure disorders. In Hathaway WE and others, editors: *Current pediatric diagnosis and treatment,* ed 10, Stamford, Conn, 1991, Appleton & Lange.
‡Modified from Tomlanovich MC, Yee AS: Seizure. In Rosen P, editor: *Emergency medicine,* ed 2, St Louis, 1988, Mosby.
*a,* Adult; *c,* child; *GI,* gastrointestinal.

*Comment:* Most epileptics require long-term drug therapy to minimize the recurrence of seizures (Table 21-2). The ideal anticonvulsant would be long acting, nonsedating, easy to tolerate, useful in many types of seizures, and without substantive effect on vital organs as it restores the electroencephalogram to normal. Such an ideal drug does not exist.

A basic principle in the use of anticonvulsants is to select a single drug (monotherapy), rather than a combination (polytherapy), and use it either until it becomes ineffective or until toxic signs become evident.[52] If seizure control proves effective (that is, no seizures for at least 4 years), the patient usually asks about drug therapy termination. Some physicians withdraw anticonvulsant medications gradually over a period of weeks to months, one drug at a time, if the patient is free of seizures for 2 to 4 years.

However, recurrences occur in many such cases. Sudden withdrawal of anticonvulsant therapy is a common cause of status epilepticus. In a study of 68 children who were free of seizures for 4 years, more than two-thirds successfully terminated drug therapy without seizure recurrence.[53] Callaghan[9] reported that only 33% of patients—both adults and children—relapsed after being free of seizures for 2 years. (The patients were followed for 3 years after discontinuation of drug therapy.) Withdrawal rarely is attempted in patients at the age of puberty, especially females, who usually continue drug therapy through adolescence.

## DIALOGUE HISTORY

In response to a positive history of convulsive seizures, the following information should be sought:

### What type of seizures (epilepsy) do you suffer?
### How often do you experience (acute) seizures? When was your last seizure?

*Comment:* Generalized tonic-clonic seizures are controlled effectively in many patients. Proper drug therapy helps prevent seizures in more than 70% of epileptics. Such patients may be free of seizures for several years, or seizures may occur only infrequently (for example, once or twice per year). Others, however, may suffer seizures several times per week or even daily. Petit mal seizures may occur as frequently as every several days or in clusters of 100 or more per day. If an individual experiences seizures frequently (decreased seizure control), the likelihood that a seizure may develop during dental treatment is increased.

### What signals the onset of your seizures? (What is your aura?)

*Comment:* Patients with grand mal epilepsy have a specific aura, or premonition, that heralds the onset of the seizure. The aura commonly lasts a few seconds and relates to the specific region of the brain in which the abnormal electrical discharge originates. The aura may be stereotyped for a particular patient. Some common auras include an odd sensation in the epigastric region; an unpleasant taste or smell; various visual or auditory hallucinations; a sense of fear; strange sensations, such as numbness in the limbs; and motor phenomena, such as turning of the head or eyes or the spasm of a limb. Because the aura is part of the seizure, the signs may alert the dental team to the onset of a seizure, enabling them to initiate proper management quickly.

### How long do your seizures normally last?

*Comment:* Seizures, except for status epilepticus, are self-limiting. The clonic phase of a GTCS usually lasts not more than 2 to 5 minutes; the immediate recovery period lasts about 10 to 15 minutes, with a complete return to preictal cerebral function in about 2 hours.[12] The duration of the convulsive phase has important implications in clinical management. Once completed, seizures do not normally recur during the immediate postseizure period; however, recurrent seizures may occur (as in status epilepticus).

### Have you ever been hospitalized as a result of your seizures?

*Comment:* This question helps determine whether status epilepticus ever occurred and whether previous seizures resulted in serious injury. In addition, most epileptics most likely have been hospitalized on one or more occasions when bystanders in a public area summoned emergency medical personnel. Paramedical personnel must follow strict treatment protocol; when the postictal epileptic patient does not meet certain recovery criteria, a brief period of hospitalization is required.

## PHYSICAL EXAMINATION

If an epileptic is examined between seizures, no specific clinical signs or symptoms exist that lead to a diagnosis of epilepsy; however, more than 50% of patients with recurring seizures demonstrate electroencephalogram abnormalities during the interictal period. No specific dental treatment modifications are indicated, aside from possible psychosedation necessitated by obvious anxiety. Because most anticonvulsants are CNS depressants, such as barbiturates (for example, pentobarbital, secobarbital, and hexobarbital) and benzodiazepines (for example, diazepam, oxazepam, and midazolam), special care must be taken to avoid oversedation when psychosedative techniques are used.

## PSYCHOLOGIC IMPLICATIONS OF EPILEPSY

Folklore and myths have tried to connect epilepsy to violent behavior.[54] Although little evidence exists to support this link, many physicians and lay individuals believe that epileptics are dangerous, potentially violent people.[55] The incidence of epilepsy among prisoners in U.S. jails is approximately 1.8%, compared with an incidence between 0.5% and 1% in the general population.[56,57] Patients with psychomotor or grand mal seizures may exhibit signs of fright and in fact struggle irrationally with any individual who tries to help during the seizure.

Most patients with recurrent seizures can and do adapt in the work force and society despite occasional periods of disability because of seizures and their immediate consequences. The most serious feature of epileptic disability is social ostracism, which is especially damaging to the school-age child who is embarrassed by seizures and may be set apart from other children due to fear and ignorance.[58] Many such epileptics feel rejected and subsequently withdraw from others. This withdrawal, combined with the prejudice that many such children and adolescents may experience, can lead to inadequate educational, matrimonial, and employment opportunities. Because

| table 21-3 | *Physical status classification of seizure disorders* | |
|---|---|---|
| | **PHYSICAL STATUS (ASA)** | **CONSIDERATIONS** |
| History of seizures well controlled by medications (no acute seizures within past 3 months) | II | Usual ASA II considerations |
| History of seizure activity controlled by medication, yet seizures occurring more often than once per month | III | ASA III considerations, including preparation for seizure management |
| History of status epilepticus | III-IV | Medical consultation before treatment |
| History of seizure activity poorly controlled by medication; frequency of acute seizures (more than once per week) | IV | Medical consultation and better control of seizures before routine dental treatment |

*ASA*, American Society of Anesthesiologists.

of low self-esteem, many epileptics may choose companions with emotional, physical, or mental handicaps of their own. Alcoholism and substance abuse may follow.

The overall risk of death among epileptics ranges from that of the general population to a rate 200% greater; this rate is significantly higher for the poorly controlled epileptic. Various factors contribute to the increased risk to the life and health of the epileptic, including ictal brain injury, medication side effects, trauma during seizure episodes, and an increased rate of suicide.[59]

## DENTAL THERAPY CONSIDERATIONS

The major consideration in the dental treatment of epileptics is preparation in case the patient does suffer a seizure. Specific modifications in dental treatment should be considered only if the situation warrants them. Psychologic stress and fatigue tend to increase the chance that an individual may develop a seizure. If the individual exhibits dental-related fear, psychosedation should be considered during treatment.

**Psychosedation**   Inhalation sedation with nitrous oxide and oxygen is a highly recommended route of sedation for the apprehensive epileptic because it allows the administrator a great degree of control over its actions. When administered with at least 20% $O_2$, no medical contraindications exist to the administration of nitrous oxide.[60] Oral medications may also be used effectively in the sedation of the less-apprehensive epileptic patient. Benzodiazepines (for example, diazepam, oxazepam, triazolam, flurazepam) are highly recommended for adult patients, whereas chloral hydrate, promethazine, hydroxyzine, and midazolam are suggested for children.

More profound levels of sedation (deep sedation) may be employed safely via intravenous or intramuscular routes of administration in the more fearful epileptic patient. The usual precautions associated with parenteral sedation techniques must be applied. Hypoxia or anoxia can induce seizures in any patient but is more likely to do so in those with preexisting seizure disorders. The use of supplemental $O_2$ during treatment, the pulse oximeter, and a pretracheal stethoscope are strongly suggested whenever deeper levels of sedation are used.[60]

The use of alcohol is definitely contraindicated in epileptic patients because it may precipitate seizures.[61] Therefore epileptic patients should not undergo dental treatment if recent alcohol ingestion is obvious. In addition, the doctor should not consider the use of alcohol as a sedative agent for an epileptic.

Table 21-3 lists the physical status classifications for epileptic patients based on the American Society of Anesthesiologists' (ASA) Physical Status Classification System. The typically well-controlled epileptic represents an ASA II risk, whereas less well-controlled patients may represent ASA III or IV risks.

# Clinical Manifestations

## PARTIAL SEIZURES

Partial seizures begin in a localized area of the brain and involve only one hemisphere. The seizure is called a *simple partial seizure* when consciousness is unaltered. For example, a focal motor seizure is a simple partial seizure during which the individual remains fully alert and conscious while a limb jerks for several seconds.

However, if the abnormal neuronal discharge spreads to the opposite hemisphere, consciousness is altered and the ability to respond is impaired. This is called a *complex partial seizure* and is associated with complex behavior patterns called *automatisms*. An example of a typical complex partial seizure is the sudden onset of a bad taste in the mouth (the aura), followed by a lack of responsiveness, fumbling of the hands, and smacking of the lips. The patient slowly becomes reoriented in about 1 minute and is back to normal except for slight lethargy within 3 minutes.

The automatic behavior that occurs is associated with impaired consciousness and a loss of higher voluntary control. The nature of the automatic behavior is related to the degree and duration of the confusion and to the psychologic and environmental conditions existing at the time of the episode. Primitive, uncoordinated, purposeless activities, such as lip smacking or chewing and sucking movements, occur in patients with moderate levels of impaired consciousness. On the other hand, the automatism may manifest as a mechanical continuation of activities initiated before the onset of the seizure in mildly confused patients. The patient may continue to move a spoon toward the mouth in an eating movement or pace around a room if either activity began before the seizure began. The entire seizure lasts a few minutes, and the individual experiences only momentary postictal confusion and amnesia for ictal events.[62]

Focal status epilepticus, a rare condition, resists anticonvulsant drug therapy. Characteristically, seizure activity lasts over a period of weeks despite vigorous treatment. Fortunately, this type of seizure is does not threaten the individual's life. Both simple and complex partial seizures may progress to generalized tonic-clonic seizures.

## PETIT MAL (ABSENCE ATTACKS)

Absence attacks occur primarily in children, with an onset between 3 and 15 years. The seizure has an abrupt onset, characterized by a complete suppression of all mental functions and manifested by sudden immobility and a blank stare. The individual also may exhibit simple automatisms and minor facial clonic movements, such as intermittent blinking at three cycles per second and mouthing movements. Such attacks may last 5 to 30 seconds, whereas petit mal status may persist for hours or days. Individuals exhibit no prodromal or postictal periods, and the episodes terminate as abruptly as they began. The blank stare is followed by the immediate resumption of normal activity. If the attack occurs during conversation, the patient may miss a few words or break off in midsentence for a few seconds; however, the impairment of external awareness is so brief that the patient is un-

aware of it. Amnesia for ictal events is common, and the individual may experience a subjective sense of lost time.[63]

Commonly, a young child may be diagnosed informally with petit mal epilepsy when the child first enters school. After a few weeks or months, the child's teacher may advise the parents that the child daydreams frequently or goes off into "another world" for brief periods of time. Medical evaluation usually provides definitive evidence of petit mal epilepsy.

## GENERALIZED TONIC-CLONIC SEIZURE

The generalized tonic-clonic seizure may be divided into three distinct clinical phases—a prodromal phase, including a preictal phase; a convulsive, or ictal, phase; and a postseizure, or postictal, phase.

### Prodromal phase

For a variable period of time (several minutes to several hours) before a GTCS occurs, the epileptic exhibits subtle to obvious changes in emotional reactivity, including increases in either anxiety or depression. These changes are usually not evident to dental staff members, but a close friend or relative may notice them. If such changes appear in an epileptic patient before a dental appointment, dental treatment should be postponed and preparation for a seizure is warranted.

The immediate onset of a GTCS is marked in most patients by the appearance of an aura. The aura is not really a warning sign; instead, it is an actual part of the seizure. Most epileptics exhibit the same recurrent aura before each episode. The aura usually lasts only a few seconds, and its clinical manifestations relate to the specific area of the brain in which the seizure originates. The aura itself, which may be olfactory, visual, gustatory, or auditory in nature, may be considered a simple partial seizure that progresses to a GTCS.

Unfortunately, many patients are unaware of their auras due to the amnesia that occurs during this period. Most patients with GTCS remember nothing from the time immediately preceding the onset of the seizure until they fully recover, perhaps 15 or more minutes. To explain their own auras, patients must seek bystanders who can relate to them the specific manifestations.

### Preictal phase

Soon after the appearance of the aura, the individual loses consciousness and, if standing, falls to the floor. It is at this time that most seizure-related injuries are sustained. Simultaneously, a series of generalized bilateral, major myoclonic jerks occur, usually in flexion, and last for several seconds. The so-called epileptic cry occurs at this time. This is a sudden vocalization produced as air is expelled through a partially closed glottis while the diaphragmatic muscles go into spasm. Autonomic changes are associated with this initial phase, including an increase in the heart rate and blood pressure up to twice the baseline value, a marked increase in bladder pressure, cutaneous vascular congestion and piloerection, glandular hypersecretion, superior ocular deviation with mydriasis, and apnea.[50]

### Ictal phase

*Tonic component.* A series of sustained generalized skeletal muscle contractions occur, first in flexion, which then progress to a tonic extensor rigidity of the extremities and trunk (Figure 21-1). During the ictal phase of the seizure the muscles of respiration are also involved, and dyspnea and cyanosis may be evident, indicating inadequate ventilation. This period of tonic rigidity usually lasts from 10 to 20 seconds.

*Clonic component.* The tonic phase evolves into the clonic component, which is characterized by generalized clonic movements of the body accompanied by heavy, stertorous breathing. Alternating muscular relaxation and violent flexor contractions characterize clonic activity (Figure 21-2). During this phase the patient may froth at the mouth because air and saliva are mixed. Blood may also appear in the mouth because the victim may bite the lateral side of the tongue and cheek during the clonic portion of the seizure, injuring intraoral soft tissues.[64] This activity usually lasts about 2 to 5 minutes, after which clonic movements become less frequent, the relaxation portions become prolonged, and the individual exhibits a final flexor jerk. The ictal phase ends as respiratory movements return to normal and tonic-clonic movements cease.

### Postictal phase

When tonic-clonic movements cease and breathing returns to normal, the patient enters the postictal phase, during which consciousness gradually returns. The clinical manifestations of this phase largely depend on the severity of the ictal phase.

In the first several minutes of the immediate postictal phase the patient exhibits a momentary period of muscular flaccidity during which urinary and/or fecal

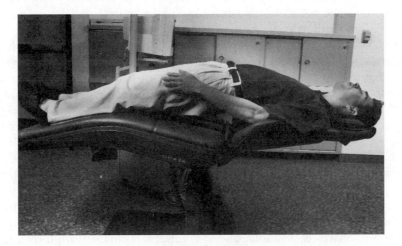

**Figure 21-1**  A victim during the tonic phase of a generalized tonic-clonic seizure (grand mal).

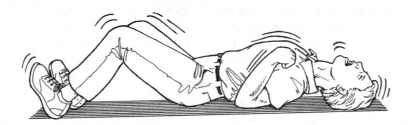

**Figure 21-2**  A victim during the clonic phase of a generalized tonic-clonic seizure (grand mal).

incontinence may occur because of sphincter relaxation. With the termination of seizure, the patient relaxes and sleeps deeply. If the seizure was severe, the patient may initially be comatose or nonresponsive. As consciousness gradually returns, the patient is initially disoriented and confused, unaware of the surroundings or the day of the week and unable to count backward from 10 to 1 or complete other simple mathematical calculations. Alertness increases with time. Patients may then fall into a deep, but rousable, recuperative sleep and complain of headache and muscle soreness when they awaken.

After most episodes of GTCS individuals usually exhibit almost total amnesia of the ictal and postictal phases. Some, however, may retain memory of the prodromal phase. Full recovery of preseizure cerebral functioning takes approximately 2 hours.[11]

### Grand mal status (GTCS status)

Status epilepticus is defined as a continuous seizure or the repetitive recurrence of any type of seizure without recovery between attacks.[21,22] In this discussion, it is considered to be a direct continuation of the GTCS previously described. Grand mal status is a life-threatening situation. Patients in status epilepticus exhibit the same clinical signs and symptoms as those in the convulsive phase of a GTCS; the one major difference is duration. Tonic-clonic seizures normally last from 2 to 5 minutes. Grand mal status may persist for hours or days and is the major cause of mortality directly related to seizure disorders. Mortality figures range from 3% to 23%, depending on the study cited.[65,66] The incidence of grand mal status has increased since the introduction of effective anticonvulsants; most cases result from drug or alcohol withdrawal (barbiturate withdrawal being particularly severe), severe head injury, or metabolic derangements.[23,24,67]

Clinically, any continuous GTCS that lasts 5 or more minutes is classified as grand mal status.[22] The patient is nonresponsive (unconscious), cyanotic, and diaphoretic and demonstrates generalized clonic contractions with a brief or entirely absent tonic phase. As grand mal status progresses, the patient becomes hyperthermic, the body temperature rising to 106 degrees Fahrenheit or above. The cardiovascular system is overworked, with tachycardia and dysrhythmias noted, and the blood pressure is elevated, with measurements of 300/150 mmHg not infrequently reported. Unterminated grand mal status may progress until one of the following occurs:

- Death as a result of cardiac arrest
- Irreversible neuronal damage from cerebral hypoxia, which occurs secondary to inadequate

ventilation and the increased metabolic requirements of the entire body (the CNS in particular)
- A decrease in cerebral blood flow in response to increased intracranial pressure
- A significant decrease in blood glucose levels as the brain uses large volumes for metabolism

## Pathophysiology

Epilepsy is not a disease; it is a symptom that normally represents a primary form of brain dysfunction. However, detection of such a lesion is not possible in approximately 75% of patients with recurrent seizure disorders (idiopathic epilepsy). Epileptics should be viewed as individuals with brains that malfunction periodically.

Although initial examination may fail to demonstrate it, adult-onset epilepsy most often occurs in response to the presence of a structural brain lesion. Small tumors may take considerable time to enlarge to a size at which they become detectable. Epileptics should undergo periodic medical examination (every 4 to 6 months), and annual electroencephalograms are recommended. The use of the computed tomography scan and magnetic resonance imaging have aided significantly in the detection of previously undetectable lesions.

Experimental drug models of epilepsy presume that intrinsic intracellular and extracellular metabolic disturbances exist in the neurons of epileptics and produce excessive and prolonged membrane depolarization. The common denominator among epileptics is an increased permeability of the neuronal cell membrane with changes in sodium and potassium movement that affect the resting membrane potential and membrane excitability.[35,68] These hyperexcitable neurons are located in aggregates in an epileptogenic focus (the site of origin of the seizure) somewhere within the brain and tend toward recurrent, high-frequency bursts of action potentials.

Clinical seizure activity develops if the abnormal discharge is propagated along neural pathways or if local neuron recruitment occurs (if additional neighboring neurons are stimulated to discharge). Once a critical mass of neurons is recruited and a sustained excitation occurs, the seizure is propagated along conducting pathways to subcortical areas and thalamic centers. If this discharge remains localized within the focal area, a partial seizure develops, with clinical signs and symptoms related to the specific focal area. If the discharge continues to spread through normal neuronal tissue and recruitment continues, generalized seizures occur. Clinical manifestations of the seizure depend on the focus of origin and the region of the brain into which the discharge subsequently spreads.

Clinical seizures caused by systemic metabolic and toxic disorders provide evidence that seizures also can arise in normal neurologic tissues. Deficiencies in $O_2$, as in the hypoxia that develops during vasodepressor syncope; or of glucose, which result in hypoglycemia; or in calcium ions, which result in hypocalcemia, create a membrane instability that predisposes otherwise normal neurons to paroxysmal discharge. Adequate electrical stimulation may also produce clinical seizures in normal neurologic tissues (for example, electroconvulsive therapy).

Significant alterations occur in both cerebral and systemic physiology during generalized motor seizures. Cerebral changes include marked increases in blood flow, $O_2$ and glucose use, and carbon dioxide production. These changes are associated with cerebral hypoxia and carbon dioxide retention, resulting in acidosis and lactic acid accumulation.[50,69] After 20 minutes of continuous seizure activity, cerebral metabolic demands may exceed the available supply, leading to potential neuronal destruction.[70]

The systemic effects of prolonged seizures are believed to be secondary to the massive autonomic discharge that produces tachycardia, hypertension, and hyperglycemia.[71] Other adverse systemic effects are produced secondary to massive skeletal muscle metabolism and disturbances in pulmonary ventilation leading to lactic acidosis, hypoxia, hypoglycemia, and hyperpyrexia.[72,73]

# Management

Management of a patient during the tonic-clonic phase of a GTCS focuses on the prevention of injury and the maintenance of adequate ventilation. In almost all cases, there is no need for administration of anticonvulsant drugs because most seizures are self limiting. If a seizure persists for an unusually long period of time (>5 minutes), however, anticonvulsant drug therapy must be seriously considered.

After the convulsive phase ends, the patient exhibits varying degrees of CNS, cardiovascular, and respiratory depression, all of which may require additional supportive management. There will almost always be a prior knowledge of seizure activity in this patient, so it is highly unlikely that the dental office staff will be surprised if a seizure occurs.

## PETIT MAL AND PARTIAL SEIZURES

Management of petit mal and partial seizures is protective in nature; the rescuer acts to protect the victim from injury. In each of these seizure types, there is little or no danger to the victim; even without assistance from staff members, death seldom occurs. Indeed many such seizures last such a short time that staff members may be unaware that an episode even occurred. However, if these seizures persist for a significant length of time (average petit mal episode being 5 to 30 seconds; average partial seizure lasting 1 to 2 minutes), emergency medical assistance should be summoned immediately.

Diagnostic clues to the presence of a petit mal or partial seizure are as follows:
- Sudden onset of immobility and blank stare
- Simple automatic behavior
- Slow blinking of eyelids
- Short duration (seconds to minutes)
- Rapid recovery

*Step 1: termination of the procedure.*

*Step 2: **P** (position).* In most cases of petit mal or simple partial seizure, neither the time nor the need exists to alter patient positioning.

*Step 3: reassurance of the patient.* After the seizure, the doctor should speak with the patient to determine the level of alertness and seek to determine whether the episode was related to the dental treatment. If the seizure was triggered by such factors, appropriate steps in the stress-reduction protocol should be used for all future appointments (see Chapter 2).

In addition, consultation with the patient's primary-care physician is indicated if seizures have increased recently in either frequency or severity. In most cases no need exists to seek outside emergency medical assistance or administer anticonvulsant drugs.

*Step 4: discharge of the patient and subsequent dental care.* The patient who suffers seizures is unlikely to be permitted to operate a motor vehicle. All states maintain requirements that prohibit epileptics from operating motor vehicles until they can document control over seizures for at least 1 year (each state varying on time requirements).[74] Therefore such patients are usually discharged from the office in the care of an adult companion or guardian.

Any dental-related factors that may have helped precipitate the episode should be taken into consideration and steps taken to prevent a recurrence in future

**box 21-3**  *Management of petit mal and partial seizures*

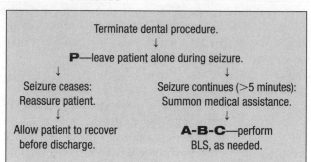

Terminate dental procedure.
↓
**P**—leave patient alone during seizure.
↓                              ↓
Seizure ceases:              Seizure continues (>5 minutes):
Reassure patient.            Summon medical assistance.
↓                              ↓
Allow patient to recover     **A-B-C**—perform
before discharge.            BLS, as needed.

**P,** Position; **A,** airway; **B,** breathing; **C,** circulation; *BLS,* basic life support.

treatments. Box 21-3 outlines the steps to follow in the management of petit mal and partial seizures.

## GENERALIZED TONIC-CLONIC SEIZURES (GRAND MAL)

Diagnostic clues that may prompt a suspicion of GTCS are as follows[75]:

- Presence of aura prior to loss of consciousness
- Loss of consciousness
- Tonic-clonic muscle contraction
- Clenched teeth; tongue biting
- Incontinence

### Preictal (prodromal) phase

*Step 1: termination of the procedure.* When a patient with a prior history of GTCS exhibits the aura, treatment should cease immediately. A variable period of time is available for the removal of as much dental equipment from the patient's mouth as possible before the individual loses consciousness and progresses to the ictal phase. In addition, any dental appliances should be removed from the patient's mouth. Documented reports exist of individuals aspirating removable dental appliances during seizures.[76]

### Ictal phase

*Step 2:* **P** *(position).* When the seizure develops while the victim is not seated in the dental chair, the individual should be placed on the floor in the supine position. When it occurs while the victim is in the dental chair, moving the patient may prove to be difficult. The patient should remain in the dental chair, which should be placed in the supine position.

*Step 3: summoning of medical assistance.* Although most generalized tonic-clonic seizures last only a short time (<5 minutes), I believe that med-

ical assistance should be sought at the onset, for the following two reasons:

1. If the patient is suffering the seizure when emergency personnel arrive, a patent vein and IV administration of anticonvulsant drug therapy may be easier to achieve.
2. If the seizure is terminated by the time emergency personnel arrive (a more common occurrence), the emergency workers can help evaluate the patient's postictal state, including the need for possible hospitalization or discharge.

That said, there are also occasions when it might be more prudent to delay in seeking medical assistance. For example, when the epileptic patient is accompanied by a spouse, parent or guardian, that individual may be able to provide guidance about the nature of the patient's seizures. However, if ever the doctor believes that the summoning of emergency medical assistance is warranted, it should be done immediately.

*Step 4:* **A-B-C** *(airway-breathing-circulation), or BLS, as needed.* During the seizure, especially during the tonic phase, respiration may be inadequate. Indeed, brief periods of apnea may occur in conjunction with obvious cyanosis. Secretions may also accumulate in the oral cavity and, if in large-enough amounts, produce a degree of airway obstruction. Saliva and blood are the most common secretions. During the clonic phase, respiration improves but may still require the rescuer's assistance via airway maintenance (for example, the head tilt–chin lift technique). The heart rate and blood pressure are significantly elevated above baseline values.

The victim's head should be extended (head tilt) to ensure airway patency, and, if possible, the oral cavity suctioned carefully to remove excessive secretions. However, suctioning is a difficult task and fortunately not always necessary. Soft rubber or plastic suction catheters are preferable to metal ones, which produce more soft and hard tissue damage (bleeding, trauma). In either case the suction apparatus should be inserted between the buccal surface of the teeth and the cheek (Figure 21-3), not between the teeth of the patient.

*Step 5:* **D** *(definitive care):*
*Step 5a: prevention of injury.* The prevention of injury is the next concern. If the victim is on a bed or a well-padded, carpeted floor in an area devoid of hard objects that may cause injury, the rescuer may permit the patient to seize with little risk of injury to the victim. Gently restraining the victim's arms and legs from gross movements (allowing for minor movements) prevents injury resulting from joint

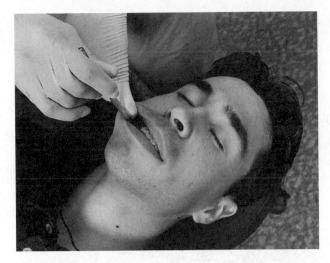

**Figure 21-3** The suction apparatus should be inserted between the buccal surface of the teeth and the cheek.

overextension or dislocation. No attempt should be made to hold the patient's extremities in a fixed position because of the risk of bony fractures.[22,50] If the floor is not padded, however, the head must be protected from traumatic injury through placement of a thin, soft item (a blanket or jacket) beneath the head, ensuring that the head is not flexed forward, obstructing the airway.

In addition, when the victim has a seizure in the dental chair, the danger is that the victim may fall off the chair or be injured by nearby dental equipment. Fortunately, the typical dental chair is a good site on which to have a seizure. The headrests on most dental units are normally well padded so that no additional protection is necessary for the head. Any additional pillow or doughnut devices atop the headrest should be removed, leaving a bare but padded headrest. The doughnut or pillow may throw the patient's head forward, increasing the likelihood of partial or complete airway obstruction. Removing the headrest permits extending the neck, lifting the tongue, and creating greater airway patency (Figure 21-4).

Our concern is that the patient not impale the arms or legs on equipment, such as burs and hand instruments. One member of the office emergency team should move as much equipment as possible away from the victim while two other members stand by the patient to minimize the risk of injury. In addition, one member should be positioned at the victim's chest to protect the head and arms; the second member should stand astride the feet (Figure 21-5).

NOTE: Placement of any object in the oral cavity is usually not indicated during a GTCS. Many dentists, physicians, and nurses have been trained to attempt to place

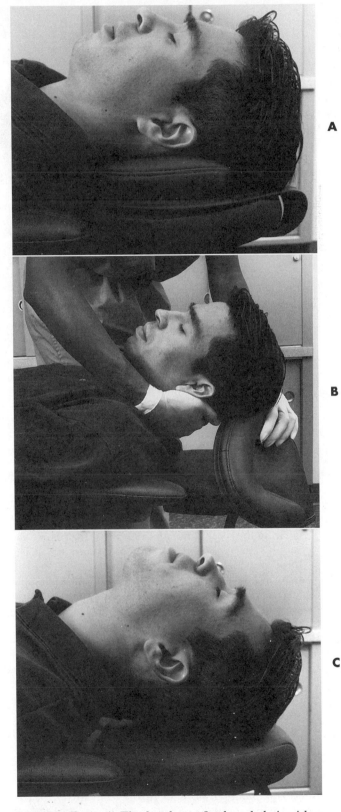

**Figure 21-4** **A,** The headrest of a dental chair with a doughnut or pillow; head thrown forward results in partial or complete airway obstruction. **B,** A bare headrest. **C,** Head extended; increased airway patency.

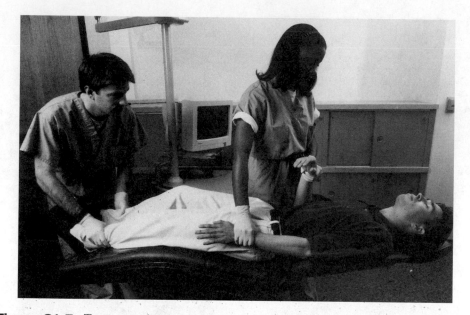

**Figure 21-5** To prevent the victim from injury, one dental office team member should be positioned at the patient's chest while the second member should stand astride the victim's feet.

objects into the mouth of the convulsing patient to prevent injury to the intraoral tissues and prevent the patient from "swallowing the tongue." Soft items, such as handkerchiefs, towels, and gauze pads, have also been recommended, as have ratchet-type (Molt) and rubber mouth props, wooden tongue depressors wrapped in gauze, and even teaspoons. The forcible insertion of these objects into the patient's mouth does not improve airway maintenance. Indeed the patient's muscles of mastication are in tetany during the seizure, and the patient's mouth must be forced open, greatly increasing the risk of injury to both the soft and hard tissues. Teeth have been fractured and aspirated during these attempts at helping seizing patients.[77] The possibility of injury to the rescuer also exists when attempts are made to place protective objects into the convulsing patient's mouth. Under no circumstances should a rescuer place the fingers between the teeth of a convulsing patient.

In most grand mal seizures, little to no bleeding occurs. Roberge and Maciera-Rodriguez[64] studied the incidence of seizure-related intraoral lacerations in 100 patients. They found that 44% of seizing patients suffered intraoral lacerations, primarily on the lateral border of the tongue. Only two of these 44 patients subsequently required surgical repair of the laceration. My experience is that the rescuer usually need not place any object into the mouth of a patient during the ictal phase of a GTCS. In addition, tight, binding clothes should be loosened to prevent possible injury by the straining patient and to aid in breathing.

*Step 5b: administration of O₂.* If available, $O_2$ may be administered to a patient suffering a seizure.

*Step 5c: monitoring of vital signs.* Throughout the seizure the patient's blood pressure, heart rate, and respiratory rate should be monitored and recorded. As mentioned previously, the blood pressure and heart rate are elevated significantly, and respiratory movements may be absent during the tonic phase. During the subsequent clonic phase the patient exhibits heavy, stertorous breathing.

## Postictal phase

With the cessation of seizures the patient enters the postictal phase, a period of generalized depression involving the central nervous, cardiovascular, and respiratory systems; the degree of depression is related to the degree of stimulation experienced during the preceding ictal phase. During the postictal phase, significant morbidity and even mortality may occur. The ictal phase of a seizure is a highly dramatic and emotionally charged event for eyewitnesses, and attention is quickly focused on the patient. Once the convulsive phase ends, the patient relaxes and so, unfortunately, do the rescuers. This response is premature because the patient may demonstrate significant CNS and respiratory depression during the postictal phase to a degree that respiratory depression and airway obstruction may become evident.

*Step 6: **P** (position).* The victim should remain in the supine position with the feet elevated slightly.

*Step 7:* **A-B-C,** *or BLS, as needed.* Postseizure patients almost always require airway maintenance; on rare occasions they also require assisted or controlled artificial ventilation. $O_2$ may be administered via a full mask or nasal cannula, if indicated. Airway maintenance and adequacy of ventilation remain the prime considerations at this time.

*Step 8: monitoring of vital signs.* Vital signs should be monitored and recorded at regular intervals (at least every 5 minutes). The blood pressure and respiration may be depressed in the immediate postictal period; their return to baseline values is gradual. The heart rate may be near the baseline level, slightly depressed, or slightly elevated.

*Step 9: reassurance of the patient and recovery.* Recovery from the seizure occurs slowly, with the patient initially somnolent, but rousable, and gradually becoming increasingly alert. Return to normal preseizure cerebral functioning may require as long as 2 hours. The patient also experiences significant confusion and disorientation. At this point the patient should be reassured that all is right. For example, I tell my patients the following: "This is Doctor Malamed. You are in the dental office. You had a seizure, and everything is all right." Many patients respond more promptly when a familiar voice speaks to them. If a spouse, family member, relative, or friend is available, that individual should be asked to reassure the patient. Recovery includes a return of the vital signs to approximately baseline levels and a disappearance of the confusion and disorientation of the early postictal period.

*Step 10: discharge.* This step is very difficult for me and represents the primary reason that I consider seeking medical assistance at the onset of the seizure. After a seizure, should the patient be hospitalized, sent to the primary-care physician, or sent home, and, if so, how?

Paramedical personnel follow strict protocol established for the management of specific emergency situations. In many jurisdictions, criteria for hospitalization of the postseizure victim who has a history of epilepsy include a lack of orientation to space and time. Emergency personnel make this decision quickly and, if necessary, transport the patient to the hospital for additional evaluation. If the patient recovers more completely and hospitalization is not warranted, discharge from the dental office occurs in the custody of a responsible adult relative or close friend.

Box 21-4 outlines the protocol for the management of a GTCS:

---

| box **21-4** | *Management of GTCS (grand mal)* |

**Prodromal stage**
Terminate dental procedure.
↓

**Ictal stage**
**P**—position patient supine with the legs elevated slightly.
↓
Summon emergency medical assistance.
↓
**A-B-C**—assess and perform BLS, as needed.
↓
**D**—definitive care
Protect patient from injury.
Administer $O_2$.
Monitor vital signs.
↓

**Postictal stage**
**P**—keep patient supine with the feet elevated slightly.
↓
**A-B-C**—perform BLS, as needed.
↓
**D**—definitive care
↓
Monitor vital signs.
↓
Reassure patient and permit recovery.
↓
Discharge patient:
↓           ↓           ↓
to hospital   to home    to physician

*P*, Position; *A*, airway; *B*, breathing; *C*, circulation; *D*, definitive care; *GTCS*, generalized tonic-clonic seizure; $O_2$, oxygen; *BLS*, basic life support.

---

## Grand mal status

If the GTCS persists for unusually long periods (>5 minutes), the use of anticonvulsant drugs may become necessary to terminate the seizure.

## Preictal phase
*Step 1: termination of the dental procedure.*

## Ictal phase
*Step 2:* **P**
*Step 3: summoning of medical assistance*
*Step 4:* **A-B-C** *(BLS) as needed*
*Step 5:* **D**
*Step 5a: protection of the patient from injury*
*Step 5b: administration of $O_2$*
*Step 5c: monitoring of vital signs*

The previous steps detailed the management of a patient with a GTCS. Although the overwhelming majority of seizures cease spontaneously within 5 minutes, prolonged seizures are possible and associated with a significantly increased risk of mortality and morbidity. Treatment options include (1) the continuation of BLS and protection of the patient until medical assistance is available and (2) definitive management of the seizure through the administration of anticonvulsant drugs. The first option is the most viable in most dental offices, in which drugs, equipment, and training for IV drug administration usually are not available. The administration of anticonvulsant drugs should be considered only when both the doctor and the office staff members are well versed in the pharmacology of these drugs and in artificial ventilation and possess the knowledge, ability, and equipment necessary to perform venipuncture.

*Step 6: venipuncture and administration of the anticonvulsant drug.* Various anticonvulsant drugs are used to terminate seizures. The ideal drug should produce a rapid onset of action and last only briefly.[50] Effectiveness depends on IV administration; the intramuscular route is too slow and unpredictable, and the oral route is contraindicated in unconscious, convulsing patients. An IV infusion should be established or the drug injected directly into the patient's vein. Because the blood pressure is elevated significantly during the seizure, superficial peripheral veins usually are visible, which makes injection relatively easy for an experienced doctor who has an assistant to restrain the arm. However, IV injections should not be performed if proper equipment and adequately trained staff members are not immediately available; in such instances supportive care should be continued until more highly trained personnel arrive.

The anticonvulsant drug of choice for the management of GTCS is a benzodiazepine, either diazepam (Valium)[51,78] or midazolam. Diazepam is more than 90% effective in instances of primary convulsive status.[79,80] A 10-mg dose should be administered at a rate of 5 mg per minute and repeated every 10 minutes, as necessary.[50] Children receive diazepam in doses of 0.3 mg/kg, a dose that should be repeated every 10 minutes, as necessary.[81] Potentially serious side effects of diazepam are related to excessively rapid injection and include transient hypotension, bradycardia, respiratory depression, and cardiac arrest.[82] If the drug is titrated slowly, such side effects occur only rarely. In general, the total dose should not exceed 0.5 mg/kg for acute therapy.[83]

Other benzodiazepines are also used to manage acute GTCSs. Lorazepam may be as effective as diazepam, but its onset is slower and its effect longer.[84] Midazolam, a water-soluble benzodiazepine, has also proven its effectiveness as an anticonvulsant when administered either via an IV or intramuscular route.[85-88]

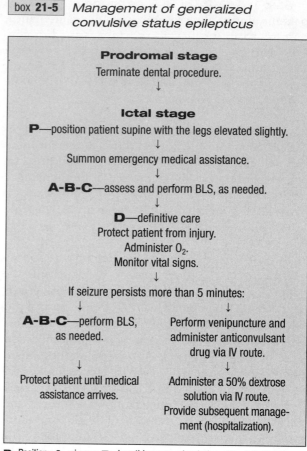

box **21-5**   *Management of generalized convulsive status epilepticus*

**Prodromal stage**
Terminate dental procedure.
↓

**Ictal stage**
**P**—position patient supine with the legs elevated slightly.
↓
Summon emergency medical assistance.
↓
**A-B-C**—assess and perform BLS, as needed.
↓
**D**—definitive care
Protect patient from injury.
Administer O₂.
Monitor vital signs.

If seizure persists more than 5 minutes:

| | |
|---|---|
| **A-B-C**—perform BLS, as needed. | Perform venipuncture and administer anticonvulsant drug via IV route. |
| Protect patient until medical assistance arrives. | Administer a 50% dextrose solution via IV route. Provide subsequent management (hospitalization). |

**P,** Position; **A,** airway; **B,** breathing; **C,** circulation; **D,** definitive care; $O_2$, oxygen; *BLS,* basic life support; *IV,* intravenous.

Until the introduction of benzodiazepines in the 1960s, barbiturates were the drugs of choice for seizure control. Pentobarbital (Nembutal), injected IV at a rate of 50 mg every 2 minutes, is an effective anticonvulsant. However, barbiturates also produce significant CNS and respiratory depression when used in anticonvulsant doses; thus the level of postictal CNS depression will be intensified. In addition, respiratory depression and apnea are frequent side effects of barbiturates when used as anticonvulsants. Effective airway maintenance and artificial ventilation must be provided until the patient recovers.

*Step 7: administration of a 50% dextrose solution.* The IV administration of 25 to 50 ml of a 50% dextrose solution is recommended to rule out hypoglycemia as a possible cause of the seizure. This solution also helps the patient maintain blood sugar levels because the brain uses large quantities of glucose during the ictal state.[50,51]

*Step 8: subsequent management.* All patients with grand mal status require hospitalization after the

table **21-4** *Possible causes of seizure disorders*

| CAUSE | FREQUENCY | TEXT DISCUSSION |
|---|---|---|
| Epilepsy (GTCS) | Most common | Seizures (Section Five) |
| Local anesthetic overdose reaction | Less common | Drug-related emergencies (Section Six) |
| Hyperventilation | Rare | Respiratory distress (Section Three) |
| CVA | Rare | Altered consciousness (Section Four) |
| Hypoglycemic reaction | Rare | Altered consciousness (Section Four) |
| Vasodepressor syncope | Rare | Unconsciousness (Section Two) |

*CVA*, Cerebrovascular accident.

episode for neurologic evaluation and initiation of a treatment protocol to minimize further episodes. If the previously mentioned drugs do not terminate the seizure, other agents may be required. These include phenytoin (15 mg/kg) for long-term seizure control, phenobarbital (10-15 mg/kg) for continuing seizures, and neuromuscular blockade (paralysis) with a non-depolarizing neuromuscular blocking agent such as pancuronium.[86]

Box 21-5 outlines the management of patients suffering GTCS status epilepticus. In addition, the following information may prove useful:

- **Drugs used in management:** $O_2$ may be used to manage any seizure. If status epilepticus occurs, an anticonvulsant, preferably diazepam or midazolam, may be used.
- **Medical assistance required:** Treatment of patients with seizures frequently requires the summoning of emergency personnel.

## Differential Diagnosis

Seizures are not easily confused with other systemic medical conditions. However, seizures may be part of the clinical manifestations of several systemic disorders (Table 21-4). This section is designed to aid in the diagnosis of the possible causes of seizure activity.

Vasodepressor syncope is the most common cause of unconsciousness in the dental office. If hypoxia or anoxia persist, brief periods of seizure activity may occur. One distinguishing factor that indicates vasodepressor syncope is the presence of a definite precipitating factor, such as fear. Individuals suffering vasodepressor syncope usually exhibit prodromal signs, such as lightheadedness, nausea, or vomiting and diaphoresis, before losing consciousness; epileptics do not exhibit such signs. The duration of unconsciousness in cases of vasodepressor syncope normally is quite brief, and recovery begins once blood flow to the brain increases. Muscles are flaccid, and no convulsive movements are present initially. Blood pres-

sure and heart rate are also depressed, and bladder and bowel incontinence are rare. When syncopal patients regain consciousness, they do not experience disorientation or confusion; they are alert and can perform simple mental calculations. The primary cause of seizure activity in vasodepressor syncope is hypoxia, which is reversible with airway management.

Cerebrovascular accident may also lead to the loss of consciousness and possible convulsions. Aids in differential diagnosis include the possible presence of an intense headache before the loss of consciousness and of signs of neurologic dysfunction (for example, muscle weakness or paralysis).

Lastly, hypoglycemia may progress to the loss of consciousness, and seizures may develop. The patient's medical history and clinical signs and symptoms can usually provide evidence (see Chapter 17). Additional management in this situation requires the administration of IV dextrose.

## REFERENCES

1. Taylor J, editor: *Selected writings of John Hughlings Jackson,* vol 1, On epilepsy and epileptiform convulsions, London, 1931, Hodder and Stoughton (reprinted 1958, New York, Basic Books).
2. Gastaut H: *Dictionary of epilepsy,* Geneva, 1973, World Health Organization.
3. Sutherland JM, Eadie MJ: The epilepsies: modern diagnosis and treatment, ed 3, Edinburgh, 1980, Churchill Livingstone.
4. Delgado-Escueta AV, Treiman DM, Walsh GO: The treatable epilepsies: (2 parts), *N Engl J Med* 308:1508, 1983.
5. Hauser WA, Kurland LT: The epidemiology of epilepsy in Rochester, Minnesota, 1935 through 1967, *Epilepsia* 61:1, 1975.
6. Hauser WA: Epidemiology of epilepsy. In Schonberg BS, editor: *Advances in neurology,* vol 19, New York, 1978, Raven Press.
7. Camfield PR and others: Epilepsy after a first unprovoked seizure in childhood, *Neurology* 35:1657, 1985.

8. Shinnar S and others: Discontinuing antiepileptic medication in children with epilepsy after two years without seizures: a prospective study, *N Engl J Med* 313:976, 1985.

9. Callaghan N, Garrett A, Goggin T: Withdrawal of anticonvulsant drugs in patients free of seizures for two years: a prospective study, *N Engl J Med* 318:942, 1988.

10. Epilepsy Foundation of America: *Basic statistics on the epilepsies,* Philadelphia, 1975, FA Davis.

11. Gastaut H and others: Generalized convulsive seizures without local onset. In Vinken PJ, Bruyn GW, editors: *Handbook of clinical neurology,* vol 15, Amsterdam, 1974, Elsevier.

12. Gastaut H: *Epileptic seizures,* Springfield, Ill, 1972, Charles C Thomas.

13. Milichap J, Aymat F: Treatment and prognosis of petit mal epilepsy, *Pediatr Clin North Am* 14:905, 1967.

14. Livingston S and others: Classification and clinical features of epileptic seizures, *Pediatr Ann* 8:176, 1979.

15. Gastaut H and others: Generalized non-convulsive seizures without local onset. In Vinken PJ, Bruyn GW, editors: *Handbook of clinical neurology,* vol 15, Amsterdam, 1974, Elsevier.

16. Vick N: *Grinker's neurology,* ed 7, Springfield, Ill, 1976, Charles C Thomas.

17. Feindel W: Temporal lobe seizures. In Vinken PJ, Bruyn GW, editors: *Handbook of clinical neurology,* vol 15, Amsterdam, 1974, Elsevier.

18. Niedermeyer E: *Compendium of the epilepsies,* Springfield, Ill, 1974, Charles C Thomas.

19. Rasmussen T: Seizures with local onset and elementary symptomatology. In Vinken PJ, Bruyn GW, editors: *Handbook of clinical neurology,* vol 15, Amsterdam, 1974, Elsevier.

20. Gastaut H: Clinical and electroencephalographical classification of epileptic seizures, *Epilepsia* 11:114, 1970.

21. Hauser A: Status epilepticus: frequency, etiology and neurological sequelae. In Delgado-Escueta AV and others, editors: *Advances in neurology,* vol 34, New York, 1983, Raven Press.

22. American Academy of Orthopedic Surgeons: *Emergency care and transportation for the sick and injured,* ed 4, Orco, Ill, 1987, The Academy.

23. Celesia G, Messert B, Murphy M: Status epilepticus of late onset, *Neurology* 22:1047, 1972.

24. Aminoff MJ, Simon RP: Status epilepticus: causes, clinical features and consequences in 98 patients, *Am J Med* 69:657, 1980.

25. Delgado-Escueta AV and others: Current concepts in neurology: management of status epilepticus, *N Engl J Med* 306:1337, 1982.

26. Oxbury J, Whitty C: Causes and consequences of status epilepticus in adults, *Brain* 94:733, 1971.

27. Treiman DM and others: Predictable sequence of EEG changes during generalized convulsive status epilepticus in man and three experimental models of status epilepticus in the rat, *Neurology* 37(suppl 1):244, 1987.

28. Gumnit RJ, Sell MA, editors: *Epilepsy: a handbook for physicians,* ed 4, Minneapolis, 1981, University of Minnesota Comprehensive Epilepsy Program.

29. Janz D: Etiology of convulsive status epilepticus. In Delgado-Escueta AV and others, editors: *Advances in neurology,* vol 34, New York, 1983, Raven Press.

30. Andermann F, Robb J: Absence status: a reappraisal review of thirty-eight patients, *Epilepsia* 13:177, 1972.

31. Robb P, McNaughton F: Etiology of epilepsy: introduction. In Vinken PJ, Bruyn GW, editors: *Handbook of clinical neurology,* vol 15, Amsterdam, 1974, Elsevier.

32. Wilkinson DS, Prockop LD: Hypoglycemia: effects on the central nervous system. In Vinken PJ, Bruyn GW, editors: *Handbook of clinical neurology,* vol 15, Amsterdam, 1974, Elsevier.

33. Earnest MP, Yarnell PR: Seizure admissions to a city hospital: the role of alcohol, *Epilepsia* 17:387, 1976.

34. Newton R: Physostigmine salicylate in the treatment of tricyclic antidepressant overdosage, *JAMA* 231:941, 1975.

35. Tower DB: Neurochemistry of epilepsy. In Vinken PJ, Bruyn GW, editors: *Handbook of clinical neurology,* vol 15, Amsterdam, 1974, Elsevier.

36. Myers JA, Earnest MP: Generalized seizures and cocaine abuse, *Neurology* 34:675, 1984.

37. Jennett WB: *Epilepsy after non-missile head injuries,* Chicago, 1975, Mosby.

38. Jennett WB: Posttraumatic epilepsy. In Thompson RA, Green JP, editors: *Advances in neurology,* vol 22, New York, 1979, Raven Press.

39. Friedlander WJ: Epilepsy, *Prog Neurol Psychiatry* 27:133, 1972.

40. Holmes GL: *Diagnosis and management of seizures in childhood,* Philadelphia, 1987, WB Saunders.

41. LeBlanc FE, Rasmussen T: Cerebral seizures and brain tumors. In Vinken PJ, Bruyn GW, editors: *Handbook of clinical neurology,* vol 15, Amsterdam, 1974, Elsevier.

42. Ketz E: Brain tumors and epilepsy. In Vinken PJ, Bruyn GW, editors: *Handbook of clinical neurology,* vol 16, Amsterdam, 1974, Elsevier.

43. Scheehan S: 1,000 cases of late onset epilepsy, *Ir J Med Sci* 6:261, 1958.

44. Schold C, Yarnell PR, Earnest MP: Origin of seizures in elderly patients, *JAMA* 238:1177, 1977.

45. Bauer G, Niedermeyer E: Acute convulsions, *Clin Electroenceph* 10:127, 1979.

46. Juul-Jensen P: Epilepsy: a clinical and social analysis of 1020 adult patients with epileptic seizures, *Acta Neurol Scand* 40(suppl 5):1, 1964.

47. Dahlquist NR, Mellinger JF, Klass DW: Hazard of video games in patients with light-sensitive epilepsy, *JAMA* 249:776, 1983.

48. Millett CJ, Fish DR, Thompson PJ: A survey of epilepsy-patient perceptions of video-game material/electronic screens and other factors as seizure precipitants, *Seizure* 6(6):457-459, 1997.

49. Annegars J: Factors prognostic of unprovoked seizures after febrile convulsions, *N Engl J Med* 316:493, 1987.

50. Tomlanovich MC, Yee AS: Seizure. In Rosen P, editor: *Emergency medicine,* ed 2, St Louis, 1988, Mosby.

51. Aminoff MJ: Epilepsy. In Schroeder SA and others, editors: *Current medical diagnosis and treatment,* Stamford, Conn, 1990, Appleton & Lange.

52. Porter RJ: How to use antiepileptic drugs. In Levy RH and others, editors: *Antiepileptic drugs,* ed 3, New York, 1989, Raven Press.

53. Emerson R and others: Stopping medication in children with epilepsy: predictors of outcome, *N Engl J Med* 304:1125, 1981.

54. Vinson T: Towards demythologizing epilepsy, *Med J Aust* 2:663, 1975.

55. Lewis JA: Violence and epilepsy, *JAMA* 232:1165, 1975.

56. Gunn JC, Fenton G: Epilepsy in prisons: a diagnostic survey, *Br Med J* 4:326, 1969.

57. King LN, Young QD: Increased prevalence of seizure disorders among prisoners, *JAMA* 239:2674, 1978.

58. Living with epilepsy, New York Times, p ??, February 23, 1982.

59. Elwes R and others: The prognosis for seizure control in newly diagnosed epilepsy, *N Engl J Med* 311:944, 1984.

60. Malamed SF: *Sedation: a guide to patient management,* ed 3, St Louis, 1995, Mosby.

61. Shaw G: Alcohol and the nervous system, *Clin Endocrinol Metab* 7:385, 1978.

62. Walter R: Clinical aspects of temporal lobe epilepsy, *Calif Med* 110:325, 1969.

63. Livingston S and others: Medical treatment of epilepsy, *South Med J* 71:298, 1978.

64. Roberge RJ, Maciera-Rodriguez L: Seizure-related oral lacerations: incidence and distribution, *J Am Dent Assoc* 111:279, 1985.

65. Nicol CF: Status epilepticus, *JAMA* 234:419, 1975.

66. Maytal J: Low morbidity and mortality of status epilepticus in children, *Pediatrics* 83:323, 1989.

67. Rowan A, Scott D: Major status epilepticus, *Acta Neurol Scand* 46:573, 1970.

68. Reynolds EH: Water, electrolytes and epilepsy, *J Neurol Sci* 11:327, 1970.

69. Chapman AG, Meldrum BS, Siesjo BK: Cerebral metabolic changes during prolonged epileptic seizures in rats, *J Neurochem* 28:1025, 1977.

70. Kreisman NR and others: Cerebral oxygenation during recurrent seizures. In Delgado-Escueta AV and others, editors: *Advances in neurology,* vol 34, New York, 1983, Raven Press.

71. Laidlaw J, Richens A: *A textbook of epilepsy,* Edinburgh, 1976, Churchill Livingstone.

72. Orringer CE and others: Natural history of lactic acidosis after grand mal seizures, *N Engl J Med* 297:796, 1977.

73. Meldrum BS, Vigouroux RA, Brierly JB: Systemic factors and epileptic brain damage: prolonged seizures in paralyzed artificially ventilated baboons, *Arch Neurol* 29:82, 1973.

74. Krumholz A and others: Driving and epilepsy: a review and reappraisal, *JAMA* 265(5):622-626, 1991.

75. Pollakoff J, Pollakoff K: EMT's guide to treatment, Los Angeles, 1991, Jeff Gould.

76. Giovannitti JA Jr: Aspiration of a partial denture during an epileptic seizure, *J Am Dent Assoc* 103:895, 1981.

77. Scheuer ML, Pedley TA: The evaluation and treatment of seizures, *N Engl J Med* 323:1468, 1990.

78. Browne T: Drug therapy reviews: drug therapy of status epilepticus, *Am J Hosp Pharm* 35:915, 1978.

79. Browne T, Penry J: Benzodiazepines in the treatment of epilepsy, *Epilepsia* 14:277, 1973.

80. Tassinari C and others: Benzodiazepines: efficacy in status epilepticus. In Delgado-Escueta AV and others, editors: *Advances in neurology,* vol 34, New York, 1983, Raven Press.

81. Aicardi J, Chevrie JJ: Convulsive status epilepticus in infants and children: a study of 239 cases, *Epilepsia* 11:187, 1970.

82. Physicians' Desk Reference, ed 53, Oradell, NJ, 1999, Medical Economics Data.

83. Tintinalli J: Status epilepticus, *JACEP* 5:896, 1976.

84. Homan R, Walker J: Clinical studies of lorazepam in status epilepticus. In Delgado-Escueta AV and others, editors: *Advances in neurology,* vol 34, New York, 1983, Raven Press.

85. Jaimovich DG and others: Intravenous midazolam suppression of pentyl–enetetrazol-induced epileptogenic activity in a porcine model, *Crit Care Med* 18(3):313-316, 1990.

86. Nordt SP, Clark RF: Midazolam: a review of therapeutic uses and toxicity, *J Emerg Med* 15(3):357-365, 1997.

87. Chamberlain JM and others: A prospective, randomized study comparing intramuscular midazolam with intravenous diazepam for the treatment of seizures in children, *Pediatr Emerg Care* 13(2):92-94, 1997.

88. Kendall JL, Reynolds M, Goldberg R: Intranasal midazolam in patients with status epilepticus, *Ann Emerg Med* 29(3):415-417, 1997.

# DRUG-RELATED EMERGENCIES

# 22

## Drug-Related Emergencies

### General Considerations

**T**HE administration of drugs is commonplace in the practice of dentistry. Local anesthetics are an integral part of the dental treatment plan whenever potentially painful procedures are considered. Analgesic drugs are prescribed for the relief of preexisting pain or the alleviation of potential postoperative discomfort, antibiotics are prescribed for the treatment of infections, and, increasingly, antianxiety drugs are prescribed for all phases of the dental treatment (before, during, and after). These four drug categories constitute the overwhelming majority of all drugs used in the practice of dentistry (Table 22-1).[1]

Whenever a drug is administered to a patient a rational purpose should exist for its use. The indiscriminate administration of drugs is one of the major reasons why the number of serious incidents of drug-related, life-threatening emergencies reported in the medical and dental literature has increased.[2-5] Most drug-related emergencies are classified as one aspect of iatrogenic disease, a category that encompasses an entire spectrum of adverse effects that physicians or dentists produce unintentionally during patient management.

The high incidence of reports of adverse drug reactions (ADRs) in medical literature accounts for 3% to 20% of all hospital admissions.[5-7] An additional 5% to 40% of patients hospitalized for other reasons also experience ADRs during their hospitalization. Furthermore, 10% to 18% of those patients

333

table **22-1** *Prescription habits in a U.S. dental school—1983 to 1985*

| DRUG CATEGORY | | NUMBER OF PRESCRIPTIONS |
| --- | --- | --- |
| Analgesics | | 5730 |
| Nonnarcotic | (1139) | |
| Combined with codeine | (4570) | |
| Narcotic | (21) | |
| Antibiotics | | 3931 |
| Penicillin | (2977) | |
| Erythromycin | (637) | |
| Tetracycline | (187) | |
| Cephalosporin | (130) | |
| Minor tranquilizers | | 219 |
| Sedative-hypnotics | | 65 |
| Other categories | | 1500 |
| **Total prescriptions filled** | | **11,445** |

Data from Department of Pharmacology, University of Southern California School of Dentistry, Los Angeles.

box **22-1** *General principles of toxicology*

1. No drug ever exerts a single action.
2. No clinically useful drug is entirely devoid of toxicity.
3. The potential toxicity of a drug rests in the hands of the user.

admitted to the hospital because of an ADR have yet another ADR during their time in the hospital, resulting in the length of hospitalization being doubled.[6] In most cases, careful prescribing habits or care in the administration of drugs might have prevented the occurrence of an ADR. A recent report noted than more than 106,000 individuals died in U.S. hospitals because of ADRs to drugs they received while undergoing medical treatment for a primary disorder. An additional 2.2 million suffered serious but nonfatal ADRs.[8]

Some general principles of toxicology are presented at this time so that the following material may be better understood (Box 22-1). Toxicology is the study of the harmful effects of chemicals (drugs) on biologic systems. These harmful effects range from those that may prove inconsequential to the patient and are reversible entirely once the chemical is withdrawn, to those that prove uncomfortable but are not seriously harmful, to those that seriously may incapacitate the patient or cause death.[9] Whenever a drug is administered, two types of reactions may be noted—desirable drug actions, or those that are sought clinically and usually are beneficial, and side effects, which are often undesirable drug actions.

An example of a desired drug action is the relief of anxiety through the administration of diazepam to a fearful dental patient. A side effect of diazepam that is normally not desired but does not usually harm the patient is drowsiness. However, drowsiness may prove beneficial under certain circumstances, such as when the patient is extremely apprehensive. However, the same degree of drowsiness while that patient is driving an automobile may prove hazardous. A side effect or undesirable drug action may also prove harmful to the patient. Respiratory and cardiovascular depression, although they rarely accompany proper administration of diazepam, can occur after either parenteral (intramuscular [IM] or intravenous [IV]) or oral administration.[10]

A general principle of toxicology is that no drug ever exerts a single action. All chemicals exert many actions, some desirable and others undesirable. Ideally, the correct drug is administered in the correct dose via the correct route to the correct patient at the correct time for the correct reason, and this drug does not produce unwanted effects.[9] This clinical situation rarely if ever occurs because no drug is so specific that it produces only the desired effects in all patients. No clinically useful drug is entirely devoid of toxicity. In addition, ADRs may occur when the wrong drug is administered to the wrong patient in the wrong dose via the wrong route at the wrong time for the wrong reason.

## Prevention

Although the preceding discussion may seem unduly pessimistic, it has not been presented with the intention of scaring dental practitioners away from administering drugs to their patients. Indeed, my firm conviction is that drug use is absolutely essential in dentistry for the safe and proper management of many patients. Thus it is important that the doctor become familiar with the pharmacologic properties of all drugs that doctor uses and prescribes. Several excellent references may serve as readily available sources of information.[11-14]

Pallasch[9] stated the following:

In most cases it is possible with sound clinical and pharmacological judgment to prevent serious toxicity from occurring. The aim of rational therapeutics is to maximize the therapeutic and minimize the toxic effects of a given drug. No drug is "completely safe" or "completely harmful." All drugs are capable of producing harm if handled improperly, and conversely, any drug may be handled safely if proper precautions are observed. The potential toxicity of a drug rests in the hands of the user.

Another factor in the safe use of drugs is a consideration of the patient who is to receive the drug. Individuals may react in very different ways to the same stimulus; it should not be surprising that patients will vary markedly in their reactions to drugs. Before administering any drug or prescribing any medication, the doctor must ask specific questions about the patient's past and present drug history.

## Medical History Questionnaire

**Question 6: Have you taken any medicine or drugs during the past 2 years?**

*Comment:* An accurate assessment of drugs and medications that a patient is taking or has taken recently must be obtained to prevent the occurrence of potential drug interactions and side effects.

**Question 7: Are you allergic to (that is, experience itching, rash, swelling of hands, feet, or eyes) or made sick by penicillin, aspirin, codeine, or any drugs or medications?**

*Comment:* Common signs and symptoms of allergy are presented in this section along with the names of three drugs that commonly are associated with ADRs. An alleged history of allergy to any drug should prompt the doctor to perform an in-depth dialogue history with the patient (see Chapters 23 and 24).

**Question 9: Circle any of the following that you have had or have at present:**

Allergy or hives
Chemotherapy (cancer, leukemia)
Cortisone medicine

*Comment:* All affirmative responses should be followed with thorough dialogue histories to determine the drugs used, the reason for their administration, and the nature of any ADRs.

## DIALOGUE HISTORY

If the patient responds positively to an allergy or ADR (question 7) the doctor should obtain the following information from the patient concerning the incident:

**What drug did you take?**
**Were you taking any other medications at the time of the allergic reaction or ADR?**
**Did the individual who administered the drug record your vital signs?**
**What was the time sequence of events during the reaction?**
**Where were you when the reaction occurred (for example, at home or in a medical or dental office)?**
**What clinical manifestations (signs and symptoms) did you exhibit?**

**What acute treatment did you receive?**
**Have you received the offending agent or any chemical related to it since the incident; if so, what was your reaction?**

Most patients respond affirmatively to the allergy question if they have ever experienced any adverse reaction to a drug. (This fact will be discussed in detail in the remaining chapters in this section.) Actually, the incidence of allergic phenomena is low, despite the high incidence of reports of allergy in dental and medical histories. The reason for this variance lies in the fact that to the patient, any ADR is an allergy; the lay individual often is not familiar with the classification of drug reactions.

Thus such notations as "allergy to Novocain" and "allergy to codeine" are commonly found on medical history questionnaires. Although allergies to these drugs are not impossible, the patient's ADR most likely was not due to an allergy. Careful questioning via the dialogue history usually reveals that the "allergy to Novocain" was a psychogenic reaction, such as hyperventilation or vasodepressor syncope, or a mild overdose (toxic) reaction to the drug. The "allergy to codeine" most likely consisted of stomach upset, nausea or vomiting, all of which are undesirable side effects of the drugs, not allergic reactions.

Questions that help reveal the precise nature of the ADR are vital. However, patients may often provide vague answers, which do not allow the doctor to distinguish a harmless ADR from a true allergic reaction. At such times the doctor should attempt to locate and speak to the individual who observed or managed the "allergic" reaction, who may be able to provide more precise details of the event.

In addition, reactions often thought of as ADRs in fact may be unrelated to the drug administered. In an article entitled "Adverse Nondrug Reactions," Reidenberg and Lowenthal[15] demonstrated the occurrence of common drug side effects in individuals who had not received any medications for 2 weeks. If these individuals had been taking medications at the time that the reaction occurred, they may have reported experiencing ADRs.

Whenever doubt remains concerning the safety of a drug, it is prudent to initially assume that the patient *is* allergic and avoid its use until the question of allergy can be answered definitively. This process may require referral of the patient to an allergist. In most cases, however, alternative drugs may be administered that possess the same beneficial clinical properties but lack the same potential for allergy as the drug in question. These "safe" alternatives should be used until allergy is ruled out conclusively.

Even in the absence of a history of ADR, it is still recommended that the patient be questioned directly before any new drugs are administered. Therefore the doctor may ask the patient: "Have you ever taken Valium before?" If the answer is yes, the next question may be: "What effect did it produce?" Common, proprietary names should also be used (for example, Valium) because few nonhealth professionals are familiar with the generic names of drugs (for example, diazepam). If the individual does not report any ADRs, the doctor may feel more confident administering the drug but always being aware that adverse reactions (including allergy) may still occur despite prior administration of the same drug without complication.

## CARE IN DRUG ADMINISTRATION

About 85% of ADRs are related to the administration of a drug overdose.[6] Drug overdose (also known as a *toxic reaction*) may be absolute (too many milligrams) or relative (a normal therapeutic dose proving an overdose in a particular patient). Regardless of the type of overdose, most such reactions can be prevented through careful dose determination (oral or IM administration) or careful administration (titration via IV and inhalation routes). Most clinical responses to drugs are related to the dose (dose dependent); however, even minute quantities of a drug may precipitate a severe allergic reaction (anaphylaxis) in a previously sensitized individual.

The route of drug administration also influences the number and severity of ADRs. Two major routes—enteral and parenteral—are considered. Enteral routes of administration are those in which the drug is administered in the gastrointestinal (GI) tract and subsequently absorbed into the circulatory system; it includes the oral and rectal routes. In parenteral administration the drug bypasses the GI tract; techniques of parenteral drug administration include IM, intranasal, transdermal, submucosal, subcutaneous, IV, intraspinal, and intracapsular injections. Inhalation and topical application comprise additional routes of administration that may be classified as parenteral.

In general, serious ADRs occur more frequently after parenteral drug administration than after administration via enteral routes. IV drug administration is the most effective route because it provides a rapid onset and a high degree of reliability; it also carries a great potential for serious ADRs. However, when used properly, the IV route remains a safe and important option in the practice of dentistry. ADRs that occur after enteral drug administration are usually less serious. The clinical effectiveness of enterally administered drugs is diminished significantly compared with those administered parenterally. A general rule in drug administration states that if a drug is clinically effective when administered enterally, this route is preferable to its parenteral administration.

In drug administration the route of administration must be considered carefully. Not all drugs may be administered via every route, and the degree of effectiveness for some drugs may vary considerably based on the route. For example, 10 mg diazepam administered via an IV route usually provides a level of sedation adequate to permit a fearful patient to tolerate dental treatment; the level of sedation achieved through oral administration of 10 mg diazepam most likely is inadequate to permit comfortable dental treatment for the same patient. On the other hand, antibiotic prophylaxis for the patient with rheumatic heart disease may be achieved with either intramuscular injection or oral administration of penicillin or amoxicillin 1 hour before treatment. In both instances the antibiotic blood level is adequate to prevent a transient bacteremia from producing bacterial endocarditis. In this instance, however, the oral route is preferred over the parenteral route. Penicillin has a high potential to provoke allergy, and the route of its administration has significant bearing on the severity of any reaction that might arise.

Most drug-related emergency situations are preventable. Careful questioning of the patient regarding any prior exposure and subsequent reaction to a drug before its administration, careful selection of the most appropriate route of administration, use of the proper technique, and familiarity with the pharmacology of all drugs prescribed to patients or used in the dental office can significantly reduce the incidence of ADRs.

## Classification

Classifying ADRs has become confusing. In the past a variety of terms, such as *side effect, adverse experience, drug-induced disease, disease of medical progress, secondary effect,* and *intolerance* described such a reaction. Today's approach is simpler; most reactions are classified simply as ADRs.

The classification proposed by Pallasch[9] represents a simplified approach to the classification of ADRs (Box 22-2). This classification presents the following three major methods by which drugs may produce ADRs:

1. Direct extension of a drug's pharmacologic actions
2. Deleterious effect on a chemically, genetically, metabolically, or morphologically altered recipient (the patient)
3. Initiation of an immune (allergic) response

Approximately 85% of ADRs result from the pharmacologic effects of the drug, whereas 15% result from immunologic reactions.[6]

---

box 22-2    *Classification of ADRs*

**Toxicity resulting from direct extension of pharmacologic effects**
Side effects
Abnormal dose (overdose)
Local toxic effects

**Toxicity resulting from altered recipient (patient)**
Presence of pathologic processes
Emotional disturbances
Genetic aberrations (idiosyncrasy)
Teratogenicity
Drug-drug interactions

**Toxicity resulting from drug allergy**

---

Modified from Pallasch TJ: *Pharmacology for dental students and practitioners,* Philadelphia, 1980, Lea & Febiger.
*ADR,* Adverse drug reaction.

Most ADRs are merely annoying and do not pose a threat to the patient's life. However, several potential responses to drugs exist that are life-threatening and require immediate effective management if the patient is to fully recover to full function. Such responses include the overdose reaction (a direct extension of the usual pharmacologic properties of the drug) and the allergic reaction. (Because of the critical nature of these responses and their importance in dentistry, subsequent chapters will discuss these responses in more detail.) Idiosyncrasy, the last of the critical drug-related situations, is discussed fully in this chapter.

## OVERDOSE REACTION

Overdose reaction (toxic reaction) is a condition that results from exposure to toxic amounts of a substance that does not cause adverse effects when administered in smaller amounts.[16] It refers to those clinical signs and symptoms resulting from an absolute or a relative overadministration of a drug that leads to elevated blood levels of the drug in various target organs and tissues. Clinical signs and symptoms of overdose are related to a direct extension of the normal pharmacologic actions of the drug. For example, with therapeutic blood levels in the central nervous system (CNS) achieved, barbiturates mildly depress the CNS, resulting in sedation or hypnosis (both desirable effects). Barbiturate overdose (higher blood levels of the barbiturate in the CNS) produces a more profound CNS depression, increasing the possibility of respiratory and cardiovascular depression.

Further elevations in barbiturate blood levels can result in the loss of consciousness (general anesthesia or a medical emergency) and increasing degrees of respiratory depression, resulting eventually in respiratory arrest. Local anesthetics are also CNS-depressants. When these drugs are administered properly and in therapeutic doses, little or no evidence of CNS depression is evident; however, increased blood levels (in the CNS and myocardium) produce signs and symptoms of selective CNS depression (see Chapter 23).

## ALLERGY

*Allergy* is defined as a hypersensitive response to an allergen to which the individual has been previously exposed and to which that individual has developed antibodies.[16] Clinically, an allergy can manifest itself in a variety of ways, including drug fever, angioedema, urticaria, dermatitis, depression of blood-forming organs, photosensitivity, and anaphylaxis (the latter being an acute systemic reaction that may result in respiratory distress and cardiovascular collapse). Certain drugs and substances are much more likely than others to cause allergic reactions (for example, penicillin, aspirin, latex, bisulfites, nuts, and bee stings). An allergic reaction is a possibility with any drug or chemical.

In marked contrast to the overdose reaction, in which clinical manifestations relate directly to the normal pharmacology of the drug, the observed clinical response in allergy is always a result of an exaggerated response by the body's immune system. The degree of heightened response determines the acuteness and severity of the observed reaction.

Allergic responses to a barbiturate, a local anesthetic, and an antibiotic are caused by the same mechanism and clinically may appear identical. Indeed allergic responses to nuts, bananas, shellfish, and bee stings are similar to each other and to those produced by drug allergy. All responses require the same basic management, whereas overdose reactions to the same three items are clinically dissimilar, requiring entirely different modes of treatment.

A third factor when comparing overdose and allergic reactions is the amount, or dose, of the drug administered. An overdose reaction requires that a dose of the drug or substance be adequate to produce a blood level high enough to produce an ADR. Overdose reactions are dose related. Allergy, in contrast, is not dose dependent. If an individual is not allergic to penicillin, that person can tolerate extremely large doses safely; however, if the individual is allergic, exposure to even a minute volume (<1 mg) could result in death. Consider the volume of venom injected into an individual by a stinging insect, such as a bee. Acutely allergic individuals may experience clinical death (cardiopulmonary arrest) within seconds of the bite.

## IDIOSYNCRASY

*Idiosyncrasy,* or an idiosyncratic reaction, may be defined alternatively as an individual's unique hypersensitivity to a particular drug, food, or other substance;[16] ADRs that cannot be explained by any known pharmacologic or biochemical mechanism; or any ADR that is neither an overdose nor an allergic reaction. An example of idiosyncratic reaction is CNS stimulation (for example, excitation or agitation) that occurs after the administration of a known CNS depressant, such as a barbiturate or histamine blocker.

Idiosyncratic reactions cover an extremely wide range of clinical expression. Virtually any type of reaction may be seen. Examples include depression that follows the administration of a stimulant, stimulation that follows the administration of a depressant, and hyperpyrexia (markedly elevated body temperature) that follows the administration of a muscle relaxant, such as succinylcholine. It is difficult to predict which persons may experience idiosyncratic reactions or the nature of the resulting reactions.

### Management of idiosyncratic reactions

Because of the unpredictability of the nature and occurrence of idiosyncratic reactions, their management is of necessity symptomatic. The essentials of basic life support—**P-A-B-C** (position-airway-breathing-circulation)—are vital.

If an idiosyncratic reaction manifests itself as a seizure, the treatment protocol for seizures should be followed (see Chapter 21). Prevention of injury and airway management are the primary considerations. Knowledge of the steps of basic management for the various emergency situations in this text should enable the doctor to successfully treat most idiosyncratic reactions.

Current wisdom proposes that virtually all instances of idiosyncrasy are associated with underlying genetic mechanisms. Such genetic aberrations remain undetected until the individual receives a specific drug, which then produces the bizarre (nonpharmacologic) clinical expression. For example, an idiosyncratic reaction to succinylcholine may produce malignant hyperthermia.

# Drug-Related Emergencies

Before the primary drugs used in dentistry and the major adverse reactions associated with each of them

are discussed, it is important to discuss a factor responsible for more drug-related emergencies than any other. In the preceding discussion of ADRs, all responses were related directly to the action of a drug on a biologic system. However, many "drug" reactions are associated with the administration of the drug, not produced by the actions of that drug. The major cause of drug-related emergency situations in the dental office is the *administration* of local anesthetics. Although true ADRs may occur in response to local anesthetics, most ADRs associated with local anesthetics are related to the act of administering the drug.

Psychogenic reactions, most notably vasodepressor syncope and hyperventilation, are the most common forms of drug-related emergencies that occur in dentistry. Both usually result from the extreme emotional stress occurring when a person receives a local anesthetic injection, not from the drug itself. Psychogenic reactions may also occur with the parenteral administration of any drug. The potential for a psychogenic reaction increases whenever a needle and syringe are involved. Only rarely do individuals exhibit psychogenic reactions in response to enteral drug administration.

## DRUG USE IN DENTISTRY

Dental practitioners use four major categories of drugs in patient management to the virtual exclusion of all others (see Table 22-1). The major categories include analgesics, antibiotics, and antianxiety drugs. To these categories a fourth—local anesthetics—must be added. Local anesthetics are dentistry's most commonly used drugs, administered routinely whenever a dental procedure might produce pain. This chapter discusses examples of commonly prescribed or administered drugs and their potential for ADRs. It is recommended that the reader also consult a pharmacology textbook when considering the use of any drug.

**Local anesthetics**  Local anesthetics, the most widely used drugs in dentistry (an estimated 300 million dental cartridges injected in the United States each year), are also among the safest drugs available when used properly. Table 22-2 lists the more commonly used local anesthetics in the United States, Canada, Europe, and Asia today. Lidocaine, mepivacaine, prilocaine, articaine, bupivacaine, and etidocaine are amide local anesthetics, whereas benzocaine, tetracaine, propoxycaine, and procaine are ester-type drugs.

Before lidocaine's introduction in the late-1940s, esters were used exclusively. Although they are effective local anesthetics, esters carry a significant risk for allergy.[17] This potential was one of the reasons for the development and introduction of amide local anes-

| table 22-2 | *Commonly used local anesthetics* | |

| GENERIC | PROPRIETARY | GROUP |
| --- | --- | --- |
| Articaine | Ultracaine, Astracaine, Septanest | Amide |
| Benzocaine | — | Ester |
| Bupivacaine | Marcaine | Amide |
| Etidocaine | Duranest | Amide |
| Lidocaine | Octocaine, Xylocaine | Amide |
| Mepivacaine | Carbocaine, Isocaine, Polocaine, Scandonest | Amide |
| Prilocaine | Citanest | Amide |

thetics. Allergy to amide local anesthetics, although not impossible,[18,19] is extremely rare.[20] Reports occasionally appear in the medical and dental literature of an allergic reaction to an amide local anesthetic. However, careful documentation proves that most incidents are psychogenic or idiosyncratic reactions or the result of overdose or allergy to some other component of the injected solution.[20] (Chapter 24 will discuss in detail allergy to local anesthetics.)

The most commonly observed ADRs to amide local anesthetics are associated with their administration. Psychogenic responses, such as vasodepressor syncope and hyperventilation, comprise the greatest number of local anesthetic reactions observed today. The next most common cause (a very distant second) of ADRs to local anesthetics is the overdose (toxic) reaction, which in many instances is produced by a relative overdose (secondary to inadvertent intravascular injection) of the drug rather than by absolute overdose (secondary to administration of too large a total dose).[21] Documented and reproducible allergy is an extremely rare and unlikely cause of an ADR resulting from an amide local anesthetic.

Topically applied local anesthetics may also produce ADRs. Psychogenic responses rarely occur; indeed topical anesthetics are usually used to minimize the occurrence of psychogenic responses during the injection of local anesthetics. However, topical anesthetics do produce two ADRs with disturbing frequency. The first, allergy, occurs because most topical anesthetics, in addition to being ester-type local anesthetics (for example, benzocaine), also contain many other ingredients (for example, methylparaben), which possess a relatively high degree of allergenicity. Allergic responses, such as erythema or angioedema of the mucous membranes and lips, are not uncommon after topical application of these drugs. The second, much less common, ADR associated with topically applied local anesthetics is the overdose reaction, which relates to the rapid absorption of some topical

anesthetics through mucous membranes of the oral cavity. When the drugs are absorbed rapidly, the local anesthetic blood level rises rapidly.[22]

I highly recommend the use of topical anesthetics before the injection of any local anesthetic.[23] The benefits of these drugs clearly outweigh any associated risks. Safer use of topical anesthetics may be achieved through the use of either benzocaine or the amide-type topical anesthetics combined with their judicious administration to mucous membranes.

**Antibiotics**    Dental practitioners also prescribe antibiotics frequently to treat established active infections. Antibiotics should not be prescribed prophylactically to prevent the development of infections except in special circumstances, such as the prevention of bacterial endocarditis. Because of the potential for development of resistant bacterial strains and allergy, antibiotics should be used only when therapeutic indications exist. As a group, antibiotics possess a low incidence of adverse effects, a fact that most likely is responsible for their current overadministration and the subsequent development of antibiotic-resistant bacterial strains (for example, tubercular bacilli and penicillin-resistant gonococcus). In addition, medical and dental practitioners are also developing an increasing unease when administering parenteral antibiotics because of their high allergic potential.

Within the practice of dentistry, there is little need for the parenteral administration of antibiotics (Table 22-3). Most protocols for the prophylactic administration of antibiotics recommend enteral administration.[24] If the dose and sequence of administration are monitored closely, the blood levels and therapeutic efficacy of these drugs should appear similar following either parenteral or oral administration. One major advantage of oral administration is the decreased likelihood of ADRs. If ADRs do occur after oral administration, they are more likely to be less acute than those that follow parenteral administration; however, serious reactions can develop in either case.[25] If parenteral administration of antibiotics, particularly penicillin, is required, the drug should not be administered in the dental office but rather in the emergency department of a nearby hospital, where the patient can be observed for about 1 hour. The major ADR for which the doctor must be prepared when antibiotics are administered is allergy.

**Analgesics**    Pain-relieving drugs comprise a significant portion of prescriptions written by dentists. Two major categories of analgesics are considered: mild (nonopioid) and strong (opioids) analgesics (Table 22-4).

table **22-3** *Commonly prescribed antibiotics*

| GENERIC | PROPRIETARY |
|---------|-------------|
| Penicillin G | Pentids |
| | Pfizerpen |
| Penicillin V | Pen-vee K |
| | Deltapen-VK |
| | V-Cillin K |
| | Ledercillin-VK |
| | Uticillin-VK |
| | Betapen-VK |
| | Penapar-VK |
| | Robicillin-VK |
| Ampicillin | Amcill |
| | D-Amp |
| | Pfizerpen-A |
| | Principen |
| | Omnipen-N |
| | Polycillin-N |
| | Totacillin-N |
| Erythromycin | E-Mycin |
| | ERYC |
| | Ery-Tab |
| | Ilotycin |
| | Robimycin |
| | Ilosone |
| | Erythrocin |
| | Wyamycin |
| Clindamycin | Cleocin |
| | Dalacin C |
| Cephalosporin | Keflin |
| | Seffin |
| | Keflex |
| | Novolexin |
| Amoxicillin | Augmentin |
| | Larotid |
| | Polymox |
| | Sumox |
| | Trimox |
| | Utimax |
| | Wymox |

table **22-4** *Common analgesic drugs used in dentistry*

| GENERIC | PROPRIETARY |
|---------|-------------|
| Acetylsalicylic acid (aspirin) | Numerous |
| Acetaminophen | Anacin-3 |
| | Datril |
| | Tempra |
| | Tylenol |
| Ibuprofen | Advil |
| | Medipren |
| | Motrin |
| | Nuprin |
| | Rufen |
| Mefenamic acid | Ponstel |
| Naproxen | Anaprox |
| | Naprosyn |
| Meclofenamate | Meclomen |

Nonsteroidal antiinflammatory drugs (NSAIDs), such as ibuprofen and naproxen, have become extremely popular and are relatively safe. Most ADRs to NSAIDs are related to the GI tract; examples include GI upset, nausea, and constipation. Other ADRs include headache, dizziness, and pruritus.[26]

Aspirin, acetaminophen, and codeine remain the most commonly prescribed analgesics in dentistry. The major ADRs associated with aspirin include a significant potential for allergy, with symptoms ranging from mild urticaria to bronchospasm to fatal anaphylaxis (see Chapter 24), and overdose (salicylism). Acetaminophen is most often associated with CNS depression or excitation, allergy, and overdose.[27]

Codeine is an opioid agonist analgesic; however, it is a mild analgesic compared with other opioids, such as morphine and meperidine. Although allergy to codeine is possible, its actual incidence is quite low. Primary ADRs to codeine include nausea, vomiting, drowsiness, and constipation, all of which occur more often in ambulatory than in nonambulatory patients.[27] After a 60-mg oral dose, approximately 22% of patients become nauseated. A significantly lower incidence of nausea accompanies smaller doses, such as 30 mg. If codeine is administered in large amounts or to sensitive (hyperresponsive) patients, it may produce the same clinical signs and symptoms of severe overdose—respiratory and cardiovascular depression—as other, more potent opioids. Generally, 30 mg administered orally is a highly effective analgesic dose of codeine associated with a minimal incidence of ADRs. The most likely ADR noted with codeine is GI upset, almost always a dose-related response.

Meperidine (Demerol), hydromorphone (Dilaudid), hydrocodone (Vicodin) and other opioid agonists occasionally are used to manage more severe dental pain. As with codeine, the major ADRs to these drugs are more often annoying than life threatening; most frequently, they include nausea and vomiting, dizziness, ataxia, sweating, and orthostatic hypotension.[27] Again, these ADRs are more likely to occur in ambulatory patients than in nonambulatory patients (most dental patients being ambulatory). Overdose may occur and, as with all opioids, results in respiratory and cardiovascular depression. Allergy, although possible, is rare.

**Antianxiety drugs** The use of drugs for the relief of anxiety during all phases of dental treatment has increased significantly in recent years. Although the enteral routes were almost the exclusive modes of administration in the past and still are used frequently today, parenteral routes of drug administration (inhalation, IM, and IV) have gained popularity. With this trend has come an increased potential for ADRs because of the increased effectiveness of parenterally administered drugs. Although a wide variety of drugs are available for use in the management of dental anxiety, those most frequently used are barbiturates (administered orally and parenterally), nonbarbiturate antianxiety agents (administered orally and parenterally), and inhalation agents (primarily nitrous oxide and oxygen).

*Barbiturates.* Excluding alcohol, barbiturates are the oldest group of antianxiety drugs available (Table 22-5). Effective via oral and parenteral administration, barbiturate sedative-hypnotics were the most frequently prescribed drugs in dentistry for the management of fear and anxiety until the introduction of benzodiazepines in the 1960s. Barbiturates commonly produce undesirable side effects. One of the most annoying side effects of barbiturate administration is the "hangover" effect, which consists of lassitude, inebriation, and vertigo.[28] Allergy associated with barbiturate use may also occur and represents an absolute contraindication to the use of such drugs.

Probably the major factor behind the growing disenchantment with barbiturates, however, is the potential for overdose reactions, both accidental and intentional.[29] Before the 1980s, barbiturates represented the leading cause of drug-induced suicide. This trend decreased after barbiturates were reclassified as schedule II, III, and IV drugs and as benzodiazepines gained popularity.[30] Barbiturate overdose causes CNS depression to the degree that respiratory function is depressed and eventually ceases.[31] Cardiovascular and CNS collapse follow, leading to death unless basic life support and more definitive measures are initiated immediately.

*Nonbarbiturate antianxiety agents.* Nonbarbiturate antianxiety agents were developed to manage anxiety effectively without the unpleasant and dangerous ADRs associated with barbiturates. Table 22-5 lists the major nonbarbiturate antianxiety and sedative-hypnotic agents. The benzodiazepines represented a major advance in the management of anxiety. The first—chlordiazepoxide (Librium)—was introduced in 1960. Others—diazepam (Valium), oxazepam (Serax), and clorazepate (Tranxene)—are among the most prescribed drugs in the western

| table 22-5 | Common antianxiety agents and sedative-hypnotics |

| GENERIC | PROPRIETARY |
|---|---|
| **Barbiturates** | |
| Hexobarbital | Presed |
| Pentobarbital | Nembutal |
| Secobarbital | Seconal |
| **Benzodiazepines** | |
| Midazolam | Versed |
| Diazepam | Valium |
| Oxazepam | Serax |
| Lorazepam | Ativan |
| Triazolam | Halcion |
| Flurazepam | Dalmane |
| **Others** | |
| Chloral hydrate | Cohidrate |
| | Noctec |
| Hydroxyzine | Atarax |
| | Durrex |
| | Orgatrax |
| | Vistaril |
| Promethazine | Pentazine |
| | Phenergan |
| | Provigan |

world and the most effective and most widely used antianxiety drugs in dentistry.

Benzodiazepines, which may be administered orally or parenterally, are a decided improvement over barbiturates because of their remarkably lower incidence of side effects and overdose. Most likely because of the ease of their availability, benzodiazepines are associated with more overdoses than any other class of drugs. However, there are extremely few well-documented reports of death associated solely with the ingestion of benzodiazepines.[32]

An overdose reaction to benzodiazepines (even when administered IV) usually consists of oversedation, drowsiness, and ataxia. Respiratory depression, although possible, is infrequent. Flurazepam (Dalmane) and triazolam (Halcion) are benzodiazepines marketed as nonbarbiturate sedative-hypnotics. They are highly effective substitutes for barbiturates when used as "sleeping pills." Although the long-term administration of triazolam has been criticized, the use of either drug for specific indications in dentistry (for example, pretreatment sedation both the evening before and the morning of treatment) is recommended.[33]

*Inhalation sedation.* Nitrous oxide and oxygen inhalation sedation is another method of anxiety control that has garnered increasing interest among dental practitioners. An estimated 35% of dentists in the United States use this method.[34] Discovered in 1776 and first used clinically in 1844, nitrous oxide is a highly effective antianxiety drug that, when properly administered, is remarkably free of unpleasant and potentially dangerous ADRs. Unwanted side effects associated with inhalation sedation include nausea, vomiting, and oversedation. If inhalation sedation is administered with less than 20% oxygen, unconsciousness may ensue, with cellular damage resulting from hypoxia (but not from nitrous oxide).

With the development of a new generation of inhalation-sedation machines and the increased awareness of dental educators and manufacturers, safety features have been incorporated into current sedation units that make administration with less than 20% oxygen difficult.[35] In addition, no reports exist of allergy to nitrous oxide. Overdose consists of oversedation, which may manifest as rousable sleep or the loss of consciousness; however, the latter is extremely unlikely. Management of oversedation focuses on a decrease in the percentage of nitrous oxide through an increase in the volume flow of oxygen, coupled with the steps of basic life support—P-A-B-C (position-airway-breathing-circulation)—until the patient regains consciousness.

Table 22-6 lists the drug categories most frequently used in dentistry and the most common ADRs associated with them. Most important in drug use is the realization that all drugs can produce virtually any of the three serious ADRs—allergy, overdose, and idiosyncrasy.

---

**table 22-6**  *Drugs commonly used in dentistry and their most common ADRs*

| DRUG | ALLERGY | OVERDOSE | SIDE EFFECTS |
|---|---|---|---|
| **Local anesthetics** | | | |
| Esters | Common, especially with topical anesthetics; manifested as localized erythema and edema | Unlikely with esters unless genetic deficiency present (for example, atypical pseudocholinesterase) | Rare; sedation (drowsiness) most common |
| Amides | Rare, virtually nonexistent; most clinical reports prove alleged allergy to be overdose or allergy to other component of solution | Most common ADR; CNS depression; manifested as drowsiness, tremor, tonic-clonic seizures | Rare; sedation most common |
| **Antibiotics** | | | |
| | Common; high allergic potential to many antibiotics; manifested clinically over entire range of allergic phenomena | Rare; virtually nonexistent with penicillin | Rare; GI upset most common |
| **Analgesics** | | | |
| Nonopioid | Common; high allergic potential (aspirin) | Common; salicylism | Common |
| Opioid | Uncommon | Common; manifested as CNS depression (drowsiness) or respiratory depression | Most common ADR; manifested clinically as nausea or vomiting, orthostatic hypotension |
| **Antianxiety agents** | | | |
| Barbiturates | Uncommon | Most common ADR; CNS depression; manifested as oversedation, loss of consciousness, respiratory and cardiovascular depression | Common; "barbiturate hangover" |
| Benzodiazepines | Uncommon | Uncommon; CNS depression; manifested as oversedation | Drowsiness most common |
| Nitrous oxide | Rare; never reported to date | Common; manifested as oversedation | Most common ADR; manifested as nausea or vomiting |

*ADR*, Adverse drug reaction; *CNS*, central nervous system; *GI*, gastrointestinal.

# REFERENCES

1. Department of Pharmacology, University of Southern California School of Dentistry: name of source material, Los Angeles, 1986, The University.

2. Caranasos GJ, Stewart RB, Cluff LE: Drug-induced illness leading to hospitalization, *JAMA* 228:713, 1974.

3. Caranasos GJ and others: Drug-associated deaths in hospital inpatients, *Arch Intern Med* 136:872, 1976.

4. Koch-Weser J: Fatal reactions to drug therapy, *N Engl J Med* 291:302, 1974.

5. McKeney JM, Harrison WL: Drug-related hospital admissions, *Am J Hosp Pharm* 33:792, 1976.

6. Caranasos GJ: Drug reactions. In Schwartz GR and others, editors: *Principles and practice of emergency medicine*, Philadelphia, 1978, WB Saunders.

7. Hallas J and others: Drug-related admissions to a department of medical gastroenterology: the role of self-medicated and prescribed drugs, *Scand J Gastroenterol* 26(2):174, 1991.

8. Lazarou L, Pomeranz BH, Corey PN: Incidence of adverse drug reactions in hospitalized patients: meta-analysis of prospective studies, *JAMA* 279:1200-1205, 1998.

9. Pallasch TJ: *Pharmacology for dental students and practitioners*, Philadelphia, 1980, Lea & Febiger.

10. Forster A and others: Respiratory depression by midazolam and diazepam, *Anesthesiology* 53:494, 1980.

11. Olin BR, editor: *Facts and Comparisons*, St Louis, 1992, Facts and Comparisons.

12. *Physician's Desk Reference*, Oradell, NJ, 1999, Medical Economics Data.

13. American Medical Association: *Drug evaluations annual*, Chicago, 1992, The Association.

14. American Dental Association: *ADA Guide to Dental Therapeutics*, Chicago, 1998, The Association.

15. Reidenberg MM, Lowenthal DT: Adverse nondrug reactions, *N Engl J Med* 279:678, 1968.

16. *Mosby's Medical, Nursing, and Allied Health Dictionary*, St Louis, 1998, Mosby.

17. Criep LH, Castilho-Ribeiro C: Allergy to procaine hydrochloride with three fatalities, *JAMA* 151:1185, 1955.

18. Brown DT, Beamish D, Wildsmith JA: Allergic reaction to an amide local anesthetic, *Br J Anaesth* 53:435, 1981.

19. Bateman PP: Multiple allergies to local anesthetics including prilocaine, *Med J Aust* 2:449, 1974.

20. Aldrete JA, Johnson DA: Allergy to local anesthetics, *JAMA* 207:356, 1969.

21. Adatia AK: Intravascular injection of local anesthetics, *Br Dent J* 138:328, 1975.

22. Adriani J: Reactions to local anesthetics, *JAMA* 196:405, 1955.

23. Malamed SF: *Handbook of local anesthesia*, ed 4, St Louis, 1997, Mosby.

24. Dajani AS and others: Prevention of bacterial endocarditis: recommendations by the American Heart Association, *JAMA* 277(22):1794-1801, 1997.

25. Gill CJ, Michaelides PL: Dental drugs and anaphylactic reactions: report of a case, *Oral Surg* 50:30, 1980.

26. Anaprox drug package insert, 1990, Syntex Puerto Rico, Inc.

27. Tylenol with codeine drug package insert, 1990, McNeil Pharmaceutical Products.

28. Harvey SC: Hypnotics and sedatives: the barbiturates. In Goodman IS and Gilman A, editors: *Pharmacological basis of therapeutics*, ed 6, New York, 1980, Macmillan.

29. Baltarowich LL: Sedative-hypnotics. In Rosen P and others, editors: *Emergency medicine*, ed 2, St Louis, 1988, Mosby.

30. National Institute on Drug Abuse: *Data from the Drug Abuse Warning Network—1980 and 1984*, Rockville, Md, 1986, U.S. Department of Health and Human Resources.

31. McCarron NM and others: Short-acting barbiturate overdosage, *JAMA* 248:55, 1982.

32. Iserson KV: Tranquilizer overdose. In Rosen P and others, editors: *Emergency medicine*, ed 2, St Louis, 1988, Mosby.

33. Gorman C: The dark side of Halcion (banned in Britain), *Time* 138:65, Oct 4, 1991.

34. ADA Survey Center: Nitrous oxide use, *ADA News* 28(17): 6, Sept 15, 1997.

35. American Dental Association Council on Dental Materials, Instruments, and Equipment: *Dentists' desk reference materials, instruments, and equipment*, Chicago, 1981, The Association.

# 23

# Drug Overdose Reactions

**D**RUG overdose reactions have been defined previously as those clinical signs and symptoms that result from overly high blood levels of a drug in various target organs and tissues. Overdose reactions, also called *toxic reactions,* are the most common of all adverse drug reactions (ADRs), accounting for up to 85% by some estimates.[1] Overdose reactions are direct extensions of the normal pharmacologic properties of the involved drug. For an overdose to occur, the drug must gain access to the body's circulation in quantities sufficient to produce adverse effects on various tissues.

Under normal circumstances there is a constant absorption of the drug from its site of administration (for example, gastrointestinal tract [oral], muscles [intramuscular (IM)]) into the body's circulation, and steady removal of the same drug from the blood as it undergoes redistribution (for example, to skeletal muscle) and biotransformation (also known as *metabolism* and *detoxification*) in other parts of the body, primarily the liver. In this situation overly high blood levels of drugs seldom develop (Figure 23-1). However, a number of ways exist in which this steady state may be altered, leading to either a rapid elevation in blood level of the drug, which produces a sudden onset of the signs and symptoms of an overdose reaction, or a more gradual elevation of a drug's blood level, producing a slower onset of signs and symptoms. In either case an overdose reaction is caused by a blood (plasma) level of a drug sufficiently high to produce adverse

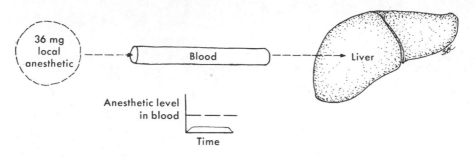

**Figure 23-1**  Under normal circumstances the body constantly absorbs the local anesthetic from the site of deposition while the liver removes the agent from the blood. Thus local anesthetic levels in the blood remain low. (From Malamed SF: *Handbook of local anesthesia,* ed 4, St Louis, 1997, Mosby.)

effects in the various organs and tissues of the body, which are influenced by the administered drug. The clinical reaction continues only as long as the blood level remains above the threshold for overdose in that target organ or tissue.

In dentistry, four commonly used drug categories possess significant potentials for overdose—local anesthetics; vasoconstrictors, such as epinephrine; sedative-hypnotics; and opioid analgesics. Of these, local anesthetics are by far the most frequently used drugs. A severe overdose reaction to a local anesthetic manifests as either a generalized tonicoclonic seizure or unconsciousness. The most commonly observed overdose reaction to sedative-hypnotics and opioid analgesics is varying degrees of central nervous system (CNS) and respiratory depression, whereas vasoconstrictor overdose produces an anxiety reaction accompanied by significant increases in cardiovascular function (blood pressure and heart rate).

Because the usual route of administration of these drugs and the clinical nature and management of the overdose reaction differ so markedly between these groups, this chapter divides overdose reactions into the following three sections:

1. Overdose reaction from local anesthetics
2. Overdose reaction from vasodepressor drugs
3. Overdose reaction from sedative-hypnotic and opioid analgesic drugs

## Local Anesthetic Overdose Reaction

Local anesthetics are the most commonly used drugs in dentistry. The number of local anesthetic cartridges injected by dentists in the United States is conservatively estimated at 6 million per week, or more than 300 million per year. Actual numbers probably greatly exceed this figure. In addition, many physicians and podiatrists also administer local anesthetics. Considering the frequency of administration, the fact that more ADRs are not reported is remarkable.

In all probability, however, a great many ADRs go unreported because they were transitory and innocuous enough that the doctor either did not recognize the reaction or deem it serious enough to report. Patients and all too frequently doctors most commonly label any ADR to a local anesthetic an *allergic reaction;* however, on careful scrutiny most reactions to local anesthetics are revealed to be either overdose reactions or, more likely, psychogenic responses.[2]

## Predisposing Factors

An overdose reaction to a local anesthetic is related to the blood level of the local anesthetic in certain tissues and organs (the myocardium and CNS). Several factors may profoundly influence the rate at which this blood level increases and the length of time for which it remains elevated. The presence of one or more of these factors predisposes the patient to the development of an overdose reaction. The first group of factors is related to the patient receiving the drug, whereas the second group relates to the drug itself and the area into which it is administered.

### PATIENT FACTORS

#### Normal distribution curve
Predisposing patient factors are those that modify the patient's response to the usual dose of a drug. This occurrence is referred to commonly as *biologic,* or *individual variation.* The normal distribution curve illustrates this variable response to drugs (Figure 23-2). For a given "normal" or "usual" dose of a drug, approximately 68%

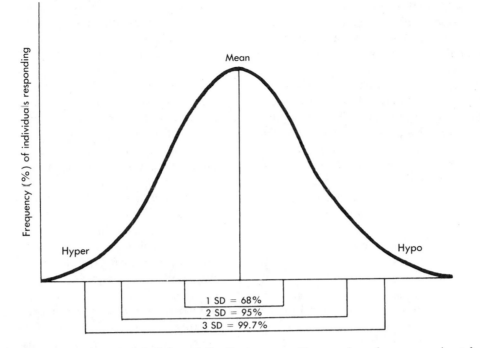

**Figure 23-2** A normal, bell-shaped distribution curve. For any given drug, approximately 68% of patients experience desirable clinical effects with the usual adult dose, and 95% exhibit desirable effects with a slightly lower or higher dose. A small percentage of patients are hyporesponsive (right side of curve), requiring doses that exceed the "normal" before clinically desirable results occur. More important, however, are those hyperresponsive individuals (left side of curve) who exhibit clinically desirable results at lower-than-normal doses. Such patients are more likely to experience drug overdoses. (From Pallasch TJ: *Pharmacology for dental students and practitioners*, Philadelphia, 1980, Lea & Febiger.)

of patients respond appropriately; 16% are less responsive (hyporesponsive), and 16% are overly responsive (hyperresponsive). Additional predisposing patient factors that influence drug responsiveness include age, body weight, pathologic processes, genetics, attitude and environment, and sex.

**Age**   At either end of the age spectrum, individuals experience a higher incidence of ADRs. Many reasons exist for this finding, several of which are relevant to this discussion. Drug absorption, metabolism, and excretion may be imperfectly developed in younger age-groups or be diminished in older age-groups. Under-developed or decreased liver functioning may result in higher blood levels of drugs because the individual cannot biotransform the local anesthetic into an inactive substance. In addition, renal dysfunction may prohibit the patient from excreting the local anesthetic. In patients 61 to 71 years, the half-life of lidocaine increased by approximately 70% over a control group composed of patients 22 to 26 years.[3] As a general rule of thumb, drug doses should be decreased for patients under 6 years and over 65 years.

**Body weight**   In general, the greater the lean body weight (within limits), the greater is the dose of a drug the individual can tolerate before an overdose develops. This relates primarily to the greater blood volume in larger, heavy, nonobese individuals. This relationship does not apply to obese individuals because the blood supply to adipose tissues is sparse compared with that supplying muscle. Therefore a 200-pound obese patient usually cannot tolerate the same dose of local anesthetic as safely as a 200-pound muscular individual. Because most drugs are distributed evenly throughout the body, the larger the individual, the greater is the blood volume and the lower the blood level of the drug per milliliter of blood. For example, a dose of a local anesthetic administered to a 67.5-kg (150-pound) adult produces a lower blood level than the same dose administered to a 22.5-kg (50-pound) child. Drug doses are normally calculated on the basis of milligrams of drug per kilogram or pound of body weight. Such considerations are especially important in pediatric and frail older patients; a lack of consideration of body weight is one of the major causes of overdose reactions.

Drug doses calculated in terms of milligrams per pound or per kilogram of body weight are based on the response of the normal responding patient, which is calculated from the responses of large numbers of patients. Thus individual patient responses to drug administration may demonstrate significant variations, a fact that the normal distribution curve plainly illustrates (see Figure 23-2). The usual blood level of lidocaine in the brain required to induce seizure activity is 7.5 μg lidocaine per milliliter of blood (μg/ml). Hyporesponsive patients may not exhibit seizures until the brain's blood level attains a significantly higher level of lidocaine, whereas hyperresponsive patients may exhibit seizures at a brain blood level of lidocaine considerably below 7.5 μg/ml.[4] Therefore a drug overdose reaction may occur even when the dose is within the normal range for that patient.

**Pathologic process**   The presence of preexisting disease may alter the body's ability to biotransform a drug into a biologically inactive substance. Most amide local anesthetics undergo biotransformation in the liver, with a small percentage of the drug excreted unchanged through the kidneys. Any disease state that reduces or increases hepatic blood flow is likely to alter various pharmacokinetic parameters of the amide local anesthetics.[5] However, renal dysfunction appears to have little effect on local anesthetic toxicity.

Patients with cardiovascular disease, especially congestive heart failure, demonstrate blood levels of local anesthetics almost twice those found in healthy patients receiving the same doses.[6,7] This difference is a result of several factors, including a reduced blood volume for drug distribution and a diminished hepatic blood flow secondary to low cardiac output. Pulmonary disease states, especially those associated with carbon dioxide retention, lead to an increased risk of local anesthetic overdose. Carbon dioxide retention (>$PaCO_2$) leads to respiratory acidosis, which results in a decrease in the seizure threshold for a local anesthetic.[8,9] An increase in $PaCO_2$ from 25-40 torr to 65-81 torr lowers the convulsive threshold for lidocaine by 53%.[8]

**Genetics**   It has been reported with increasing frequency that certain individuals possess genetic deficiencies that alter their responses to certain drugs. A genetic deficiency in the enzyme serum cholinesterase is an important example. Produced in the liver, this enzyme circulates in the blood and is responsible for the biotransformation of two important drugs—succinylcholine[10] and the ester-type local anesthetics.[11,12] Succinylcholine is a short-acting, neuromuscular-blocking agent frequently administered during the induction of general anesthesia to produce skeletal muscle relaxation (as well as respiratory arrest) during tracheal intubation. In normal individuals the action of succinylcholine is approximately 3 minutes, the drug being metabolized by serum cholinesterase. In contrast, individuals with deficient or atypical serum cholinesterase biotransform succinylcholine at an extremely slow rate, and the ensuing period of apnea may persist up to several hours.[10] This same enzyme is responsible for the biotransformation of the ester local anesthetics. If an individual possesses atypical or deficient serum cholinesterase, the blood level of the ester local anesthetic increases and remains elevated longer than normal, increasing the likelihood of an overdose reaction.[12]

**Attitude and environment**   The psychologic attitude of a patient greatly influences the ultimate effect of a drug. This factor is considerably important with sedative-hypnotic and opioid analgesics; what an individual expects a drug to do greatly influences the clinical efficacy of that agent. This expectation is called the *placebo response* and may be of benefit to the doctor. With regard to local anesthetics, it has been shown that the local anesthetic convulsive threshold is lowered in patients who are overly stressed (frightened). In addition, a patient's psychologic attitude affects the response to stimulation. All dental practitioners have encountered apprehensive patients who overreact to stimuli, noting pain when only gentle pressure is applied to tissues. Additional local anesthetic is then administered, increasing the total dose received.

**Sex**   Differences between men and women regarding drug distribution, response, and metabolism have been described in animals that are not of major importance to humans. The only instance of sexual difference in the human species occurs in the pregnant female. During pregnancy, renal function may be altered, leading to the impaired excretion of certain drugs and their accumulation in the blood, leading to an increased risk of overdose. Although this is normally not clinically significant, this disturbance of renal function is a potential cause of local anesthetic overdose.

## DRUG FACTORS

The second group of factors that may predispose an individual to overdose relates to the drugs themselves and to the site of administration. The drug's vasoactivity, dose and route of administration, speed of administration, vascularity of the injection site, and the presence of vasoconstrictors influence the risk of overdose.

**Vasoactivity**  Several factors relating to the physicochemical properties of local anesthetics may help determine whether the drug's blood level after injection is low or high. These include lipid solubility, protein binding, and vascular activity.

Local anesthetics that are more lipid soluble and more highly protein bound, such as etidocaine and bupivacaine, are retained in the fat and tissues at the site of injection and therefore exhibit a slower net systemic absorption rate compared to lidocaine and mepivacaine. This slower systemic absorption rate is associated with increased margins of safety. The rate of absorption of local anesthetics also depends on their direct actions on blood vessels at the injection site. All local anesthetics, with the notable exception of cocaine, have vasodilating properties.[13] Bupivacaine and etidocaine produce more vasodilation than do prilocaine, lidocaine, or mepivacaine. Vascular regulation of absorption appears to be a more important factor for the shorter-acting agents, such as lidocaine, mepivacaine, and prilocaine, whereas tissue binding is of greater significance for the longer-acting drugs, bupivacaine and etidocaine. Table 23-1 compares the lipid solubility, protein binding, and vasodilating properties of commonly used local anesthetics. The greater the degree of vasodilation that a local anesthetic produces, the more rapid its absorption into the circulation.

**Dose**  For many years it was thought that the concentration of an injected solution was of major importance in determining overdose potential, even though the total milligram dose remained the same.

This thinking is incorrect. Braid and Scott[14] demonstrated that 2% and 3% solutions of prilocaine yield the same blood level as an equivalent dose of a 1% solution if the same number of milligrams is administered. Jebson[15] proved the same theory, using 10% and 2% lidocaine.

Dosage, on the other hand, is a highly significant factor. Within the clinical dose range for most local anesthetics, a linear relationship exists between dose and peak blood concentration. The larger the dose of local anesthetic injected, the higher the peak blood level of the drug (Table 23-2).

**Route of administration**  Local anesthetics used to control pain produce their clinical actions at the site of administration. Unlike most other drugs, local anesthetics (when used for pain prevention or control) need not enter the circulation and reach a certain minimal therapeutic blood level. The greater the length of time a local anesthetic remains in the area where pain control is desired and the greater its concentration at that site, the longer is its duration of action. As the drug is absorbed into the circulatory system it becomes less effective for pain control. When sufficient volume has been removed from the area, the individual may again experience painful stimuli. At the same time, the more rapidly the local anesthetic is removed from the site of injection, the more rapidly the blood level of the drug increases (toward overdose levels).

One factor frequently noted in overdose reactions to local anesthetics is inadvertent intravascular injection. In this instance extremely high blood levels may be achieved in a brief period, producing acute overdose reactions; the peak anesthetic blood level is dependent on the rate of intravascular administration. Absorption of (some) topical anesthetics through the oral mucous membrane and absorption of solutions

| table 23-1 | *Comparison of phsyicochemical properties of local anesthetics* |

| DRUG | LIPID OR BUFFER PARTITION COEFFICIENT* | PROTEIN BINDING (%)* | RELATIVE VASODILATING VALUES† |
|---|---|---|---|
| Articaine | 0.0 | 95 | 1.0 |
| Procaine | 0.6 | 5.8 | >2.5 |
| Prilocaine | 0.8 | 55 | 0.5 |
| Mepivacaine | 1.0 | 77 | 0.8 |
| Lidocaine | 2.9 | 64 | 1.0 |
| Bupivacaine | 28 | 95 | 2.5 |
| Etidocaine | 141 | 94 | 2.5 |

*The body absorbs more lipid-soluble drugs slower; slower action is associated with an increased margin of safety.
†The greater the degree of vasodilation a drug produces, the more rapidly the drug is absorbed into the circulatory system.

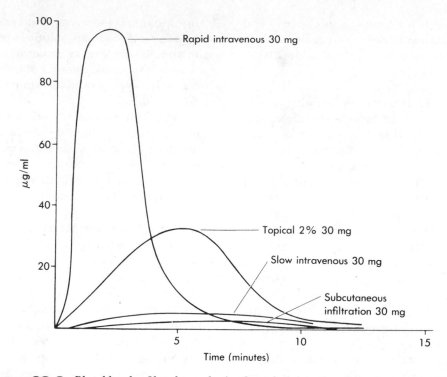

**Figure 23-3**　Blood levels of local anesthetic after administration via various routes. Note particularly the blood levels after the rapid and slow IV administrations. *IV,* Intravenous. (From Adriani J, Campbell B: *JAMA* 162:1527, 1956.)

table **23-2**　*Concentrations of commonly used local anesthetics*

| DRUG | GROUP | AVAILABLE CONCENTRATIONS (%) |
|------|-------|------------------------------|
| Lidocaine | Amide | 2 |
| Mepivacaine | Amide | 2 (with vasoconstrictor) |
|  |  | 3 (without vasoconstrictor) |
| Prilocaine | Amide | 4 |
| Bupivacaine | Amide | 0.5 |
| Etidocaine | Amide | 1.5 |
| Articaine | Amide | 4 |

from multiple intraoral injection sites may also produce overdose reactions (some topical anesthetics are absorbed rapidly through the oral mucous membrane).

**Rate of injection**　The rate of injection is vital in the cause or prevention of overdose reactions to all drugs. Intravenous (IV) injection of a local anesthetic drug may or may not produce signs and symptoms of overdose. Indeed lidocaine is frequently administered via the IV route in doses of 1.0 to 1.5 mg per kg (70 mg to 105 mg in the typical 70-kg male) to manage several ventricular dysrhythmias. A major

deciding factor in whether intravascular administration is clinically safe or hazardous is the rate at which the drug is injected. A 36-mg dose of lidocaine (one dental cartridge in the United States) administered via an IV route in less than 15 seconds produces markedly elevated blood levels and a virtual guarantee of a serious overdose reaction. On the other hand, 100 mg of lidocaine administered IV over several minutes (as recommended in the management of cardiac dysrhythmias*), produces a significantly lower lidocaine blood level (because greater distribution and biotransformation have occurred) and a subsequent decreased risk of overdose.

Figure 23-3 illustrates representative blood levels following administration of 30 mg of tetracaine via various routes. The blood levels for the slow and rapid IV administration of tetracaine are especially significant.[17] Many local anesthetic overdose reactions result from the combination of inadvertent intravascular injection, combined with too rapid a rate of injection. Both causes are virtually 100% preventable.

**Vascularity of injection site**　The greater the vascularity at the site of injection, the more rapidly the

---

*The drug-package insert for intravenous cardiac lidocaine administration recommends 0.5 to 1.0 mL every minute.[16]

box **23-1**   *Predisposing factors for drug overdose*

**Patient factors**

Age (under 6 years; over 65 years)
Body weight (lower body weight increasing risk)
Pathologic processes (for example, liver disease, congestive heart failure, pulmonary disease)
Genetics (for example, atypical plasma cholinesterase)
Mental attitude (anxiety decreasing seizure threshold)
Sex (slight increase in risk during pregnancy)

**Drug factors**

Vasoactivity (vasodilation increasing risk)
Dose (higher dose increasing risk)
Route of administration (intravascular route increasing risk)
Rate of injection (rapid injection increasing risk)
Vascularity of injection site (increased vascularity increasing risk)
Presence of vasoconstrictor (decreasing risk)

drug is absorbed into circulation. Although rapid absorption is desirable with most parenterally administered drugs when therapeutic blood levels are required, it is a decided disadvantage in the use of local anesthetics administered for pain control. Local anesthetics must remain in the area of injection in order to block nerve conduction. Unfortunately for dentistry (at least as far as local anesthetic administration is concerned), the oral cavity is one of the more highly vascular areas of the body. A drug injected into the oral cavity is usually absorbed into the blood more rapidly than the same drug injected elsewhere in the body. This factor, plus the inherent vasodilating properties of most local anesthetics, are the major reasons for the addition of vasoconstrictors to most local anesthetics.

**Presence of vasoconstrictors**   The addition of a vasoconstrictor to a local anesthetic results in a decrease in the rate of systemic absorption of the drug. The use of vasoconstrictors, along with proper injection technique, has greatly reduced the clinical toxicity of local anesthetics. Box 23-1 summarizes risk factors for local anesthetic overdose.

# Prevention

Almost all overdose reactions to local anesthetics are preventable. Careful evaluation of the patient before the start of treatment along with careful drug administration can minimize the risk of overdose in all but a few situations. Two sets of predisposing factors were presented in the previous section. The first set, patient factors, are those that cannot be eliminated but which,

when present, may require specific modifications in dental care to prevent drug-related problems from developing. The second set of factors are related to the drugs themselves or to their administration. These factors are usually avoidable through proper drug selection and local anesthetic injection technique.

## MEDICAL HISTORY QUESTIONNAIRE AND DIALOGUE HISTORY

The only questions directly related to the use of local anesthetics are included in the questionnaire's general drug use discussion (see Figure 2-2). The doctor should carefully examine any ADRs to a local anesthetic to determine their precise nature. (Chapter 24 will present a detailed dialogue history for this type of questioning.)

In the absence of a history of ADRs to local anesthetics, a series of questions about past experiences with dental injections should be posed to that patient. Questions 2 and 3, which focus on prior dental experiences in general, may provide relevant information about drug use and be useful in an evaluation of the patient's psychologic status. A thorough medical history evaluation enables the doctor to eliminate two potential causes of local anesthetic overdose—unusually slow biotransformation of the local anesthetic and unusually slow elimination of the drug from the body.

## CAUSES OF OVERDOSE REACTIONS

Consideration of the various mechanisms by which blood levels of local anesthetics may become increased is necessary before a discussion about prevention can commence. Moore[18] stated that high blood levels of local anesthetics may occur in one or more of the ways listed in Box 23-2. These factors form the basis for a discussion of the methods through which overdose reactions to local anesthetics may be prevented. As in any discussion of prevention, the patient-completed medical history questionnaire is a vital element.

**Biotransformation and elimination**   Ester local anesthetics undergo rapid biotransformation in the blood and liver. The major portion of this biotransformation process occurs within the blood through hydrolysis to paraaminobenzoic acid by the enzyme pseudocholinesterase.[19] A patient with a familiar history of atypical pseudocholinesterase cannot biotransform ester-type local anesthetics at a normal rate, thereby increasing the likelihood of elevated local anesthetic blood levels.[12] Atypical pseudocholinesterase is believed to occur in 1 of 2820 individuals.[20] Any patient with a questionable history should be referred to a physician for diagnostic tests, which may confirm or deny its existence. Atypical pseudocholinesterase, if

box **23-2** *Causes of high blood levels of local anesthetics*

Biotransformation of the drug is unusually slow.
Drug is slowly eliminated from the body through the kidneys.
Total dose of local anesthetic administered is too large.
Absorption of the local anesthetic from the site of injection is unusually rapid.
Local anesthetic is inadvertently administered intravascularly.

Modified from Moore DC: *Complications of regional anesthesia,* Springfield, Ill, 1955, Charles C Thomas.

present, is a relative contraindication to administration of an ester local anesthetic.

Amide local anesthetics may be administered to patients with atypical plasma cholinesterase without increased risk of overdose. Microsomal enzymes in the liver biotransform these anesthetics.[5] A history of liver disease (for example, previous or present hepatitis or cirrhosis) does not absolutely contraindicate the use of amides but it may indicate that a degree of residual hepatic dysfunction exists, which may alter the ability of the liver to biotransform amide local anesthetics.

An ambulatory patient with a history of liver disease may receive amide local anesthetics; however, these drugs should be used judiciously (hepatic dysfunction is a relative contraindication to their administration). Minimal volumes should be employed for local anesthesia, bearing in mind that one cartridge may be able to produce an overdose in this patient if liver function is compromised significantly. In my experience, however, such degrees of compromised liver function are more commonly present in hospitalized than in ambulatory patients. Whenever doubt exists, medical consultation should be sought before any drugs are injected. When a greater degree of liver function is present (ASA IV or V), the use of an ester local anesthetic is also relatively contraindicated because the liver produces the hydrolytic enzyme cholinesterase, and liver dysfunction may also disturb the biotransformation of the esters as well.

A small percentage of an administered local anesthetic dose is eliminated from the blood unchanged, in its active form, through the kidneys. Reports have cited values for urinary excretion as 3% for lidocaine,[21] less than 1% for prilocaine,[22] 1% for mepivacaine,[23] less than 1% for etidocaine,[24] and less than 1% for bupivacaine.[25] Renal dysfunction does not usually result in excessive blood levels of local anesthetics. As with liver dysfunction, however, the dose of anesthetic should be limited to the absolute minimum required for clinically effective pain control.

The patient requiring renal dialysis also represents a relative contraindication to the administration of large doses of local anesthetics. Such patients are ambulatory between dialysis appointments and can visit the dental office for treatment. Undetoxified local anesthetic may accumulate in the blood of the patient, producing clinical signs and symptoms (usually mild) of local anesthetic overdose.

**Too large a total dose**    Administered to excess, any drug can produce signs and symptoms of overdose. The precise milligram dose at which the individual experiences toxic effects is impossible to predict consistently. The principle of biologic variability greatly influences the manner in which individuals respond to drugs. Most parenterally administered drugs are commonly administered in doses based on many factors, including age and physical status. A third consideration in dose determination is weight, a factor especially important in lighter-weight patients. Usually the larger the individual receiving the drug (within certain limits), the greater is the drug distribution; therefore the resulting blood level of the drug is lower, and the milligram dose for "safe" administration is larger.*

In the recent past, manufacturers of local anesthetic cartridges for dental use did not indicate maximum doses based on body weight. Instead, generations of dentists were taught, for example, that the maximum dose of lidocaine was 300 mg (without epinephrine) or 500 mg (with epinephrine) for any adult patient.[26] Unfortunately, instances arose in which these maximum doses proved too high for an individual patient's ability to tolerate, leading to morbidity or even mortality. Such arbitrary doses for adult patients are meaningless; one adult may weigh 200 pounds, whereas another may weigh 100 pounds. According to the old way of thinking, both patients could tolerate safely the same dose of local anesthetic.

It becomes obvious that such thinking is erroneous. Distribution of the local anesthetic throughout the circulatory system of a muscular 200-pound adult results in a lower blood concentration than the same drug in a 100-pound adult. When all other potential factors are equal, the smaller adult has a greater risk of overdose than the larger adult when both receive the same dose. Overdose develops when the rate of absorption of the local anesthetic into the cardiovascular system exceeds the rate at which the body removes that drug. Maximum doses of local anesthetics should be calculated on a milligram-per-weight basis (Table 23-3).[27]

---

*Although generally valid, exceptions to this rule do exist. Biologic variability and pathologic states may dramatically alter a patient's responsiveness to a drug; therefore doctors must use special care when administering any drug.

table **23-3**  *Maximum recommended doses of commonly used local anesthetics\**

| PATIENT WEIGHT (LB) | LIDOCAINE 2% WITH OR WITHOUT VASOCONSTRICTOR; 2.0 MG/LB TO 300 MG (MAXIMUM) | | MEPIVACAINE 2% OR 3%; 2.0 MG/LG TO 300 MG (MAXIMUM) | | | PRILOCAINE 4% WITH OR WITHOUT VASOCONSTRICTOR; 2.7 MG/LB TO 400 MG (MAXIMUM) | | ARTICAINE (ADULTS) 4% WITH VASOCONSTRICTOR; 3.2 MG/LB TO 500 MG (MAXIMUM) | | ARTICAINE (CHILDREN) 4% WITH VASOCONSTRICTOR; 2.3 MB/LB TO 500 MG (MAXIMUM) | |
|---|---|---|---|---|---|---|---|---|---|---|---|
| | MG | NO. OF CARTRIDGES | MG | NO. OF CARTRIDGES | | MG | NO. OF CARTRIDGES | MG | NO. OF CARTRIDGES | MG | NO. OF CARTRIDGES |
| | | | | **2%** | **3%** | | | | | | |
| 20 | 40 | 1.1 | 40 | 1.1 | 0.8 | 54 | 0.75 | 64 | 0.9 | 46 | 0.6 |
| 40 | 80 | 2.2 | 80 | 2.2 | 1.5 | 108 | 1.5 | 128 | 1.8 | 92 | 1.3 |
| 60 | 120 | 3.3 | 120 | 3.3 | 2.0 | 162 | 2.25 | 192 | 2.7 | 138 | 1.9 |
| 80 | 160 | 4.4 | 160 | 4.4 | 3.0 | 216 | 3.0 | 256 | 3.6 | 184 | 2.5 |
| 100 | 200 | 5.5† | 200 | 5.5 | 3.5 | 270 | 3.75 | 320 | 4.4 | 230 | 3.0 |
| 120 | 240 | 6.5 | 240 | 6.5 | 4.0 | 324 | 4.5 | 384 | 5.33 | | |
| 140 | 280 | 7.5 | 280 | 7.5 | 5.0 | 378 | 5.0 | 448 | 6.2 | | |
| 160 | 300 | 8.0 | 300 | 8.0 | 5.5 | 400 | 5.0 | 500 | 7.0 | | |
| 180 | 300 | 8.0 | 300 | 8.0 | 5.5 | 400 | 5.5 | 500 | 7.0 | | |
| 200 | 300 | 8.0 | 300 | 8.0 | 5.5 | 400 | 5.5 | 500 | 7.0 | | |

Modified from Malamed SF: *Handbook of local anesthesia,* ed 4, St Louis, 1997, Mosby.
*Indicated doses are recommended for normal, healthy patients and should be decreased for debilitated or older individuals.
†The 0.2-mg epinephrine dose is a limiting factor for 1:50,000 epinephrine.

It is highly unlikely that the doses indicated in Table 23-3 will be reached. Conservative dental treatment rarely calls for the administration of more than four or five cartridges. Indeed full-mouth anesthesia (palatal, maxillary, and mandibular) may be achieved in the adult with fewer than six cartridges of local anesthetics. Exceptions do exist, however, such as with surgical procedures and prolonged treatments.

It is strongly suggested that the doctor think in terms of milligrams of local anesthetic injected instead of the number of cartridges. Therefore reviewing the relationship between percent solution and number of milligrams contained in that solution becomes necessary (Table 23-4). A 1% solution contains 10 mg/ml; 2% solution, 20 mg/ml, 3% solution, 30 mg/ml, 4% solution, 40 mg/ml, and so on. If a typical dental cartridge in the United States contains 1.8 ml of solution, the number of milligrams of anesthetic is the volume of solution (1.8 ml) multiplied by the number of milligrams per milliliter of solution (for example, 20 for a 2% solution). The result (36) is the number of milligrams of anesthetic in the dental cartridge. Cartridges in some countries contain 2.2 ml of anesthetic; thus a cartridge of a 2% solution would contain 44 mg of anesthetic drug.

## Rapid absorption of drug into circulation

The addition of various vasoconstrictors to local anesthetics has proved to be of great benefit. Not only do vasoconstrictors increase the duration of action of many local anesthetics by enabling them to remain at the site of injection for a greater length of time in adequate concentration to produce conduction blockade,[28] but they also reduce the systemic toxicity of these drugs by retarding their absorption into the cardiovascular system (Table 23-5).[29] Peak local anesthetic blood levels of nonvasoconstrictor-containing solutions ("plain" drugs) occur 5 to 10 minutes after the injection. When a vasopressor, such as epinephrine, is added to the anesthetic solution, peak blood levels do not occur for approximately 30 minutes and they are lower.[30] Indeed decreasing in local anesthetic toxicity is the primary reason for the addition of vasoconstrictors to local anesthetic solutions. Vasoconstrictors are integral components of all local anesthetic solutions whenever depth and duration of anesthesia are important. There are but few indications in dentistry in which local anesthetics should be used without vasoconstrictors.

The addition of vasoconstrictors to local anesthetics has brought with it a potential problem—vasoconstrictor overdose.[31] Because in most instances the vasoconstrictor in question is epinephrine, this potential toxic reaction cannot be taken lightly. (Vasoconstrictor overdose will be discussed later in this chapter.)

Clinical experience with vasoconstrictors has led to the use of more and more dilute solutions with equally effective clinical applications. Early local anes-

table **23-4**  *Milligrams of local anesthetic per cartridge*

| CONCENTRATION (%) | = | MG/ML | × 1.8 ML = | TOTAL CARTRIDGE (USA) | × 2.2 ML = | TOTAL CARTRIDGE (UK) |
|---|---|---|---|---|---|---|
| 0.5 | | 5 | | 9 | | 11 |
| 1 | | 10 | | 18 | | 22 |
| 1.5 | | 15 | | 27 | | 33 |
| 2 | | 20 | | 36 | | 44 |
| 3 | | 30 | | 54 | | 66 |
| 4 | | 40 | | 72 | | 88 |

table **23-5**  *Effect of vasoconstrictor (epinephrine 1:200,000 on peak local anesthetic level in blood)*

| LOCAL ANESTHETIC | DOSE (MG) | PEAK LEVEL ($\mu$G/ML) | |
|---|---|---|---|
| | | NO VASOCONSTRICTOR | VASOCONSTRICTOR |
| Mepivacaine | 500 | 4.7 | 3.0 |
| Lidocaine | 400 | 4.3 | 3.0 |
| Prilocaine | 400 | 2.8 | 2.6 |
| Etidocaine | 300 | 1.4 | 1.3 |

Modified from Malamed SF: *Handbook of local anesthesia,* ed 4, St Louis, 1997, Mosby.

thetics (procaine) contained epinephrine concentrations of 1:50,000. Later combinations were produced with 1:80,000 and 1:100,000 concentrations. The most recent dental local anesthetic additions—prilocaine, etidocaine, bupivacaine, and articaine—all contain epinephrine in 1:200,000 concentrations. Mepivacaine is available in some countries in a 1:200,000 epinephrine concentration, and lidocaine with a 1:200,000 epinephrine concentration recently became available in dental cartridges in some countries (not in the United States as of 1999). Use of the minimum effective concentrations of both the local anesthetic and the vasoconsrictor increase the safety of any drug.

Topical application of some local anesthetics to the oral mucous membrane may also produce a rapid uptake of the drug. Absorption of some local anesthetics into the circulation after topical application is rapid, exceeded only by direct IV injection (see Figure 23-3).[17] Another important factor that increases the overdose potential of topically applied local anesthetics is the need for administration in higher concentrations than the injectable doses of the same drugs in order to anesthetize the mucous membrane adequately. For example, injectable lidocaine is effective as a 2% solution, whereas lidocaine for topical application requires a 5% or 10% concentration for effectiveness. Thus the imprudent use of topical anesthetics may produce signs and symptoms of local anesthetic overdose.

Fortunately, many topical anesthetics are used as the base form of the drug (for example, lidocaine, not lidocaine HCl), which is relatively insoluble in water and poorly absorbed into the circulation, thereby increasing the safety of this topical form of the drug. An example is the recently introduced DentiPatch,* a topical anesthetic bandage. It contains 46.1 mg of the base form of lidocaine, more than a single cartridge of injectable lidocaine HCl. The maximum blood level of lidocaine after a 15-minute application is 12.8 μg/ml, compared with 220 μg/ml after injection of 36 mg of lidocaine HCl.[32]

Other local anesthetics commonly used topically include benzocaine and tetracaine, both of which are esters and rapidly detoxified by plasma pseudocholinesterase. Tetracaine is absorbed rapidly from mucous membranes, whereas benzocaine is poorly absorbed.[17] Overdose reactions to benzocaine are virtually unknown.[33] Tetracaine, on the other hand, has a significant toxicity potential and must therefore be used judiciously. In addition, as esters, both drugs are

more likely to produce allergic reactions and localized tissue reactions (irritation) than are the amide topical anesthetics.

Topical anesthetics are important components in the management of pain and anxiety. They are applied commonly to the site of needle penetration before intraoral injections. When used in small, localized areas, topical anesthetics carry only a small chance for significant increases in anesthetic blood levels. Unfortunately, these anesthetics are also commonly applied over large areas (quadrants, or whole arches) before soft tissue procedures, such as scaling and curettage, when the injection of local anesthetic is not planned. Used in this manner, some topical anesthetics may produce significant blood levels, increasing the possibility of clinical overdose, particularly if this topical application is followed by the injection of local anesthetics.

This information must not be used to justify discontinuance of topical anesthetic use. Indeed, I feel that topical anesthetics are extremely important components of every local anesthetic procedure. However, the dentist and dental hygienist must be aware of the potential complications and take care to prevent them. The following suggestions are offered to aid in the wise administration of topical anesthetics:

- Amide-type topical anesthetics should be used whenever possible. Although the potential for overdose exists with all local anesthetics, other ADRs (for example, local tissue reaction and allergy) occur more frequently with ester-type topical anesthetics, such as benzocaine and tetracaine.

- The area of application should be small. Only rarely is application over a full quadrant warranted. The application of topical anesthetics to a full quadrant requires larger drug quantities and increases the risk of overdose. I think that whenever larger areas (for example, three or more teeth) require soft tissue anesthesia, an injection of a local anesthetic should be given serious consideration.

- Metered dose forms of topical anesthetics should be used. Local anesthetics in the form of ointments and especially sprays are difficult to monitor during application, and overdose may occur inadvertently. A spray form of an amide anesthetic (for example, lidocaine 10%) is available that delivers a metered 10-mg dose with each application is recommended (Figure 23-4).[34]

**Intravascular injection**    Intravascular injections are possible with any intraoral injection but is more likely to occur in certain anatomic areas (Table 23-6). Nerve-block techniques usually possess the greatest potential for intravascular injection; 11% of

---

*DentiPatch, Noven Pharmeceuticals, Miami, Fla.

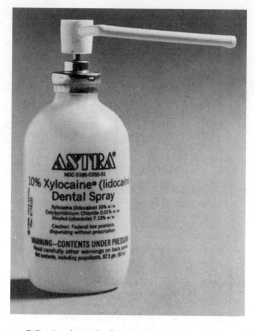

**Figure 23-4** A topical anesthetic spray with a metered applicator. Depression of the nozzle releases a 10-mg dose of lidocaine.

aspiration tests were positive in inferior alveolar nerve block, 5% in mental nerve block, and 3% in posterior superior alveolar nerve block, indicating that the needle bevel lay within the lumen of a blood vessel (vein or artery).[35]

Both IV and intraarterial administration may produce overdose reactions. Past wisdom stated that only IV injection of a local anesthetic could produce an overdose reaction and that intraarterial injection would not elevate blood levels since arterial blood travels away from the heart, not toward it, like venous blood. Aldrete[36,37] theorized that intraarterial administration of local anesthetics may produce an overdose as rapidly as (or more rapidly than) IV injection. The suggested mechanism for this reaction is a reversal of blood flow within the artery when the local anesthetic is injected rapidly. If such a mechanism occurred during an inferior alveolar nerve block, blood would flow retrograde from the inferior alveolar artery to the internal maxillary artery, back to the external carotid, then to the common carotid, and finally to the internal carotid and to the brain, a distance of only several inches in a human.

Intravascular injection of local anesthetics in the practice of dentistry should almost never occur. Careful injection technique and a knowledge of the area to be anesthetized should minimize the occurence of overdose reactions. Factors necessary to prevent this complication include the use of an aspirating syringe, use of a needle no smaller than 27

| table **23-6** | Percentage of positive aspiration for various intraoral injections |

| INJECTION | % POSITIVE ASPIRATION |
| --- | --- |
| Inferior alveolar block | 11.7 |
| Mental block | 5.7 |
| Posterior superior alveolar block | 3.1 |
| Anterior superior alveolar block | 0.7 |
| (Long) Buccal block | 0.5 |

From Barlett SZ: Clinical observations on the effects of injections of local anesthetics preceded by aspiration, *Oral Surg* 33:520, 1972.

gauge, aspiration in at least two planes before injection, and slow administration of the local anesthetic.

Recommending the use of an aspirating syringe for all injections should seem unnecessary; all North American dental schools teach its use to their students. However, in a survey of the injection practices of dentists, 21% of those surveyed voluntarily admitted using nonaspirating syringes.[27] No justification exists for the use of such devices for any local anesthetic injection because a nonaspirating syringe makes impossible aspiration to determine the location of the needle bevel.

Needle gauge is important in the determination of whether a needle is located within a vessel before drug injection. The needles most commonly available in dentistry are 25-, 27-, and 30-gauge, with the 27-gauge being used most frequently.[27] Needle gauge is of importance in several respects during local anesthetic injection. Accuracy in injection technique is one critical point. For a local anesthetic to control pain, it must be deposited near the nerve. As the needle passes through tissue toward the target nerve, it is deflected to varying degrees by its bevel. The extent of deflection has been tested and is related to the caliber or gauge of the needle. Needles with greater rigidity (that is, larger gauge) deflect less when passed through tissues to the depth required for an inferior alveolar nerve block.[38]

The second critical point relating to needle gauge concerns the reliability of aspiration. In other words, if a needle is located within the lumen of a blood vessel, do aspiration tests always prove positive? Several studies have demonstrated that it is not possible to aspirate consistently with a needle gauge smaller than 25.[39,40] However, Trapp and Davies[41] reported that in vivo human blood may be aspirated through 23-, 25-, 27-, and 30-gauge needles without clinically significant differences in flow resistance.

Small-gauge needles occlude more easily with tissue plugs or with the wall of the blood vessel than do larger needles, leading to false-negative aspirations. For injection technique with a greater likelihood of

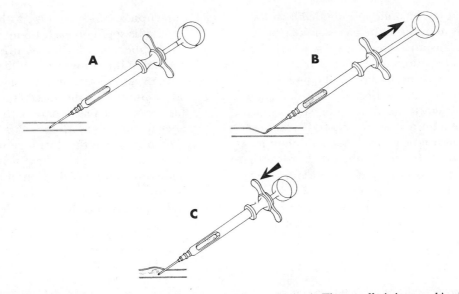

**Figure 23-5** Intravascular injection of a local anesthetic. **A,** The needle is inserted in the lumen of the blood vessel. **B,** An aspiration test should then be performed. Negative pressure pulls the vessel wall against the bevel of the needle; therefore no blood enters the syringe, indicating a negative aspiration. **C,** The drug is injected. Positive pressure on the plunger of the syringe forces the local aesthetic solution out via the needle. The wall of the vessel is forced from the bevel, and the anesthetic solution is deposited directly into the lumen of the blood vessel.

positive aspiration, a 25-gauge needle should always be used. These techniques include all block injections, especially inferior alveolar nerve block. Unfortunately, the majority of practicing dentists surveyed favor the 27-gauge needle for inferior alveolar nerve block (64% using the 27-gauge needle and 34% using the 25-gauge needle).[27]

The method through which aspiration is carried out is yet another factor of importance in the prevention of intravascular injection. All local anesthetic needles are beveled at the tips (Figure 23-5, *A*). The bevel of the needle may lie against the inner wall of a blood vessel. When negative pressure is created in the aspirating syringe (harpoon-type or self-aspirating syringe), the wall of the vessel may be sucked up against the bevel of the needle, preventing entry of blood into the needle and cartridge (see Figure 23-5, *B*). Clinically, the absence of blood return is interpreted as a negative aspiration, and the injection of the anesthetic solution proceeds. Injection of the local anesthetic requires that positive pressure be placed on the plunger to expel the anesthetic from the cartridge through the needle and into the tissues. However, where the bevel of the needle lies against the inner wall of the vessel, the positive pressure of the anesthetic solution pushes the vessel wall away from the needle bevel and the local anesthetic is then deposited intravascularly following a negative aspiration test (see Figure 23-5, *C*).

Therefore a single aspiration test may prove inadequate in the prevention of intravascular injection. Two or three tests should be performed before and during drug injection. During each test orientation of the needle bevel should be changed. The hand holding the syringe should be turned approximately 45 degrees to reorient the needle bevel relative to the vessel wall. Return of blood into the anesthetic cartridge is considered a positive aspiration and mandates repositioning of the needle and reaspiration. A negative result should be obtained before the local anesthetic is administered. Only 60% of dentists surveyed indicated that they always aspirate before mandibular block; 25% said they rarely aspirate, and 15% said they never aspirate.[27]

The last factor related to prevention of overdose from intravascular injection concerns the rate of injection. Rapid intravascular injection of a full cartridge (1.8 ml) of a 2% local anesthetic solution (36 mg) produces anesthetic blood levels that significantly exceed those required for overdose. In addition, the anesthetic blood level is elevated rapidly so that the onset of signs and symptoms is immediate. Rapid injection may be defined as the administration of the contents of a dental anesthetic cartridge in 30 seconds or less. The same quantity of anesthetic injected intravascularly at a slower rate (at least 60 seconds) produces blood levels below the minimum for overdose (see Figure 23-3).[17]

In the event that the ensuing anesthetic blood level does exceed this minimum, the onset of the reaction is slower, with signs and symptoms less severe than those observed after rapid injection.

Slow injection of drugs is perhaps the most important factor in the prevention of ADRs. It is difficult to inject a drug too slowly, but it is quite easy to inject too rapidly. The administration of a full 1.8-ml cartridge of local anesthetic should take a minimum of 60 seconds.[27] Such efforts significantly reduce the risk of a serious overdose reaction from intravascular injection. Of doctors surveyed, 46% administered a full cartridge of solution for the inferior alveolar nerve block in fewer than 30 seconds. Only 15% responded that they spent 60 seconds or longer on the same injection.[27]

## ADMINISTRATION TECHNIQUE

Overdose reactions and indeed all ADRs related to local anesthesia, may be minimized through proper administration of local anesthetics, described as follows:

1. A preliminary medical evaluation should be completed before local anesthetic administration.
2. Anxiety, fear, and apprehension should be recognized and managed before administration of a local anesthetic.
3. Whenever possible, the patient should receive injections while in a supine or semisupine position. An upright position should only be used if necessary, as with patients suffering severe cardiorespiratory diseases.
4. Topical anesthetics should be applied to the site of needle penetration for at least 1 minute before all injections.
5. The weakest effective concentration of local anesthetic solution should be injected in the smallest volume compatible with successful anesthesia.
6. The anesthetic solution should be appropriate for the patient and for the planned dental treatment (for example, appropriate duration of effect).
7. Vasoconstrictors should be included in all local anesthetics, if not specifically contraindicated.
8. Aspirating syringes must always be used for all local anesthetic injections.
9. Needles should be disposable, sharp, rigid, capable of reliable aspiration, and of adequate length for the contemplated injection technique. Most nerve blocks require the use of long (1⅝-inch) 25-gauge needles. Short 27-gauge needles (1-inch) may be used for other injection techniques.
10. Aspiration should be performed in at least two planes before injection.
11. Injection should be slow; at least 60 seconds should be spent on each 1.8-ml dental cartridge.
12. A member of the dental office staff who is trained in the recognition of life-threatening situations should remain with the patient after the administration of the anesthetic. Most local anesthetic overdose reactions occur 5 or more minutes after the injection. All too often incidents are reported in which the doctor returns to the treatment room only to find the patient in the throes of a life-threatening ADR. Continuous observation permits prompt recognition and management with a high probability of complete recovery.

NOTE: Variations may exist in needle selection for some regional nerve blocks. Textbooks on local anesthesia should be consulted for more specific information.

# Clinical Manifestations

Signs and symptoms of overdose appear whenever the local anesthetic blood level in an organ, such as the brain or heart (myocardium), rises above the critical level at which adverse effects of the drug develop. The brain responds to the concentration of local anesthetic delivered by the circulatory system regardless of the way in which the local anesthetic initially entered into the blood. The blood or plasma level of local anesthetic dictates the degree of severity and the duration of the response. The rate of onset of signs and symptoms corresponds to the blood level. Various causes of local anesthetic overdose produce a range of rates of onset.

## ONSET, INTENSITY, AND DURATION

Rapid intravascular injection produces clinical signs and symptoms of overdose rapidly, with unconsciousness and seizures appearing within seconds. The duration of this form of overdose reaction, assuming that the patient receives adequate management, is usually shorter than other forms because of drug redistribution (lowering cerebral blood levels) and to a lesser extent the continued biotransformation of the local anesthetic by the liver or by serum cholinesterase while the reaction continues. Overdose reaction due to rapid intravascular injection may occur with all types of local anesthetics (Table 23-7).

Signs and symptoms of local anesthetic overdose resulting from too large a total dose or unusually rapid absorption into the cardiovascular system do not develop as rapidly as those produced by intravascular injection. In these two situations, signs and symptoms usually appear approximately 5 to 10 minutes after

**table 23-7** Comparison of forms of local anesthetic overdose

| METHOD OF OVERDOSE | LIKELIHOOD OF OCCURENCE | ONSET OF SIGNS AND SYMPTOMS | INTENSITY OF SIGNS AND SYMPTOMS | DURATION OF SIGNS AND SYMPTOMS | PRIMARY PREVENTION | DRUG GROUPS |
|---|---|---|---|---|---|---|
| Rapid intravascular | Common | Most rapid (seconds); intraarterial faster than IV | Usually most intense | 2-3 minutes | Aspiration; slow injection | Amides and esters |
| Too large a total dose | Most common | 5-30 minutes | Gradual onset with increased intensity; may prove severe | Usually 5-30 minutes (depends on dose and ability to metabolize or excrete) | Administration of minimal doses | Amides; esters only rarely |
| Rapid absorption | Likely with "high normal" doses if no vasoconstrictors used | 5-30 minutes | Gradual onset with increased intensity; may prove severe | Usually 5-30 minutes (depends on dose and ability to metabolize or excrete) | Use of vasoconstrictor; limit on topical anesthetic use or use of nonabsorbed type (base) | Amides; esters only rarely |
| Slow biotransformation | Uncommon | 1-3 hours | Gradual onset with slow increase in intensity | Potential for longest duration because of inability to metabolize agents | Adequate pretreatment physical evaluation of patient | Amides and esters |
| Slow elimination | Least common | Several hours | Gradual onset with slow increase in intensity | Potential for longest duration because of inability to excrete agents | Adequate pretreatment physical evaluation of patient | Amides and esters |

*IV,* Intravenous.

drug administration if the anesthetic solution does not contain a vasopressor or approximately 30 minutes after injection if vasopressors are included; such signs and symptoms are initially mild.[30] Signs and symptoms may manifest as obvious agitation and increase in intensity and progression over the next few minutes or longer if the blood level continues to rise. Clinically, the severity of these reactions may be as great as those associated with direct intravascular injection or may not progress beyond mild reactions. These reactions are also self limiting because of the continued redistribution and biotransformation of the local anesthetic, but they tend to last significantly longer than the intravascular responses.

In two cases that I have witnessed the patients received adequate mandibular anesthesia (after multiple injections) and were undergoing restorative procedures for 20 and 25 minutes, respectively, when clinical manifestations of overdose became obvious. These included mild tremor, which progressed slowly into a mild convulsion over the next 30 minutes.

Unusually slow biotransformation or elimination of local anesthetics rarely produces signs and symptoms of overdose while the patient is still in the dental office. In situations in which the patient has received a large dose of local anesthetic, signs and symptoms of mild overdose may develop 90 or more minutes later. In most situations this patient has usually left the dental office.

## SIGNS AND SYMPTOMS

Local anesthetics depress excitable membranes. The cardiovascular system, in particular, and CNS are especially sensitive. The usual clinical expression of local anesthetic overdose is one of apparent stimulation followed by a period of depression.

**Minimal to moderate blood levels**    The initial signs of CNS overdose are usually excitatory. At low overdose blood levels the patient usually becomes confused, talkative, apprehensive, and excited; speech may be slurred. A generalized stuttering follows, which may lead to muscular twitching and tremor, commonly occurring in the muscles of the face and the distal parts of the extremities. The patient may also exhibit nystagmus. The blood pressure, heart rate, and respiratory rate increase.[42]

Headache may also be a symptom of overdose. In addition, many patients initially report feeling a generalized feeling of lightheadedness and dizziness, one different than that produced by alcohol. These symptoms then lead to visual and auditory disturbances (for example, difficulty in focusing, blurred vision, and ringing in the ears [tinnitus]). Numbness of the tongue and perioral tissues commonly develops, as does a feeling of being either flushed or chilled. As the reaction progresses and if the anesthetic blood level rises, the patient experiences drowsiness and disorientation and eventually may lose consciousness. Signs and symptoms of mild local anesthetic overdose may resemble psychomotor or temporal lobe epilepsy (see Chapter 21).

**Moderate to high blood levels**    As the local anesthetic blood level continues to rise, the clinical manifestations of an overdose reaction progress to a generalized convulsive state with tonic-clonic seizures. After this stimulatory phase, a period of generalized CNS depression ensues, characteristically of a degree of severity related to the degree of stimulation that preceded it. Therefore if the patient suffered intensive tonicoclonic seizures, postictal depression is more profound, characterized by probable unconsciousness and respiratory depression and possible respiratory arrest. If the stimulatory phase was mild (for example, talkativeness or agitation), the depressant phase will also be mild, perhaps consisting of only a period of disorientation and lethargy. The blood pressure, heart rate, and respiratory rate are usually depressed during this phase, again to a degree proportionate to the degree of previous stimulation (Box 23-3).

Although the sequence just described is the usual clinical expression of local anesthetic overdose, the excitatory phase of the reaction may be extremely brief or even absent entirely. This is especially true with lidocaine and mepivacaine, in which overdose may appear initially as drowsiness and nystagmus, leading directly to either unconsciousness or generalized tonic-clonic seizure activity.[43] Etidocaine and bupivacaine do not cause drowsiness before seizures;[44] progression from the preseizure state of alertness to seizures with these drugs is much more abrupt.

The overdose reaction continues until the cerebral blood level of the local anesthetic falls below the minimal blood level for overdose or until the reaction is terminated through appropriate management, including possible drug therapy.

## Pathophysiology

Local anesthetic overdose is produced by overly high blood levels of a drug in various target organs and tissues. In instances in which the drug's entry into the blood exceeds its rate of removal, overdose levels may be reached. The period of time required for clinical signs and symptoms to appear varies considerably depending on the cause of the elevated blood level.

box 23-3    *Clinical manifestations of local anesthetic overdose*

**SIGNS**

**Low to moderate overdose levels**

Confusion
Talkativeness
Apprehension
Excitedness
Slurred speech
Generalized stutter
Muscular twitching and tremor of the face and extremities
Nystagmus
Elevated blood pressure
Elevated heart rate
Elevated respiratory rate

**Moderate to high blood levels**

Generalized tonicoclonic seizure, followed by:
    Generalized CNS depression
    Depressed blood pressure, heart rate, and respiratory rate

**SYMPTOMS**

Headache
Lightheadedness
Dizziness
Blurred vision, inability to focus
Ringing in ears
Numbness of tongue and perioral tissues
Flushed or chilled feeling
Drowsiness
Disorientation
Loss of consciousness

table 23-8    *Overdose thresholds*

| AGENT | USUAL THRESHOLD FOR CNS SIGNS AND SYMPTOMS |
|---|---|
| Bupivacaine, etidocaine | 1-2 µg/ml |
| Prilocaine | 4 µg/ml |
| Lidocaine, mepivacaine | 5 µg/ml |

*CNS,* Central nervous system.

Drugs do not merely affect a single organ or tissue, and all drugs have multiple actions. Local anesthetics are typical of all drugs in this regard.

Although the primary pharmacologic action of a local anesthetic is the inhibition of the excitation conduction process in peripheral nerves, its ability to stabilize membranes is not limited solely to peripheral nerves. Any excitable membranes, such as those in the heart, brain, and neuromuscular junction, are altered by local anesthetics if they reach a sufficient tissue concentration.[45] The following section discusses both the desirable and the undesirable systemic actions of local anesthetics.

The term *blood level,* or *plasma level,* refers to the amount of a drug that is absorbed into circulation and transported in the blood plasma throughout the body. A sample of blood may be drawn from the patient to determine the amount of local anesthetic present per milliliter of blood. This amount is referred to commonly as the *blood level,* or *plasma level,* of a local anesthetic. Blood levels of drugs are measured in micrograms (µg) per milliliter (1000 µg = 1 mg).

An additional factor to consider when discussing blood levels of drugs is that, although ranges are mentioned for various systemic actions, patients will differ in their responses to drugs. Even though seizure activity may occur at a blood level of 7.5 µg/ml of lidocaine for most individuals, others may exhibit seizures at lower blood levels, whereas still others may be able to tolerate blood levels that are greatly in excess of those listed without experiencing ADRs. In addition, different local anesthetics have different threshold levels at which the signs and symptoms of overdose usually appear (Table 23-8). Drugs associated with higher plasma levels for overdose are not necessarily less toxic because these drugs are usually less potent as local anesthetics and must therefore be injected at higher concentrations to be effective. For example, the ratio of CNS toxicity of bupivacaine, etidocaine, and lidocaine is approximately 4:2:1, which is similar to the relative potency of these drugs for the production of regional anesthesia in humans.[46]

## LOCAL ANESTHETIC BLOOD LEVELS

After intraoral injection the drug slowly enters the blood. Circulating blood levels of lidocaine have been monitored and recorded after such injections; these documented levels form the basis of this chapter's discussion (Figure 23-6). Blood levels of other anesthetics differ from those reported for lidocaine. Cannell and others[47] demonstrated that blood levels rise to a maximum of approximately 1.0 µg/ml after the administration of 40 mg to 160 mg lidocaine via intraoral injection. No ADRs were reported at those levels.

As the lidocaine blood level increases, systemic actions are noted, some of which have considerable therapeutic value. When lidocaine blood levels reach 4.5 to 7.0 µg/ml, signs of CNS irritability are noticeable. When this level increases to 7.5 µg/ml or greater, tonicoclonic seizure activity occurs. A level of 10 µg/ml is characterized by marked CNS depression. In addition, at overdose levels adverse actions on the cardiovascular

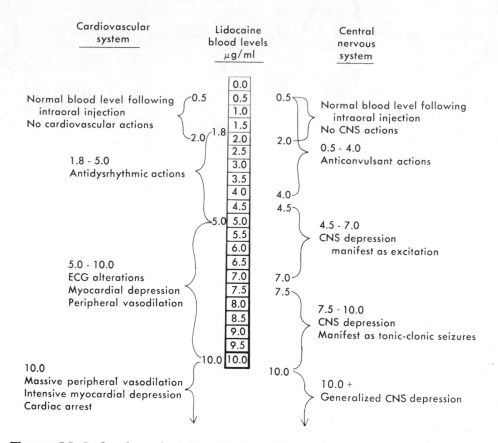

**Figure 23-6**   Local anesthetic blood levels and their actions on cardiovascular and CNS systems. (*CNS*, Central nervous system.)

system are noted. Most adverse effects on the cardiovascular system do not develop until high overdose levels for the CNS occur. (See Figure 23-3 for the effect of the various routes of administration on the blood level of the anesthetic.)

## SYSTEMIC ACTIVITY OF LOCAL ANESTHETICS

Local anesthetics inhibit the function of any excitable membrane. In the practice of dentistry these drugs are normally applied to a very specific region of the body where they perform their primary function—a reversible blockade or depression of peripheral nerve conduction. Other actions of local anesthetics relate to the absorption of the drugs into circulation and their systemic activities on various excitable membranes, including smooth muscle, the myocardium, and the CNS. Although high blood levels of local anesthetics produce undesirable systemic responses, some desirable actions may occur at nonoverdose levels.

**Cardiovascular actions**   Local anesthetics, particularly lidocaine, are frequently used in the man-

agement of various ventricular dysrhythmias, especially ventricular extrasystole (PVCs) and ventricular tachycardia. Considerable data today illustrate the alterations that occur in the myocardium as blood levels of lidocaine increase.[49,50] In general, the minimal effective blood level of lidocaine for antidysrhythmic activity is 1.8 µg/ml.[48] In the range from approximately 2 to 5 µg/ml, the action of lidocaine on the myocardium includes electrophysiologic changes only. These include a prolongation or abolition of the slow phase of depolarization during diastole in Purkinje fibers and a shortening of the action potential duration and of the effective refractory period. At this therapeutic level no alterations in myocardial contractility, diastolic volume, intraventricular pressure, or cardiac output are evident.[44,50] The healthy as well as the diseased myocardium can both tolerate mildly elevated blood levels of local anesthetic without deleterious effects.

When used to treat dysrhythmias, lidocaine is administered IV (slowly!) in a 50- to 100-mg bolus (1.0 to 1.5 mg/kg).[51] Overdose is a potential problem at this time, but the benefit-to-risk ratio allows for the judicious use of IV lidocaine. Further elevation of the lidocaine blood level (5 to 10 μg/ml) produces a prolongation of conduction time through various portions of the heart and an increase in the diastolic threshold. This may be noted on the electrocardiogram as an increased P-R interval and QRS duration and sinus bradycardia. In addition, decreased myocardial contractility, increased diastolic volume, decreased intraventricular pressure, and decreased cardiac output are evident.[49,52] Peripheral vascular effects observed at this level include vasodilation, which produces a drop in blood pressure and occurs as a result of the direct relaxant effect of lidocaine on peripheral vascular smooth muscle.[53]

Further increases in blood levels of lidocaine (>10 μg/ml) lead to an accentuation of the aforementioned electrophysiologic and hemodynamic effects, in particular a massive peripheral vasodilation, marked reduction in myocardial contractility, and slowed heart rate, which may ultimately result in cardiac arrest.[49,53]

**CNS actions**    The CNS is extremely sensitive to the actions of local anesthetics.[54] As cerebral blood levels of local anesthetics increase, clinical signs and symptoms develop. Local anesthetics readily cross the blood-brain barrier, depressing CNS function.[45] At nonoverdose levels of lidocaine (<5 μg/ml), no clinical signs of adverse effects on the CNS exist; however, a CNS-depressant action that has potential therapeutic value is observed. At cerebral blood levels between 0.5 and 4.0 μg/ml, lidocaine can terminate various forms of seizure.[55,56] Most clinically useful local anesthetics possess this anticonvulsant property (both procaine and lidocaine having been used to terminate or decrease the duration of grand mal or petit mal seizures). This anticonvulsant action may be related to a depression of hyperexcitable cortical neurons present in epileptic patients.

As the blood level of lidocaine increases above 4.5 μg/ml, initial signs and symptoms of CNS alteration appear. These are usually related to increased cortical irritability (for example, agitation, talkativeness, and tremor). Numbness of the tongue and perioral tissues may result from the rich blood supply to these tissues, allowing the drugs to produce a blockade of the nerve endings.[52]

With a further increase in the cerebral blood level to 7.5 μg/ml or greater (lidocaine), generalized tonic-clonic seizures develop. Following this period of CNS stimulation, a further increase in cerebral blood level of the local anesthetic results in termination of seizure activity and an electroencephalographic pattern consistent with generalized CNS depression.[52] Respiratory depression and arrest are also noted.

The fact that local anesthetics are CNS depressants on the one hand but that CNS stimulation is the first clinical manifestation of this depression seems contradictory. The stimulation and subsequent depression produced by high blood levels of local anesthetics result solely from depression of neuronal activity. The cerebral cortex receives inhibitory and facilitory (stimulatory) impulses. If it is considered that these two groups of neurons are depressed selectively by different blood levels of local anesthetics explains this seeming contradiction is explained. At anesthetic blood levels capable of producing seizures, the inhibitory pathways in the cerebral cortex are depressed, not the stimulatory pathways. This depression of inhibitory pathways allows facilitory neurons to function unopposed, leading to increased excitation of the CNS and ultimately to seizures.[57] As the local anesthetic blood level increases further, stimulatory neurons are depressed along with inhibitory neurons, producing a state of generalized CNS depression.

The duration of the seizure, although primarily dependent on the local anesthetic blood level, can be further modified by the acid-base status of the patient. The higher the $PaCO_2$, the lower the local anesthetic blood level required to precipitate generalized seizures. In contrast, the lower the $PaCO_2$, the greater the drug blood level required to produce seizures.[8] Lowering a patient's $PaCO_2$ through hyperventilation raises the cortical seizure threshold to local anesthetics and lessens the chance that a drug may cause seizures.

Drug-induced seizures, in and of themselves, are not necessarily fatal. However, the mortality rate in untreated animals is more than 60%.[58] The duration of the seizure appears to be a critical factor in determining the degree of morbidity. The convulsing brain requires greatly elevated oxygen ($O_2$) and glucose levels to continue functioning. To a degree, the body's own mechanisms can compensate for this; however, respiratory and circulatory support can enhance the chances of survival significantly. If blood levels of the local anesthetic elevate even further, cardiovascular depression is produced and respirations are increasingly impaired by uncoordinated muscle spasm during the seizure. Brain function is affected even more through reduced cerebral blood flow and hypoxia (see Figure 23-6).[59]

## Management

Management of a local anesthetic overdose is based on its severity. In most cases the reaction is mild and transitory, requiring little or no specific treatment. However, when the reaction is more severe and of longer duration prompt management is necessary. Most local anesthetic overdoses are self limiting; the blood level of the local anesthetic decreases as the reaction progresses because of redistribution (primarily) and biotransformation (secondarily) of the drug. Rare indeed is the occasion on which drugs other than $O_2$ need to be administered to terminate a local anesthetic overdose.

Overtreatment of a local anesthetic overdose is a potential problem. In the rush of excitement that follows this unexpected reaction, emergency drugs, such as anticonvulsants, may be administered too freely. All anticonvulsants are CNS depressants and will delay the return of consciousness. The time for aggressive IV management of the local anesthetic overdose comes when simpler measures fail to terminate the seizure. However, by ending the seizure, anticonvulsants may give the rescuer a false sense of accomplishment; no anticonvulsant is wholly innocuous.

It is well worth repeating that during and after administration of a local anesthetic the patient should be observed continuously. Careful observation for any change in behavior after the administration of a local anesthetic permits prompt recognition and management and helps minimize potential hazard for the patient.

## MILD OVERDOSE REACTION WITH RAPID ONSET

An overdose reaction developing within 5 to 10 minutes of drug administration is considered rapid in onset. Possible causes include intravascular injection, unusually rapid absorption, or administration of too large a total dose. If clinical manifestations do not progress beyond mild CNS excitation and consciousness is retained, definitive care is not necessary. The local anesthetic undergoes redistribution and biotransformation, and the blood level falls below the overdose level in a short time.

The following are diagnostic clues to the presence of mild local anesthetic overdose:

- Onset 5 to 10 minutes or longer after drug administration
- Talkativeness
- Increased anxiety
- Facial muscle twitching
- Increased heart rate, blood pressure, and respiration

*Step 1: termination of the dental procedure.*

*Step 2:* **P** *(position).* The conscious patient is placed in a comfortable position.

*Step 3: reassurance of the patient.*

*Step 4:* **A-B-C** *(airway-breathing-circulation), basic life support (BLS), as needed.* The patency of the airway, breathing, and circulation must be assessed and implemented, as needed. In mild local anesthetic overdose, the victim's airway, breathing, and circulation remain adequate, and no intervention is necessary.

*Step 5:* **D** *(definitive care):*
*Step 5a: administration of $O_2$.* At this point the fact that a lowered $PaCO_2$ level elevates the local anesthetic seizure threshold may be used to the patient's advantage. The patient should be asked to hyperventilate by deep breathing on room air or $O_2$ via a full-face mask or nasal hood. This will usually prevent the development of seizures.
*Step 5b: monitoring of vital signs.* The stage of postexcitation depression is mild in this form of reaction, and little or no therapy is required to manage it. $O_2$ may be administered and the patient's vital signs monitored and recorded regularly.
*Step 5c: administration of an anticonvulsant drug, if needed.* The administration of an anticonvulsant, such as diazepam or midazolam, usually is not indicated in the mild overdose described here. However, if the doctor is trained in venipuncture and has little difficulty in accessing a vein, diazepam or midazolam may be administered via an IV route and titrated slowly until the clinical reaction abates. IV drugs should always be titrated to clinical effect (in this case the cessation of muscular twitching). Small doses of IV diazepam or midazolam may prove effective.[60] As little as 2.5- to 5-mg doses of diazepam have been known to terminate seizures. It must be emphasized, however, that a mild reaction to a local anesthetic, anticonvulsant drug therapy normally is not indicated.
*Step 5d: summoning of emergency medical assistance.* If the doctor deems emergency assistance necessary, such assistance should be sought immediately. The decision to seek help is based solely on the doctor's instinct. My feeling is that emergency assistance should be sought whenever an anticonvulsant drug has been administered to terminate the reaction. In addition, if signs and symptoms appear to be increasing in intensity and venous access is not available, emergency assistance is indicated.

*Step 6: recovery and discharge.* The patient should be permitted to recover for as long as is necessary. The scheduled treatment may continue or be postponed after a thorough evaluation of the patient's physical and emotional status. If the treating doctor harbors any doubts or concerns about the patient's condition following the reaction, medical evaluation, preferably by an emergency room physician, is indicated before that patient is discharged. If an anticonvulsant drug was administered, the patient should receive medical evaluation before discharge and must not leave the office unescorted.

Box 23-4 outlines the steps in the management of a mild local anesthetic overdose with rapid onset.

## MILD OVERDOSE REACTION WITH DELAYED ONSET (>10 MINUTES)

If the patient exhibits signs and symptoms of a mild overdose after the local anesthetic has been administered in the recommended manner, if adequate pain control has resulted, and if dental treatment has begun, the most likely causes are unusually rapid absorption and administration of too large a total dose of the drug.

*Step 1: termination of the procedure.*

*Step 2:* **P** *(position).* The patient should be allowed to assume a comfortable position.

*Step 3: reassurance of the patient.*

*Step 4:* **A-B-C** *(airway, breathing, circulation) or BLS, as needed.* If the patient is conscious, the steps of BLS are not necessary.

*Step 5:* **D** *(definitive care):*

box **23-4** | *Management of mild local anesthetic overdose with rapid onset*

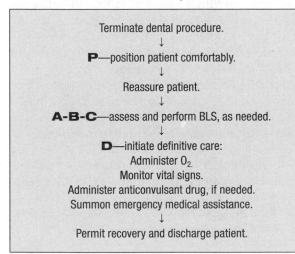

Terminate dental procedure.
↓
**P**—position patient comfortably.
↓
Reassure patient.
↓
**A-B-C**—assess and perform BLS, as needed.
↓
**D**—initiate definitive care:
Administer O₂
Monitor vital signs.
Administer anticonvulsant drug, if needed.
Summon emergency medical assistance.
↓
Permit recovery and discharge patient.

**P,** Position; **A,** airway; **B,** breathing; **C,** circulation; **D,** definitive care; *BLS,* basic life support; *O₂,* oxygen.

*Step 5a: administration of O₂ and instruction to hyperventilate.*

*Step 5b: monitoring of vital signs.*

*Step 5c: administration of anticonvulsant, if needed.* Overdose reactions resulting from either unusually rapid absorption or administration of too large a total dose of the drug usually progress in intensity gradually and last longer than those caused by intravascular drug administration. If venous access is possible, an IV infusion may be established and an anticonvulsant, such as diazepam or midazolam, administered via titration until clinical signs and symptoms abate.

*Step 5d: summoning of medical assistance (optional).* When venipuncture is not practical, medical assistance should be sought immediately.

Post-excitement depression is relatively mild after a mild excitement phase. The use of an anticonvulsant to help terminate the reaction may increase the level of post-excitation depression—but only a little. Monitoring the patient and adhering to the steps of BLS are normally entirely adequate to successfully manage a mild overdose reaction with delayed onset. In addition, O₂ should be administered. Whenever an anticonvulsant is administered, medical assistance should be sought.

*Step 5d: medical consultation.* After successful management of a mild overdose with slow onset, a physician should evaluate the patient to seek possible causes of the reaction.

*Step 6: recovery and discharge.* The patient should be allowed to recover for as long as necessary and escorted to a local hospital or the primary-care physician's office by an adult companion, such as a spouse, relative, or friend. When emergency personnel are present, a decision on patient disposition will be suggested by them.

*Step 7: subsequent dental treatment.* Before scheduling further dental treatment in which local anesthetics may be necessary, a complete evaluation of the patient should be performed to help determine the cause of the overdose reaction.

Box 23-5 outlines the protocol for the management of a mild local anesthetic overdose with delayed onset.

## SEVERE OVERDOSE REACTION WITH RAPID ONSET

If signs and symptoms of overdose appear almost immediately after local anesthetic administration (for example, while the anesthetic syringe is still in the patient's mouth or within a few seconds after the in-

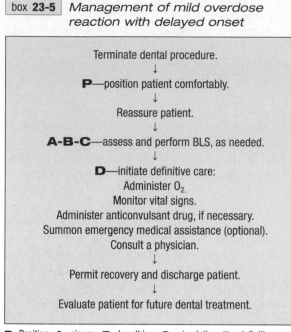

**box 23-5** *Management of mild overdose reaction with delayed onset*

Terminate dental procedure.
↓
**P**—position patient comfortably.
↓
Reassure patient.
↓
**A-B-C**—assess and perform BLS, as needed.
↓
**D**—initiate definitive care:
Administer O₂.
Monitor vital signs.
Administer anticonvulsant drug, if necessary.
Summon emergency medical assistance (optional).
Consult a physician.
↓
Permit recovery and discharge patient.
↓
Evaluate patient for future dental treatment.

*P,* Position; *A,* airway; *B,* breathing; *C,* circulation; *D,* definitive care; *BLS,* basic life support; *O₂,* oxygen.

jection), intravascular injection—either IV or intraarterial—is the most likely cause of the overdose reaction. Because of the extremely rapid increase in anesthetic blood level, clinical manifestations are likely to be severe. Unconsciousness, possibly accompanied by seizures, may mark the initial clinical manifestation.

The following are diagnostic clues to the presence of severe overdose to a local anesthetic:

- Signs and symptoms appearing either during injection or seconds after its completion
- Generalized tonic-clonic seizures
- Loss of consciousness

*Step 1:* **P** *(position).* The syringe should be removed from the patient's mouth (if applicable) and the patient placed in the supine position with the feet elevated slightly. Subsequent management is based on the presence or absence of seizures.

*Step 2: summoning of emergency medical assistance.* When the patient develops a seizure either during or after local anesthetic injection, emergency assistance should be sought immediately.

When the loss of consciousness is the sole clinical sign present, the patient should be placed in the supine position with the feet elevated slightly and managed as described in Chapter 5. If consciousness rapidly returns, vasodepressor syncope was the likely cause and medical assistance is usually not required.

If the patient does not respond rapidly, emergency assistance should be sought as soon as possible.

*Step 3:* **A-B-C** *(airway, breathing, circulation) or BLS, as needed.*

*Step 4:* **D** *(definitive care):*
*Step 4a: administration of O₂.* Adequate oxygenation and ventilation during local anesthetic-induced seizures is extremely important in the termination of seizures and in minimizing the associated morbidity. O₂ should be administered as soon as it becomes available.

Maintenance of adequate ventilation—the removal of carbon dioxide and the administration of O₂—helps to minimize and prevent hypercarbia and hypoxia and to maintain the seizure threshold of the anesthetic drug (local anesthetic seizure threshold is lowered if the patient becomes acidotic). In most instances of local anesthetic-induced seizures, airway maintenance and assisted ventilation are necessary **(A+B)**, but the heart should remain functional (blood pressure and heart rate are present).

*Step 4b: protection of the patient.* If seizures occur, which are common, management should follow the protocol outlined in the discussion on seizures (see Chapter 21). Recommended management includes the prevention of injury through protection of the arms, legs, and head. Do not attempt to place any object between the teeth of a convulsing patient. Tight, binding articles of clothing, such as ties, collars, and belts, should be loosened. Prevention of injury is the primary aim of seizure management.

*Step 4c: monitoring of vital signs.* The blood level of the local anesthetic decreases as it undergoes redistribution. Assuming ventilation of the victim is adequate, the anesthetic blood level should fall below the seizure threshold and the seizure cease (unless the patient has become acidotic). In most cases of local anesthetic-induced seizures, definitive drug therapy to terminate the seizure is unnecessary.

*Step 4d: venipuncture and IV anticonvulsant administration.* IV anticonvulsant administration should not be considered unless the doctor is well trained in venipuncture, has available the appropriate drugs, and can manage an apneic patient during the postseizure period. If possible, diazepam or midazolam should be titrated slowly until the seizure ends. In certain cases, however, securing of a vein in a convulsing patient may prove difficult. In such situations BLS should continue until assistance arrives.

*Step 5: postictal management.* Following the seizure a period of generalized CNS depression occurs that is usually equal in intensity to the previous degree of excitation. During this period the patient may be drowsy or even unconscious, breathing may be shallow or absent, the airway may be partially or totally obstructed, and the blood pressure and heart rate may be depressed or absent. Management is predicated upon the signs and symptoms present.

The use of anticonvulsants to terminate seizures only increases postictal depression. Barbiturates have a greater depressant effect than benzodiazepines, such as diazepam and midazolam, although all are equally effective as anticonvulsants; thus benzodiazepines are the drugs of choice in seizure management.

*Step 5a:* **A-B-C** *(airway, breathing, circulation), or BLS, as needed.*

*Step 5b: monitoring of vital signs.* Management in the postictal period requires adherence to the steps of BLS. A patent airway must be maintained and $O_2$ or artificial ventilation administered, as needed. In addition, vital signs should be monitored and recorded. If the blood pressure or heart beat is absent, chest compressions is started immediately (see Chapter 30). Most commonly, however, the blood pressure and heart rate generally are depressed in the immediate postictal period, gradually returning toward baseline levels as the patient recovers.

*Step 5c: additional management considerations.* If the patient's blood pressure remains depressed for an extended period (>30 minutes) and medical assistance is not yet available, the administration of a vasopressor should be considered to elevate blood pressure. Once again, this step should be considered only when the doctor is well trained in the administration of such drugs and in the management of all the complications associated with their administration. A vasopressor, such as 20 mg IM methoxamine, produces a mild elevation in blood pressure, the effect lasting 1 hour or more. Administration of 1000 ml of either normal saline or a 5% dextrose and water solution via IV infusion is another method by which a patient's blood pressure may be elevated.

*Step 6: recovery and discharge.* Emergency medical personnel will stabilize the patient's condition before transferring that patient via ambulance to the emergency department of a local hospital for definitive management, observation, and recovery.

> NOTE: As previously discussed, the first clinical sign of a rapid rise in the local anesthetic blood level may be unconsciousness. When this occurs, management follows the protocol outlined in Chapter 5. Follow-up therapy is identical to that suggested for the postseizure patient.

## SEVERE OVERDOSE REACTION WITH SLOW ONSET

Local anesthetic overdose reactions that evolve slowly over 10 or more minutes are unlikely to progress to the point at which the patient develops severe clinical signs and symptoms develop if that individual is observed continuously and prompt management initiated. Clinical signs and symptoms of overdose usually progress from mild to tonic-clonic seizures over a relatively brief period of time (5 minutes); in some cases the progression may be much less pronounced. In all cases dental treatment must cease as soon as signs and symptoms of overdose become evident.

*Step 1: termination of dental treatment.* Treatment is likely to have begun before the signs and symptoms of overdose become evident. Immediately cease the procedure and initiate emergency care.

*Step 2:* **P** *(positioning).* Positioning depends on the status of the patient. If the patient is conscious, initial positioning is based on comfort; however, the unconscious patient should be placed in the supine position with the legs elevated slightly.

*Step 3:* **A-B-C** *(airway, breathing, circulation), or BLS, as needed.*

*Step 4:* **D** *(definitive care):*
*Step 4a: summoning of medical assistance.*
*Step 4b: protection of the patient.*
*Step 4c: administration of $O_2$.*
*Step 4d: monitoring of vital signs.*
*Step 4e: venipuncture and administration of IV anticonvulsant.* If symptoms are mild at the onset but become more severe, the administration of an anticonvulsant drug should be considered. IV titration of a suitable anticonvulsant is indicated.

*Step 5: postictal management:*
*Step 5a:* **A-B-C** *(airway, breathing, circulation), or BLS, as needed.*
*Step 5b: monitoring of vital signs.* Management in the postictal period of CNS, respiratory, and cardiovascular depression requires adherence to the steps of BLS. A patent airway must be maintained and $O_2$ or artificial ventilation administered, as needed. Vital signs must continue to be monitored and recorded. If the blood pressure or heart rate is absent, chest compression should be initiated immediately (see Chapter 30). In general, the blood pressure and heart rate are depressed in the immediate postictal period but gradually return toward baseline levels as the patient recovers.

*Step 5c: additional management considerations.* A mild vasopressor (for example, methoxamine) or infusion of IV fluids may be necessary if the blood pressure remains depressed for a prolonged period.

*Step 6: recovery and discharge.* Emergency personnel stabilize the patient and prepare for transport to the emergency room of a local hospital for definitive management, recovery, and discharge.

Local anesthetic–induced seizures need not lead to significant morbidity or death if the patient is properly prepared for the injection, if the individual administering the local anesthetic is well trained in the recognition and management of complications, including seizures, and if appropriate resuscitation equipment is readily available. Administration of local anesthetics without such precautions is contraindicated.

Box 23-6 outlines the protocol for the management of severe local anesthetic drug overdose with slow or rapid onset.

- **Drugs used in management:** $O_2$, anticonvulsants (for example, diazepam or midazolam), and vasopressors, such as methoxamine (optional) may be administered in the management of an overdose reaction.

**box 23-6** *Management of a severe local anesthetic overdose with slow or rapid onset*

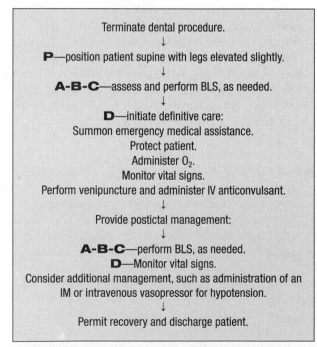

Terminate dental procedure.
↓
**P**—position patient supine with legs elevated slightly.
↓
**A-B-C**—assess and perform BLS, as needed.
↓
**D**—initiate definitive care:
Summon emergency medical assistance.
Protect patient.
Administer $O_2$.
Monitor vital signs.
Perform venipuncture and administer IV anticonvulsant.
↓
Provide postictal management:
↓
**A-B-C**—perform BLS, as needed.
**D**—Monitor vital signs.
Consider additional management, such as administration of an IM or intravenous vasopressor for hypotension.
↓
Permit recovery and discharge patient.

**P,** Position; **A,** airway; **B,** breathing; **C,** circulation; **D,** definitive care; *BLS,* basic life support; *O₂,* oxygen; *IV,* intravenous.

- **Medical assistance required:** If the reaction is mild, assistance is recommended but not necessary; if, however, the reaction is severe or if an anticonvulsant is administered to terminate the episode, emergency personnel should be sought immediately.

## Epinephrine (Vasoconstrictor) Overdose Reaction

## Precipitating Factors and Prevention

The increasing use of vasoconstrictors in local anesthetic solutions has introduced a potentially new ADR—vasoconstrictor overdose. Although a variety of vasoconstrictors currently are used in dentistry (Table 23-9), the most effective and widely used is epinephrine (Adrenalin). Overdose reactions with drugs other than epinephrine are uncommon because of the lower potencies of the other drugs. These reactions are more likely to occur when greater concentrations of epinephrine are used (Table 23-10).

The optimum concentration of epinephrine for the prolongation of anesthesia with lidocaine is a 1:250,000 dilution.[61] No apparent reason exists for the use of the 1:50,000 dilution so frequently used today for pain control; it contains twice as much epinephrine per milliliter as a 1:100,000 dilution and four times the amount in a 1:200,000 dilution while not providing the anesthetic with any positive attributes. The only benefit of the 1:50,000 concentration of epinephrine over other concentrations is the control of bleeding (hemostasis). However, when used for this purpose, epinephrine must be applied directly at the site where the bleeding occurs or may occur. Only small volumes of the solution are necessary, and only small quantities are feasible in many surgical areas because larger volumes may actually interfere with the procedure. Overdose reactions from this use of 1:50,000 epinephrine are rare.

Another form of epinephrine used in dentistry is more likely to produce an overdose reaction or precipitate other life-threatening situations. Many doctors use racemic epinephrine gingival retraction cord before impressions for crown and bridge procedures are taken. The currently available epinephrine-impregnated retraction cord contains from 310 to

1000 µg of racemic epinephrine per inch of cord.[62] Racemic epinephrine is a combination of the levorotatory and dextrorotatory forms of epinephrine, the latter being about one-twelfth to one-eighteenth as potent as the former.

Because of the high concentration of epinephrine in this preparation, retraction cords are potential dangers to all patients, especially at-risk cardiovascular patients. The gingival epithelium, already disturbed (that is, abraded) by dental procedures such as cavity preparation, absorbs the epinephrine in the retraction cord rapidly, whereas the intact oral epithelium absorbs little of the drug into the systemic circulation. Studies have demonstrated that from 24% to 92% of the applied epinephrine is absorbed into the CVS[62]; the extreme variability is believed to result from the degree of vascular exposure (bleeding) and the length of time of the exposure.

When gingival retraction is necessary, as occurs frequently, other, nonvasoactive retraction materials should be used. Effective hemostatics that do not possess the cardiovascular actions of epinephrine are available and recommended. Commercial preparations of hemostatics that do not contain vasoactive substances include Hemodent and Retreat (containing aluminum chloride); Gingi-Aid Z-Twist, Pascord, R-Cord, Sil-Trax AS (with aluminum sulfate); GingiBraid, GingiKnit, Gingi-Tract, Sil-Trax, Sulpak, Sultan Ultra, and uniBraid (containing potassium aluminum sulfate); and Sultan (containing zinc chloride). The American Dental Association states that "epinephrine cord is contraindicated in patients with a history of cardiovascular diseases, diabetes and hyperthyroidism, and in those taking monoamine-oxidase inhibitors, rauwolfias, and ganglionic blocking agents."[62]

# Clinical Manifestations and Pathophysiology

The clinical manifestations of epinephrine (vasoconstrictor) overdose appear to be similar in many ways to an acute anxiety response. Indeed most signs and

**table 23-9**  *Vasoconstrictors commonly used in dentistry*

| AGENT | AVAILABLE CONCENTRATIONS | MAXIMUM DOSE | LOCAL ANESTHETICS USED WITH AGENT |
|---|---|---|---|
| Epinephrine | 1:50,000 | Healthy adult: 0.2 mg | Lidocaine 2% |
|  | 1:100,000 | Cardiac patient: 0.04 mg | Articaine 4% |
|  |  |  | Lidocaine 2% |
|  | 1:200,000 |  | Articaine 4% |
|  |  |  | Lidocaine 2%* |
|  |  |  | Prilocaine 4% |
| Levonordefrin (Neo-Cobefrin) | 1:20,000 | Healthy adult: 1.00 mg  Cardiac patient: 0.2 mg | Mepivacaine 2% |

*Available in Europe

**table 23-10**  *Dilutions of vasoconstrictors used in dentistry*

| DILUTIONS | AVAILABLE DRUG | MG/ML | MG PER CARTRIDGE (1.8 ML) | MAXIMUM NO. OF CARTRIDGES |
|---|---|---|---|---|
| 1:1000 | Epinephrine (emergency kit) | 1.0 | N/A | Not available in local anesthetic cartridge |
| 1:10,000 | Epinephrine (emergency kit) | 0.1 | N/A | Not available in local anesthetic cartridge |
| 1:20,000 | Levonordefrin | 0.5 | 0.09 | 10 (H), 2 (C) |
| 1:50,000 | Epinephrine | 0.02 | 0.036 | 5 (H), 1 (C) |
| 1:100,000 | Epinephrine | 0.01 | 0.018 | 10 (H), 2 (C) |
| 1:200,000 | Epinephrine | 0.005 | 0.009 | 20 (H), 4 (C) |

*N/A,* Not applicable; *H,* healthy patient; *C,* cardiac patient.

symptoms of the acute anxiety response are produced by the large increase in endogenous catecholamine release (epinephrine and norepinephrine) from the adrenal medulla. As with all drug overdose reactions, clinical signs and symptoms relate to the normal pharmacology of the administered drug (Box 23-7). The patient may voice complaints, such as "My heart is pounding" or "I feel nervous." Signs of epinephrine overdose include a sharp rise in both the blood pressures—especially the systolic—and following heart rate. The rise in blood pressure creates potential hazards, especially when it follows inadvertent intravascular injection. Epinephrine overdose may produce cerebral hemorrhage and cardiac dysrhythmias.

Cases of subarachnoid hemorrhage have been recorded after subcutaneous administration of 0.5 mg epinephrine, and blood pressures of more than 400/300 mm Hg have been recorded for short periods.[63] Epinephrine, a powerful cardiac stimulant, may predispose a patient to ventricular dysrhythmias. The heart rate increases (>140 to 160 beats per minute being common), and the rhythm may be altered. Premature ventricular contractions occur first and are followed by ventricular tachycardia. Ventricular fibrillation may follow and usually is fatal unless immediate recognition and management ensue (see Chapter 30). Patients with preexisting cardiovascular disease are at greater risk for such adverse actions. Increasing the workload of an already impaired cardiovascular system is likely to precipitate an acute exacerbation of the preexisting problem, such as

---

box **23-7** | *Clinical manifestations of epinephrine overdose*

**Signs**
Elevated blood pressure
Elevated heart rate

**Symptoms**
Fear
Anxiety
Tenseness
Restlessness
Throbbing headache
Tremor
Perspiration
Weakness
Dizziness
Pallor
Respiratory difficulty
Palpitations

---

anginal pain, myocardial infarction, heart failure, or cerebrovascular accident.[64,65]

Epinephrine overdose reactions are transitory, the acute phase rarely lasting for more than a few minutes; however, the patient may feel tired and depressed ("washed out") for prolonged periods after the episode. The normally short duration of an epinephrine reaction is related to the body's rapid biotransformation of the drug. The liver produces the enzymes monoamine oxidase and catecholamine-O-methyltransferase necessary for the biotransformation of epinephrine. Patients receiving monoamine-oxidase inhibitors to manage depression cannot eliminate epinephrine from their bodies at the normal rate and are more susceptible to epinephrine overdose.

In addition, drug-drug interactions between epinephrine and noncardioselective β-blockers may create another risky situation for overdose.[66,67] Propranolol (Inderal) is a commonly used example of this group, the reaction being a hypertensive crisis. Both the systolic and the diastolic blood pressures elevate dramatically, with a compensatory decrease in the heart rate (bradycardia). Although usually a dose-related response requires a considerably large dose of epinephrine, it has occurred in individuals who received small doses (for example, 1 or 2 cartridges of local anesthetic with epinephrine 1:100,000).

## Management

Most instances of epinephrine overdose last for such short periods that little or no formal management is necessary. On occasion, however, the reaction may last longer and thus require some action. Management parallels that of a cerebrovascular accident associated with markedly elevated blood pressure (see Chapter 19).

The following signs and symptoms provide diagnostic clues to the presence of an overdose of vasoconstrictor:

- Increased anxiety after injection
- Tremor of limbs
- Diaphoresis (sweating)
- Headache
- Florid appearance
- Possible increased or decreased heart rate (tachycardia [palpitation] and bradycardia, respectively)
- Elevated blood pressure

*Step 1: termination of the procedure.* As soon as clinical manifestations of overdose appear, the procedure should be halted and the source of epinephrine removed. Obviously, removal is impossible after injection of a local anesthetic; however, gingival retraction cord should be removed immediately.

*Step 2:* **P** *(position).* The conscious patient should be positioned comfortably (patient determining the position). However, the supine position is not recommended because it accentuates the cardiovascular effects of epinephrine, particularly increased cerebral blood flow. A semiseated or upright position minimizes the elevation in cerebral blood pressure to a slight degree.

*Step 3:* **A-B-C** *(airway, breathing, circulation) (BLS), as needed.* The patient's airway, breathing, and circulation should be assessed and implemented, as needed. Assessment demonstrates a patient who is conscious with a patent airway and adequate circulation.

### Step 4: **D** *(definitive care):*

*Step 4a: reassurance of the patient.* Patients experiencing this reaction usually demonstrate increased anxiety and restlessness accompanied by other signs and symptoms, such as palpitation and respiratory distress, which increase apprehension further and may exacerbate the clinical problem. The doctor should attempt to reassure these patients.

*Step 4b: monitoring of vital signs.* The patient's blood pressure and heart rate should be monitored and recorded every 5 minutes during the episode. Striking elevations may be noted in both, but they should decline gradually toward baseline levels over time. This statement is especially true when the epinephrine-impregnated retraction cord has been applied and removed from the gingival tissues.

*Step 4c: summoning of medical assistance.* When a patient exhibits a markedly elevated blood pressure and heart rate and signs and symptoms associated with cerebrovascular problems (for example, headache and flushing), medical assistance should be sought immediately.

*Step 4d: administration of $O_2$.* If necessary $O_2$ may be administered. If the patient complains of difficulty in breathing, a nasal cannula, nasal hood, or full-face mask should be used.

*Step 4e: recovery.* Vital signs gradually return to baseline levels. The patient's blood pressure and heart rate should be monitored and recorded every 5 minutes during this time, and the patient should remain seated in the dental chair for as long as necessary after the episode. Patients invariably feel fatigued and depressed for considerable lengths of time after epinephrine overdose.

*Step 4f: administration of a vasodilator (optional).* If the patient's blood pressure does not begin to return toward the baseline level, administration of a drug designed to lower blood pressure may become necessary. Nitroglycerin, available in the office emergency drug kit, is a potent vasodilator used primarily in the management of anginal pain. However, a side effect of the drug is postural hypotension; the administration of a dose (2 sprays transligually) to a patient who is seated upright takes advantage of this fact. The blood pressure should be monitored continually at this time.

*Step 5: discharge.* When emergency personnel arrive, they can more completely evaluate the patient's cardiovascular status through use of an electrocardiogram. When blood pressure is still considerably elevated, IV antihypertensive drugs, such as labetalol or atenolol, may be administered. A decision is then made as to the patient's disposition after consultation with the emergency medical team, dentist, and emergency room physicians. In most situations in which the intensity of cardiovascular symptoms and signs was not great, the patient will not require hospitalization. However, when signs and symptoms of cardiovascular stimulation persist, a period of hospitalization for evaluation will be recommended.

Box 23-8 outlines the steps in the protocol for the management of an epinephrine overdose.

- **Drugs used in management:** $O_2$ is used to manage this reaction.
- **Medical assistance required:** If the reaction is minor, no assistance is necessary. If, however, the reaction proves severe, emergency personnel should be summoned.

## Central Nervous System Depressant Overdose Reactions

Whenever CNS depressant drugs are administered, the possibility exists that an exaggerated degree of CNS depression may develop. Clinically, this reaction may be noted in a range from slight oversedation to unconsciousness and respiratory arrest. Many experts believe that barbiturates are the most likely drug group to produce an overdose.[68] The barbiturates

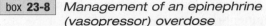

box **23-8**    *Management of an epinephrine (vasopressor) overdose*

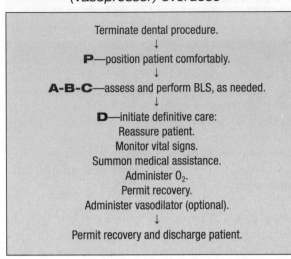

Terminate dental procedure.
↓
**P**—position patient comfortably.
↓
**A-B-C**—assess and perform BLS, as needed.
↓
**D**—initiate definitive care:
Reassure patient.
Monitor vital signs.
Summon medical assistance.
Administer O₂.
Permit recovery.
Administer vasodilator (optional).
↓
Permit recovery and discharge patient.

**P,** Position; **A,** airway; **B,** breathing; **C,** circulation; **D,** definitive care; *BLS,* basic life support; *O₂,* oxygen.

represented the first major breakthrough in drug management of anxiety, and because of this, many associated ADRs, such as allergy, addiction, and overdose, were tolerated. However, with the introduction of newer antianxiety drugs, such as benzodiazepines, that do not possess the same potential for abuse and overdose, barbiturate use has declined.[68]

Although the barbiturates possess the greatest potential for ADR, opioid agonist analgesics are responsible for a greater number of clinically significant episodes of overdose and respiratory depression in dentistry. This is simply because opioids are used today to a much greater extent than barbiturates. The administration of opioids is popular in the management of uncooperative or precooperative pediatric patients.[69] In addition, opioids are often used IV in conjunction with other sedative drugs to help achieve sedation and pain control in fearful patients. Goodson and Moore[70] reported 14 cases in pediatric dentistry in which the administration of opioids and other drugs led to 7 deaths and 3 cases of brain damage. Several opioids were implicated in these reactions—alphaprodine (7 cases), meperidine (6 cases), and pentazocine (1 case).

## Predisposing Factors and Prevention

Because barbiturates and opioids are used commonly in the preoperative management of anxiety, they are most often administered orally or IM. The clinical efficacy of a drug depends in large part on its absorption into the cardiovascular system and its subsequent blood level in different organs of the body. In the case of CNS depressants the brain is the target organ. Only the inhalation and IV routes of drug administration, with their rapid onsets of action, permit titration of the drug to a precise clinical effect.[71] Drug absorption via oral and IM administration is erratic, demonstrated by a wide range of variability in clinical effectiveness.

The normal distribution curve becomes important when drugs are administered via routes in which titration is not possible. Average drug doses are based on this curve. For example, an oral dose of 100 mg secobarbital, or 5 mg diazepam, produces a desired effect (drowsiness for secobarbital; anxiolysis for diazepam) in the majority of patients (about 70%). For some patients (about 15%), however, these doses are ineffective. Such individuals require larger doses to attain the same clinical level of sedation. Patients like this, termed *hyporesponders,* are not at risk for overdose when they receive average doses because the clinical result of their condition is a lack of adequate sedation. The potential danger in the use of drugs lies with the remaining 15% of patients for whom average doses of secobarbital or diazepam are too great. These individuals are sensitive (a term that differs in meaning greatly with the term *allergy*) to the drug, requiring smaller doses to obtain clinically effective sedation and are known as *hyperresponders.*

Normally, predicting a patient's response to a drug is impossible; only a previous history of an ADR can provide a clue. The medical history questionnaire should be examined carefully regarding all drug reactions. If the patient reports a history of drug sensitivity, great care must be exercised whenever the administration of a CNS depressant, especially a barbiturate or opioid, is considered. The administration of lower-than-usual doses or the substitution of different drug categories, such as nonbarbiturate sedative-hypnotics, benzodiazepines, and opioid agonist/antagonist, should be considered.

Although the nature of the overdose cannot be predicted easily in advance, one method through which overdose reactions may occur is preventable; it relates to the clinical goal that the doctor seeks through drug administration. Some doctors use barbiturates or opioids to achieve deep levels of sedation in fearful patients. When these drugs are administered for this purpose via oral or IM routes, the potential for overdose increases. Most doctors who use barbiturates for sedation have encountered patients who became uncooperative (less inhibited) after receiving these drugs. Because of the difficulty en-

| table 23-11 | *Routes of drug administration* |

| ROUTE OF ADMINISTRATION | CONTROL | | RECOMMENDED SAFE SEDATIVE LEVELS |
| | TITRATION | RAPID REVERSAL | |
| --- | --- | --- | --- |
| Oral | No | No | Light only |
| Rectal | No | No | Light only |
| IM | No | No | Adults: light, moderate |
| | | | Children: light, moderate, deep |
| IV | Yes | No (most drugs) | Adults and children: light, moderate, deep* |
| | | Yes (opiods, benzodiazepines) | |
| Inhalation | Yes | Yes | Any sedation level |

*IM,* Intramuscular; *IV,* intravenous.
*Usually, little need exists for IV sedation in normal, healthy children. Most children who can tolerate venipuncture can also receive intraorally administered local anesthetics. IV sedation, however, remains important in the management of disabled children and adults.

countered in attempts to manage this patient, the planned dental treatment could not be completed. Larger doses of barbiturates administered to an anxious patient to produce deep levels of sedation result in even greater degrees of CNS depression accompanied by respiratory depression and the possible loss of consciousness.

Therefore the use of a CNS depressant to obtain deep sedation via a route of administration in which titration is not possible is an invitation to overdose and cannot be recommended. Only those techniques that permit titration—IV and inhalation—can be safely employed to achieve deeper levels of sedation, and then only when the doctor is thoroughly familiar with both the technique of administration and the drugs to be administered and is prepared to manage all possible complications associated with the procedure. One point worth stressing, however, is that absorption of drugs administered via inhalation and IV sedation into the systemic circulation occurs rapidly so that drug responses, both therapeutic and adverse, may occur suddenly. Therefore titration remains the greatest safety feature that these techniques possess (Table 23-11).

# Clinical Manifestations

## BARBITURATE AND NONBARBITURATE SEDATIVE-HYPNOTICS

Barbiturates depress a number of physiologic properties, including nerve tissue; respiration; and skeletal, smooth, and cardiac muscle. The mechanism of action (sedation and hypnosis) is depression at the level of the hypothalamus and ascending reticular activating system, which decreases the transmission of impulses to the cerebral cortex. Further increases of barbiturates in the blood level of barbiturates produce depression at other CNS levels, including profound cortical depression, depression of motor function, and depression of the medulla.[72] The following diagram illustrates this decline:

Sedation (calming) → hypnosis (sleep) → general anesthesia (unconsciousness with progressive respiratory and cardiovascular depression) → respiratory arrest

**Sedation and oversedation**   At low (therapeutic) blood levels, the patient appears calm and cooperative (sedated). As the barbiturate blood level increases, the patient begins to fall into a rousable sleep (hypnosis). The doctor then notices the patient's inability to keep the mouth open in spite of constant reminders. In addition, patients at this level of barbiturate-induced CNS depression tend to overrespond to stimulation, especially noxious stimulation. The unsedated adult patient may grimace in response to pain, but the oversedated (with barbiturates) adult exhibits an exaggerated response, perhaps yelling or jumping. This reflects the loss of self-control over emotion produced by the generalized CNS-depressant action of the barbiturate.[72]

**Hypnosis**   As the barbiturate blood level continues to increase, hypnosis (sleep) ensues and the patient experiences a minor depression of respiratory function (decreased depth and increased rate of ventilation). This barbiturate blood level produces virtually no adverse action on the cardiovascular system, only a slight decrease in blood pressure and heart rate similar to that of normal sleep. However, dental treatment cannot be continued at this level of CNS depression because the patient cannot cooperate in keeping the mouth open and may require assistance in the maintenance of a patent airway (for example, the head-tilt method). The patient can still respond to noxious stimulation but in a sluggish, but still exaggerated manner.

**General anesthesia**   A further increase in barbiturate blood level broadens the degree of CNS depression to the point at which the patient loses consciousness (that is, is incapable of responding to sensory stimulation, loses protective reflexes, and cannot maintain a patent airway). Spontaneous respiratory movements remain; however, further increases in barbiturate blood levels result in medullary depression, clinically evident as respiratory and cardiovascular depression. Respiratory depression is clinically evident as shallow breathing movements at slow or more commonly rapid rates. Expansive movements of the chest do not guarantee that air is entering or leaving the lungs, only that the patient is attempting to bring air into the lungs. Airway obstruction may occur as the muscular tongue relaxes and falls into the hypopharynx.

Cardiovascular depression is notable as a continued decrease in blood pressure, caused by medullary depression, direct depression of the myocardium and vascular smooth muscle, and an increased heart rate. The patient develops a shocklike appearance, with a weak and rapid pulse and cold, moist skin.

**Respiratory arrest**   If the barbiturate blood level continues to increase or the patient does not receive adequate treatment in the general anesthesia stage, respiratory arrest may occur. This condition can be diagnosed readily and managed through assessment of the airway and breathing. However, delays in management or inadequate management will cause the condition to progress to cardiac arrest.

Other nonbarbiturate sedative-hypnotic drugs, such as hydroxyzine, chloral hydrate, and promethazine, also possess the potential to produce overdose; however, overdoses are not as likely to occur as with the barbiturates.[73,74] The potential for overdose varies significantly from drug to drug, but all sedative-hypnotics harbor this potential to some degree.

## OPIOID AGONISTS

Meperidine, morphine, and fentanyl (and its congeners alfentanil, sufentanil, and remifentanil) are the most frequently used parenteral opioids. Meperidine and fentanyl are the most popular in dentistry. For many years alphaprodine (Nisentil), because of its rapid onset and short duration of action, was extremely popular as a sedative in pediatric dentistry. However, alphaprodine no longer is marketed in the United States; it was withdrawn in 1986 after reports surfaced of fatalities associated with its administration during dental treatment.[70,75-77]

Meperidine, like most opioid agonists, exerts its primary pharmacologic actions on the CNS. Therapeutic doses of meperidine produce analgesia, sedation, euphoria, and a degree of respiratory depression. Of principle concern is the respiratory depressant effect of opioid agonists; these drugs directly depress the medullary respiratory center. Individuals demonstrate respiratory depression from opioid agonists even at doses that do not disturb the level of consciousness. The degree of respiratory depression produced by opioids is dose dependent—the greater the dose of the drug, the more significant the level of respiratory depression.[71] The newer opioid agonist/antagonist—nalbuphine and butorphanol—offer the prospects of analgesia and sedation with minimal respiratory depression.[78,79]

Death from opioid overdose almost always is the result of respiratory arrest.[80] All phases of respiration are depressed—rate, minute volume, and tidal volume.[81] Respiratory rate may fall below 10 breaths per minute; rates of 5 to 6 breaths per minute are common. The cause of the decreased respiratory activity is a reduction in the responsiveness of the medullary respiratory centers to increases in $PaCO_2$ and a depression of the pontine and medullary centers responsible for respiratory rhythm.[80]

The cardiovascular effects of meperidine are not clinically significant when the drug is administered within the usual therapeutic dose range. After IV administration of meperidine, however, the heart rate normally increases, produced by the atropine-like, vagolytic properties of meperidine. At overdose levels the blood pressure remains stable until late in the course of the reaction, when it drops, primarily as a result of hypoxia. At this point the administration of $O_2$ will produce an increase in blood pressure despite continued medullary depression. Overly high blood levels of opioid agonists may lead to the loss of consciousness (general anesthesia).

Overdose reactions to both the sedative-hypnotic drugs and opioid agonists are produced by a progressive depression of the central nervous system that is manifested by alterations in the level of consciousness and as respiratory distress that ends, ultimately, in respiratory arrest. The loss of consciousness produced by barbiturates or opioid agonists is not always due to overdose; in other words, loss of consciousness is sometimes desirable. For example, these drugs are administered commonly as the primary agents in general anesthesia. However, when sedation is the goal, the loss of consciousness and respiratory depression must be considered to be serious, though not always preventable, complications of drug administration.

The duration and degree of this clinical reaction varies according to the route of administration, the dose, and the patient's individual sensitivity to the drug. In most situations oral and rectal administration result in less CNS depression; however, this depression tends to last longer. IM and submucosal administration result in more profound levels of CNS depression that last relatively long periods of time, whereas IV administration produces a rapid onset of a profound level of depression that lasts for a shorter period than the levels produced by other routes. The onset of respiratory depression after IV administration may be rapid, whereas the level after oral or rectal administration is slower. Onset is intermediate for IM and subcutaneous drug administration.

## Management

### SEDATIVE-HYPNOTIC DRUGS

Management of an overdose to sedative-hypnotic drugs is predicated on correction of the clinical manifestations of CNS depression. Of primary importance is the management of respiratory depression through the administration of BLS. Unfortunately, no effective antagonist exists to reverse the CNS-depressant properties of the barbiturate sedative-hypnotics. Benzodiazepines, however, can be reversed through administration of flumazenil.

Diagnostic clues to an overdose of a sedative-hypnotic drug include the following[82]:

- Recent administration of sedative-hypnotic drug
- Decreased level of consciousness

Sleepy → unconscious

- Respiratory depression (rapid rate, shallow depth)
- Loss of motor coordination (ataxia)
- Slurred speech

*Step 1: termination of the dental procedure.* The rate at which clinical signs and symptoms of overdose develop varies with route of administration. Onset occurs within minutes after IV administration; within 10 to 30 minutes after IM administration; and within 45 minutes to 1 hour after oral administration.

*Step 2:* **P** *(position).* The semiconscious or unconscious patient should be placed in the supine position with the legs elevated slightly (Figure 23-7). The goal in this situation, regardless of the level of consciousness, is the maintenance of adequate cerebral blood flow.

*Step 3:* **A-B-C** *(airway, breathing, circulation), (BLS), as needed.* A patent airway must be ensured and the adequacy of breathing assessed. Head–tilt or head tilt–chin lift may be required to maintain airway patency (Figure 23-8). The rescuer must next assess the presence or adequacy of the patient's spontaneous ventilatory efforts by placing the ear 1 inch from the patient's mouth and nose and listening and feeling for exhaled air while looking at the patient's chest to determine whether spontaneous respiratory efforts are present. Maintenance of a patent airway is the most important step in management of this patient. Step 4b, the provision of adequate oxygenation, is contingent on successful maintenance of a patent airway.

*Step 4:* **D** *(definitive care):*

*Step 4a: summoning of medical assistance, if needed.* In a situation in which the patient loses consciousness after the administration of a barbiturate, medical assistance should be sought immediately. The requirement for medical assistance varies, depending upon the doctor's training in airway management and anesthesiology. When the patient remains conscious but overly sedated, seeking medical assistance is more of a judgment call by the doctor. When in doubt it is always wiser to seek assistance sooner rather than later.

*Step 4b: administration of $O_2$.* The patient may exhibit different types of breathing. They may be conscious but overly sedated, responding slowly to painful stimuli. In this situation the patient most likely can maintain the airway and breathe spontaneously and somewhat effectively. The rescuer need only monitor the patient, assist with airway maintenance (for example, the head tilt–chin lift procedure) and administer $O_2$ through a demand valve or nasal cannula, if desired.

However, the patient may be more deeply sedated and barely responsive to stimulation, with a partially or totally obstructed airway. In this situation assisted ventilation is essential in addition to airway maintenance. With airway patency ensured, the patient should receive $O_2$ via full-face mask. If spontaneous breathing is present but shallow, assisted positive-pressure ventilation is indicated. Such ventilation is accomplished through activation of the positive-pressure

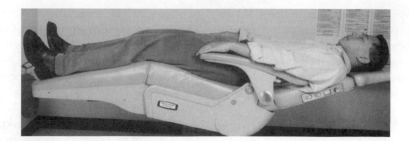

**Figure 23-7**   The unconscious patient should be placed in the supine position with the legs elevated slightly.

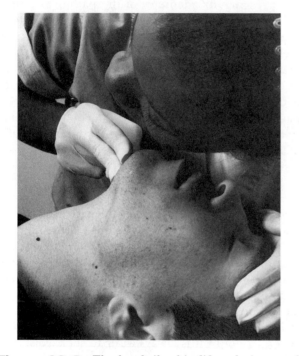

**Figure 23-8**   The head tilt–chin lift technique and "Look-listen-feel."

mask just as the patient begins each respiratory movement (as the chest begins to expand). The positive-pressure mask is activated by pressing the button on top of the mask until the patient's chest rises, at which point the button is released (Figure 23-9). When a self-inflating bag-valve-mask device is used, the bellows bag is squeezed at the start of each inhalation. An air-tight seal and head tilt must be maintained at all times when either device is used.

If respiratory arrest has occurred, controlled artificial ventilation must be started immediately. The recommended rate for the adult is one breath every 5 seconds (12 per minute). For the child 1 to 8 years and the infant, one breath every 3 seconds (20 per minute) is recommended.[83] Expansion of the patient's chest with every ventilation is the only sure

sign of a successful ventilation. Overinflation is to be avoided because this leads to abdominal distention, resulting in inadequate ventilation and increased risk of regurgitation.

*Step 4c: monitoring of vital signs.* The patient's vital signs must be monitored throughout the episode. A member of the office emergency team should monitor and record the blood pressure, heart rate and rhythm, and respiratory rate every 5 minutes. If the blood level of the sedative-hypnotic drug increases significantly, the blood pressure decreases as the heart rate increases.[84] If the blood pressure and pulse disappear, cardiopulmonary resuscitation **(P+A+B+C)** must be instituted immediately.

In most cases of barbiturate or nonbarbiturate sedative-hypnotic drug overdose, the patient can be maintained in this manner until the cerebral blood level of the drug decreases and the patient recovers consciousness or emergency assistance arrives. Recovery occurs as a result of redistribution of the drug within compartments in the body, not because of biotransformation. The patient appears more alert and responsive, breathing improves (becomes deeper), and the blood pressure returns to near baseline levels. The length of time for recovery depends on the drug administered (short acting versus long acting) and its route of administration.

*Step 4d: establishment of an IV line, if possible.* If an IV infusion has not previously been established, one should be set up at this time if proper training and equipment are available. Although no effective antidotal drugs exist for sedative-hypnotic drug overdoses, hypotension may be treated effectively through intravenously administered fluids or drugs. As blood pressure decreases, however, veins become progressively more difficult to locate and cannulate. Establishing venous access at the earliest possible time may prove invaluable later.

Only the doctor who possesses the necessary training and equipment and can ensure that the patient continues to receive adequate care from other per-

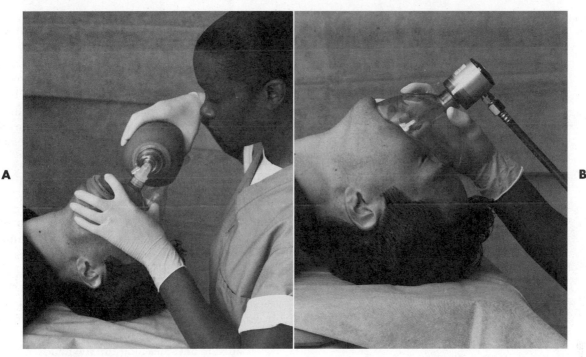

**Figure 23-9**    The use of positive-pressure ventilation. **A,** bag-valve-mask; **B,** positive-pressure oxygen.

sonnel should attempt venipuncture. *A patent airway is more important than a patent vein.*

*Step 4e: definitive management.* Definitive management of sedative-hypnotic overdose produced by a barbiturate is based on maintenance of a patent airway and adequacy of ventilation until the patient recovers. Signs and symptoms of hypotension are checked by monitoring vital signs and determining the adequacy of tissue perfusion.*

The IV administration of flumazenil, a specific benzodiazepine antagonist, will reverse benzodiazepine overdose. Flumazenil is administered IV in a 0.2 mg-dose over 15 seconds, then waiting 45 seconds to evaluate recovery. If recovery is not adequate at 1 minute, an additional dose of 0.2 mg may be administered. This is repeated every 5 minutes until recovery occurs or a dose of 1.0 mg is administered.[85]

*Step 5: recovery and discharge.* If the overdose is profound and requires the assistance of emergency personnel, the patient may require stabilization and transportation to a hospital for observation and full recovery. If hospitalization is necessary, the doctor always should accompany the patient to the hospital.

Box 23-9 outlines the steps in the management of sedative-hypnotic overdose.

- **Drugs used in management:** $O_2$, flumazenil— for benzodiazepine overdose.
- **Medical assistance required:** If the patient's level of consciousness is altered, the training and experience of the doctor dictates the need for assistance. If the patient is unconscious, assistance should be sought.

In most cases, however, sedative-hypnotic overdose is significantly less severe, with diminished responsiveness and minimal respiratory depression. Management consists of positioning, airway maintenance, and assisted ventilation until the individual recovers. Emergency medical assistance is usually not required. Before being discharged into the custody of a responsible adult, the patient must be able to stand and walk without assistance. Under no circumstances should the patient be discharged alone or before adequate recovery has occurred.

## OPIOID ANALGESICS

Oversedation and respiratory depression are the primary clinical manifestations of opioid overdose.

---

*Adequacy of tissue perfusion may be determined by pressing on a nail-bed or skin and releasing pressure. Adequate perfusion is present when color returns in not more than 3 seconds. If 4 or more seconds are required, tissue perfusion is inadequate and consideration must be given to the immediate infusion of intravenous fluids.

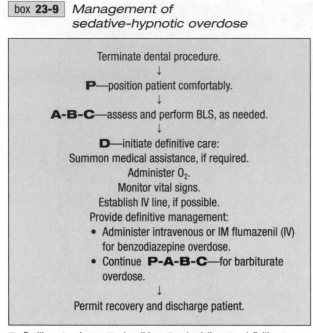

box **23-9**  *Management of
sedative-hypnotic overdose*

Terminate dental procedure.
↓
**P**—position patient comfortably.
↓
**A-B-C**—assess and perform BLS, as needed.
↓
**D**—initiate definitive care:
Summon medical assistance, if required.
Administer O₂.
Monitor vital signs.
Establish IV line, if possible.
Provide definitive management:
- Administer intravenous or IM flumazenil (IV) for benzodiazepine overdose.
- Continue **P-A-B-C**—for barbiturate overdose.
↓
Permit recovery and discharge patient.

**P,** Position; **A,** airway; **B,** breathing; **C,** circulation; **D,** definitive care; *BLS,* basic life support; *O₂,* oxygen; *IV,* intravenous.

Cardiovascular depression normally does not develop until late in the overdose reaction, especially in a supine patient. Management of the patient who has received an absolute or relative overdose of an opioid is the same as that described for the sedative-hypnotic drugs with one major addition—specific antagonists are available that reverse the clinical actions of opioid agonists. The clinical picture may vary from minor alterations in consciousness with minimal respiratory depression to unconsciousness and apnea.

Diagnostic clues to the presence of an opioid overdose include the following[82]:

- Altered level of consciousness
- Respiratory depression (slow rate; normal to deep depth)
- Miosis (contraction of pupils of the eyes)

*Step 1: termination of the dental procedure.*

*Step 2:* **P** *(position).* The patient should be placed in the supine position with the legs elevated slightly.

*Step 3:* **A-B-C** *(airway, breathing, circulation), (BLS), as needed.* A patent airway must be ensured and breathing monitored. Opioids produce decreased rates of respiration with little change in tidal volume, therefore the depth of ventilation is increased.[81]

In most cases of opioid overdose the patient remains conscious though not fully alert and responsive.

Assistance in airway maintenance may be desirable (for example, the head tilt–chin lift technique). When more profound depression is present, unconsciousness and respiratory arrest may occur, necessitating assessment of the airway and breathing. Because the cardiovascular system is relatively unaffected by opioid overdose, the blood pressure and heart rate will remain close to baseline values if the patient receives adequate oxygenation (especially if the patient remains in the supine position).[86]

*Step 4:* **D** *(definitive care):*

*Step 4a: summoning of medical assistance, if needed.* Depending on the level of consciousness, the degree of respiratory depression, the training of the doctor in emergency care and anesthesiology, and the availability of equipment and drugs, the summoning of emergency medical assistance may be indicated at this time. When the patient is unconscious and in respiratory arrest, emergency medical assistance should be summoned immediately if the doctor is not well trained in anesthesiology. In the hands of a doctor well trained in emergency care and anesthesiology (for example, general anesthesia), management may continue to include the administration of antidotal drugs.

*Step 4b: administration of O₂.* O₂ and/or artificial ventilation should be administered, if necessary. The administration of O₂ is especially important in the early management of opioid overdose. Minimal cardiovascular depression is normally present and, when present, occurs as a result of hypoxia secondary to respiratory depression. The administration of O₂ to a patient with a patent airway prevents or reverses opioid-induced cardiovascular depression.[87]

*Step 4c: monitoring and recording of vital signs.* Vital signs should be monitored every 5 minutes and entered on a record sheet. If the pulse and blood pressure are absent, cardiopulmonary resuscitation **(P+A+B+C)** must be initiated immediately.

*Step 4d: establishment of an IV line, if possible.* Because the cardiovascular system is minimally affected by opioid overdose (with the patient in the supine position), the establishment of an IV infusion is possible in most patients. The availability of an IV access expedites definitive therapy.

*Step 4e: antidotal drug administration.* Definitive management is available when an opioid is the likely cause of the overdose. Even when what normally is considered a small opioid dose is administered (in a hyperresponding patient), an opioid antagonist should be administered if excessive respiratory depression or apnea develops. However, no drug should be administered until airway patency and adequate ventilation are ensured and vital signs monitored **(P, A, B, C).**

At this time an opioid antagonist should be administered. The drug of choice, naloxone, should be administered via an IV route, if possible, to take advantage of the more rapid onset of action.

If the IV route is unavailable, IM administration is acceptable. The onset of action is slower, but naloxone will be just as effective if an opioid is responsible for the respiratory depression. Regardless of the route of administration, the emergency team must continue to provide the necessary steps of BLS from the time of naloxone administration until its onset of action, a point that becomes evident through increased patient responsiveness and more adequate and rapid ventilatory efforts. After IV administration, naloxone begins to work within 1 to 2 minutes (if not faster), and within 10 minutes after IM administration if the blood pressure is near its baseline value.

Naloxone is available in a 1-ml ampule containing 0.4 mg (adult) and 0.02 mg (pediatric). The drug is loaded into a plastic disposable syringe, and when the IV route is available, 3 ml of diluent (any IV fluid) is added to the syringe, producing a final concentration of 0.1 mg/ml of naloxone (adult) or 0.005 mg/mL (pediatric). The drug then is administered via an IV route to the adult at a rate of 1 ml per minute until the ventilatory rate and alertness increase. In children the IV dose is 0.01 mg/kg.[88] If administered via the IM route, a dose of 0.4 mg (adult) or 0.01 mg/kg (pediatric) is injected into a suitable muscle mass, such as the middeltoid (adult) or vastus lateralis (child or adult); if the patient is unconscious, the drug may also be administered sublingually.

One potential problem with naloxone is that its duration of clinical activity may be shorter than that of the opioid it is used to reverse. This fact is especially true in cases in which longer-acting opioid agonists, such as morphine, are administered; it is less likely to occur with meperidine and even less likely with fentanyl and its anologues alfentanil,[89] sufentanil,[90] and remifentanil.[91] When the opioid action is of greater duration than the naloxone administered via an IV route, the doctor and staff would notice an initial improvement in the patient's clinical picture as the naloxone begins to act and then see a recurrence of CNS depression approximately 10 or more minutes later, (after IV administration of naloxone). Because the opioid producing the overdose continues to undergo redistribution and biotransformation during this time, if such a rebound effect does occur, the effect is more likely to be much less intense than the initial response.

In cases in which longer-acting opioids, such as morphine, are administered via an IM or submucosal route, the initial IV dose of naloxone should be followed with an IM dose (0.4 mg [adult] or 0.01 mg/kg [pediatric]). In this way, as the clinical action of the IV naloxone dose wanes, the level of naloxone from the IM dose reaches a peak, minimizing the likelihood of a relapse of significant respiratory or CNS depression. The availability of naltrexone, a longer-acting opioid antagonist, further minimizes the risk of relapse. The administration of naloxone in opioid overdose is important but not the most critical step in overall patient management.

*Step 5: permit recovery.* The patient is continuously observed and monitored after naloxone administration. The patient may be transported to a recovery area within the dental office but should remain under constant supervision for at least 1 hour. On the other hand, the planned dental treatment may continue if the doctor deems it safe. Once again, whether to continue dental care is a judgment that can only be made by the doctor after both the status of the patient and the level of expertise of the doctor and staff in recognizing and managing this problem are considered. If any doubt exists, treatment should not continue. Vital signs should be recorded every 5 minutes during the recovery period; $O_2$ and suction must be available; and trained personnel must be present.

*Step 6: discharge.* Patient discharge may require transport to a hospital facility for observation or follow-up care. Usually, hospitalization is unnecessary. After an adequate period of recovery (minimum of 1 hour observation) in the dental or medical office, the patient may be discharged into the custody of a responsible adult companion through use of the same recovery criteria established for parenteral sedation and general anesthesia.[71]

Box 23-10 outlines the steps to follow in management of opioid overdose.

- **Drugs used in management:** $O_2$ and naloxone are used to manage opioid overdose.
- **Medical assistance required:** In cases in which the patient's level of consciousness is altered or is unconscious, the doctor's training and expertise should determine whether emergency personnel are necessary.

## Summary

The previous discussions dealt with overdose reactions of varying degrees of severity that occur after the administration of a single drug. Although single-drug overdose can and does occur, especially after IM or submucosal administration (for example, because of the inability to titrate to effect), a majority of overdose reactions involve the administration of more than one drug. In many of these cases, for example, an antianxiety drug may be combined with an opioid to provide a level of sedation and some analgesia. To these, a local anesthetic is added for pain control. Drugs in all three categories are CNS depressants. Added to this combination, in many cases, is nitrous oxide and $O_2$, yet another CNS depressant.

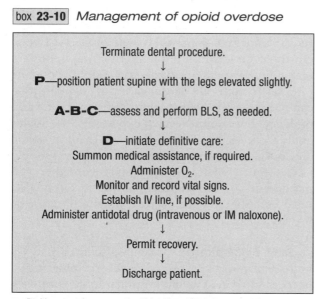

box **23-10**    *Management of opioid overdose*

Terminate dental procedure.
↓
**P**—position patient supine with the legs elevated slightly.
↓
**A-B-C**—assess and perform BLS, as needed.
↓
**D**—initiate definitive care:
Summon medical assistance, if required.
Administer $O_2$.
Monitor and record vital signs.
Establish IV line, if possible.
Administer antidotal drug (intravenous or IM naloxone).
↓
Permit recovery.
↓
Discharge patient.

**P**, Position; **A**, airway; **B**, breathing; **C**, circulation; **D**, definitive care; *BLS*, basic life support; $O_2$, oxygen; *IV*, intravenous.

Whenever more than one CNS-depressant drug is administered, the doses of both drugs must be reduced to prevent exaggerated, undesirable clinical responses. As Table 23-12 illustrates, most of the cases reported by Goodson and Moore[70] did not take this step, with disastrous consequences.

Another factor must be considered, one to which most health professionals do not, as a rule, give much thought in the use of sedative techniques. Local anesthetics themselves are CNS depressants and may produce additive actions when administered in conjunction with the drugs commonly used for sedation. The maximum dose of local anesthetic administered to any patient, but especially to a child or lighter-weight or older adult, should be based on body weight in kilograms or pounds. When no other CNS depressants are administered, this maximum dose may usually be administered without adverse effects if the patient is an ASA I and falls within the normal responding range on the bell-shaped curve. Table 23-13 lists the maximum recommended doses of the most commonly used local anesthetics. When administered in conjunction with other CNS depressants, the dose of the local anesthetic should be minimized.

Ensuring a cooperative patient who still maintains the protective reflexes (for example, swallowing, coughing, and maintaining the airway) is the primary goal of sedation. Whenever possible, this goal should be achieved through use of the simplest technique available and the fewest number of drugs possible. Polypharmacy, the combination of several drugs, is necessary in many patients to achieve the desired

table **23-12**    *Dose administered relative to recommended maximum dose*

| CASE | OPIOID ANALGESICS (%)* | ANTIMETIC SEDATIVES (%)* | LOCAL ANESTHETICS | | |
|------|------------------------|--------------------------|-------------------|--------|--------|
| | | | %* | $N_2O$-$O_2$ | RESULT |
| 1 | 216 | 36 | 172 | — | Fatality |
| 2 | 173 | 145 | 237 | — | Fatality |
| 3 | 336 | 0 | 342 | — | Fatality |
| 4 | 127 | 27 | 267 | + | Fatality |
| 5 | 309 | 372 | 230 | + | Brain damage |
| 6 | 436 | ? | ? | — | Fatality |
| 7 | 100 | 136 | 107 | — | Fatality |
| 8 | 167 | 300 | 219 | + | Brain damage |
| 9 | 66 | 0 | 60 | — | Recovery |
| 10 | 66 | 92 | ? | + | Recovery |
| 11 | 183 | 0 | ? | — | Recovery |
| 12 | 200 | 558 | 0 | — | Recovery |
| 13 | 250 | 136 | 127 | — | Brain damage |
| 14 | 50 | 0 | 370 | + | Fatality |

From Goodsen JM, Moore PA: *J Am Dent Assoc* 107:239, 1983.
*Expressed as percentage of maximal recommended dose for that patient.

level of sedation or analgesia; however, if reaching this desired effect is possible with one drug, the combination should not be used. The use of drug combinations simply increases the opportunity for ADRs as well as making it less obvious which drug may be responsible for the problem, thereby making management more difficult.

Single-drug regimens are preferable to combinations of drugs. Rational drug combinations are available for use in cases in which they are specifically indicated. Severe ADRs should not develop after IV drug administration if the technique of titration is strictly adhered to at all times. Titration is not possible with the IM and oral routes of administration, and the doctor must modify individual drug doses prior to their administration. Serious ADRs are more likely to occur in techniques where titration is not possible.

Consideration also must be given to the use of multiple techniques of sedation, as opposed to multiple drugs via one technique of administration. During the course of treatment a hard-to-manage patient may receive oral antianxiety drugs for pretreatment, followed by IM, submucosal or IV sedation as well as inhalation sedation and local anesthesia during the course of treatment. Whenever oral sedation with CNS depressants has been used, the doses of all subsequent CNS depressants should be carefully evaluated before their administration. This step is critical when either the IM or submucosal routes are used because they do not permit titration. With inhalation and IV sedation, careful titration of CNS-depressant drugs to the patient who has previously received oral premedication usually produces the desired level of clinical sedation with a minimal risk of ADRs.

How, then, may overdose reactions best be prevented? Goodson and Moore[70] made the following recommendations on the use of sedative techniques in which opioids are being administered:

table **23-13**   *Maximum recommended doses of local anesthetics*

| DRUG | DOSE | | ABSOLUTE MAXIMUM DOSE |
|---|---|---|---|
| | **MG/KG** | **MG/LB** | |
| Articaine | 7.0 | 3.2 | 500 |
| Lidocaine | 4.4 | 2.0 | 300 |
| Mepivacaine | 4.4 | 2.0 | 300 |
| Prilocaine | 6.0 | 2.7 | 400 |
| Bupivacaine | 2.0 | 0.9 | 90 |
| Etidocaine | 8.0 | 3.6 | 400 |

- Be prepared for emergencies. Continuous monitoring of the cardiovascular and respiratory systems is necessary. An emergency kit containing epinephrine, $O_2$, naloxone, and flumozenil should be readily available, as should equipment and trained personnel. In their article Goodson and Moore[70] state that "because multiple sedative drug techniques can easily induce unconsciousness, respiratory arrest, and convulsions, practitioners should be prepared and trained to recognize and control these occurrences."

- Individualize the drug doses. When drugs are used in combination, the dose of each drug must be selected carefully. The toxic effects of drug combinations appear to be additive. Drug selection must be based on the patient's general health history. The presence of systemic disease (ASA II, III, or IV) usually indicates the need for a dose reduction. Because most sedative drugs are available in concentrated forms and because children require such small doses, extreme care must be taken when these drugs are prepared for administration. Fixed-dose administration of drugs based on a range of ages (for example, children 4 to 6 years all receiving 50 mg) is not recommended. Doses should be based on the patient's body weight or surface area or on whenever possible.[92]

If the selected drug dose is inadequate to produce the desired effect, it is prudent to consider a change in the sedation technique or in the drug (at a subsequent appointment), rather than increasing the drug dose to a higher and potentially more dangerous level at the same visit.

- Recognize and expect adverse drug effects. When combinations of CNS depressants are administered, the potential for excessive CNS and respiration depression is increased and should be expected.

The Dentists Insurance Company, in a retrospective study of deaths and morbidity in dental practices over a 3-year period, concluded that in most of those incidents related to drug administration, three common factors were present:[93]

1. Improper preoperative evaluation of the patient
2. Lack of knowledge of drug pharmacology by the doctor
3. Lack of adequate monitoring during the procedure

These three factors increased the risk of serious ADRs significantly, with a negative outcome as the usual result.

An overdose reaction to the administration of CNS-depressant drugs may not always be preventable; however, proper care on the part of the doctor will minimize the incidence of these events, with a successful outcome almost every time. With techniques such as intravenous and inhalation sedation, in which titration is possible, overdosage should be rare. With oral, IM, and submucosal drug administration, the doctor has little control over the drug's ultimate effect because of the inability to titrate and must exercise greater care in the preoperative evaluation of the patient, determination of the appropriate drug dose, and monitoring throughout the procedure.

When oral, submucosal, or IM routes of administration are used, the onset of adverse reactions may be delayed. The adverse reaction may not develop until after the rubber dam is in place and the dental procedure has begun. Monitoring throughout the procedure therefore becomes extremely important in patient safety. As of August 1999, my preferences in monitoring during parenteral sedation are as follows[71]:

CNS
    Direct verbal contact with patient
Respiratory system
    Pretracheal stethoscope
    Pulse oximetry
Cardiovascular system
    Continuous monitoring of vital signs
    Electrocardiogram

## REFERENCES

1. Caranasos GJ: Drug reactions. In Schwartz GR and others, editors: *Principles and practice of emergency medicine,* Philadelphia, 1978, WB Saunders.
2. Aldrete JA, Johnson DA: Evaluation of intracutaneous testing for investigation of allergy to local anesthetic agents, *Anesth Analg* 49:173, 1970.
3. Nation RL, Triggs EJ, Selig M: Lignocaine kinetics in cardiac patients and aged subjects, *Br J Clin Pharmacol* 4:439, 1977.
4. Demetrescu M, Julien RM: Local anesthesia and experimental epilepsy, *Epilepsia* 15:235, 1974.
5. Arthur GR: Pharmacokinetics of local anesthetics. In Strichartz GR, editor: *Local anesthetics, handbook of experimental pharmacology,* vol 81, Berlin, 1987, Springer-Verlag.
6. Bax ND, Tucker GT, Woods HF: Lignocaine and indocyanine green kinetics in patients following myocardial infarction, *Br J Clin Pharmacol* 10:353, 1980.
7. Sawyer DR, Ludden TM, Crawford MH: Continuous infusion of lidocaine in patients with cardiac arrhythmias: unpredictability of plasma concentrations, *Arch Intern Med* 141:34, 1981.
8. Englesson S: The influence of acid-base changes on central nervous system toxicity of local anaesthetic agents. I. An experimental study in cats, *Acta Anaesthesiol Scand* 18:79, 1974.
9. DeJong RH, Wagman IH, Prince DA: Effect of carbon dioxide on the cortical seizure threshold to lidocaine, *Exp Neurol* 17:221, 1982.
10. Lear E and others: Atypical pseudocholinesterase: a clinical report, *Anesth Analg* 55:243, 1976.
11. Lanks KW, Sklar GS: Pseudocholinesterase levels and rates of chloroprocaine hydrolysis in patients receiving adequate doses of phospholine iodide, *Anesthesiology* 52:434, 1980.
12. Zsigmond EK, Eilderton TE: Survey of local anesthetic toxicity in the families of patients with atypical plasma cholinesterase, *J Oral Surg* 33:833, 1975
13. Lindorf HH, Ganssen A, Mayer P: Thermographic representation of the vascular effects of local anesthetics, *Electromedica* 4:106, 1974.
14. Braid DP, Scott DB: The systemic absorption of local analgesic drugs, *Br J Anaesth* 37:394, 1965.
15. Jebson PR: Intramuscular lignocaine 2% and 10%, *Br Med J* 3:566, 1971.
16. Drug package insert, lidocaine hydrochloride, *Physician's GenRx,* St Louis, 1996, Mosby.
17. Adriani J, Campbell B: Fatalities following topical application of local anesthetics to mucous membranes, *JAMA* 162:1527, 1956.
18. Moore DC: *Complications of regional anesthesia,* Springfield, Ill, 1955, Charles C Thomas.
19. DuSouich P, Erill P: Altered metabolism of procainamide and procaine in patients with pulmonary and cardiac disease, *Clin Pharmacol Ther* 21:101, 1977.
20. Downs JR: Atypical cholinesterase activity: its importance in dentistry, *J Oral Surg* 24:256, 1966.
21. Keenaghan JB, Boyes RN: The tissue distribution, metabolism and excretion of lidocaine in rats, guinea pigs, dogs and man, *J Pharmacol Exp Ther* 180:454, 1972.
22. Mather LE, Tucker GT: Pharmacokinetics and biotransformation of local anesthetics, *Anesthesiol Clin* 16:23, 1978.
23. Meffin P and others: Neutral metabolites of mepivacaine in humans, *Xenobiotica* 3:191, 1973.
24. Thomas J, Morgan D, Vine J: Metabolism of etidocaine in man, *Xenobiotica* 6:39, 1976.
25. Friedman GA and others: Evaluation of the analgesic effect and urinary excretion of systemic bupivacaine in man, *Anesth Analg* 61:23, 1982.
26. Monheim LM: *Local anesthesia and pain control in dental practice,* St Louis, 1957, Mosby.
27. Malamed SF: *Handbook of local anesthesia,* ed 4, St Louis, 1997, Mosby.
28. Bieter RN: Applied pharmacology of local anesthetics, *Am J Surg* 34:500, 1936.
29. Vandam LD: Some aspects of the history of local anesthesia. In Strichartz GR, editor: *Local anesthetics: handbook of experimental pharmacology,* vol 81, Berlin, 1987, Springer-Verlag.
30. Jastak JT, Yagiela JA, Donaldson D: *Local anesthesia of the oral cavity,* Philadelphia, 1995, WB Saunders.
31. Larsen LS, Larsen A: Labetalol in the treatment of epinephrine overdose, *Ann Emerg Med* 19(6):680-682, 1990.
32. Houpt MI and others: An evaluation of intraoral lidocaine patches in reducing needle-insertion pain, *Compendium* 18(4):309-318, 1997.

33. Marcovitz PA, Williamson BD, Armstrong WF: Toxic methemoglobinemia caused by topical anesthetic given before transesophageal echocardiography, *J Amer Soc Echocardiog* 4(6):615-618, 1991.

34. Xylocaine 10% oral spray, drug package insert, 1996, Astra Pharmaceutical Products, Westboro, Mass.

35. Bartlett SZ: Clinical observations on the effects of injections of local anesthetics preceded by aspiration, *Oral Surg* 33:520, 1972.

36. Aldrete JA, Narang R, Sada T: Untoward reactions to local anesthetics via reverse intracarotid flow, *J Dent Res* 54:145, 1975.

37. Aldrete JA and others: Reverse carotid blood flow—a possible explanation for some reactions to local anesthetics, *J Am Dent Assoc* 94:142, 1977.

38. Jeske AH, Boshart BF: Deflection of conventional versus nondeflecting dental needles in vitro, *Anesth Prog* 32:62, 1985.

39. Foldes FF, McNall PG: Toxicity of local anesthetics in man, *Dent Clin North Am* July: 257, 1961.

40. Kramer H, Mitton V: Dental emergencies, *Dent Clin North Am* 17:443, 1973.

41. Trapp LD, Davies RO: Aspiration as a function of hypodermic needle internal diameter in the in-vivo human upper limb, *Anesth Prog* 27:49, 1980.

42. Covino BG, Vassallo HG: *Local anesthetics: mechanisms of action and clinical use,* New York, 1976, Grune & Stratton.

43. Scott DB, Cousins MJ: Clinical pharmacology of local anesthetic agents. In Cousins MJ, Bridenbaugh PO, editors: *Neural blockade,* edition 3, Philadelphia, 1998, Lippincott-Raven.

44. Munson ES and others: Etidocaine, bupivacaine, and lidocaine seizure thresholds in monkeys, *Anesthesiology* 42:471-478, 1975.

45. Covino BG: Toxic and systemic effects of local anesthetic agents. In Strichartz GR, editor: *Local anesthetics, handbook of experimental pharmacology,* vol 81, Berlin, 1987, Springer-Verlag.

46. Liu PL and others: Comparative CNS toxicity of lidocaine, etidocaine, bupivcaine, and tetracaine in awake dogs following rapid IV administration, *Anesth Analg* 62:375, 1983.

47. Cannell H and others: Circulating levels of lignocaine after peri-oral injections, *Br Dent J* 138:87, 1975.

48. Harrison DC, Alderman FL: Relation of blood levels to clinical effectiveness of lidocaine. In Scott DB, Julian DC, editors: *Lidocaine in the treatment of ventricular arrhythmias,* Edinburgh, 1971, E & S Livingstone.

49. Block A, Covino BG: Effects of local anesthetic agents on cardiac conduction and contractility, *Reg Anaesth* 6:55, 1982.

50. Liu PL and others: Acute cardiovascular toxicity of intravenous amide anesthetics in anesthetized ventilated dogs, *Anesth Analg* 61:317, 1982.

51. American Heart Association: *Textbook of Advanced Cardiac Life Support,* Dallas, 1997, The Association

52. Strichartz GR, Covino BG: Local anesthetics. In Miller RD, editor: *Anesthesia,* ed 2, New York, 1990, Churchill-Livingstone.

53. Liu PL and others: Acute cardiovascular toxicity of procaine, chloroprocaine, and tetracaine in anesthetized ventilated dogs, *Reg Anaesth* 7:14, 19, 1982.

54. Scott DB: Toxicity caused by local anaesthetic drugs, *Br J Anaesth* 53:553-554, 1981.

55. Julien RM: Lidocaine in experimental epilepsy: correlation of anticonvulsant effect with blood concentration, *Electroencephalogr Clin Neurophysiol* 34:639, 1973.

56. Julien RM, Demetrescu M: A neutral local anesthetic for research in experimental epilepsy, *J Life Sci* 4:27, 1974.

57. Wagman IH, DeJong RH, Prince DA: Effects of lidocaine on the central nervous system, *Anesthesiology* 28:155, 1967.

58. Adatia AK: Intravascular injection of local anesthetics, *Br Dent J* 138:328, 1975.

59. Ingvar M, Siesjo BK: Local blood flow and glucose consumption in the rat brain during sustained bicuculline-induced seizures, *Acta Neurol Scand* 68:129, 1983.

60. Jaimovich DG and others: Intravenous midazolam suppression of pentylene tetrazol-induced epileptogenic activity in a porcine model, *Crit Care Med* 18(3):313, 1990.

61. Jakob W: Local anaesthesia and vasoconstrictive additional components, *Newslett Int Fed Dent Anesthesiol Soc* 2(1):3, 1989.

62. American Dental Association: *ADA Guide to Dental Therapeutics,* Chicago, 1998, The Association.

63. Verrill PJ: Adverse reactions to local anesthetics and vasoconstrictor drugs, *Practitioner* 214:380, 1975.

64. Alexander RE: Epinephrine is safe for heart patients, *Med Times* 99:132, 1971.

65. Campbell RL: Cardiovascular effects of epinephrine overdose: case report, *Anesth Prog* 24:190, 1977.

66. Merck S: Adverse effects of epinephrine when given to patients taking propranolol (Inderal) *J Emerg Nurs* 21(1):27-32, 1995.

67. Wynn RL: Epinephrine interactions with beta-blockers, *Gen Dent* 42(2):116-117, 1994.

68. Baltarowich LL: Sedative-hypnotics. In Rosen P, editor: *Emergency medicine,* ed 2, St Louis, 1988, Mosby.

69. Braham RL: *Textbook of pediatric dentistry,* Baltimore, 1985, Williams & Wilkins.

70. Goodson JM, Moore PA: Life-threatening reactions after pedodontic sedation: an assessment of opioid, local anesthetic, and antiemetic drug interaction, *J Am Dent Assoc* 107:239, 1983.

71. Malamed SF: *Sedation: a guide to patient management,* ed 3, St Louis, 1995, Mosby.

72. Harvey SC: Hypnotics and sedatives: the barbiturates. In Goodman IS, Gilman A, editors: *Pharmacological basis of therapeutics,* ed 6, New York, 1980, Macmillan.

73. Zendell E: Chloral hydrate overdose: a case report, *Anesth Prog* 19:6, 1972.

74. Benusis KP, Kapuan D, Furnam LJ: Respiratory depression in a child following meperidine, promethazine and chlorpromazine premedication: report of a case, *J Dent Child* 46:50, 1979.

75. Del Vecchio PJ Jr: 20/20, *Am Dent Assoc News* 14:4, 1983 (letter).

76. Hine CH, Pasi A: Fatality after use of alphaprodine in analgesia for dental surgery: report of a case, *J Am Dent Assoc* 84:858, 1972.

77. Okuji DM: Hypoxic encephalopathy after the administration of alphaprodine hydrochloride, *J Am Dent Assoc* 103:50, 1981.

78. Gal TJ, DiFazio CA, Moscicki J: Analgesic and respiratory depressant activity of nalbuphine: a comparison with morphine, *Anesthesiology* 57:367, 1982.

79. Heel RC and others: Butorphanol: a review of its pharmacological properties and therapeutic efficacy, *Drugs* 16:473, 1978.

80. Jaffe JH, Martin WR: Opioid analgesics and antagonists. In Goodman L, Gilman A, editors: *The pharmacological basis of therapeutics,* ed 6, New York, 1980, Macmillan.

81. Allen T: Opioids. In Rosen P, editor: *Emergency medicine,* ed 2, St Louis, 1988, Mosby.

82. Pollakoff J, Pollakoff K: *EMT's guide to signs and symptoms,* Los Angeles, 1991, Jeff Gould.

83. American Heart Association and National Academy of Sciences, National Research Council: Standards for cardiopulmonary resuscitation (CPR) and emergency cardiac care (ECC), *JAMA* 255:2905, 1986.

84. Matthew H: Barbiturates, *Clin Toxicol* 8:495, 1975.

85. Romazicon drug package insert, Roche Laboratories, October 1994.

86. Lowenstein E: Morphine anesthesia in perspective, *Anesthesiology* 35:563, 1971.

87. Duberstein JL, Kaufman DM: A clinical study of an epidemic of heroin-induced pulmonary edema, *Am J Med* 51:704, 1971.

88. Narcan drug package insert, DuPont Pharmaceuticals, July 1996.

89. Janssens F, Torremans J, Janssen PA: Synthetic 1,4-disubstituted-1,4-dihydro-5H-tetrazol-5-one derivatives of fentanil: alfentanil (R 39209), a potent, extremely short-acting opioid analgesic, *J Med Chem* 29:2290, 1986.

90. Clotz MA, Nahata MC: Clinical uses of fentanyl, sufentanil, and alfentanil, *Clin Pharmacy* 10(8):581-593, 1991.

91. Servin F: Remifentanil: when and how to use it. *Eur J Anaesthesiol* 15(suppl):41-44, 1997.

92. Done AK: In Modell W, editor: *Drugs of choice 1972-1973,* St Louis, 1972, Mosby.

93. deJulien LE: Causes of severe morbidity/mortality cases, *J Cal Dent Assoc* 11:45, 1983.

# 24

# *Allergy*

**A**LLERGY has previously been defined as a hypersensitive state acquired through exposure to a particular allergen, reexposure to which produces a heightened capacity to react.[1] Allergic reactions cover a broad range of clinical manifestations, from mild, delayed reactions that develop as long as 48 hours after exposure to the antigen, to immediate and life-threatening reactions developing within seconds of exposure. A classification of allergic reactions is presented in Table 24-1.[2] Although all allergic phenomena are important, two forms of allergy are of particular consequence in the practice of dentistry. The type I, or anaphylactic (immediate), reaction may present the dental office staff with the most acutely life-threatening situation of any discussed in this textbook. The type IV, or delayed, allergic reaction, seen clinically as contact dermatitis, is particularly relevant because of the significant number of dental personnel who develop this form of allergy. Allergic reactions to latex among health workers are being reported with increasing frequency,[3] as are reports of allergy in patients to latex gloves worn by their doctors.[4]

Immediate allergic reactions are of primary concern and receive major emphasis in the following discussion. The type I reaction may be subdivided into several forms of response, including generalized and localized anaphylaxis.[2] A list of type I allergic reactions follows:

Type I immediate hypersensitivity:

    Generalized (systemic) anaphylaxis

    Localized anaphylaxis

table **24-1** *Classification of allergic diseases (after Gell and Coombs)*

| TYPE | MECHANISM | PRINCIPAL ANTIBODY OR CELL | TIME OF REACTIONS | CLINICAL EXAMPLES |
|------|-----------|----------------------------|-------------------|-------------------|
| I | Anaphylactic (immediate, homocytotrophic, antigen-induced, antibody-mediated) | IgE | Seconds to minutes | Anaphylaxis (drugs, insect venom, antisera) Atopic bronchial asthma Allergic rhinitis Urticaria Angiodema Hay fever |
| II | Cytotoxic (antimembrane) | IgG IgM (activate complement) | — | Transfusion reactions Goodpasture's syndrome Autoimmune hemolysis Hemolytic anemia Certain drug reactions |
| III | Immune complex (serum sickness–like) | IgG (form complexes with complement) | 6 to 8 hours | Membraneous glomerulonephrosis Serum sickness Lupus nephritis Occupational allergic alveolitis Acute viral hepatitis |
| IV | Cell-mediated (delayed) or tuberculin-type response | — | 48 hours | Allergic contact dermatitis Infectious granulomas (tuberculosis, mycoses) Tissue graft rejection Chronic hepatitis |

Modified from Krupp MA, Chatton MJ: *Current medical diagnosis and treatment,* Los Altos, Calif, 1984, Lange Medical.

---

**allergen** An antigen that can elicit allergic symptoms.

**anaphylactic** From the Greek *ana* = against or backward; phy-lax = guard or protect, meaning "without protection"; to be distinguished from prophylaxis, as in "for protection."[5]

**anaphylactoid** Anaphylactoid reactions, which mimic true IgE-mediated anaphylaxis, are idiosyncratic reactions that occur generally when the patient is first exposed to a particular drug or agent. Although not immunologically mediated, their emergency management is the same as that of immunologically mediated reactions.

**angioedema (angioneurotic edema)** Noninflammatory edema involving the skin, subcutaneous tissue, underlying muscle, and mucous membranes, especially those of the gastrointestinal and upper respiratory tracts; occurs in response to exposure to an allergen; the most critical area of involvement is the larynx (laryngeal edema).

**antibody** Those substances found in the blood or tissues that respond to the administration of, or react with, an antigen; they differ in structure (e.g., IgE and IgG) and are capable of eliciting distinctly different responses (e.g., anaphylaxis or serum sickness).

**antigen** Any substance foreign to the host that is capable of activating an immune (e.g., allergic) response by stimulating the development of a specific antibody.

**atopy** A "strange disease"; a clinical hypersensitivity state subject to hereditary influences; examples include asthma, hay fever, and eczema.

**pruritus** Itching.

**urticaria** A vascular reaction of the skin marked by the transient appearance of smooth, slightly elevated patches that are redder or paler than the surrounding skin and are often accompanied by severe itching.

---

Urticaria (in the skin)
Bronchospasm (in the respiratory tract)
Food allergy (in the gastrointestinal tract and other organs)

Terms relevant to allergy are listed in the box above.

All allergic reactions are mediated through immunologic mechanisms that are similar, regardless of the specific antigen responsible for initiating the reaction. Therefore it is possible, and likely, that an allergic reaction to the venom of a stinging insect, such as a wasp, may be identical to the reaction to eating a strawberry, or after aspirin or penicillin administration to a previously sensitized individual. This must be differentiated from the overdose or toxic drug reaction that

represents a direct extension of the normal pharmacologic properties of the drug involved.

Overdose reactions are much more frequently encountered than are allergic drug reactions (85% of adverse drug reactions [ADRs] result from the pharmacologic actions of a drug; 15% are immunologic reactions[6]), even though to the nonmedical individual *any* ADR is usually thought to be allergy. It is hoped that following the discussions in this section, the reader will be able to fully evaluate a history of alleged allergy to determine what really occurred and will be able to differentiate between these two important ADRs—allergy and overdose.

Chapter 25 presents a differential diagnosis of the several ADRs and other clinically similar reactions.

Allergy is a frightening word to those health professionals who are involved in primary patient care. In the dental profession many drugs that have a significant potential for producing allergy are regularly administered or prescribed. Although the concept of prevention has been emphasized repeatedly throughout this book, in no other situation is this concept of greater importance than it is in allergy.

Although not the most common ADR, allergy is frequently involved with the most serious of these reactions. Emphasis will be placed on the more immediate allergic reaction and on those specific drugs and chemicals in common use in dental practice.

## Predisposing Factors

The number of persons with significant allergy is not small. Of the population in the United States, 15% have allergic conditions severe enough to require medical management. Thirty-three percent of all chronic disease in children is allergic in nature.[7,8] Individuals with allergy problems represent a potentially serious risk when they receive drugs during their dental care. Although never without risk, the administration of drugs is normally accomplished without any significant frequency of adverse reactions (indeed, if ADRs occurred with greater frequency, dentists would avoid using many drugs in dental practice). However, in an individual with a genetic predisposition to allergy (e.g., the atopic patient), great care must be taken when considering the use of any drug. The patient with multiple allergies (e.g., hay fever, asthma, or allergy to numerous foods) is much more likely to have an allergic response to drugs used in dentistry than is a patient with no prior history of allergy.

Although the patient's prior history is the major factor in determining the risk of allergy, the specific drug to be employed is also of extreme importance.

In allergy, as opposed to overdose, prior contact (a sensitizing dose) is almost always necessary for the allergy to develop. Such is not the case in anaphylactoid reactions, however. In the "usual" allergic reaction, signs and symptoms appear only after a subsequent (challenge) dose is administered. Without the sensitizing and challenge doses, allergy will not occur.

Various drug groups are more highly allergenic than others. In one survey barbiturates, penicillins, meprobamate, codeine, and thiazide diuretics were responsible for over 70% of the allergic reactions encountered.[9] Laryngeal edema, acute bronchospasm with respiratory failure, and circulatory collapse, occurring alone or in combination, are responsible for 400 to 800 anaphylactic deaths annually in the United States.[10] Leading causes of death from anaphylaxis are parenterally administered penicillin (100 to 500 deaths per year) and *Hymenoptera* (bees, wasps, hornets, and yellow jackets) stings (40 to 100 deaths per year).[11,12] Medications frequently involved in anaphylactoid deaths include radiopaque contrast media (up to 50 deaths per year)[13] and the iatrogenic administration of common medications such as aspirin and other nonsteroidal antiinflammatory drugs.[14,15] Recent additions to the list of leading causes of death from anaphylaxis are peanuts[16] and latex.[17]

Box 24-1 lists the more commonly used drugs in dental practice that possess a significant potential for allergy.

## ANTIBIOTICS

Probably the most significant ADR associated with antibiotics is the ability of many of them to produce allergic reactions. Some antibiotics, such as erythromycin, are associated with a very low incidence of allergy, whereas others, particularly the sulfonamides and penicillins, frequently produce allergic responses. In virtually all cases the allergic reaction associated with antibiotic therapy is not life threatening. The penicillins, the most commonly used antibiotics in dentistry, are a major exception. The first anaphylactic-induced fatality caused by penicillin was reported in 1949.[18] Penicillin has remained the leading cause of fatal anaphylaxis since that time.[19,20]

It has been estimated that the incidence of allergy to penicillin ranges anywhere from 0.7% to 10% of those receiving the drug.[11] Approximately 2.5 million persons in the United States are allergic to penicillin. Of patients receiving penicillin, 0.015% to 0.04% will develop anaphylaxis, with a fatality rate of 0.0015% to 0.002%.[11] This accounts for 100 to 500 deaths per year.

box 24-1

### Antibiotics
Penicillins
Cephalosporins
Tetracyclines
Sulfonamides

### Analgesics
Acetylsalicylic acid (ASA-aspirin)
Nonsteroidal antiinflammatory drugs (NSAIDs)

### Opioids
Morphine
Meperidine
Codeine

### Antianxiety drugs
Barbiturates

### Local anesthetics
Esters
   Procaine
   Propoxycaine
   Benzocaine
   Tetracaine
Antioxidant
   Sodium (meta)bisulfite
Parabens
   Methylparaben

### Other agents
Acrylic monomer (methyl methacrylate)

In a survey on the nature and extent of penicillin side reactions, 150 cases of anaphylaxis were studied. Of the patients observed, 14% had a history of other allergies, 70% had previously received penicillin, and over 33% had experienced a prior immediate allergic reaction to the drug. When death occurred, it normally occurred within 15 minutes.[21] Allergy to penicillin may be induced by any mode of administration. The topical route is probably the most likely to sensitize (5% to 12% sensitized) and the oral route is the least likely (0.1% sensitized). However, it is also possible to be sensitized to penicillin without knowledge of prior exposure because penicillin is a natural contaminant of our environment. The penicillin mold is airborne and may be found in bread, cheese, milk, and fruit. Parenterally administered penicillin is responsible for the vast majority of severe anaphylactic reactions, with only six fatalities reported from oral penicillin.[9] Cephalosporins, structurally similar to penicillin, have been reported to be cross-allergenic in 5% to 16% of patients.[22]

## ANALGESICS

Allergy may develop to any of the pain-relieving drugs commonly used in dentistry. This is somewhat true regarding the opioid agonist analgesics, such as codeine and meperidine, but the incidence of true allergy to these drugs is quite low, even though "allergic to codeine" is frequently listed on medical history questionnaires. A thorough dialogue history is required to determine the precise nature of the ADR. In most instances allergy to codeine turns out to be merely annoying (dose-related) side effects such as nausea, vomiting, drowsiness, dysphoria (restlessness), or constipation.

The incidence of allergy to aspirin is relatively high (estimated to be from 0.2% to 0.9%), with symptoms ranging from mild urticaria to anaphylaxis.[23,24] Previous ingestion of aspirin without ill effect is no guarantee against subsequent allergic reaction to the drug. Allergic reactions to aspirin also take the form of angioedema and bronchospasm. Bronchospasm is the chief allergic manifestation in most persons sensitive to aspirin, but especially in the middle-aged woman who also has nasal polyps, pansinusitis, and rhinitis.[25,26] Anaphylaxis may also occur.[27] Other NSAIDs also carry a risk of allergy.[14,15,28]

## ANTIANXIETY DRUGS

Of the many drugs commonly used for the management of fear in dentistry, the barbiturates probably possess the greatest potential for sensitization of patients. Although not as common as allergy to penicillin or aspirin, allergy to barbiturates usually manifests itself in the form of skin lesions such as hives and urticaria or, less frequently, in the form of blood dyscrasias such as agranulocytosis or thrombocytopenia.[29] Allergy to barbiturates occurs much more frequently in persons with a history of asthma, urticaria, and angioedema. A history of allergy to any of the barbiturates represents an absolute contraindication to the use of any other barbiturate.

## LOCAL ANESTHETICS

Local anesthetics are the most commonly used drugs in dentistry and the most important. Without their availability dentistry would revert back to the days when all dental procedures were associated with pain.

Adverse drug reactions, although uncommon, are seen with the use of local anesthetics. The overwhelming majority of these ADRs are not allergic in nature, but are related to a direct effect of the drug.[30,31] Allergy to local anesthetics does occur; however, the incidence of such reactions has dramatically decreased since the introduction of amide-type local anesthetics in the 1940s. Allergic manifestations of local anesthetics may range from an allergic dermatitis (commonly occurring among dental office personnel) to typical bronchospasm to fatal systemic anaphylaxis.

Allergy to local anesthetics occurs much more frequently in response to the ester local anesthetics such as procaine, propoxycaine, benzocaine, tetracaine, and compounds related to them, such as procaine penicillin G and procainamide (an antidysrhythmic drug).[30,32] Amide-type local anesthetics are essentially free of this problem, yet the frequency of reports of allergy to amide local anesthetics in the dental and medical literature and on the medical history questionnaire seems to be increasing.[33-37] This apparent contradiction may be cleared up with careful evaluation of these alleged allergies. Several investigators, most notably Aldrete and Johnson,[38] have investigated these reports and performed extensive evaluation of each case, seeking to determine the nature of the reaction. In most cases the reaction was the result of either psychogenic factors or drug overdose (see Chapter 23); in other cases, reactions were of an allergic nature. When an ester local anesthetic is administered, a true allergic reaction is frequently elicited; however, with use of an amide local anesthetic, a purported allergic reaction is frequently shown to be another type of response (e.g., overdose, idiosyncrasy, or psychogenic). Malamed[39] examined 210 patients referred for evaluation of "local anesthetic allergy." Careful dialogue history and intracutaneous testing found no patient to be allergic to an amide local anesthetic and four patients with allergy to the paraben preservative. Esters were not evaluated in these patients.

Although true allergy to amide local anesthetics is rare, patients have more frequently demonstrated true allergic reactions to components of the dental cartridge. The dental cartridge contains a number of items besides the local anesthetic (Table 24-2). Of special interest with respect to allergy are two items: methylparaben and sodium metabisulfite. The parabens—methyl, ethyl, and propyl—are bacteriostatic agents and are added to many drugs, foods, and cosmetics that are meant for multiple use. Parabens are structurally related to the ester local anesthetics,

| table **24-2** | Contents of local anesthetic cartridge |
| --- | --- |

| INGREDIENT | FUNCTION |
| --- | --- |
| Local anesthetic agent | Conduction blockade |
| Vasoconstrictor | Decrease absorption of local anesthetic into blood, thus increasing duration of anesthesia and decreasing toxicity of anesthetic |
| Sodium metabisulfite | Antioxidant for vasoconstrictor |
| Methylparaben* | Preservative to increase shelf life; bacteriostatic |
| Sodium chloride | Isotonicity of solution |
| Sterile water | Diluent |

*Methylparaben has been excluded from all local anesthetic cartridges manufactured in the United States since January, 1984. It is still found in multiple-dose vials of medications and in some local anesthetic solutions manufactured in other countries.

thus their increased allergenicity. It is difficult if not impossible to avoid contact with the parabens. Because of their increasing use, the frequency of sensitization to the parabens has greatly increased. Parabens are used increasingly in nondrug items such as skin creams, hair lotions, suntan preparations, face powder, soaps, lipsticks, toothpastes, syrups, soft drinks, and candies. In response to the increasing incidence of allergic reactions to these products, certain products have been marked as "hypoallergenic" and do not contain any parabens. Although anaphylaxis has been reported, paraben allergy is rarely systemic, most commonly appearing as a localized skin eruption or as localized edema.

Patients with a history of allergy to an amide local anesthetic were tested, using the anesthetic without methylparaben and with the preservative alone.[38,39] In every instance the patient reacted to the preservative but did not react to the same anesthetic without methylparaben. Paraben allergy is almost exclusively limited to a dermatologic-type response. In 1984 the Food and Drug Administration (FDA) ordered the removal of paraben preservatives from all single-use local anesthetic cartridges manufactured in the United States. Methylparaben is still included in dental cartridges of local anesthetics in some countries and is found in all multiple-dose containers of injectable drugs.

Allergy to sodium bisulfite or metabisulfite is being reported with increasing frequency.[40-42] Bisulfites are antioxidants and are commonly used in restaurants where they are sprayed on fruits and vegetables as a preservative and to prevent discoloration. For example, sliced apples sprayed with bisulfite do not turn brown (i.e., become oxidized). Bisulfites are also used to prevent bacterial contamination of wines, beers, and distilled beverages.[43] Persons with bisulfite allergy frequently respond to contact with bisulfite with severe respiratory allergy, commonly bronchospasm. Within the asthmatic population, reports demonstrate that up to 10% are allergic to bisulfites.[40,44] It is not known if bisulfites are triggers of anaphylaxis.[40,44] A history of bisulfite allergy should alert the doctor to the possibility of this same type of response if sodium bisulfite or metabisulfite is included in the local anesthetic cartridge. Bisulfites are present in all local anesthetic cartridges that contain a vasoconstrictor. Local anesthetic solutions not containing vasoconstrictor additives do not contain bisulfites. Common sources of exposure to bisulfites are presented in Box 24-2.

Topical anesthetics are also potential allergens. Most topical anesthetics are esters, with benzocaine and tetracaine most commonly employed. Many topical anesthetics, even amides (e.g., lidocaine), contain preservatives such as the parabens (methyl, ethyl, propyl), so that allergy must always be considered when these agents are used.

Clinical manifestations of allergy related to topical anesthetic application may span the entire spectrum of allergic responses; however, the most common response is allergic contact stomatitis, which may include mild erythema, edema, and ulcerations. If widespread and severe, the edema may lead to difficulty in swallowing and breathing.

## OTHER AGENTS

"Denture sore mouth" is a name commonly given to inflammatory changes of mucous membranes developing beneath dentures. Most frequently the palatal oral mucosa and maxillary ridges are involved, with the tissue appearing bright red and edematous and the patient complaining of soreness, rawness, dryness, and burning.

The acrylic resins used in most dentures today can produce allergy. This is much more likely to occur when self-cured acrylics are used instead of heat-cured acrylics. In addition, dental personnel and laboratory technicians may develop contact dermatitis to these materials. These reactions occur most frequently on the fingers and hands and are almost always caused by the acrylic monomer (the liquid), methyl methacrylate.

Heat-cured acrylics are less frequently associated with allergy because the monomer is used more completely in the polymerization process. In cold-cured or self-cured acrylics, it is likely that small amounts of monomer remain unpolymerized, and it is this that produces the allergic response in the previously sensitized individual. Cold-curing or self-curing acrylics are employed in denture repair and relining procedures, as well as in the fabrication of temporary crowns, bridges, and splints.

# Prevention

## Medical History Questionnaire

The medical history questionnaire contains several questions relating to allergy.

7. **Are you allergic to (i.e., experience itching, rash, swelling of hands, feet, or eyes) or made sick by penicillin, aspirin, codeine, or any drugs or medications?**

9. **Circle any of the following that you have had or have at present:**
   **Asthma**
   **Hay fever**
   **Sinus trouble**
   **Allergies or hives**

   *Comment:* These questions seek to determine if ADRs have occurred. Adverse drug reactions are not uncommon;

---

box **24-2**  *Sulfite-containing agents*

Restaurant salads (e.g., lettuce, tomatoes, carrots, peppers, dressings)
Fresh fruits
Dried fruits
Wine, beer, cordials
Alcohol
All sparkling grape juices, including nonalcoholic
Potatoes (e.g., french fries, chips)
Sausage meats
Cider and vinegar
Pickles
Dehydrated vegetables
Cheese and cheese mixtures
Bottled lemon and lime juice
Gelatin
Corn bread or muffin mix
Shrimp and other seafood
Fresh fish
Avocados (e.g., guacamole)
Soups (canned or dried)
Sauces and gravies used on meats and fish

those most frequently reported are usually labeled "allergy." Any positive response to these questions must be thoroughly evaluated through the dialogue history. In all instances in which the possibility of allergy does exist, it is prudent for the doctor to assume that the claim of allergy is valid and to continue to do so until the exact nature of the reaction can be determined. The dialogue history is a vital part of this determination process, as is possible medical consultation in the event that any doubt remains concerning the allergy following the dentist's evaluation of the patient. The drug or drugs in question, as well as any closely related drugs, should not be used until the alleged allergy has been thoroughly evaluated and disproved.

Fortunately, substitute drugs exist and may be employed in place of most of those that commonly cause allergy. These substitute drugs possess most of the same desirable clinical actions as the primary drugs, but are not as allergenic. The only group in which substitute drugs are not as effective clinically as the primary agents is local anesthetics. Because these are also the most important drugs employed in dentistry, much of the following discussion is related to the problem of local anesthetic allergy.

## DIALOGUE HISTORY

Following an affirmative response to the question about a previous adverse drug reaction, the doctor should seek as much information as possible directly from the patient. The following questions should be asked, modified where appropriate, in the evaluation of an alleged drug allergy.

### What drug was used?

*Comment:* A patient who is truly allergic to a drug should be told the exact generic name of that drug. Many persons with documented allergic histories wear a Medic Alert bracelet (Fig. 24-1) that lists those items to which they are allergic as well as other medical conditions that might exist. However, the most common responses to this question are, "I'm allergic to local anesthetics," "I'm allergic to Novocain," or "I'm allergic to all '-caine' drugs." Novocain (procaine), an ester, is infrequently used today as a local anesthetic in dentistry, the amides having virtually replaced the esters. Yet patients routinely refer to the local anesthetics they receive as "shots of Novocain." There are two reasons for this: first, the name Novocain has become virtually synonymous with dental injections. Second, despite the fact that most doctors do not use procaine or procaine-propoxycaine, many doctors themselves still refer to all local anesthetics as Novocain, even though they are using amide local anesthetics exclusively. Therefore the usual response to the question remains, "I'm allergic to Novocain." This response, if received from a patient who has truly been managed properly (see text that follows) in the past after an adverse reaction to a local anesthetic, indicates that the patient was sensitive to an ester local anesthetic but not to the amide local anesthetic. However, the answers received are usually too general and too vague to permit conclusions to be drawn without further questioning.

### What amount of drug was administered?

*Comment:* This question seeks to determine whether or not there was a definite dose-response relationship, as might, or might not, be seen in an overdose reaction. The problem is that the patient rarely knows these clinical details and can provide little or no assistance.

### Did the solution contain vasoconstrictors or preservatives?

*Comment:* The reaction may have been an overdose or overreaction to the vasoconstrictor in the solution. If an allergic reaction did occur, perhaps it was related to the preservative and not to the local anesthetic. Unfortunately, however, most patients are unable to furnish this information.

### Were you taking any other medication at the time?

*Comment:* This question seeks to determine the possibility that drug interaction or another drug was responsible for the reported adverse reaction.

### What was the time sequence of events?

*Comment:* When, in relation to the administration of the drug, did the reaction occur? Most ADRs associated with local anesthetic administration occur during or immediately following their injection. Syncope, hyperventilation, overdose, and anaphylaxis are most likely to develop at the time of injection,

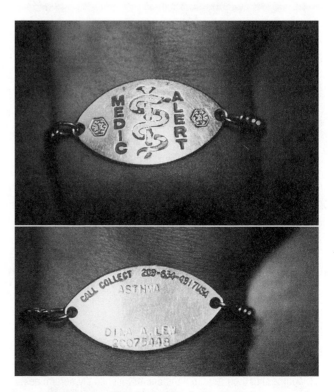

**Figure 24-1**   Medical alert bracelet.

although any of these reactions might also occur later during dental therapy. Try to determine how long the episode lasted. How long was it until the patient was discharged from the office? Was dental treatment continued after the episode?

Dental treatment that continued following the episode indicates that the reaction was probably not an allergic response.

**What position were you in when the reaction took place?**

*Comment:* Injection of local anesthetics with the patient in an upright position is most likely to produce a psychogenic response (e.g., vasodepressor syncope). This does not exclude the possibility that other reactions might have occurred; however, if the patient was in a supine position during injection, vasodepressor syncope seems less likely to be the cause of the reaction, even though loss of consciousness may occur on rare occasion in these circumstances.

**How did the reaction manifest itself?**
**What happened?**

*Comment:* This is a very important question because it asks the patient to describe what actually occurred. The allergy in many instances is explained by the answer to this question. The signs and symptoms described by the patient should be recorded and evaluated to make a tentative diagnosis of the ADR. See the chapters on overdose reaction (Chapter 23), vasodepressor syncope (Chapter 6), and the differential diagnosis of drug reactions (Chapter 25), as well as this chapter for complete listings of clinical signs and symptoms of each of these responses.

**Did the patient lose consciousness?**
**Did seizures occur?**
**Was there a skin reaction or respiratory distress?**

*Comment:* Allergic reactions normally involve one or more of the following systems: skin (e.g., itching, edema, rash), the gastrointestinal system (e.g., diarrhea, nausea and vomiting, cramping), exocrine glands (e.g., running nose, watery eyes), respiratory system (e.g., bronchospasm, laryngeal edema), and cardiovascular (e.g., hypotension, tachycardia) and/or genitourinary system. Most often, patients describe their allergic reaction as one in which they suffered palpitations, severe headache, sweating, and mild shaking (tremor). Such reactions are usually of psychogenic origin or are related to the administration of large doses of vasoconstrictors and are not allergenic. Hyperventilation, an anxiety-induced response in which the patient loses control of his or her breathing—breathing rapidly and deeply—leads to signs and symptoms of dizziness, light-headedness, and peripheral (e.g., fingers, toes, lips) paresthesias.

**What treatment was given?**

*Comment:* Where the patient is able to describe the management of their reaction, the doctor can usually determine its cause. Were drugs administered? If so, what drugs? Epi-

nephrine, anticonvulsants, aromatic ammonia? Knowledge of definitive management of each of these situations can lead to an accurate diagnosis.

Drugs employed in the management of allergy include three drug types or categories: epinephrine (Adrenalin); histamine blockers, including diphenhydramine (Benadryl) or chlorpheniramine (Chlor-Trimeton); and corticosteroids, including hydrocortisone sodium succinate (Solu-Cortef). The use of one or more of these drugs greatly increases the likelihood that an allergic reaction did occur.

Anticonvulsants such as diazepam (Valium), midazolam (Versed, Hypnovel, Dormicum), and the injectable barbiturates, including pentobarbital (Nembutal), are administered to manage seizures, either generalized tonic-clonic or those induced by local anesthetics. Aromatic ammonia is frequently used in the treatment of syncopal episodes. Oxygen may be administered in any or all of these reactions.

**Were the services of a physician or paramedical personnel required? Were you hospitalized?**

*Comment:* A positive response indicates that a more serious reaction occurred. Most psychogenic responses can be ruled out in this instance.

**What is the name and address of the doctor (dentist, physician, or hospital) who was treating you at the time the adverse reaction took place?**

*Comment:* Whenever possible, it is usually valuable to speak to the doctor who managed the previous acute episode. He or she is, in most instances, able to locate the patient's records and to describe in detail what really happened. Direct discussion with the dentist or physician normally provides a wealth of information with which the knowledgeable practitioner can determine the precise nature of the previous reaction.

It is quite unlikely that a health professional will ever forget a case of anaphylaxis that occurred during the management of a patient. It is much more likely that details of a syncopal episode will be forgotten with time.

## MEDICAL CONSULTATION

If doubt remains in the doctor's mind after completion of the dialogue history, allergy must still be considered a possibility and the drugs in question not used. At this point, referral of the patient should be considered, looking for a doctor who will be able to more fully evaluate the nature of the previous reaction. Physicians, primarily allergists and anesthesiologists, and some dentists (dentist anesthesiologists) are likely to be willing and able to completely evaluate this patient. This doctor will also be able to perform certain tests that will prove more reliable in assessing the patient's alleged local anesthetic allergy.

Among the more commonly used tests are skin testing, passive transfer methods, and blood tests, such as the basophil degranulation test.[45]

Skin testing is still the primary means of testing for local anesthetic allergy. Although several types of skin test are used, the *intracutaneous test* is considered to be among the most reliable.[38] Intracutaneous testing involves the injection of 0.1 mL of the test solution and is thought to be 100 times more sensitive than the cutaneous test. It is, however, more unpleasant because it requires multiple needle punctures. Other problems associated with its use involve false-positive results produced by the localized release of histamine in response to skin puncture by the needle. However, intracutaneous testing is clinically useful because a negative response probably means that the patient can safely receive the local anesthetic tested. No instance of an immediate allergic reaction has been reported in a patient with a previously negative intracutaneous response for a given agent.[38,39]

In all instances in which skin testing is employed, the anesthetic solutions should not contain any preservative. Tests for allergy to methylparaben may be done separately, if considered necessary (parabens are no longer found in dental local anesthetic cartridges). If a positive response to paraben occurs, local anesthetics to which the patient is not allergic should be used during the patient's dental treatment, provided they do not contain any preservative. Dental cartridges manufactured in the United States since January, 1984, do not contain methylparaben.

The protocol for intracutaneous testing for local anesthetic allergy currently in use at the University of Southern California School of Dentistry is summarized as follows: After an extensive dialogue history, review of the patient's medical history, informed consent, and establishment of an intravenous line, 0.1 mL of each of the following is deposited intracutaneously: 0.9% normal saline solution, 1% or 2% lidocaine, 3% mepivacaine, and 4% prilocaine, all without methylparaben, followed, if considered necessary, by 0.1 mL of bacteriostatic water and/or one or more local anesthetics containing methylparaben. The patient's vital signs (blood pressure, heart rate and rhythm, PaO$_2$) are monitored throughout the procedure. After successful completion of this phase of the testing (60 minutes), 1 mL of one of the preceding local anesthetic solutions that tested negative is administered intraorally by means of supraperiosteal (infiltration) injection, atraumatically, but without using a topical anesthetic, above a maxillary anterior tooth. This is called the *challenge test,* and it frequently provokes the so-called allergic reaction, that is, signs and symptoms of a psychogenic response.[39]

After having completed more than 215 local anesthetic allergy test procedures, I have encountered four allergic responses to the paraben preservative (all in the early 1980s) but none to the local anesthetic itself. Numerous psychogenic responses have developed during either the intracutaneous or the intraoral testing procedures.

Skin testing is not without risk. Severe, immediate allergic reactions may be precipitated by the administration of as little as 0.1 mL of a drug to a sensitized patient. Emergency drugs, equipment, and personnel for resuscitation must always be readily available when allergy testing is contemplated.

## ALLERGY TESTING IN THE DENTAL OFFICE

It is occasionally suggested that in an emergency situation (such as a toothache or infection) the doctor should carry out the aforementioned testing procedure in the dental office. It is my firm conviction that dental office allergy testing should not be considered for the following reasons. First, skin testing, although potentially valuable, is not foolproof. Localized histamine release (false-positive reactions) may result from the trauma of the needle insertion. A negative reaction, although commonly taken to indicate that a drug may be injected safely, may also prove unreliable. In some cases the drug itself is not the agent to which the patient is sensitive. Instead, a metabolite resulting from biotransformation of the drug may be responsible. The skin test would be negative or a positive response would be delayed for many hours under these circumstances. A second and even more compelling factor for not using skin testing in the dental office is the possibility (although remote) that even the minute quantity of local anesthetic being employed (0.1 mL) might precipitate an immediate and acute systemic anaphylaxis in a truly allergic patient. Drugs, equipment, and personnel needed for the management of anaphylaxis and cardiopulmonary arrest must always be available when allergy testing is undertaken.

## DENTAL THERAPY MODIFICATIONS

### Allergy to drugs other than local anesthetics
When a patient is proved to be truly allergic to a drug, precautions must be taken to prevent the individual from receiving that substance. The outside of the dental chart should be marked with a medical alert sign that is easily visible, alerting dental office staff to look at the medical history carefully. Inside the chart it should be noted that the patient

"is allergic to."* For all of the more highly allergenic drugs prescribed in dentistry, substitute drugs are available that are usually equipotent in therapeutic effect but that pose less of a risk of allergy.

Penicillin allergy may be circumvented through the use of erythromycin; it is a drug possessing virtually the same clinical spectrum of effectiveness as penicillin G, but with a lower incidence of allergy. Sensitization reactions to erythromycin, including skin lesions, fever, and anaphylaxis, have been reported but are much less frequent than penicillin allergy.[46] Erythromycin remains the classic substitute drug for penicillin G.

Acetaminophen is the drug employed in cases of allergy to aspirin. Although as effective an analgesic as aspirin, acetaminophen is not as effective an antipyretic. However, it is not cross-allergenic with aspirin and may be administered to the salicylate-sensitive patient. NSAIDs may also be substituted for aspirin if non-cross-sensitivity exists.

Allergy to opioid analgesics is rare, with the unpleasant side effects of nausea and vomiting the most commonly encountered adverse reactions. However, in the presence of true opioid allergy, no opioid should be used because cross-allergenicity occurs. Nonopioid analgesics may be of some value in this situation.

Barbiturate allergy represents an absolute contraindication to the use of any barbiturate because cross-allergenicity exists among all group members. However, the chemical structures of the nonbarbiturate sedative-hypnotics are sufficiently different so that cross-allergenicity does not occur. These drugs may safely be employed in patients with barbiturate allergy. Included in this group of drugs are the benzodiazepines flurazepam, diazepam, midazolam, oxazepam, and triazolam, as well as chloral hydrate, and hydroxyzine.

Allergy to methyl methacrylate monomer is most readily avoided by not employing acrylic resins. If, however, acrylic resins must be used, heat-cured acrylic is much less allergenic than cold-cured or self-cured acrylic.

Another potential cause of allergy involves the (bi-)-sulfites. Sulfites are included, as antioxidants, in every dental local anesthetic cartridge that contains a vasopressor. Although sulfite allergy can occur in any person, it is the allergic-type asthmatic who is most likely to exhibit this problem. When sulfite allergy is present, local anesthetics not containing a vasopressor should be substituted (e.g., prilocaine "plain" and mepivacaine "plain").

Latex sensitivity has grown to become a significant problem among all health professionals and their patients. The use of vinyl as a latex substitute has minimized the occurrence of allergic reactions. When latex allergy exists, the use of local anesthetic cartridges should be avoided. The thin diaphragm through which the needle enters the cartridge is latex. Although unlikely, it is potentially possible for this latex to be injected into the sensitive patient, inducing a serious allergic reaction.[47-49]

Table 24-3 summarizes the substitute drugs discussed here. In all cases it is possible for a patient to

*Patient confidentiality laws preclude writing a patient's medical information on the outside of the chart where it may be seen by other persons. A general notice on the outside, "Medical Alert," is adequate to alert the staff to check the patient's medical history prior to the start of treatment.

table **24-3**  *Allergenic drugs and possible substitutes*

| CATEGORY | DRUG | USUAL SUBSTITUTE | |
| --- | --- | --- | --- |
| | | GENERIC | PROPRIETARY |
| Antibiotics | Penicillin | Erythomycin | Ilosone |
| | | | Erythrocin |
| Analgesics | Acetylsalicylic acid (aspirin) | Acetaminophen | Tylenol |
| | | | Tempra |
| | | | Datril |
| | Opioid | NSAIDs | Many available |
| Sedative-hypnotics | Barbiturates | Flurazepam | Dalmane |
| | | Diazepam | Valium |
| | | Triazolam | Halcion |
| | | Chloral hydrate | Noctec |
| | | Hydroxyzine | Atarax, Vistaril |
| Acrylic | Methyl methacrylate | Avoid use if possible, otherwise use heat-cured acrylic | |
| Antioxidants | Sodium bisulfite | Non–vasopressor-containing local anesthetic | Mepivacaine Prilocaine |

be allergic to one of the substitute drugs. Therefore the doctor must specifically question the patient about any drug before it is administered. When considering the use of these or any other drugs, several additional factors must be considered. The likelihood of an allergic reaction to a drug increases with the duration and the number of courses of drug therapy. One remarkable example is a patient who had received 16 courses of penicillin therapy without adverse reaction over many years but developed anaphylactic shock with the seventeenth. Although long-term drug therapy is rarely necessary in dentistry, acute allergic reactions may occur even in the absence of a previous history of allergy.

The route of drug administration is also important. Allergic symptoms can arise with any route of administration. The site of administration is frequently the main target area for the allergic symptoms, especially after topical application of drugs. Of significance, however, is the finding that anaphylactic reactions occur much less commonly after enteral rather than parenteral administration of drugs. The frequency of other types of allergy may also be decreased through the use of the oral route. It is important therefore to consider the route of drug administration and, if possible, to administer the drug orally rather than parenterally. Penicillin is an example of a highly allergenic drug. There are few, if any, indications today for the parenteral administration of this drug in the dental office because oral administration has been shown to result in therapeutic blood levels of penicillin in a relatively short time.[50] However, anaphylaxis has been reported after the oral administration of penicillin.[9,51] Drugs for the management of anxiety may require parenteral administration when used in the fearful patient. The risk of allergy to the drug must be weighed against the potential benefit to be gained from its use by this route. Local anesthetics, however, are a drug group that must be administered parenterally to be effective. Allergic reactions observed after parenteral drug administration tend to occur more rapidly and to become more intense than those following enteral administration.

# Management

## ALLEGED ALLERGY TO LOCAL ANESTHETICS

**Elective dental care**   When there is a questionable history of allergy, local anesthetics should not be administered to the patient. Elective dental care requiring local anesthesia (e.g., topical or injectable)

may need to be postponed until a thorough evaluation of the patient is completed by a competent individual. Dental care not requiring injectable or topical anesthesia may be carried out during this period.

**Emergency dental care**   The patient in pain or with an oral infection presents a more difficult situation. In many cases the patient will be new to the office, has a tooth requiring extraction or pulpal extirpation, and has a satisfactory medical history except for an alleged allergy to Novocain. After questioning the patient, the allergy seems most likely to have been of psychogenic origin (e.g., vasodepressor syncope), but a degree of doubt remains. How might this patient be managed?

*Option 1: Consultation.*   The most practical approach to this patient is an immediate consultation with a person able to test the patient for allergy to local anesthetics. Dental treatment should be postponed if at all possible. If pain is present, it may be managed orally with various analgesics; infection can be controlled with antibiotics. These are temporary measures only. After evaluating the patient's claim of allergy, definitive dental care may proceed.

*Option 2: General anesthesia.*   A second approach might be to use general anesthesia in place of local anesthesia to manage the dental emergency. Although highly useful and a relatively safe technique when properly performed, there are complications and problems associated with the use of general anesthesia, not the least of which is the fact that it is unavailable in most dental offices. However, general anesthesia remains a viable alternative to local anesthesia in the management of the "allergic" patient, provided adequate facilities and well-trained personnel are available.

*Option 3: Histamine blocker.*   A third option to consider when emergency treatment is necessary and general anesthesia is not available is the use of a histamine blocker, such as diphenhydramine, as a local anesthetic for the management of pain during treatment. Most injectable histamine blockers possess local anesthetic properties. Several are more potent local anesthetics than procaine. Diphenhydramine has been the most commonly used histamine blocker in this regard. Used as a 1% solution with 1:100,000 epinephrine, diphenhydramine produces pulpal anesthesia of up to 30 minutes' duration.[52,53] An unwanted side effect frequently noted during the intraoral administration of diphenhydramine is a burning or stinging sensation. The use of nitrous oxide and oxygen along with diphenhydramine minimizes discomfort. Another possible unwanted result of the use of a histamine blocker as a local anesthetic is postoperative tissue swelling and soreness. These unpleasant actions must be considered before using these agents. For these reasons the use of diphenhydramine as a local anesthetic is usually limited to those circumstances in which there is a questionable history of local anesthetic allergy, the patient has a dental emergency requiring immediate physical intervention, and general anesthesia is not a reasonable alternative. It must again be kept in mind that allergy may develop to any drug, including the histamine blockers.[54] The patient should be questioned concerning prior exposure to histamine blockers or other drugs before they are used.

It is also important to remember that there are almost no dental emergency situations (short of hemorrhage and infection involving airway obstruction) in which immediate physical intervention is absolutely required. Appropriate drug therapy with immediate medical consultation (option 1) probably remains the most reasonable mode of action in these cases of alleged local anesthetic allergy coupled with a dental emergency.

## CONFIRMED ALLERGY TO LOCAL ANESTHETICS

Management of the patient with a true, documented, and reproducible allergy to local anesthetics varies according to the nature of the allergy. If the allergy is limited to the ester drugs (e.g., procaine, propoxycaine, benzocaine, or tetracaine), the amides (e.g., articaine, lidocaine, mepivacaine, or prilocaine) may be used because cross-allergenicity, although possible, is quite rare. If the local anesthetic allergy was actually an allergy to the paraben preservative, an amide local anesthetic may be injected if it does not contain any preservative. Dental cartridges in the United States have not contained parabens since 1984; however, if the local anesthetic was administered by a non–dental health care professional, it is possible that the drug contained paraben because multiple-dose vials of local anesthetics (all of which contain paraben) are frequently used by medical personnel outside of dentistry. Documented sulfite allergy mandates the use of a local anesthetic that does not contain a vasopressor.

On occasion, however, it is reported that a patient is allergic to all "-caine" drugs. The author recommends that this report undergo careful scrutiny and that the method by which this conclusion was reached be reexamined (What tests, if any, were carried out? By whom? Were pure solutions used? Or were preservatives present?). All too often patients are labeled allergic to all local anesthetics when in reality they are not. These patients often have their dental treatment carried out in a hospital setting under general anesthesia, when proper evaluation might have prevented this, saving the patient much time and money in addition to decreasing both the operative and anesthetic risk.

The following statement on local anesthetic allergy by Aldrete and Johnson[38] concludes this important section on the prevention of allergy:

> A strong plea is made for a thorough evaluation of the circumstances surrounding an adverse reaction to a local anesthetic before the label of "allergic to procaine," "allergic to lidocaine," or "allergic to all 'caine' drugs" is entered on the front of the patient's chart. We believe that untoward reactions observed during the use of local anesthetic agents are quite frequently the result of overdosage. . . . The benefits obtained from the use of local anesthetic agents should not be denied to a patient just because of an untoward response during a previous exposure to one of them. Instead, details of the circumstances surrounding the incident, such as sequence of events, other drugs administered, and the type of procedure, must be evaluated.

# Clinical Manifestations

The various forms that allergic reactions may take are listed in Table 24-1. In addition to this classification, it is also possible to list reactions according to the length of time that elapses between contact with the antigen and the appearance of clinical signs and symptoms. The two categories in this grouping are immediate and delayed reactions.

Immediate allergic reactions are those that occur within seconds to hours of exposure and include types I, II, and III of the Gell and Coombs classification system (Table 24-1). Delayed allergic reactions occur hours to days after antigenic exposure. The type IV reaction is an example of delayed response.

Of greatest significance to the dentist are immediate reactions, in particular the type I, or anaphylactic, reaction. Most allergic drug reactions are immediate. A number of organs and tissues are affected during immediate allergic reactions, particularly the skin, cardiovascular system, respiratory system, eyes, and gastrointestinal tract. Generalized (systemic) anaphylaxis by definition affects all of these systems. When hypotension occurs as a part of the reaction, resulting in the loss of consciousness, the term *anaphylactic shock* is employed.

Immediate allergic reactions also manifest themselves through any number of combinations involving these systems. Reactions involving one organ system are referred to as *localized anaphylaxis*. Examples include bronchial asthma, in which the respiratory system is the target, and urticaria, in which skin is the target organ. Skin and respiratory reactions are discussed individually, followed by a description of generalized anaphylaxis.

## ONSET

The time elapsing between antigenic exposure of the patient and development of clinical symptoms is of great importance. In general, the more rapidly signs and symptoms of allergy occur after exposure to an allergen, the more intense the ultimate reaction.[55] Conversely, the greater the amount of time elapsing between exposure and onset, the less intense the reaction. However, rare cases have been reported of systemic anaphylaxis developing up to several hours after antigenic exposure.[56] Of importance, too, is the rate at which signs and symptoms progress once they appear. If they appear and rapidly increase in intensity, the reaction is more likely to be life threatening than is one that progresses slowly or not at all once initial signs and symptoms appear. These time factors have a bearing on the management of allergic reactions.

> NOTE: The more rapidly signs and symptoms of allergy occur after exposure, the more intense is the ultimate reaction and the more aggressive its management.

## SKIN REACTION

Allergic skin reactions are the most common sensitization reaction to drug administration. Many types of allergic skin reaction may occur; the three most important types are localized anaphylaxis, contact dermatitis, and drug eruption. Drug eruption constitutes the most common group of skin manifestations of drug allergy. Included in this category are urticaria (itching, hives), erythema (rash), and angioedema (localized swelling measuring several centimeters in diameter). Urticaria is associated with wheals

(smooth, slightly elevated patches of skin) and frequently with intense itching (pruritus). In angioedema, localized swelling occurs in response to an allergen. Several forms of angioedema exist, but they are clinically similar.[57,58] Skin is usually of normal temperature and color, unless the reaction is accompanied by urticaria and/or erythema. Pain and itching are uncommon. The areas most frequently involved include the periorbital, perioral, and intraoral regions of the face, as well as the extremities. Of special interest in dentistry is the potential involvement of the lips, tongue, pharynx, and larynx, which can lead to significant airway obstruction.

The preceding group of signs and symptoms are most often noted in *hereditary angioneurotic edema*. Angioedema is observed most frequently after the administration of topical anesthetics (e.g., ester local anesthetics or methylparaben) to the oral mucosa. Within 30 to 60 minutes the tissue in contact with the allergen appears quite swollen and erythematous.

Allergic skin reactions, if they are the sole manifestation of an allergic response, are normally not considered life threatening. Yet a skin reaction developing rapidly after drug administration may be only the first indication of a more generalized reaction to follow.

Contact dermatitis is an allergic reaction more often observed in members of the dental profession than in dental patients. The sensitization process may require years of constant exposure to the allergen before clinical symptoms occur. These include erythema, induration (hardness), edema, and vesicle formation. Chronic exposure to a specific antigen results in dry, scaly lesions resembling eczema. Signs and symptoms related to allergic skin reactions are presented in Table 24-4.

## RESPIRATORY REACTIONS

Clinical signs and symptoms of allergy may be limited exclusively to the respiratory tract, or signs and symptoms of respiratory tract involvement may occur along with other systemic responses. In a slowly evolv-

table **24-4**   *Clinical manifestations of allergic skin reactions*

| REACTION | SYMPTOMS | SIGNS | PATHOPHYSIOLOGY |
|---|---|---|---|
| Urticaria | Pruritus, tingling and warmth, flushing, hives | Urticaria, diffuse erythema | Increased vascular permeability, vasodilation |
| Angioedema | Nonpruritic extremity, periorbital and perioral swelling | Nonpitting edema, frequently asymetric | Increased vascular permeability, vasodilation |

From Lindzon RD, Silvers WS: Anaphylaxis. In Rosen P, Baker FJ, Barkin RM, and others, editors: *Emergency medicine*, ed 4, St Louis, 1998, Mosby.

ing generalized allergic reaction, respiratory reactions normally follow skin, exocrine, and gastrointestinal responses, but precede cardiovascular signs and symptoms. *Bronchospasm* is the classic respiratory manifestation of allergy. It represents the clinical result of bronchial smooth muscle constriction. Signs and symptoms of an acute episode of allergic asthma are identical to nonallergic asthma. They include respiratory distress, dyspnea, wheezing, flushing, possible cyanosis, perspiration, tachycardia, greatly increased anxiety, and the use of accessory muscles of respiration. Asthma is described fully in Chapter 13.

A second respiratory manifestation of allergy may be the extension of angioedema to the larynx, which produces swelling of the vocal apparatus with subsequent obstruction of the airway. Clinical signs and symptoms of this acutely life-threatening situation include little or no exchange of air from the lungs (*look* to see if the chest is moving; *listen* for wheezing, indicative of a partial airway obstruction, or no sound, indicating complete airway obstruction; *feel* that there is little or no air exchange).

The occurrence of significant angioedema represents an ominous clinical sign. Acute airway obstruction leads rapidly to death unless corrected immediately. Laryngeal edema represents the effects of allergy on the upper airway. Asthma represents the actions of allergy on the lower airway.

Table 24-5 summarizes the clinical signs and symptoms of allergy on the respiratory system.

## GENERALIZED ANAPHYLAXIS

Generalized anaphylaxis is a most dramatic and acutely life-threatening allergic reaction and may cause death within a few minutes. Most fatalities from anaphylaxis occur within the first 30 minutes after antigenic exposure, although many victims succumb up to 120 minutes after the onset of the anaphylactic reaction.[59] It may develop after the administration of

an antigen by any route, but is most likely to occur after parenteral administration. The time from antigenic challenge to the onset of signs and symptoms is quite variable, but typically the reaction develops rapidly, reaching a maximal intensity within 5 to 30 minutes. Delayed responses of an hour or more have also been reported. It is thought that this results from the rate at which the antigen enters the circulatory system.

Signs and symptoms of generalized anaphylaxis are highly variable.[10] Four major clinical syndromes are recognized: skin reactions, smooth muscle spasm (gastrointestinal and genitourinary tracts and respiratory smooth muscle), respiratory distress, and cardiovascular collapse (Box 24-3). In typical generalized anaphylaxis, the symptoms progressively evolve through these four areas; however, in cases of fatal anaphylaxis, respiratory and cardiovascular disturbances predominate and are evident early in the reaction. In a typical generalized anaphylactic reaction the first involvement is with the skin. The patient experiences a generalized warmth and tingling of the face, mouth, upper chest, palms, soles, or the site of antigenic exposure. Pruritus is a universal feature and may be accompanied by generalized flushing and urticaria, whereas nonpruritic angioedema may also be evident initially. Other reactions noted during the early phase of the reaction include conjunctivitis, va-

box **24-3**   *Usual progression of anaphylaxis*

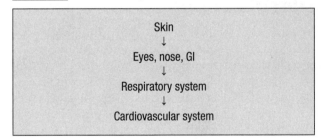

Skin
↓
Eyes, nose, GI
↓
Respiratory system
↓
Cardiovascular system

table **24-5**   *Clinical manifestations of respiratory allergic reactions*

| REACTION | SYMPTOMS | SIGNS | PATHOPHYSIOLOGY |
|---|---|---|---|
| Rhinitis | Nasal congestion, nasal itching, sneezing | Nasal mucosal edema, rhinorhea | Increased vascular permeability, vasodilation, stimulation of nerve endings |
| Laryngeal edema | Dyspnea, hoarseness, throat tightness, hypersalivation | Laryngeal stridor, supraglottic and glottic edema | As above, plus increased exocrine gland secretions |
| Bronchospasm | Cough, wheezing, retrosternal tightness, dyspnea | Cough, wheeze (bronchi), tachypnea, respiratory distress, cyanosis | As above, plus bronchiole smooth muscle contraction |

From Lindzon RD, Silvers WS: Anaphylaxis. In Rosen P, Baker FJ, Barkin RM, and others, editors: *Emergency medicine*, ed 4, St Louis, 1998, Mosby.

somotor rhinitis (inflammation of the mucous membranes of the nose, marked by increased mucous secretion), and pilomotor erection (the feeling of "hair standing on end"). Cramping abdominal pain with nausea, vomiting, diarrhea, and tenesmus (persistent, ineffectual spasms of the rectum or bladder, accompanied by the desire to empty the bowel or bladder), incontinence, pelvic pain, headache, a sense of impending doom, or a decrease in the level of consciousness also occur.

These manifestations may soon be followed by mild to severe respiratory distress. The patient may describe a cough, a sense of pressure on the chest, dyspnea, and wheeze from bronchospasm, or throat tightness, odynophagia (a severe sensation of burning, squeezing pain while swallowing), or hoarseness associated with laryngeal edema or oropharyngeal angioedema. In a rapidly developing reaction, all symptoms may occur within a very short time with considerable overlap. In particularly severe reactions, respiratory and cardiovascular symptoms may be the only signs present.

Signs and symptoms of cardiovascular involvement occur next and include pallor, lightheadedness, palpitation, tachycardia, hypotension, and cardiac dysrhythmias, followed by the loss of consciousness and cardiac arrest. With loss of consciousness the anaphylactic reaction may more properly be called anaphylactic shock.

Cardiovascular signs and symptoms of allergy are summarized in Table 24-6. Any of these patterns may occur singly or in combination.[10] The duration of the anaphylactic reaction or any part of it may vary from minutes to a day or more. With prompt and appropriate therapy the entire reaction may be terminated rapidly; however, the two most serious sequelae, hypotension and laryngeal edema, may persist for hours or days despite therapy. Death may occur at any time, the usual cause (from autopsy reports) being upper airway obstruction secondary to laryngeal edema.

# Pathophysiology

The clinical manifestations of allergy result from an antigen-antibody reaction. Such reactions are a part of the body's defense mechanisms (i.e., immune system), described in the following material to provide a better understanding of the processes involved in allergy.

For acute, immediate allergy or for anaphylaxis to occur, three conditions must be met[10]:

1. An antigen-induced stimulation of the immune system with specific IgE antibody formation
2. A latent period after the initial antigenic exposure for sensitization of mast cells and basophils
3. Subsequent reexposure to that specific antigen

Anaphylactoid reactions are similar to anaphylaxis, but do not require an immunologic mechanism. Anaphylactoid reactions may occur after a single, first-time exposure to certain substances (such as drugs).

table **24-6**   *Clinical manifestations of allergic cardiovascular reactions*

| REACTION | SYMPTOMS | SIGNS | PATHOPHYSIOLOGY |
|---|---|---|---|
| Circulatory collapse | Light-headedness, generalized weakness, syncope, ischemic chest pain | Tachycardia, hypotension, shock | Increased vascular permeability, vasodilation<br>a. Loss of vasomotor tone<br>b. Increased venous capacitance |
| Dysrhythmias | As above, plus palpitations | ECG changes: tachycardia, nonspecific and ischemic ST-T wave changes, premature atrial and ventricular contractions, nodal rhythm, atrial fibrillation | Decreased cardiac output<br>a. Direct mediator-induced myocardial suppression<br>b. Decreased effective plasma volume<br>c. Decreased preload<br>d. Decreased afterload<br>e. Dysrhythmias<br>g. Iatrogenic effects of drugs used in treatment<br>h. Preexisting heart disease |
| Cardiac arrest | | Pulselessness; ECG changes: ventricular fibrillation, asytole | |

From Lindzon RD, Silvers WS: Anaphylaxis. In Rosen P, Baker FJ, Barkin RM, and others, editors: *Emergency medicine,* ed 4, St Louis, 1998, Mosby.

## ANTIGENS, HAPTENS, AND ALLERGENS

An antigen is any substance capable of inducing the formation of an antibody. Antigens are foreign to the species into which they are injected or ingested and may be harmful or harmless. Most antigens are proteins with a molecular weight between 5000 and 40,000. Materials with a molecular weight less than 5000 are usually not allergenic or antigenic. Virtually all proteins, whether of animal, plant, or microbial origin, possess antigenic potential.

Drugs, however, are not proteins and commonly possess a very low molecular weight (500 to 1000), making them unlikely antigens. The hapten theory of drug allergy explains the mechanism through which drugs may act as antigens. A hapten is a specific, protein-free substance that can combine to form a hapten-protein complex with a carrier protein—circulating albumin. The hapten itself is not antigenic; however, when coupled with the carrier protein, it may provoke an immune response. The hapten may combine with the carrier protein outside the body and then be injected into the individual, or the hapten may combine with tissue proteins of the host after administration into the body. The latter mechanism is the one by which most drugs become antigens and thus capable of inducing antibody formation and causing an allergic reaction.[10] Penicillin, aspirin, and barbiturates are examples of haptens. Haptens are also called *incomplete antigens*.

An allergen is an antigen that can elicit allergic symptoms. It is obvious that not every antigen is an allergen. An antigen or allergen may stimulate the production of several classes of immunoglobulins, each of which possesses different functions.

NOTE: All drugs must be viewed as potential antigens and should be administered only when clinically indicated.[60]

## ANTIBODIES (IMMUNOGLOBULINS)

An antibody is a substance found in the blood or tissues that responds to the administration of an antigen or that reacts with it. The molecular weights of antibodies range from 150,000 (immunoglobulin G [IgG]) to 900,000 (IgM). The basic structure of an antibody molecule consists of two heavy and two light polypeptide chains linked in a Y configuration by covalent disulfide bonds. The base of the heavy chain (called *Fc* for crystallizable unit) binds the antibody to the surface of a cell, while the arms of the antibody bind with receptor sites on the antigen.

Immunoglobulins are produced by B lymphocytes (which constitute 10% to 15% of the circulating lymphocyte population) and are classified as IgA, IgD, IgE, IgG, and IgM according to structural differences in the heavy chains. Each immunoglobulin differs in its biologic functions and in the type of allergic response it may elicit (Tables 24-1 and 24-7).[61]

IgA is found principally in the serum and in external secretions such as saliva and sputum. It represents 10% to 15% of all immunoglobulins. It plays a role in the defense mechanisms of the external surfaces of the body, including the mucous membranes. The fetus begins to produce IgA during the last 6 months in utero, and adult levels are reached by 5 years of age.

IgD is found in serum only in small amounts, representing but 0.2% of immunoglobulins. IgD is probably important as an antigen receptor on B lymphocytes.

IgE, the antibody responsible for immediate hypersensitivity, is synthesized by plasma cells in the nasal mucosa, respiratory tract, gastrointestinal tract, and lymphoid tissues. It is only found in trace amounts in the serum. It binds to tissue mast cells and basophils. When mast cell–bound IgE combines with an antigen, the mast cell releases histamine and other vasoactive substances. The half-life of IgE is approximately 2 days, serum levels normally being quite low—0.03 mg/100 mL.

IgG represents approximately 75% to 80% of antibodies in normal serum. Its chief biologic functions are the binding to and enhancement of phagocytosis of bacteria and the neutralization of bacterial toxins. IgG also crosses the placenta and imparts immune

table **24-7**  *Properties of human immunoglobulins*

|  | IgA | IgD | IgE | IgG | IgM |
|---|---|---|---|---|---|
| Molecular weight | 180,000 | 150,000 | 200,000 | 150,000 | 900,000 |
| Normal serum concentration (mg/100 mL) | 275 | 5 | 0.03 | 1200 | 120 |
| Primary function | Local or mucosal reactions and infections | Antigen receptor on B lymphocytes | Type I hypersensitivity | Infection, type III hypersensitivity | Possible role in particular antigens |

protection to the fetus, which continues for the first 6 months after birth. Shortly after birth the infant begins to synthesize IgG, and by the age of 4 to 5 years, IgG levels approach adult levels.

IgM, the heaviest antibody, is active in both agglutinating and cytolytic reactions, accounting for 5% to 10% of all immunoglobulins. Production of IgM begins during the final 6 months of fetal life, and adult levels are reached by 1 year of age.

Antibodies possess the ability to bind with the specific antigen that induces their production. This immunologic specificity is based on similarities in the structures of the antigen and antibody. Antibodies possess at least two specific antigen-binding sites per molecule (the Fab fragments). IgM possesses five, and IgA probably has more than two. Antibodies are not entirely specific, and cross-sensitivity is possible between chemically similar substances.

## DEFENSE MECHANISMS OF THE BODY

When a person is exposed to a foreign substance, the body attempts to protect itself through a number of mechanisms (Box 24-4). These include anatomic barriers, which attempt to exclude entry of the antigen into the body. Examples of barriers include the epithelium of the gastrointestinal tract, the sneeze and cough mechanisms, and the mucociliary blanket of the tracheobronchial tree. Once the foreign substance gains entry to the body, two other nonspecific defense mechanisms are brought into play. These include the mobilization of phagocytic blood cells such as leukocytes, histiocytes, and macrophages, and the production of nonspecific chemical substances such as lysozymes and proteolytic enzymes, which assist in removal of the foreign substance. A more specific defense mechanism is also employed. IgA antibody is produced by plasma cells in response to the antigen. IgA then aids in the removal or detoxification of the antigen from the host.

Through these processes of anatomic localization, phagocytosis, and destruction, the antigen is usually eliminated, resulting in little or no damage to the host. If, however, the antigen survives because of ge-

netic defects in the patient such as atopy or because of the nature of the antigen itself, additional defense mechanisms may be called into play that may ultimately prove harmful to the host. These include reactions resulting in the formation of antibodies that, on subsequent exposure to the antigen, may induce the formation of precipitates of antigen-antibody complexes within cells or blood vessels (type III response) or may result in the subsequent release of the chemical mediators of the type I allergic response.

There are at least three possible results of an antigen-antibody reaction:
1. Antibodies are produced that combine with the antigen to neutralize it or change it so that it becomes innocuous.
2. The antigen-antibody combination occurs within blood vessels in a magnitude sufficient to produce actual precipitates within small blood vessels, resulting in vascular occlusions with subsequent ischemic necrosis (e.g., the Arthus reaction type III).
3. The antigen-antibody union activates proteolytic enzymes that release certain chemicals from cells, which in turn act to produce the anaphylactic response.

The first response is of benefit to the host, leading to elimination of the foreign material; the second and third responses can produce injury and death.

## TYPE I ALLERGIC REACTION— ANAPHYLAXIS

The type I (anaphylactic or immediate) allergic reaction is of great concern to all health professionals. For any true allergic reaction to occur, the patient must have previously been exposed to the antigen. This is called the *sensitizing dose,* and the subsequent exposure to the antigen is called the *challenge dose.*

**Sensitizing dose**  During the sensitization phase the patient is initially exposed to the antigen. In response to the antigen, β lymphocytes are stimulated to develop into mature plasma cells that produce increasing amounts of immunoglobins specific for that antigen. When a susceptible (atopic) individual is exposed, antigen-specific IgE antibodies are formed, which interact only with that particular antigen (or with very closely related antigens, i.e., cross-sensitivity). IgE antibodies are cytophilic and selectively attach themselves to the cell membranes of circulating basophils and tissue mast cells.

Sensitization occurs when the complement-fixing (Fc) portion of the IgE antibody affixes to receptor sites on the cell membrane of mast cells in the interstitial space and circulating basophils in the vascular

---

box **24-4**  *Defense mechanisms of the body*

Anatomic barriers
Mobilization of phagocytic blood cells
Production of enzymes
IgA antibody production

space.[62,63] A latent period of variable duration (several days to possibly years) ensues, during which time IgE antibody continues to be produced (attaching to basophils and mast cells) while the level of antigen progressively decreases. After this latent period, antigen is no longer present, but high levels of IgE-sensitized basophils and mast cells remain. The patient is then sensitized to the specific antigen.

**Challenge (allergic) dose**   Reexposure to the antigen results in an antigen-antibody interaction thought to be initiated by the antigen bridging the antibody fixing (Fab) arms of two adjacent IgE antibodies on the surface of sensitized mast cells or basophils.[64] In the presence of calcium, this bridging initiates a complex series of intramembrane and intracellular events that culminate in structural and functional membrane changes, granule solubilization, exocytosis, and the release of preformed chemical mediators of allergy into the circulation.[65] The primary preformed mediators of allergy are histamine, eosinophilic chemotactic factor of anaphylaxis (ECF-A), high-molecular-weight–neutrophil chemotactic factor (HMW-NCF), and the kallikreins.[66] Other preformed chemical mediators include enzymatic proteases (e.g., tryptase), acid hydrolases, and proteoglycans. These preformed mediators in turn may directly produce local and systemic pharmacologic effects, cause the release of other spontaneously generated mediators, or activate reflexes that ultimately produce the clinical picture of anaphylaxis. Spontaneously generated mediators include the leukotrienes, prostaglandins, and platelet aggregating factor (PAF).[67]

**Chemical mediators of anaphylaxis**   The endogenous chemicals released from tissue mast cells and circulating basophils act on the primary target tissues, including the vascular, bronchial, and gastrointestinal smooth muscle, vascular endothelium, and exocrine glands, and are ultimately responsible for the clinical picture of allergy. That these chemicals are responsible for the signs and symptoms of allergy explains the similarity in allergic reactions regardless of the antigen inducing the response (e.g., penicillin, aspirin, procaine, shellfish, strawberries, peanuts, bisulfites, stinging insects). The level of intensity of an allergic reaction may vary greatly (e.g., anaphylaxis, mild urticaria) from patient to patient. Factors involved in determining the level of magnitude of an allergic response include (1) the amount of antigen or antibody present, (2) the affinity of the antibody for the antigen, (3) the concentration of chemical mediators, (4) the concentration of receptors for mediators, and (5) the affinity of the mediators for receptors. All these factors, except for the antigen, are endogenous, which explains the wide variation in individual susceptibility. The major chemical mediators of allergy are briefly described along with their primary biologic functions.

*Histamine.* Histamine is a widely distributed normal constituent of many tissues of the body, including the skin, lungs, nervous system, and gastrointestinal tract. In many tissues histamine is stored in preformed granules within the mast cell (a fixed-tissue cell) or in circulating blood in basophils.[68] It is stored in these sites in a physiologically inactive form and is electrostatically bound to heparin in granule form. When an IgE-induced antigen-antibody reaction occurs, these granules undergo a process in which they are activated and released from the basophils and mast cells without damaging the cell. The actions of histamine within the body (which is described in the following paragraphs) are mediated by two different tissue histamine receptors called $H_1$ and $H_2$.[69,70] The clinical manifestations of histamine are influenced by the ratio of $H_1$ and $H_2$ activation.[67]

Particularly important pharmacologic actions of histamine include those on the cardiovascular system, smooth muscle, and glands. Cardiovascular actions of histamine include capillary dilation and increased capillary permeability. The action of capillary dilation, an $H_1$ and $H_2$ effect, is probably the most important action effected by histamine. All capillaries are involved after histamine administration. The effect is most obvious in the skin of the face and upper chest, the so-called *blushing area,* which becomes hot and flushed. Increased capillary permeability also leads to an outward passage of plasma protein and fluid into extracellular spaces, resulting in the formation of edema.

Other cardiovascular responses to histamine include the *triple response.* When administered subcutaneously or released in the skin, histamine produces (1) a localized red spot extending a few millimeters around the site of injection, (2) a brighter red flush or flare that is irregular in outline and extends for about 1 cm beyond the original red spot, and (3) localized edema fluid, which forms a wheal that is noted in about 1.5 minutes and occupies the same area as the original red spot. Histamine is also the chemical mediator of pain and itch.

Because of the cardiovascular actions of histamine, there is a decrease in venous return and a significant reduction in systemic blood pressure and cardiac output. The resulting hypotension is normally of short duration because of the rapid inactivation of histamine and because of other compensatory reflexes that are activated in response to histamine release, including increased catecholamine release from the adrenal medulla. Histamine relaxes vascular smooth muscle in humans; however, most nonvascular smooth muscle is contracted ($H_1$). Smooth muscle constriction is most prominent in the uterus and bronchi. Bronchiolar smooth muscle constriction leads to the clinical syndrome of bronchospasm.

Smooth muscle of the gastrointestinal tract is moderately constricted, whereas that of the urinary bladder and gallbladder is only slightly constricted.

Actions of histamine on exocrine glands involve stimulation of secretions. Stimulated glands include the gastric, salivary, lacrimal, pancreatic, and intestinal glands. Increased secretion from mucous glands leads to the clinical syndrome of rhinitis, which is prominent in many allergic reactions.

Histamine is considered to be *the* major chemical mediator of anaphylaxis. Many of the physiologic responses to histamine may be moderated or blocked by the administration of pharmacologic doses of histamine-blockers before the release of histamine has occurred.

*Slow-reacting substance of anaphylaxis (SRS-A).* SRS-A is a spontaneously generated mediator thought to be produced from the interaction of the antigen–IgE–mast cell and the subsequent transformation of cell membrane lipids to arachidonic acid. Arachidonic acid is then metabolized to the prostaglandins, thromboxanes, and prostacyclins, or to the leukotrienes. SRS-A was recently identified as a mixture of leukotrienes ($LTC_4$, $LTD_4$, $LTE_4$).[71] Leukotrienes produce a marked and prolonged bronchial smooth muscle contraction. This effect is 6000 times as potent as that of histamine.[72] This bronchoconstrictive action is slower in onset (thus its original name, SRS-A) and longer lasting than that of histamine. Leukotrienes also increase vascular permeability and potentiate the effects of histamine.[73] The actions of leukotrienes are not diminished or reversed by histamine-blocking drugs.

*Eosinophylic chemotactic factor of anaphylaxis (ECF-A).* ECF-A is a preformed mediator that has the ability to attract eosinophils to the target organ involved in the allergic reaction.[74] Eosinophils, through their release of secondary enzymatic mediators, are major regulatory leukocytes of anaphylaxis.

Another preformed mediator, *HMW-NCF,* is released rapidly into the circulation, has a half-life of several hours, and has a second peak level that correlates with the late-phase asthmatic response.[75]

*Basophil kallikreins,* preformed mediators, are responsible for the generation of kinins. Bradykinins have been implicated as the mediators responsible for cardiovascular collapse in clinical situations where no other manifestations of anaphylaxis are present.[76] The pharmacologic actions of the bradykinins include vasodilation, increased permeability of blood vessels, and production of pain. Blood levels of bradykinin are significantly increased during anaphylaxis.

*Prostaglandins* (PGs) are spontaneously generated mediators that are metabolites of arachidonic acid. Almost all cells can produce these potent mediators. $PGD_2$ causes smooth muscle contraction and increased vascular permeability; $PGE_1$ and $PGE_2$ produce bronchodilation, whereas $PGF_2$ is a potent bronchoconstrictor.[77]

*Platelet-activating factor* (PAF) has recently been described in humans[78] and is the most potent compound known to cause the aggregation of human platelets.[79] PAF produces many important clinical findings in anaphylaxis, including cardiovascular collapse, pulmonary edema, and a prolonged increase in total pulmonary resistance.[80]

The chemical mediators described here act on the primary target organs to produce the clinical picture (signs and symptoms) of allergy and anaphylaxis.

## RESPIRATORY SIGNS AND SYMPTOMS

Vasodilation and increased vascular permeability result in transudation of plasma and proteins into interstitial spaces, which, along with increases in the secretion of mucus, laryngeal edema, and angioedema, may result in asphyxia from upper respiratory tract obstruction.[81] Bronchospasm resulting from bronchial smooth muscle constriction, respiratory mucosal edema, and increased mucus production can produce coughing, chest tightness, dyspnea, and wheezing.[10]

## CARDIOVASCULAR SIGNS AND SYMPTOMS

Decreased vasomotor tone and increases in venous capacitance secondary to vasodilation can provoke cardiovascular collapse. Circulatory collapse may develop suddenly and without prior respiratory or dermatologic manifestations.[82] Lightheadedness and syncope, tachycardia, dysrhythmia, orthostatic hypotension, and shock are all results of these cardiovascular responses.

## GASTROINTESTINAL SIGNS AND SYMPTOMS

Cramping, abdominal pain, nausea and vomiting, diarrhea, and tenesmus are produced by gastrointestinal mucosal edema and smooth muscle contraction.[83]

## URTICARIA, RHINITIS, AND CONJUNCTIVITIS

These are endpoints of increased vascular permeability and vasodilation.[10]

In cases of fatal anaphylaxis the most prominent clinical pathologic features are observed in the respiratory and cardiovascular systems and include laryngeal edema, pulmonary hyperinflation, peribronchial vascular congestion, intraalveolar hemorrhage, pulmonary edema, increased tracheobronchial secretions, eosinophilic infiltration of the bronchial walls, and varying degrees of myocardial damage.[84]

# Management

The clinical expression of allergy may be quite varied. Of special concern to the doctor are signs and symptoms of immediate allergy, which range from mild skin lesions to angioedema to generalized anaphylaxis. The speed with which symptoms of allergy appear and the rate at which they progress have a determining effect on the mode of management of the reaction.

## SKIN REACTIONS

Skin lesions may range from localized angioedema to diffuse erythema, urticaria, and pruritus. Management of these reactions is based on the speed with which they appear after antigenic challenge (e.g., drug administration).

**Delayed reactions**   Skin reactions that appear a considerable time after antigenic exposure (60 minutes or more) and do not progress may be considered, at least initially, to be non–life threatening. These include a mild skin reaction or a localized mucous membrane reaction after the application of topical anesthesia.

Diagnostic clues to the presence of an allergic skin reaction include the following[85]:
- Hives, itching
- Edema
- Flushed skin

*Step 1: termination of the dental procedure.* Stop treatment immediately on recognizing the clinical manifestations of an allergic skin reaction.

*Step 2:* **P** *(position).* Because this patient is not in distress except for a degree of discomfort produced by any itching that might be present, positioning is based on comfort.

*Step 3:* **A-B-C** *(airway-breathing-circulation), basic life support (BLS), as needed.* Assess airway, breathing, and circulation, implementing basic life support as needed. At this juncture, airway, breathing, and circulation will be adequately maintained by the patient.

*Step 4:* **D** *(definitive care):*
*Step 4a: administration of histamine-blocker.* Immediate management of a mild, delayed-onset skin reaction will be to *consider* the administration of a histamine blocker. In the presence of a very localized response, such as a small area of the lower lip appearing slightly swollen, erythematous, and itching after topical anesthetic application, observation might be considered the initial mode of treatment. The patient, or parent or guardian, should be advised to call the dental office immediately if the reaction appears to increase so that a suitable drug (histamine blocker) may be prescribed. An alternative in this case of a very mild, localized reaction is to give the patient a prescription for an oral histamine blocker and either advise the patient not to take the drug unless the reaction becomes bothersome or to begin taking the drug immediately. When taken orally, administer the histamine blocker as recommended for 2 to 3 days. The oral dose of diphenhydramine is 50 mg (for adults) three to four times a day, and 25 mg for children over 20 pounds. Chlorpheniramine (4 mg for adults, three or four times a day; for children, 2 mg every 4 to 6 hours) may be given in its place.

There is rarely an indication for summoning outside medical assistance for this type of response. When a *more generalized slow-onset skin reaction* develops, recommended management is somewhat more aggressive. This situation is most likely to occur in a patient who has received oral antibiotic prophylaxis about 1 hour before the onset of symptoms and has developed a more generalized allergic skin reaction. Examination of the patient demonstrates no involvement, as yet, of other systems. Management of this patient should involve the intravenous (IV) or intramuscular (IM) administration of a histamine blocker such as diphenhydramine (50 mg for adults;

25 mg for children) or chlorpheniramine (10 mg for adults; 5 mg for children). Onset of action of an intravenously administered histamine blocker will be within a few minutes, whereas 10 to 30 minutes might be required for the relief of symptoms after intramuscular administration. The patient is then given a prescription for either diphenhydramine or chlorpheniramine to be taken orally every 4 to 6 hours for 2 to 3 days.

Do not permit this patient to leave the dental office until the clinical signs and symptoms have resolved. In addition, do not allow a patient who has received a parenteral histamine blocker to leave the dental office alone or to operate a motor vehicle. Varying degrees of central nervous system (CNS) depression (e.g., drowsiness, fatigue, sedation) are noted after histamine blocker administration by any route, but this is much more likely when the agent is administered parenterally.

*Step 4b: medical consultation.* A consultation with the patient's physician or an allergist should follow, with a thorough evaluation of the allergic reaction completed before continuing any future dental treatment. Compile a complete list of all drugs and chemicals administered to the patient for use by the allergist.

If the skin reaction does not develop until the patient has left the dental office, request that the patient return to the office,* where one of the therapies just described will be employed.

Should the reaction occur when the patient is unable to return to the dental office, advise the patient to see his or her physician or to report to the emergency room of a local hospital.

Histamine blockers reverse the actions of histamine by occupying $H_1$ receptor sites on the effector cell (competitive antagonism). Histamine blockers thereby prevent the agonist molecules (histamine) from occupying these sites, without initiating a response themselves. The protective responses of histamine blockers include the control of edema formation and pruritus. Other allergic responses such as hypotension and bronchospasm are influenced little, if at all, by histamine blockers. It can be seen therefore that histamine blockers are of value only in mild allergic responses where small quantities of histamine have been released or in the prevention of allergic reactions in allergic individuals.

---

*Although most delayed-onset, localized skin reactions do not progress to systemic involvement and anaphylaxis, extreme caution must be observed with all allergic reactions. It is impossible to effectively evaluate a patient by telephone.

box **24-5** | *Management of delayed-onset, allergic skin reaction*

Terminate dental procedure.
↓
**P**—position patient comfortably.
↓
**A-B-C**—assess and perform BLS, as needed.
↓
**D**—initiate definitive care:

| ↓ | ↓ | ↓ |
| Observe patient. | Administer oral histamine blocker, prn. | Administer IM + oral histamine blocker q4-6h. |

↓
Begin medical consultation.

Box 24-5 outlines the steps in management of the delayed-onset, allergic skin reaction.
- **Drugs used in management:** For this, give a histamine blocker orally or parenterally.
- **Medical assistance required:** None is required.

**Rapid-onset skin reaction** Allergic skin reactions arising in less than 60 minutes should be managed more aggressively. Other allergic symptoms of a relatively minor nature included in this section are conjunctivitis, rhinitis, urticaria, pruritus, and erythema.

Diagnostic clues to the presence of an allergic skin reaction include the following[85]:
- Same as delayed skin reaction
- Conjunctivitis
- Rhinitis

*Step 1: termination of the dental procedure.* Stop treatment immediately on recognition of the clinical manifestations of allergy.

*Step 2: **P** (position).* Because this patient is not in acute distress, positioning is based on comfort.

*Step 3: **A-B-C** (airway, breathing, circulation), (BLS), as needed.* Assess airway, breathing, and circulation and implement basic life support as needed. At this juncture, airway, breathing, and circulation will be adequate.

*Step 4: **D** (definitive care):* Management of the more rapid-onset allergic reaction is predicated on the presence or absence of signs of respiratory and/or cardiovascular involvement. Allergy that appears shortly after antigenic challenge is more likely to progress rapidly and to be more intense than a delayed-onset reaction. Treatment will necessarily be more aggressive the more rapid the onset.

*Step 4a: monitoring of vital signs.* Monitor and record vital signs—heart rate and rhythm, blood pressure, and respirations—every 5 minutes.

*Step 4b: administration of histamine blocker.* In the absence of signs of cardiovascular and respiratory involvement (no tachycardia, hypotension, dizziness, lightheadedness, dyspnea, or wheezing), definitive management involves the administration of a parenteral histamine blocker. Give either diphenhydramine or chlorpheniramine intravenously or intramuscularly as described in the previous section. When the clinical signs and symptoms resolve, prescribe an oral histamine blocker for 2 to 3 days. Do not permit the patient to leave the office alone or to operate a motor vehicle. Medical evaluation should be completed before any further dental treatment.

*Step 4c: repositioning of patient.* In the presence of signs of either cardiovascular or respiratory involvement (tachycardia, hypotension, dizziness, lightheadedness, dyspnea, wheezing), additional steps are necessary. If *hypotension* is evident, reposition the patient in the supine position with legs elevated. Should *respiratory distress* be present in the absence of cardiovascular involvement, position is determined by patient comfort.

*Step 4d: oxygen and venipuncture administration, if available.* Administer oxygen via nasal cannula, nasal hood, or face mask as soon as it becomes available. In addition, if equipment and trained personnel are available, establish an IV line.

*Step 4e: administeration of epinephrine.* Recommended management of this mild anaphylactic reaction involving either the cardiovascular and/or respiratory systems requires the immediate IM administration of 0.3 mL (0.3 mg) of a 1:1000 epinephrine solution (adult), 0.15 mg (child), or 0.075 mg (infant). Epinephrine may be administered every 5 to 20 minutes as needed, to a total of three doses. If the IV route is available, administer 1 mL of 1:10,000 (0.1 mg) by slow IV push over 3 to 5 minutes. Observe the patient for either the desired therapeutic effect or the development of complications. Additional 0.1 mg (1 mL) doses may be administered over a 15- to 30-minute period to a maximum dose of 5 mL.

*Step 4f: summoning of medical assistance.* It is my firm conviction that any allergic reaction requiring the administration of epinephrine also requires additional medical assistance.

*Step 4g: administration of histamine blocker.* After resolution of the cardiovascular and/or respiratory signs and symptoms of the allergic reaction, administer a histamine blocker (diphenhydramine, 50 mg, or chlorpheniramine, 10 mg) intramuscularly. The pediatric dose of diphenhydramine is 25 mg, and chlorpheniramine is 5 mg. Histamine blockers are administered intramuscularly to provide a more prolonged duration of clinical activity.

*Step 4h: continual monitoring and recording of the cardiovascular and respiratory responses of the patient throughout the episode.* The need for additional drug therapy (e.g., epinephrine) will be based on these findings.

*Step 4i: recovery and discharge.* With the arrival of emergency medical personnel, an IV infusion will be started, if not done previously, and appropriate drug therapy administered. The patient who has had a mild anaphylactic reaction (e.g., urticaria, rhinitis, conjunctivitis, with respiratory and/or cardiovascular involvement) will be stabilized and transported to the emergency department of a hospital for observation and possible additional treatment.

Box 24-6 outlines the steps in management of a rapid-onset skin reaction.

- **Drugs used in management:** Oxygen, a histamine blocker (intramuscularly), and epinephrine (intramuscularly or intravenously).
- **Medical assistance required:** None is required if skin only; it is needed if there is respiratory and/or cardiovascular involvement.

## RESPIRATORY REACTIONS

**Bronchospasm** The most likely situations in dentistry in which an allergic reaction will manifest itself as a respiratory problem (bronchospasm) are (1) in the asthmatic patient who is allergic to bisulfites and comes into contact with them during dental care and (2) in the patient who is allergic to aspirin.

Diagnostic clues to the presence of an allergy involving bronchospasm include the following:
- Wheezing
- Use of accessory muscles of respiration

Bronchial smooth muscle constriction results in asthma-like reactions. Management of the acute asthmatic episode was described in depth in Chapter 13 and includes the following steps.

*Step 1: termination of the dental procedure.*

*Step 2: **P** (position).* An upright or semierect position is usually preferred by the conscious patient exhibiting difficulty breathing.

*Step 3: **A-B-C** (airway, breathing, circulation), or BLS, as needed.* Assessment of airway and circulation initially proves adequate. Breathing may show varying degrees of inadequacy, ranging from mild bronchospasm to almost complete obstruction, and cyanosis.

*Step 4: removal of materials from the patient's mouth.*

*Step 5: calming of the patient.* The conscious patient who experiences respiratory distress may become quite fearful. Try to allay any apprehensions.

*Step 6: **D** (definitive care):*

*Step 6a: summoning of medical assistance:* With clinically evident respiratory distress associated with wheezing and cyanosis, immediately summon emergency medical care.

*Step 6b: administration of bronchodilator.* Give epinephrine by means of an aerosol inhaler (Medihaler Epi) (Fig. 24-2), by IM or subcutaneous injection (0.3 mL of a 1:1000 dilution for adults), or intravenously (0.1 mL of 1:10,000) every 15 to 30 minutes. The potent bronchodilating actions of epinephrine usually terminate bronchospasm within a few minutes of administration. Epinephrine is the drug of choice as a bronchodilator because it effectively reverses the actions of one of the major causes of bronchospasm—histamine—but, like the histamine blockers, epinephrine does not relieve bronchospasm produced by leukotrienes.[86] Other inhaled bronchodilators, such as albuterol, may be used in the management of bronchospasm.

*Step 6c: monitoring of the patient.* Have the patient remain in the dental office for observation because a recurrence of bronchospasm is possible as the epinephrine undergoes rapid biotransformation. Should bronchospasm reappear, readminister epinephrine intramuscularly, subcutaneously, or by inhalation (aerosol).

*Step 6d: administration of histamine blocker.* The IM administration of a histamine blocker minimizes the risk of a recurrence of bronchospasm because the histamine blocker occupies the histamine

| box **24-6** | *Management of rapid-onset, allergic skin reaction* |

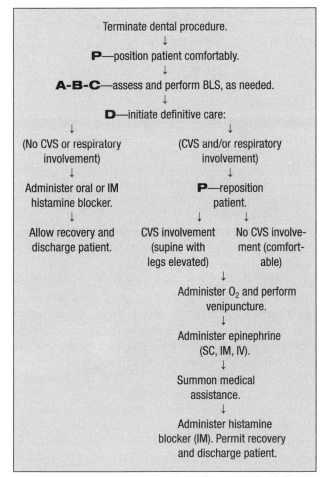

Terminate dental procedure.
↓
**P**—position patient comfortably.
↓
**A-B-C**—assess and perform BLS, as needed.
↓
**D**—initiate definitive care:
↓                                    ↓
(No CVS or respiratory              (CVS and/or respiratory
involvement)                        involvement)
↓                                    ↓
Administer oral or IM               **P**—reposition
histamine blocker.                  patient.
↓                              ↓              ↓
Allow recovery and       CVS involvement     No CVS involve-
discharge patient.       (supine with        ment (comfort-
                         legs elevated)      able)
                                ↓
                         Administer O₂ and perform
                         venipuncture.
                                ↓
                         Administer epinephrine
                         (SC, IM, IV).
                                ↓
                         Summon medical
                         assistance.
                                ↓
                         Administer histamine
                         blocker (IM). Permit recovery
                         and discharge patient.

**P,** Position; **A,** airway; **B,** breathing; **C,** circulation; **D,** definitive care; *BLS,* basic life support; *O₂,* oxygen; *IM,* intramuscular; *IV,* intravenous; *SC,* subcutaneous.

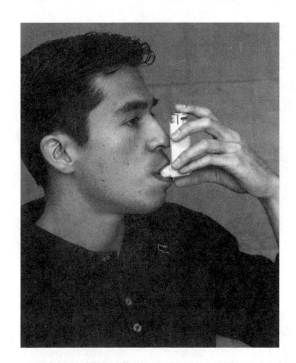

**Figure 24-2** Aerosol spray of bronchodilator for management of bronchospasm.

receptor site, preventing a relapse. Diphenhydramine, 50 mg IM (adults), or 2 mg/kg IM or IV (children), is recommended.

*Step 6e: recovery and discharge.* With arrival of emergency medical personnel the victim will be stabilized, and additional treatment started, if necessary. Additional treatment may involve the administration of one or more of the following: intravenous bronchodilators; atropine, steroids (methylprednisolone), and intubation and ventilation if bronchospasm is persistent and severe. In most cases a patient exhibiting an allergic reaction consisting primarily of respiratory signs and symptoms will require a variable period of hospitalization.

Box 24-7 outlines the steps to take in managing the respiratory allergic reaction.
- **Drugs used in management:** Oxygen; bronchodilators, specifically, epinephrine (inhalation, intravenously, intramuscularly, or subcutaneously); and a histamine blocker (intramuscularly).
- **Medical assistance required:** Assistance is needed if there is significant respiratory distress.

**Laryngeal edema**   The second and usually more life-threatening respiratory allergic manifesta-

tion is the development of laryngeal edema. It may be diagnosed when little or no air movement can be heard or felt through the mouth and nose despite exaggerated spontaneous respiratory movements by the patient, or when a patent airway cannot be obtained. A partially obstructed larynx in the presence of spontaneous respiratory movements produces the characteristically high-pitched crowing sound of stridor, in contrast to the wheezing of bronchospasm, whereas total obstruction is accompanied by silence in the presence of spontaneous chest movement. The patient soon loses consciousness from lack of oxygen (e.g., hypoxia or anoxia). Fortunately, laryngeal edema is not common, but may arise in any acute allergic reaction that involves the airway.

Diagnostic clues to the presence of laryngeal edema include the following:
- Respiratory distress
- Exaggerated chest movements
- High-pitched crowing sound—stridor (partial obstruction), no sound (total obstruction)
- Cyanosis
- Loss of consciousness

*Step 1: termination of treatment.*

*Step 2: **P**—position the patient.* An upright or semi-erect position is usually preferred by the conscious patient exhibiting difficulty breathing. If the degree of edema is severe, the patient's level of consciousness will be significantly altered and the supine position with feet elevated is most appropriate. Should the patient be unwilling or unable to tolerate the supine position, then position based on comfort is recommended.

*Step 3: **A-B-C** (airway, breathing, circulation), (BLS), as needed.* Airway will be the most critical factor in management of laryngeal edema. Initial management should include extension of the neck via head tilt–chin lift, or jaw thrust–chin lift, followed by the insertion of either a nasopharyngeal tube or an oropharyngeal airway. The conscious patient is usually able to tolerate a nasopharyngeal airway, whereas the orpharyngeal airway is likely to produce a gag reflex.

*Step 4: **D** (definitive care):*
*Step 4a: summoning of medical assistance.*
*Step 4b: administration of epinephrine.* The immediate administration of 0.3 mL of 1:1000 epinephrine intramuscularly (0.15 mL for child, 0.075 for infant) or 10 mL of 1:10,000 epinephrine IV over 5 minutes (adult), repeated every 3 to 5 min-

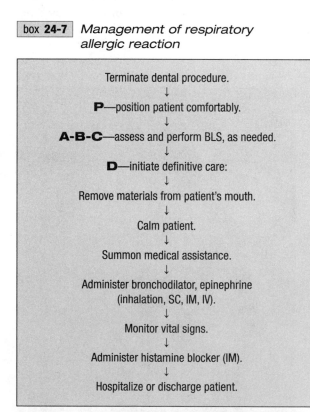

box **24-7**   *Management of respiratory allergic reaction*

Terminate dental procedure.
↓
**P**—position patient comfortably.
↓
**A-B-C**—assess and perform BLS, as needed.
↓
**D**—initiate definitive care:
↓
Remove materials from patient's mouth.
↓
Calm patient.
↓
Summon medical assistance.
↓
Administer bronchodilator, epinephrine (inhalation, SC, IM, IV).
↓
Monitor vital signs.
↓
Administer histamine blocker (IM).
↓
Hospitalize or discharge patient.

*P,* Position; *A,* airway; *B,* breathing; *C,* circulation; *D,* definitive care; *BLS,* basic life support; *IM,* intramuscular; *IV,* intravenous; *SC,* subcutaneous

utes as necessary, is recommended. Do not exceed a maximum dose for 1:10,000 epinephrine of 5.0 mL every 15 to 30 minutes.

*Step 4c: maintainance of airway.* In the presence of a partially obstructed airway, epinephrine administration may halt or even reverse the progress of laryngeal edema.

*Step 4d: administration of oxygen.* Administer oxygen as soon as it becomes available.

*Step 4e: additional drug management.* Administer a histamine blocker (diphenhydramine, 50 mg for adults, 25 mg for children) and corticosteroid (hydrocortisone, 100 mg) IM or IV after clinical recovery, as noted by airway improvement: normal, or at least improved, breath sounds; absence of cyanosis; and less exaggerated chest excursions. Corticosteroids inhibit edema and capillary dilation by stabilizing basement membranes. They are of little immediate value because of their slow onset of action, even when administered intravenously. Corticosteroids have an onset of action approximately 6 hours after their administration.[87] Corticosteroids function to prevent a relapse, whereas the function of epinephrine, a more rapidly acting drug employed during the acute phase, is to halt or reverse the deleterious actions of histamine and other mediators of allergy.

These procedures (steps 1 through 4e) are normally adequate to maintain the patient. With the arrival of medical assistance, the patient will be stabilized and transferred to a hospital for further observation and treatment.

*Step 4f: cricothyrotomy.* A totally obstructed airway may not be reopened at all or not in time by the administration of epinephrine and other drugs. In this case it becomes necessary to create an emergency airway to maintain the patient's life. Time is of the essence, and it is not possible to delay action until medical assistance arrives. A cricothyrotomy is the procedure of choice to establish an airway in this situation. (Cricothyrotomy is described in Chapter 11.) Once an airway is obtained, administer oxygen, use artificial ventilation if needed, and monitor vital signs.

Before the arrival of medical assistance, the drugs previously administered may halt the progress of the laryngeal edema and might even reverse it to a degree. The patient will require hospitalization after stabilization and transfer from the dental office by the paramedics.

Box 24-8 outlines the steps in the management of laryngeal edema.

- **Drugs used in management:** Oxygen, epinephrine (IV, IM), histamine blocker (IM), and a corticosteroid (IV, IM).

- **Medical assistance required:** Assistance is required.

## EPINEPHRINE AND ALLERGY

Epinephrine is the most important drug in the initial management of all immediate allergic reactions involving either the respiratory or cardiovascular system. Its actions effectively counteract those of histamine and other chemical mediators of allergy. Although histamine blockers reverse several allergic symptoms, especially edema and itch, they are of little value with other symptoms such as bronchospasm and hypotension. Epinephrine possesses properties to reverse all of these actions and has a more rapid onset of action than do histamine blockers. The actions of epinephrine are classified as β-adrenergic and α-adrenergic agonist effects. The β-adrenergic effects of epinephrine mimic those produced by efferent sympathetic (adrenergic) nerve activity on the heart ($\beta_1$) and lungs ($\beta_2$), whereas α-adrenergic properties mimic those of the sympathetic nerves on the peripheral vasculature. Useful β-adrenergic actions of epinephrine include bronchodilation, increased myocardial contractility, increased heart rate, and constriction of arterioles with a redistribution of blood to the systemic circulation. Useful α-adrenergic actions include cutaneous, mucosal, and splanchnic vasoconstriction, with a total increase in systemic

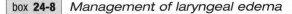

| box **24-8** | *Management of laryngeal edema* |

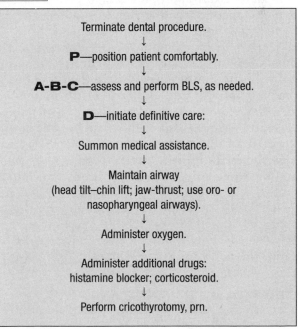

Terminate dental procedure.
↓
**P**—position patient comfortably.
↓
**A-B-C**—assess and perform BLS, as needed.
↓
**D**—initiate definitive care:
↓
Summon medical assistance.
↓
Maintain airway
(head tilt–chin lift; jaw-thrust; use oro- or nasopharyngeal airways).
↓
Administer oxygen.
↓
Administer additional drugs:
histamine blocker; corticosteroid.
↓
Perform cricothyrotomy, prn.

**P,** Position; **A,** airway; **B,** breathing; **C,** circulation; **D,** definitive care.

vascular resistance. This action, in addition to the $\beta_1$-adrenergic actions (e.g., increased heart rate and myocardial contractility), leads to an increased cardiac output. Increased cardiac output, in addition to the increased systemic vascular resistance, produces an increased systemic blood pressure. Through as yet unknown mechanisms, epinephrine also reverses rhinitis and urticaria.

Although epinephrine is rapid acting, it is also a relatively short-acting drug, owing to its rapid biotransformation. Therefore, whenever epinephrine is used in an emergency situation, the patient should be observed for a long enough period to ensure that symptoms of allergy do not recur. In addition, care must be taken when considering the re-administration of epinephrine. Epinephrine produces dramatic increases in heart rate and blood pressure (epinephrine injection has produced cerebrovascular hemorrhage) and increases the risk of developing dysrhythmias. Before re-administering epinephrine (0.3 mL of 1:1000 in adults, 0.15 mL in children, 0.0075 in infants), the cardiovascular status of the patient must be evaluated and the risk of readministration carefully weighed against its benefits.

Epinephrine is relatively contraindicated in elderly patients and in those with known coronary artery disease and hypertension, and it must be avoided in those patients with life-threatening tachydysrhythmias.[10] In these situations it may be prudent to delay the (re)adminstration of epinephrine and to administer a histamine blocker and/or corticosteroid (whichever is/are appropriate) in its place. However, in the presence of continued deterioration of the patient, epinephrine must be (re)administered.

The route of epinephrine administration depends on the severity of the clinical situation. Epinephrine may be given subcutaneously when the reaction is mild and the patient normotensive. However, when generalized urticaria or hypotension exists, subcutaneous absorption may be variable and slow and IM administration is preferred.[10] Whenever possible, the IV route should be used in more acute and life-threatening allergic reactions. It is important to remember that epinephrine 1:1000 is not meant for IV administration. One milliliter should always be diluted with 9 ml of diluent to produce a 1:10,000 concentration, which is administered IV at a rate of 1 ml (0.1 mg) per minute.

## GENERALIZED ANAPHYLAXIS

In generalized anaphylaxis a wide range of clinical manifestations may develop; however, the cardiovascular system is involved in virtually all systemic allergic reactions. In rapidly progressing anaphylaxis, cardiovascular collapse may occur within minutes of the onset of symptoms. Immediate and aggressive management of this situation is imperative if the victim is to survive. In the dental office this reaction is most likely to occur during or immediately after the administration of penicillin or aspirin to a previously sensitized patient. A more remote, although increasingly possible, cause might be latex sensitivity.

Two other life-threatening situations may develop during the injection of a local anesthetic that might on occasion mimic anaphylaxis: vasodepressor syncope and a local anesthetic overdose. In the immediate management of this situation, there must be an attempt to diagnose the actual cause of the problem.

**Signs of allergy present**    Should any clinical signs, such as urticaria, erythema, pruritus, or wheezing, be noted before or after the patient's collapse, the diagnosis is obvious—allergy—and management proceeds accordingly.

*Step 1:* **P**—*position the patient.* Place the unconscious, or conscious but hypotensive, patient into a supine position with the legs elevated slightly.

*Step 2:* **A-B-C** *(airway, breathing, circulation), (BLS), as needed.* Open the airway via head tilt, and carry out the steps of basic life support as needed.

*Step 3:* **D**—*definitive care:*
*Step 3a: summoning of medical assistance.* As soon as systemic allergy is considered a possibility, summon emergency medical care.
*Step 3b: administration of epinephrine.* The doctor should have previously called for the office emergency team. Administer epinephrine from the emergency kit (0.3 mL of 1:1000 for adults, 0.15 mL for children, 0.075 mL for infants) intramuscularly as quickly as possible. Because of the immediate need for epinephrine in this situation, a preloaded syringe of epinephrine is recommended for the emergency kit. Epinephrine is the only injectable drug that needs to be kept in a preloaded form, which minimizes confusion when looking for it in this near-panic situation.

The site for IM injection should be based on muscle perfusion in the presence of what is likely to be profound hypotension. With decreased perfusion, the absorption of epinephrine from a muscle will be delayed. It is recommended that consideration be given to the administration of epinephrine in this situation into the body of the tongue (intralingual) or the floor of the mouth (sublingual) (Fig. 24-3). The

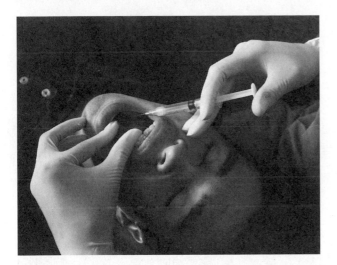

**Figure 24-3**  Sublingual epinephrine injection.

needle may enter from either an extraoral or an intraoral puncture site. The vascularity of the oral cavity, even in the presence of hypotension, will provide a more rapid onset of activity than is seen in the more traditional IM sites (mid-deltoid, vastus lateralis).

Epinephrine, in one or more doses, usually produces clinical improvement in the patient. Respiratory and cardiovascular signs and symptoms should decrease in severity; breath sounds improve as bronchospasm decreases and blood pressure increases.

Should the clinical picture fail to improve or continue to deteriorate (i.e., increasing severity of symptoms) within 5 minutes of the initial epinephrine dose, give a second dose. Subsequent doses may be administered as needed every 5 to 10 minutes, if the potential risk of epinephrine administration (e.g., excessive cardiovascular stimulation) is kept in mind and the patient is adequately monitored.

*Step 3c: administration of oxygen.*  Deliver oxygen at a flow of 5 to 6 L/minute via nasal hood or full face mask at any time during the episode.

*Step 3d: monitoring of vital signs.*  Monitor the patient's cardiovascular and respiratory status continuously. Record blood pressure and heart rate (at the carotid artery) at least every 5 minutes, and start closed chest compression if cardiac arrest occurs. During this acute, life-threatening phase of what is obviously an anaphylactic reaction, management consists of basic life support; the administration of oxygen and epinephrine; and continual monitoring of vital signs. Until an improvement in the patient's status is noted, no additional drug therapy is indicated.

*Step 3e: additional drug therapy.*  Once clinical improvement is noted (e.g., increased blood pressure,

decreased bronchospasm, return of consciousness), additional drug therapy is required. This includes the administration of a histamine blocker and a corticosteroid (both drugs IM or, if possible, IV). They function to prevent a recurrence of symptoms and to obviate the need for the continued administration of epinephrine. They are not administered during the acute phase of the reaction because they are too slow in onset and they do not do enough immediate good to justify their use while the victim's life remains in danger. Epinephrine and oxygen are the only drugs to administer during the life-threatening phase of the anaphylactic reaction.

Throughout this text it has been stressed that definitive treatment of emergencies with drugs is of secondary importance to the PABCs of basic life support. Drugs need not be administered in all emergency situations. Anaphylaxis is the exception. Once a diagnosis of acute, generalized anaphylaxis has been made, it is imperative that drug therapy (i.e., epinephrine) be initiated as soon as possible after the start of basic life support. Review of clinical reports demonstrates the effectiveness of immediate drug therapy in anaphylaxis. Recovery from anaphylaxis is related to the rapidity with which effective treatment is instituted. Delay in treatment increases the mortality rate. Eighty-seven percent of those experiencing anaphylaxis provoked by bee stings survived if treated within the first hour, but only 67% of dying patients were treated in this first hour.[88]

On arrival in the office, emergency personnel will establish intravenous access, administer appropriate drugs (histamine blocker, corticosteroid), stabilize the victim, and transport him or her to the hospital emergency department for definitive care.

Box 24-9 outlines the steps to take to manage generalized anaphylaxis.

- **Drugs used in management:**  Oxygen, epinephrine (IV, IM, or sublingually), a histamine blocker (IM), and a corticosteroid (IV, IM).
- **Medical assistance required:**  Assistance is required.

### No clinical signs of allergy present  A
second clinical picture of anaphylaxis might well be one in which the patient receiving a potential allergen loses consciousness without any obvious signs of allergy being observed.[82,89]

This picture is disturbing because in the absence of obvious clinical signs and symptoms of allergy, drug management of anaphylaxis is not indicated.

*Step 1: Termination of dental treatment.*

*Step 2: **P**—position the patient.*  Management of this situation, which might prove to result from any

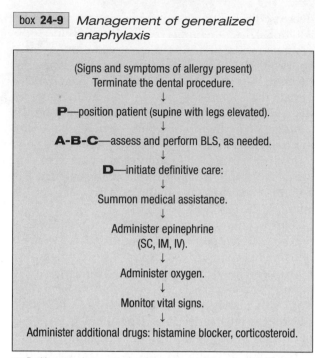

box **24-9**  *Management of generalized
           anaphylaxis*

(Signs and symptoms of allergy present)
Terminate the dental procedure.
↓
**P**—position patient (supine with legs elevated).
↓
**A-B-C**—assess and perform BLS, as needed.
↓
**D**—initiate definitive care:
↓
Summon medical assistance.
↓
Administer epinephrine
(SC, IM, IV).
↓
Administer oxygen.
↓
Monitor vital signs.
↓
Administer additional drugs: histamine blocker, corticosteroid.

**P,** Position; **A,** airway; **B,** breathing; **C,** circulation; **D,** definitive care;
*IM,* intramuscular; *IV,* intravenous; *SC,* subcutaneous.

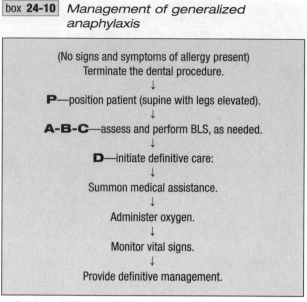

box **24-10**  *Management of generalized
            anaphylaxis*

(No signs and symptoms of allergy present)
Terminate the dental procedure.
↓
**P**—position patient (supine with legs elevated).
↓
**A-B-C**—assess and perform BLS, as needed.
↓
**D**—initiate definitive care:
↓
Summon medical assistance.
↓
Administer oxygen.
↓
Monitor vital signs.
↓
Provide definitive management.

**P,** Position; **A,** airway; **B,** breathing; **C,** circulation; **D,** definitive care.

of a number of causes, requires immediate positioning of the patient in the supine position with the legs elevated slightly.

*Step 3:* **A-B-C,** *or BLS, as needed.* Victims of vasodepressor syncope or postural hypotension rapidly recover consciousness once they are properly positioned and airway patency is ensured. Patients who do not recover at this point should continue to have the appropriate elements of BLS applied (breathing, circulation).

*Step 4:* **D**—*definitive care:*
*Step 4a: summoning of medical assistance.* If consciousness does not return rapidly after the steps of basic life support, seek emergency medical assistance immediately.
*Step 4b: administration of oxygen.*
*Step 4c: monitoring of vital signs.* Monitor blood pressure, heart rate and rhythm, and respiration at least every 5 minutes, and start the elements of basic life support at any time they are required.
*Step 4d: definitive management.* On arrival, emergency medical personnel will seek to diagnosis the cause of the loss of consciousness. If this is possible, appropriate drug therapy will be instituted, the patient stabilized, and then transferred to a local hospital emergency department.

In the absence of any definitive signs and symptoms of allergy, such as edema, urticaria, or bronchospasm, epinephrine and other drug therapies are usually not indicated. Any of a number of other situations may be the cause of the unconsciousness, for example, drug overdose, hypoglycemia, cerebrovascular accident, acute adrenal insufficiency, myocardial infarction, or cardiopulmonary arrest.

Continuing to apply the steps of BLS until medical assistance arrives is the most rational management of this situation.

Box 24-10 outlines the steps to take to manage generalized anaphylaxis without obvious signs of allergy being present.
- **Drugs used in management:** Oxygen.
- **Medical assistance required:** Assistance is required.

## LARYNGEAL EDEMA

Laryngeal edema is yet another possible development during the generalized anaphylactic reaction. Should a patent airway be difficult to maintain despite adequate head-tilt and a clear pharynx (obtained by suctioning), it may become necessary to perform a cricothyrotomy to obtain a patent airway. Laryngeal edema is a very serious manifestation of allergy. Once airway patency has been ensured by cricothyrotomy, epinephrine may be administered (0.3 mL of 1:1000 solution), followed by administration of a histamine blocker and corticosteroid, as described earlier. Once stabilized, the patient should be transferred to a hospital for definitive management and observation.

# REFERENCES

1. *Mosby's medical & nursing dictionary,* St Louis, 1998, Mosby.

2. Gell PGH, Coombs RRA: *Clinical aspects of immunology,* ed 4, Oxford & London, 1982, Blackwell Scientific.

3. Chen MD, Greenspoon JS, Long TL: Latex anaphylaxis in an obstetrics and gynecology physician, *Amer J Obstet Gynecol* 166(2):968, 1992.

4. Leynadier F, Dry J: Allergy to latex, *Clin Rev Allergy* 9(3-4):371, 1991.

5. Portier P, Richet C: De l'action anaphylactique des certain venins. *CR Soc Biol (Paris)* 54:170, 1902.

6. Caranasos GJ: Drug reactions. In Schwartz GR, editor: *Principles and practice of emergency medicine,* Philadelphia, 1992, Lea & Febiger.

7. Buisseret PD: Allergy, *Sci Am* 247:86, 1982.

8. Pascoe DJ: Anaphylaxis. In Pascoe DJ, Grossman J, editors: *Quick reference to pediatric emergencies,* ed 3, Philadelphia, 1984, JB Lippincott.

9. Anderson JA: Allergic reactions to drugs and biologic agents, *JAMA* 268:2845, 1992.

10. Lindzon RD, Silvers WS: Anaphylaxis. In Rosen P, Baker FJ, Barkin RM, and others, editors: *Emergency medicine,* ed 4, St Louis, 1998, Mosby.

11. Idsoe O, and others: Nature and extent of penicillin side-reactions, with particular reference to fatalities from anaphylactic shock, *Bull WHO* 38:159, 1968.

12. Barnard JH: Studies of 400 *Hymenoptera* sting deaths in the United States, *J Allergy Clin Immunol* 52:259, 1973.

13. Lieberman P, Siegle RL, Taylor WW Jr: Anaphylactoid reactions to iodinated contrast material, *J Allergy Clin Immunol* 62:174, 1978.

14. Settipane GA: Adverse reactions to aspirin and related drugs, *Arch Intern Med* 141:328, 1981.

15. Smith VT: Anaphylactic shock, acute renal failure, and disseminated intravascular coagulation: suspected complications of zomepirac, *JAMA* 247:1172, 1982.

16. Sampson HA, Mendelson L, Rosen JP: Fatal and near-fatal anaphylactic reactions to food in children and adolescents, *N Engl J Med* 327(6):380, 1992.

17. Simms J: Latex allergy alert, *Can Nurse* 91(2):27, 1995.

18. Waldbott GL: Anaphylactic death from penicillin, *JAMA* 139:526, 1949.

19. Sogn DD: Penicillin allergy, *J Allergy Clin Immunol* 74:589, 1984.

20. Erffmeyer JE: Adverse reactions to penicillin: a review, *Ann Allergy* 47:288, 1981.

21. Spark RP: Fatal anaphylaxis to oral penicillin, *Am J Clin Pathol* 56:407, 1971.

22. Levine BB: Antigenicity and cross-reactivity of penicillins and cephalosporins, *J Infect Dis* 128:8364, 1974.

23. Samter M, Beers RF Jr: Intolerance to aspirin: clinical studies and consideration of its pathogenesis, *Ann Intern Med* 68:975, 1968.

24. Yurchak AM, Wicher K, Arbesman CE: Immunologic studies on aspirin: clinical studies with aspiryl-protein conjugates, *J Allergy* 46:245, 1970.

25. Spector SL, Farr RA: Aspirin idiosyncrasy: asthma and urticaria. In Middleton E Jr, Reed CE, Ellis FF, editors: *Allergy: principles and practice,* ed 2, St Louis, 1983, Mosby.

26. Lowell FC: "Asthma," "rhinitis," and "atopy," reconsidered (editorial), *N Engl J Med* 300:669, 1979.

27. Ross JE: Naproxen-induced anaphylaxis: A case report. *Am J Forensic Med Pathol* 15(2):180, 1994.

28. Moore ME, Goldsmith DP: Nonsteroidal anti-inflammatory intolerance: an anaphylactic reaction to tolmetin, *Arch Intern Med* 140:1105, 1980.

29. Wasserman SI: Anaphylaxis. In Middleton E, Ellis FF, Reed CE, editors: *Allergy: principles and practice,* ed 5, St Louis, 1998, Mosby.

30. Aldrete JA, Johnson DA: Allergy to local anesthetics, *JAMA* 207:356, 1969.

31. deShazo RD, Nelson HS: An approach to the patient with a history of local anesthetic hypersensitivity: experience with 90 patients, *J Allergy Clin Immunol* 63:387, 1979.

32. Swanson JG: Assessment of allergy to local anesthetic, *Ann Emerg Med* 12:316, 1983.

33. Ogunsalu CO: Anaphylactic reaction following administration of lignocaine hydrochloride infiltration: Case report, *Aust Dent J* 43(3):170, 1998.

34. Ismail K, Simpson PJ: Anaphylactic shock following intravenous administration of lignocaine, *Acta Anaesthesiol Scand* 41(8):1071, 1997.

35. Seng GF and others: Confirmed allergic reactions to amide local anesthetics, *Gen Dent* 44(1):52, 1996.

36. Malanin K, Kalimo K: Hypersensitivity to the local anesthetic articaine hydrochloride, *Anesth Prog* 42(3-4):144, 1995.

37. Jackson D, Chen AH, Bennett CR: Identifying true lidocaine allergy, *J Am Dent Assoc* 125(10):1362, 1994.

38. Aldrete JA, Johnson DA: Evaluation of intracutaneous testing for investigation of allergy to local anesthetic agents, *Anesth Analg* 49:173, 1970.

39. Malamed SF: Evaluation of 220 patients with presumed "allergy to local anesthesia," unpublished data, 1999.

40. Vandenbossche LE, Hop WC, de Jongste JC: Bronchial responsiveness to inhaled metabisulfite in asthmatic children increases with age, *Pediatr Pulmonol* 16(4):236, 1993.

41. Stevenson DD, Simon RA: Sensitivity to ingested metabisulfites in asthmatic subjects, *J Allergy Clin Immunol* 68:26, 1981.

42. Sher TH, Schwartz HJ: Bisulfite sensitivity manifesting as an allergic reaction to aerosol therapy, *Ann Allergy* 54:224, 1985.

43. Clayton DE, Busse W: Anaphylaxis to wine, *Clin Allergy* 10:341, 1980.

44. Twarog FJ, Leung DYM: Anaphylaxis to a component of isoetharine (sodium bisulfite), *JAMA* 248:2030, 1982.

45. Sogn DD and others: Results of the National Institute of Allergy and Infectious Diseases Collaborative Clinical Trial to test the predictive value of skin testing with major and minor penicillin derivatives in hospitalized adults, *Arch Intern Med* 152:1025, 1992.

46. Kamada MM, Twarog F, Leung DY: Multiple antibiotic sensitivity in a pediatric population, *Allergy Proceed* 12(5):347, 1991.

47. Perusse R, Goulet JP, Turcotte JY: Contraindications to vasoconstrictors in dentistry: Part II. Hyperthyroidism, diabetes, sulfite sensitivity, cortico-dependent asthma, and pheochromocytoma, *Oral Surg Oral Med Oral Pathol* 74(5):687, 1992.

48. Schwartz HJ and others: Metabisulfite sensitivity and local dental anesthesia, *Ann Allergy* 62(2):83, 1989.

49. Schwartz HJ, Sher TH: Bisulfite sensitivity manifesting as allergy to local dental anesthesia, *J Allergy Clin Immunol* 75(4):525, 1985.

50. Dajani AS and others: Prevention of bacterial endocarditis. Recommendations by the American Heart Association, *JAMA* 277(22):1794, 1997.

51. Glauda NM, Henerfer EO, Super S: Nonfatal anaphylaxis caused by oral penicillin: report of a case, *J Am Dent Assoc* 90:159, 1975.

52. Malamed SF: The use of diphenhydramine HCl as a local anesthetic in dentistry, *Anesth Prog* 20:76, 1973.

53. Uckan S and others: Local anesthetic efficacy for oral surgery. Comparison of diphenhydramine and prilocaine, *Oral Surg Oral Med Oral Pathol Oral Radiol Endod* 86(1):26, 1998.

54. Benadryl package insert, Parke-Davis, Morris Plains, NJ, 1990.

55. Ewan PW: Anaphylaxis, *BMJ* 316(7142):1442, 1998.

56. Siegel SC, Heimlich EM: Anaphylaxis, *Pediatr Clin North Am* 9:29, 1962.

57. Frank MM, Gelfand JA, Atkinson JP: Hereditary angioedema: the clinical syndrome and its management, *Ann Intern Med* 84:580, 1976.

58. Hopkinson RB, Sutcliffe AJ: Hereditary angioneurotic oedema, *Anaesthesaia* 34:183, 1979.

59. Gavalas M, Sadana A, Metcalf S: Guidelines for the management of anaphylaxis in the emergency department, *J Accid Emerg Med* 15(2):96, 1998.

60. Van Arsdel PP Jr: Drug allergy, an update, *Med Clin North Am* 65:1089, 1981.

61. Katz WA, Kaye D: Immunologic principles. In Rose LF, Kaye D, editors: *Internal medicine for dentistry,* ed 2, St Louis, 1990, Mosby.

62. Ishizaka K, Tomioka H, Ishizaka T: Mechanisms of passive sensitization. I. Presence of IgE and IgG molecules on human leukocytes, *J Immunol* 105:1459, 1970.

63. Isizaka T, Soto CS, Ishizaka K: Mechanisms of passive sensitization. III. Number of IgE molecules and their receptor sites on human basophil granulocytes, *J Immunol* 111:500, 1973.

64. Sullivan TJ, Kulcyzcki A Jr: Immediate hypersensitivity responses. In Parker CW, editor: *Clinical immunology,* vol 1, Philadelphia, 1980, WB Saunders.

65. Ishizaka T, Ishizaka K, Tomioka H: Release of histamine and slow reacting substance of anaphylaxis (SRS-A) by IgE-anti-IgE reactions on monkey mast cells, *J Immunol* 108:513, 1972.

66. Kaliner M, Austen KF: A sequence of biochemical events in the antigen-induced release of chemical mediator from sensitized human lung tissue, *J Exp Med* 138:1077, 1973.

67. Wasserman SI: Mediators of immediate hypersensitivity, *J Allergy Clin Immunol* 72:101, 1983.

68. Piper PJ: Mediators of anaphylactic hypersensitivity. In Brent L, Holborow J, editors: *Progress in immunology II,* vol 4, London, 1974, North-Holland.

69. Black JW, and others: Definition and antagonism of histamine $H_2$-receptors, *Nature* 236:385, 1972.

70. Beaven MA: Histamine, the classic histamine-blockers ($H_1$ inhibitors), *N Engl J Med* 294:320, 1976.

71. Sammuelson B: Leukotrienes: mediators of allergic reactions and inflammation, *Int Arch Allergy Appl Immunol* 66(suppl 1):98, 1981.

72. Israel E, Drazen JM: Leukotrienes and asthma: a basic review, *Curr Concepts Aller Clin Immunol* 14:11, 1983.

73. Levi R, Burke JA: Cardiac anaphylaxis: SRS-A potentiates and extends the effects of released histamine, *Eur J Pharmacol* 62:41, 1980.

74. Wasserman SI, Goetzl EJ, Austen KF: Preformed eosinophiltactic tetrapeptides of human lung tissue; identification of eosinophilic chemotactic factor of anaphylaxis (ECF-A), *Proc Natl Acad Sci USA* 72:4123, 1975.

75. Nagy L, Lee TH, Kay AB: Neutrophil chemotactic activity in antigen-induced late asthmatic reactions, *N Engl J Med* 306:497, 1982.

76. Newball HH and others: Anaphylactic release of a basophil kallikrein-like activity. I. Purification and characterization, *J Clin Invest* 64:457, 1979.

77. Schulman ES and others: Anaphylactic release of thromboxane $A_2$, prostaglandin $D_2$, and prostacyclin from human lung parenchyma, *Am Rev Respir Dis* 124:402, 1981.

78. Wanderer AA and others: Detection and management of cold urticaria patients at high risk for cold-induced systemic reactions (abstract), *J Allergy Clin Immunol* 75:114, 1985.

79. Hanahan DJ and others: Identification of platelet activating factor isolated from rabbit basophils as acetyl glyceryl ether phosphorylcholine, *J Biol Chem* 255:5514, 1980.

80. Pinkard RN and others: Intravascular aggregation and pulmonary sequestration of platelets during IgE-induced systemic anaphylaxis in the rabbit: abrogation of lethal anaphylactic shock by platelet depletion, *J Immunol* 119:2185, 1977.

81. Orange RP, Donsky GJ: Anaphylaxis. In Middleton E, Ellis FF, Reed CE, editors: *Allergy: principles and practice,* ed 5, St Louis, 1998, Mosby.

82. Lockey RF, Bukantz SC: Allergic emergencies, *Med Clin North Am* 58:147, 1974.

83. Austen KF: Systemic anaphylaxis in the human being, *N Engl J Med* 291:661, 1974.

84. Delage C, Irey NS: Anaphylactic deaths: a clinicopathologic study of 43 cases, *F Forensic Sci* 17:525, 1972.

85. Pollakoff J, Pollakoff K: *EMT's guide to signs and symptoms,* Los Angeles, 1991, Jeff Gould.

86. Brocklehurst WE: Slow reacting substance and related compounds, *Prog Allergy* 6:539, 1962.

87. Morris HG: Pharmacology of corticosteroids in asthma. In Middleton E, Ellis FF, Reed CE, editors: *Allergy: principles and practice*, ed 5, St Louis, 1998, Mosby.

88. Peters GA, Karnes WE, Bastron JA: Near fatal and fatal reactions to insect sting, *Ann Allergy* 41:268, 1978.

89. Hanashiro PK, Weil MH: Anaphylactic shock in man: report of two cases with detailed hemodynamic and metabolic studies, *Arch Intern Med* 119:129, 1967.

# 25

# Drug-Related Emergencies

## Differential Diagnosis

**T**HE use of drugs is never undertaken without risk. In this section several adverse drug reactions (ADRs) were described that are potentially life threatening. These reactions are compared here so that the doctor called on to manage them may be better able to rapidly diagnose the precise cause of the reaction and initiate appropriate therapy. Included in the differential diagnosis is vasodepressor syncope because it is a common "drug-related" reaction.

## Medical History

Past medical history is of great importance in the prevention of ADRs. Careful evaluation of a patient's prior response to drugs is a major factor in prevention of these reactions. Allergy must be documented; however, the drug or drugs producing the reaction must be avoided until the patient undergoes more definitive evaluation. When a documented allergy does exist, alternative drugs must be used. Prior history of drug exposure without adverse response does not, however, preclude the occurrence of allergy with the next exposure.

Drug overdose (or toxic) reactions are more difficult to evaluate from the medical history. Patients commonly record all ADRs as "allergy." Only a thorough dialogue history and knowledge of the pharmacology of the drug in question can lead to a diagnosis of prior overdose reaction.

Vasodepressor syncope is commonly associated with parenteral drug administration, particularly the

417

administration of local anesthetics. A history of "blacking out" whenever an injection is administered should lead the doctor to suspect vasodepressor syncope and take measures to prevent its recurrence.

## Age

Allergy and overdose may occur at any age. Children appear to have a greater potential to develop allergy than do adults; however, many children outgrow their childhood allergies, especially food allergies. Interestingly, over 90% of fatalities from anaphylaxis occur in patients over 19 years of age.[1]

Drug overdose may also develop in any patient, but patients on either end of the age spectrum, children and the elderly, represent a greater risk, especially with central nervous system (CNS)–depressant drugs such as sedative-hypnotics, opioid agonist analgesics, and local anesthetics. Adult dosages of these drugs should not be administered to children.

Vasodepressor syncope, on the other hand, is only rarely observed in younger patients or in patients over the age of 40 years. It is an axiom that "healthy children do not faint." They act like children, not keeping their fears inside, but loudly and visibly expressing them. The age span from late teens to late thirties, primarily in males, represents the high occurrence category for vasodepressor syncope.

## Sex

Drug overdose and allergy are not found more often in one sex than the other. However, vasodepressor syncope is much more common in males. The most likely candidate for vasodepressor syncope is a male under the age of 35 years.

## Position

The patient's position at the time clinical signs and symptoms appear is relevant primarily during the administration of local anesthetics. Position has no bearing on the development of allergy or overdose. Both may develop with the patient in an upright or supine position. Vasodepressor syncope, however, is rarely observed if local anesthetics are administered with the patient supine. Injection of local anesthetics into a patient seated upright is much more likely to lead to vasodepressor syncope.

Positioning of the patient once clinical symptoms develop also aids in diagnosing the cause of the reaction if unconsciousness is a clinical sign. Placing the unconscious patient into a supine position leads to rapid improvement in the case of vasodepressor syncope (assuming a patent airway), but produces no significant improvement in the patient suffering from drug overdose or allergy.

## Onset of Signs and Symptoms

Vasodepressor syncope, drug overdose, and allergy may develop immediately after drug administration, or they may develop more slowly. Vasodepressor syncope most often occurs immediately before the actual administration of a drug, but may also develop during or after its administration. Loss of consciousness (syncope) occurring *just before* drug administration is caused neither by allergy nor overdose and is most often related to fear. Clinical symptoms developing *during* drug administration may be related to any of these reactions; however, in this situation the dose of drug injected is of great importance (see text that follows). Signs and symptoms that appear *after* drug administration most probably represent drug overdose or allergy. Vasodepressor syncope may also occur at this time, but in this situation the acute precipitating factor is most probably related to a different stimulus, such as the sight of blood or of dental instruments.

## Prior Exposure to Drug

Prior exposure to a specific drug or to a closely related drug is essential for an allergic response to occur.

Vasodepressor syncope is not truly a drug-related situation except in the sense that the psychologic aspect of receiving a drug may precipitate the reaction. (The injection of sterile water might just as readily precipitate vasodepressor syncope as a local anesthetic in the fearful patient. The main factor in the reaction is the injection.)

Prior exposure to a drug is not relevant in drug overdose. It may occur with the first exposure to the drug or at any subsequent exposure.

## Dose of Drug Administered

Vasodepressor syncope is unrelated to the dose of drug administered, whereas drug overdose is, in most instances, related to the quantity of drug administered. Overdose represents an extension of the normal pharmacologic actions of a drug beyond its desired therapeutic effect and is related to elevated blood levels of that drug in specific target organs. Relative overdose may develop in patients for whom a normal therapeutic dose produces adverse effects (hyperresponders), illustrating the phenomenon of biologic variability as represented by the normal distribution curve.

Allergy is not normally related to the absolute dosage of drug administered. Allergy testing using 0.1 mL of an agent may produce fatal systemic anaphylaxis in a previously sensitized patient.

# Overall Incidence of Occurrence

Vasodepressor syncope is the most commonly occurring adverse reaction in dental offices. Of true adverse drug reactions, minor side effects (nonlethal, undesirable drug actions that develop at therapeutic levels, e.g., nausea or sedation) are encountered most frequently. Drug overdose represents the most common of the potentially life-threatening situations that occur, whereas only 15% of ADRs are truly allergic in nature.[2]

# Signs and Symptoms

## DURATION OF REACTION

Overdose reactions to local anesthetics are normally self-limiting. Inadvertent intravascular injection of one cartridge of local anesthetic may lead to acute clinical symptoms (e.g., seizures) for 1 to 2 minutes before the blood level falls below overdose levels (provided airway patency and oxygenation are maintained). Epinephrine overdose is of extremely short duration because of the rapid biotransformation of epinephrine into inactive forms.

Vasodepressor syncope is commonly self-limiting, the victim regaining consciousness once placed into a supine position.

Allergy, on the other hand, may persist for extended periods. As long as any chemical mediators, released in response to the allergen, remain in the patient's body, signs and symptoms of allergy may continue. It is not uncommon for allergic reactions to persist for hours or days despite aggressive treatment.

## CHANGES IN APPEARANCE OF SKIN

Allergy most often presents as a skin reaction. One of its clinical signs, flushing (i.e., erythema) may occur in other emergency situations, as well; however, when flushing is accompanied by urticaria, pruritus (itching), or both, a clinical diagnosis of allergy is appropriate.

Epinephrine overdose may also produce erythema, yet other clinical signs allow for the ready differentiation of this reaction from allergy. Signs of epinephrine overdose include intense headache, tremor, increased anxiety, tachycardia, and significantly elevated blood pressure.

Pallor and cold, clammy skin are observed in vasodepressor syncope and possibly in local anesthetic overdose as hypotension develops. Pallor may also be noted in the epinephrine overdose reaction. Edema is noted only in allergic reactions.

## APPEARANCE OF NERVOUSNESS

An increase in outward nervousness, described as fear, apprehension, or agitation, after completion of the injection may be observed in both local anesthetic and epinephrine overdose. The patient with vasodepressor syncope may appear nervous before and during the administration of the drug, but does not normally become progressively more nervous during the postinjection period. This patient's major complaint is one of "feeling bad" or "feeling faint." Allergic patients do not develop marked nervousness; most of these patients simply complain of "feeling terrible."

## LOSS OF CONSCIOUSNESS

Local anesthetic overdose, acute systemic anaphylaxis, and vasodepressor syncope may all lead to the loss of consciousness. All may also produce milder reactions that do not evolve to this degree.

Epinephrine overdose seldom produces unconsciousness unless serious cardiovascular complications develop (CVA, cardiac arrest).

## PRESENCE OF SEIZURES

Local anesthetic overdose is most likely to produce generalized seizures of a tonic-clonic variety, whereas milder convulsive movement (e.g., individual muscles such as a finger or facial muscle twitching) may occur in vasodepressor syncope. A mild, generalized tremor of the extremities is normally observed in epinephrine overdose. Seizures do not usually occur with allergy in the absence of hypoxia.

## RESPIRATORY SYMPTOMS

Dyspnea, or difficulty in breathing, may be present in any of these situations. Respiratory symptoms are most marked in the allergic reaction. Wheezing, a product of bronchial smooth muscle constriction, leads to a presumptive diagnosis of asthma or allergy. Because management of both of these clinical entities is identical, precise diagnosis is not immediately required.

table **25-1** *Comparison of drug-related emergencies (by common factor)*

| RELATED (COMMON) FACTORS | VASODEPRESSOR SYNCOPE | OVERDOSE: LOCAL ANESTHETIC OR EPINEPHRINE | DRUG ALLERGY |
|---|---|---|---|
| Age of patient | 18 to 40 years most common | Any age: more likely in children than in adults | Any age |
| Sex of patient | More common in males | No sexual difference in occurrence | No sexual difference in occurrence |
| Position of patient | Unlikely in supine position | Not related to position | Not related to position |
| Onset of symptoms | Before, during, or immediately after administration | During or after administration | During or after administration |
| Prior exposure to drug | Not related | May occur with any drug; any administration | Prior exposure; "sensitizing dose" required |
| Dose of drug administered | Not related | Dose-related | Not dose-related |
| Overall incidence of occurrence | Most common "drug-related" emergency | Overdose is the most common true drug-related emergency (85% of all ADRs) | Rare; represents 15% of all ADRs |

table **25-2** *Comparison of drug-related emergencies (by signs and symptoms)*

| SIGNS AND SYMPTOMS | VASODEPRESSOR SYNCOPE | OVERDOSE | | DRUG ALLERGY |
|---|---|---|---|---|
| | | LOCAL ANESTHETIC | EPINEPHRINE | |
| Duration of acute symptoms | Brief, following positioning | Self-limiting (2 to 30 minutes) | Extremely brief (usually seconds) | Long; hours to days |
| Appearance of skin | Pale, cold, moist | Not relevant | Erythematous | Erythematous, presence of urticaria, pruritus, edema |
| Appearance of nervousness | No drastic increase | Increased anxiety, agitation | Fear, anxiety present | Not present |
| Loss of consciousness | Yes—vasodepressor syncope is most common cause of loss of consciousness | Yes—in severe reaction | No—rarely, if ever | Yes—in severe reaction |
| Presence of seizures | Rare—limited to mild, localized | Yes; tonic-clonic seizure | Mild tremor | No—unless hypoxia present |
| Respiratory symptoms | Not diagnostic | Not diagnostic | Not diagnostic | Wheezing, laryngeal edema |
| **Cardiovascular symptoms** | | | | |
| Heart rate (pulse) | Initial elevation (presyncope), then depression (syncope) | Increased Weak and thready | Dramatic increase in palpitations Full and bounding | Increased Weak and thready |
| Blood pressure | Initially normal (presyncope); then depression | Initial increase; then depression | Dramatic increase | Significant depression |
| Most significant diagnostic criteria | Presyncopal manifestations; rapid recovery following positioning | CNS "stimulation" after drug administration | Palpitations; intense headache; brief duration | Erythematous, urticaria, and pruritus; bronchospasm |

Stridor, a high-pitched crowing sound, should lead the doctor to consider laryngeal obstruction. This may be produced by a foreign object in the posterior pharynx or by laryngeal edema resulting from an allergic reaction. In the absence of other signs of allergy, such as a skin reaction, the airway should be suctioned to remove any foreign material before further management is considered.

Total airway obstruction is most often produced by the tongue in an unconscious patient. If, following airway maneuvers (head tilt–chin lift) and suctioning, the obstruction persists, lower airway obstruction should be considered. Regardless of the cause (e.g., edema or foreign object), a patent airway must be established rapidly through manual thrust or cricothyrotomy.

# Vital Signs

## HEART RATE

The heart rate increases during the presyncopal phase of vasodepressor syncope, but it decreases dramatically to approximately 40 beats per minute once consciousness is lost and remains low during throughout the postsyncopal period.

Local anesthetic overdose and allergic reactions are also associated with increases in heart rate, but bradycardia does not occur when consciousness is lost. A shock reaction develops that is characterized by rapid heart rate (tachycardia) and low blood pressure (hypotension), producing a pulse that is described as "weak and thready."

Epinephrine overdose, on the other hand, produces a dramatic increase in heart rate *and* blood pressure, leading to a "full and bounding" pulse. In addition, the heart rate may become irregular during the epinephrine reaction, owing to the effects of the drug on the myocardium.

## BLOOD PRESSURE

Blood pressure remains at or near the baseline level during the presyncopal phase of vasodepressor syncope. With loss of consciousness, however, blood pressure drops significantly. In acute allergic reactions the blood pressure may fall precipitously because of massive vasodilation. Indeed, this reaction (acute systemic anaphylaxis) is one of the most likely of all the ADRs to lead to cardiovascular collapse (cardiac arrest).

During the early phase of local anesthetic overdose, blood pressure is usually slightly elevated. As the reaction progresses, blood pressure returns to baseline or falls below this level. Blood pressure during an epinephrine overdose reaction is dramatically increased. Pressures greatly in excess of 200 mmHg systolic and 120 mmHg diastolic may be observed during this reaction.

# Summary

Each of these clinical syndromes is presented with several outstanding features.

*Vasodepressor syncope* has a presyncopal phase of relatively long duration. The patient feels faint and lightheaded, the skin loses color, and perspiration is evident. Consciousness is regained rapidly after placing the victim in the supine position. This reaction commonly results from fear and is the most frequent (drug-related) emergency noted in dentistry.

*Local anesthetic overdose* is related to high blood levels of local anesthetic in its target organs: the CNS and the myocardium. It is commonly produced by the administration of too large a dose, overly rapid absorption, or rapid intravascular injection. Commonly, signs and symptoms of CNS stimulation (e.g., agitation, increased heart rate and blood pressure, and possibly seizures) are followed by depression (e.g., lethargy, cardiovascular depression, respiratory depression, and loss of consciousness).

*Epinephrine overdose* is most frequently produced by the use of excessive concentrations of epinephrine in gingival retraction cord and much less commonly by vasopressor-containing local anesthetics. The most prominent clinical signs include greatly increased nervousness; mild tremor; an intense, throbbing headache; and greatly increased blood pressure and heart rate. Epinephrine reactions are usually brief. Consciousness is seldom lost unless significant cardiovascular complications arise.

*Allergy* may manifest itself in a variety of ways. However, obvious clinical signs of allergy include the skin reactions of flushing, urticaria, and itching. Edema may also occur. The presence of wheezing with increased respiratory efforts also signifies allergy. Allergy is the least common of these three ADRs, but is potentially the most dangerous.

Tables 25-1 and 25-2 compare the different types of adverse drug reactions.

## REFERENCES

1. Parrish HM: Analysis of 460 fatalities from venomous animals in the United States, *Am J Med Sci* 245:129, 1963.
2. Caranasos GJ: Drug reactions. In Schwartz GR, Safar P, Stone JH, and others, editors: *Principles and practice of emergency medicine*, ed 2, Philadelphia, 1986, WB Saunders.

# CHEST PAIN

# 26

## Chest Pain

### General Considerations

**T**HERE are many specific causes for the clinical symptom of chest pain that are entirely noncardiac in origin. Yet the sudden onset of chest pain is invariably a frightening experience because it immediately invokes thoughts of "heart attack" in the mind of the victim. Because cardiovascular disease is *the* major cause of death in the United States today, this concern is not entirely unfounded. The almost universal presence of signs of cardiovascular disease in adults means that we all are potential victims of one or more of the clinical manifestations of cardiovascular disease. If we add to this the stresses involved in dental treatment, it becomes evident that many medically compromised patients represent an increased risk during treatment. Recognition of these potentially high-risk patients and the use of specific treatment modifications go far to diminish the chances of life-threatening situations developing.

Although chest pain is a major clue to the possible presence of ischemic heart disease (IHD), the underlying disease process has normally been present for a considerable time before the appearance of clinical symptoms. Indeed, chest pain is not always the presenting symptom of IHD. Previous chapters have discussed two other clinical expressions of cardiovascular disease: heart failure, presenting as respiratory distress (Chapter 14), and cerebrovascular ischemia and infarction (Chapter 19), presenting as an alteration in consciousness. In this section, three additional clinical manifestations of heart disease are discussed. Two of these, angina pectoris (Chapter 27) and myocardial infarction (Chapter 28), most commonly present as chest

425

pain. Another clinical syndrome, cardiac arrest, is discussed in Chapter 30. Cardiac arrest is a possible acute complication of all forms of cardiovascular disease, or it may be the initial indication of the presence of cardiovascular disease.[1]

The most common causes of acute chest pain encountered in dental situations include angina pectoris, hyperventilation, and myocardial infarction (Table 26-1). There are numerous other causes, both cardiac and noncardiac, that present as chest pain and must be differentiated from true cardiac pain. These include hiatal hernia, esophageal spasm, peptic ulcer, cholecystitis, musculoskeletal pain associated with the chest wall syndrome, pulmonary embolism, pneumothorax, mitral valve prolapse, pericarditis, and acute dissecting aortic aneurysm.[2-6] A differential diagnosis of chest pain, both cardiac and noncardiac, is presented in Chapter 29.

A major etiologic factor underlying virtually all forms of cardiovascular disease is atherosclerosis. Atherosclerosis represents a special type of thickening and hardening of medium- and large-size arteries that accounts for a very large proportion of acute myocardial infarcts (AMI or heart attack) and cases of IHD. It is also responsible for many strokes (those caused by cerebral ischemia and infarction[7]), numerous instances of peripheral vascular disease, and most aneurysms of the lower abdominal aorta, which can rupture, causing sudden fatal hemorrhage.[8] Atherosclerosis is present in approximately 90% of patients with significant noncongenital heart disease.[9] When present in arteries that supply the myocardium, the disease state is called *coronary artery disease (CAD)*. Other common names for CAD include *coronary heart disease (CHD), IHD,* and *atherosclerotic heart disease*. CAD may be defined as a narrowing or an occlusion of the coronary arteries, usually by atherosclerosis, that results in an imbalance between the requirement for and the supply of oxygen to the myocardium, leading to myocardial ischemia. An understanding of CAD and atherosclerosis leads to a greater knowledge of their clinical manifestations. The remainder of this chapter discusses the important factors of cardiovascular disease, a disease responsible for 41% of all deaths in the United States.[10]

Definitions of terms to be used in this section are listed in the box at bottom right.

## table **26-1** *Causes of chest pain*

| CAUSE | FREQUENCY | WHERE DISCUSSED |
|---|---|---|
| Angina pectoris | Most common | Chest pain (Section VII) |
| Hyperventilation | Common | Respiratory difficulty (Section III) |
| Acute myocardial infarction | Less common | Chest pain (Section VII) |

# Predisposing Factors

In 1995 diseases of the heart and blood vessels were responsible for an estimated 960,592 deaths in the United States.[11] In 1995, 1,100,000 Americans experienced myocardial infarction, with about 33% dying (366,300 approximately). The remainder succumbed to cerebrovascular accident, high blood pressure, rheumatic heart disease, and other causes such as aneurysms and pulmonary emboli (Fig. 26-1).[11]

The death rate resulting from cardiovascular disease increased in each decade in the United States until the 1970s. Since that time there has been a dramatic decline in the death rate from myocardial ischemia and its complications (see Fig. 26-1).[12] A decline of 20.7% in the death rate was noted between 1968 and 1976.[12] This decline occurred each year and was noted in both sexes, in all age-groups, and in the three major ethnic groups. This decline continues at the present time, with a 37% decline in cardiovascular deaths reported in the past 20 years.[13] Between the years 1985 and 1995 the death rate from IHD declined 28.7%.[10] Reasons for the decline in IHD mortality are not well understood, but are thought to result from factors including the following[14,16]:

- Improved detection and treatment of high blood pressure
- Decreased cigarette use by middle-age men
- A change toward a more prudent diet
- Improvements in the medical and surgical care for cardiovascular disease

These modifications in cardiovascular disease risk factors are thought to account for only half of the decline in mortality for men and a third of the decline in mortality for younger women.[12] In addition, the impact of emergency medical services and coronary artery bypass surgery is not believed to account for this decline in cardiovascular mortality.[12]

Despite these advances and the unexplained decline in cardiovascular mortality, death from cardiovascular disease is still a formidable problem. Cardiovascular disease is still the leading cause of death in the United States (see Figure 26-1). Of an estimated 2,319,679

---

**hypoxia** Reduced oxygen supply to tissue despite adequate perfusion

**anoxia** Absence of oxygen supply to tissue despite adequate perfusion

**ischemia** Oxygen deprivation accompanied by inadequate removal of metabolites consequent to inadequate perfusion

**infarction** Area of coagulation necrosis in a tissue caused by local ischemia, resulting from obstruction of circulation to the area

deaths that occurred in the United States in 1995, 41.5% were caused by cardiovascular disease, two thirds of which were caused by underlying coronary and IHD.[10]

An even more disturbing figure, however, is the overall incidence of cardiovascular disease in the United States. According to the American Heart Association,[10] more than 42 million persons have clinical evidence of one or more forms of cardiovascular disease. These persons represent a great potential risk during dental treatment. Most of these persons are ambulatory, and a significant number may be asymptomatic, perhaps even unaware of their cardiovascular disease, when appearing for routine dental care. As is evident, any procedure or incident that results in an increase in the workload of such an individual's cardiovascular system is potentially dangerous.

In 1995 it was estimated that 1.1 million persons in the United States suffered a myocardial infarction and that 305,000 (36%) died, 250,000 of those before they reached a hospital.[17] Thus more than two thirds of deaths from IHD occurred outside of the hospital, the vast majority within 2 hours of the onset of symptoms.[18] Although infrequent, it is entirely likely that such deaths will occur within the confines of the dental office.

Recent advances in emergency cardiac care have decreased mortality for patients with CAD suffering AMI who reach the hospital.[19,20] Additional decreases in mortality from acute IHD have occurred from the increased use of aspirin in the prehospital phase of AMI,[21,22] thrombolytic therapy, and/or percutaneous transluminal angioplasty.[23] Yet in those instances in which cardiopulmonary arrest occurs outside of the

hospital, the survival rate for those victims who are not resuscitated before their arrival at the hospital remains dismal.[24] The introduction of the automatic external defibrillator (AED) shows promise in increasing this rate of survival.[25,26]

CAD occurs more frequently in males, demonstrating an overall male to female incidence of 4:1. Of all deaths in men between the ages of 55 and 64, 40% are from CAD. In whites between the ages of 35 and 44 years, there is a 5.2:1 male to female ratio for CAD, which progressively falls until between the ages of 65 and 74, the male to female ratio for whites with CAD is 2.3:1. For nonwhites, these male to female ratios are 2.5:1 and 1.5:1, respectively. In general, the female rate lags behind the male rate by about 10 years in whites and by about 7 years in nonwhites.[10,24,27]

Data show that 2% of clinically significant CAD occurs before the age of 30 years. This incidence increases with age; 80% of CAD occurs between the sixth and eighth decades of life (ages 50 to 70 years), with the peak incidence in men occurring between 50 and 60 years of age and, in women, between 60 and 70 years of age.[10,28] The widespread occurrence and increasing incidence of CAD has prompted much research into its causes. In addition, possible methods are being researched to prevent CAD from progressing to the point of clinical morbidity and mortality. To date, a number of factors have been identified that, when present, increase the probability of an individual exhibiting clinical manifestations of CAD.[29] Major risk factors for heart disease are listed in Box 26-1. Although the evidence relating these factors to a significant increase in morbidity and mortality from CAD is obvious, uncertainty remains about the degree of benefit to be obtained by removing or managing these factors.[1,14,15]

## MAJOR MODIFIABLE RISK FACTORS

The following are major risk factors of heart disease that when modified result in a decrease in risk.

**Tobacco smoking**  Tobacco smoking is a major risk factor for AMI and death from CAD. Results of several studies demonstrate that total mortality (all causes), total cardiovascular morbidity and mortality, and the incidence of CAD are about 1.6 times higher in male smokers than in male nonsmokers. There is also a direct relationship between these events and the number of cigarettes smoked daily.[30,31] Fortunately, the excessive risk factor for CAD declines in ex-smokers within 1 or 2 years after they discontinue smoking, but it does remain slightly greater than the risk associated with nonsmokers.[32]

Several reasons for the increased risk caused by smoking have been postulated, including the effects of

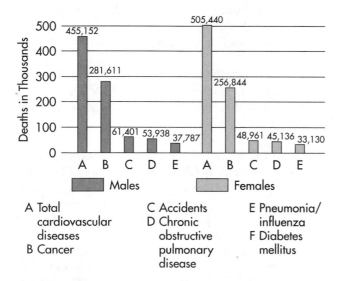

**Figure 26-1**  Leading causes of death for all males and females. (From United States, 1995 Mortality, Final Data from the National Center for Health Statistics and the American Heart Association.)

| box **26-1** | *Major risk factors of heart disease* |

**Factors that cannot be changed**
Heredity
Sex
Race
Age

**Factors that can be changed**
Tobacco smoking
High blood pressure
High blood cholesterol levels
Diabetes

nicotine and carbon monoxide on the heart, coronary arteries, and blood. Nicotine increases myocardial demand for oxygen, increases the adhesiveness of platelets, and lowers the threshold for ventricular fibrillation.[33] Carbon monoxide prevents oxygen from forming oxyhemoglobin, decreasing oxygen availability to tissues. Blood carbon monoxide levels in smokers range from 1% to 20%, compared with normal levels of 0.5% to 1.0% (blood levels from 20% to 80% occur in carbon monoxide poisoning).[34] When a person stops smoking, carbon monoxide blood levels fall, and the increased risk of CAD falls to approximately that of the nonsmoker. This factor also explains the increased incidence of cardiovascular abnormalities noted in automobile passengers on crowded Los Angeles freeways.[35] These subjects were exposed to a significantly higher level of gasoline engine exhausts, of which carbon monoxide is a major part. Carbon monoxide levels in their blood reached 1.4% to 3.0%.

**Blood lipids**    Among the recognized risk factors for the development of atherosclerosis, one of the most well documented is the relationship between blood lipid levels and CAD.[36] Evidence associating increased serum cholesterol levels with increased incidence of CAD is extensive and unequivocal.[37] Stated quite simply, persons with the highest cholesterol levels are at greatest risk of developing CAD, but even those with lower serum cholesterol levels are not completely free of risk.

Several types of lipoproteins have been identified. Low-density lipoprotein (LDL) is known to be atherogenic and is the lipoprotein most directly associated with CAD.[38] High-density lipoprotein (HDL) demonstrates an inverse association with risk of CAD (higher HDL levels equate with lower risk of development of CAD).[39] There is, however, no cutoff point in serum cholesterol levels below which there is no risk.[29] Persons with blood cholesterol levels in excess of 300

mg% have a risk of developing CAD four times greater than do those with blood cholesterol levels less than 200 mg%. Mean levels for total plasma cholesterol (mg/dL) in white males are 200 between the ages of 35 and 39, 213 between the ages of 45 and 49, and 221 between the ages of 65 and 69, whereas plasma LDL cholesterol levels in these same groups are 133, 143, and 150, respectively.[28]

**Blood pressure**    The risk of morbidity and mortality from CAD, as well as the risk of other diseases produced or exacerbated by atherosclerosis, show a smooth, direct relationship to blood pressure levels over the entire range of values. As with blood lipids, there is no cutoff point at which risk suddenly changes from low to high.[40]

Management of high blood pressure through the administration of antihypertensive drugs can decrease risk to the patient.[41] Damage that has developed within arteries over the years due to high blood pressure cannot be undone (see section on pathophysiology); however, the atherosclerotic process will be slowed if the patient's blood pressure is lowered.

**Abnormal glucose tolerance**    Hyperglycemia and glucose intolerance are associated with increased risk of developing CAD. Overt diabetes mellitus has long been recognized as a precursor of vascular disease.[42] Males with glucose intolerance have a 50% greater chance of developing CAD than do those with normal values, whereas in females the risk is doubled.[43] In non–insulin-dependent diabetes the major cause of mortality is CAD. Both non–insulin-dependent and insulin-dependent adult-onset diabetics are at increased risk for developing CAD.[42] Mortality in type I, insulin-dependent diabetes is primarily associated with renal disease.[44]

**Major unmodifiable risk factors**    Several other major risk factors of heart disease remain unmodifiable at this time. These include heredity, sex, race, and age.

*Heredity.*  Persons with either parents or siblings who were affected by CAD before the age of 50 years have a significantly greater risk of developing the disease themselves at a younger age than those who do not have such a history. This risk may be as great as 5:1.

*Sex.*  As was previously discussed, CAD remains predominantly a male disease. The premenopausal female is relatively unaffected by CAD. After menopause the incidence of CAD in females increases, but it never reaches that of males.[28]

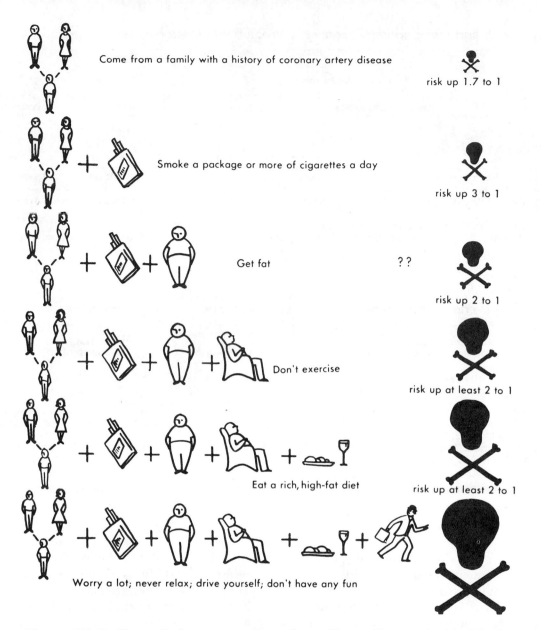

Come from a family with a history of coronary artery disease

risk up 1.7 to 1

Smoke a package or more of cigarettes a day

risk up 3 to 1

Get fat                    ??

risk up 2 to 1

Don't exercise

risk up at least 2 to 1

Eat a rich, high-fat diet

risk up at least 2 to 1

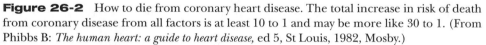

Worry a lot; never relax; drive yourself; don't have any fun

**Figure 26-2**    How to die from coronary heart disease. The total increase in risk of death from coronary disease from all factors is at least 10 to 1 and may be more like 30 to 1. (From Phibbs B: *The human heart: a guide to heart disease,* ed 5, St Louis, 1982, Mosby.)

*Race.* Nonwhite men and women have higher rates of CAD up to the age of 65 years. Among specific ethnic groups in the United States, Japanese men in Hawaii and California, and Hispanic men in Puerto Rico have been found to have about half the amount of CAD as Caucasians.[45]

*Age.* The incidence of CAD increases with age. By 55 to 64 years, 40% of deaths in males result from CAD.

**Minor risk factors**    Other factors related to increased risk of significant CAD that are not as

well supported by clinical evidence include gout,[46] menopause and oral contraceptives,[47,48] obesity,[49] physical activity,[50] and type of personality and behavior.[51,52] In addition, it is known that individuals with certain noncardiac diseases demonstrate a higher incidence of significant CAD. Hypercholesterolemia, high blood pressure, and diabetes mellitus have been mentioned previously. Another disease with significant CAD rates is uncontrolled hypothyroidism. Figure 26-2 illustrates the increased risk of death that is presented by some of these factors.

table **26-2**  *Death and major nonfatal events in untreated and treated hypertensive patients*

| | INITIAL DIASTOLIC BLOOD PRESSURE | | | |
| --- | --- | --- | --- | --- |
| | 115-129 mmHg* | | 90-114 mmHg* | |
| | 70 UNTREATED MEN† | 73 ACTIVELY TREATED MEN | 194 UNTREATED MEN | 186 ACTIVELY TREATED MEN |
| Cardiovascular deaths | 4 | 0 | 19 | 8 |
| Major nonfatal events‡ | 23 | 2 | 57 | 14 |

From Veterans Administration Cooperative Study Group on Antihypertensive Agents (1970). II. Results in patients with diastolic blood pressure averaging 90-114 mmHg, *JAMA* 213:1143, 1970.
*Average period of observation for men with diastolic blood pressure of 115 to 129 was 18 months; for men with diastolic blood pressure of 90 to 114, it was 40 months.
†Includes 20 patients whose diastolic blood pressure exceeded 124 mmHg at three separate clinic visits.
‡Includes congestive heart failure, cerebrovascular thrombosis, cerebral hemorrhage, myocardial infarction, grade 3 or 4 retinopathy, and azotemia.

table **26-3**  *Effectiveness of antihypertensive treatment in reducing death and major nonfatal events*

| INITIAL DIASTOLIC BLOOD PRESSURE | PERCENTAGE OF PATIENTS WITH EVENTS | | EFFECTIVENESS OF TREATMENT (%)* |
| --- | --- | --- | --- |
| | CONTROL | TREATED | |
| 90-114 mmHg | 33.3 | 11.8 | 70 |
| 115-129 mmHg | 33.6 | 2.7 | 93 |

From Veterans Administration Cooperative Study Group on Antihypertensive Agents (1970). II. Results in patients with diastolic blood pressure averaging 90-114 mmHg, *JAMA* 213:1143, 1970.
*Effectiveness of treatment is the difference between percentages of incidence of events in control and treated groups, divided by percentage of incidence in control group.

# Prevention

Unfortunately, primary prevention (i.e., prevention of initial development) of atherosclerosis and CAD has not yet been effectively demonstrated. Research into the known risk factors may ultimately demonstrate the feasibility of prevention of clinical CAD. To date, however, secondary prevention (i.e., prevention of death after the onset of clinical symptoms) is the norm, but in too many cases this effort proves to be too late to prevent death or the occurrence of significant morbidity.

Emphasis is currently being placed on the elimination of any known risk factors that may be present. Smoking is discouraged, optimal weight and physical fitness are encouraged, and special diets and medications are recommended for those with elevated blood cholesterol levels. Uncontrolled hyperthyroidism or diabetes mellitus is brought under control and blood pressure elevations corrected. However, conflicting evidence has been gathered concerning the effectiveness of many of these therapies in preventing morbidity and mortality.

Management of elevated blood pressure has been effectively demonstrated to produce a significant decrease in morbidity and mortality rates from CAD. The Veterans Administration studies (Tables 26-2 and 26-3) proved conclusively that reduction of elevated blood pressure leads to a highly significant decrease in the incidence of fatal and nonfatal cardiovascular events.[53] The Hypertension Detection and Follow-up Program Cooperative Group[54] demonstrated that vigorous drug management of even mild elevations in blood pressure (diastolic blood pressure 90 to 104 mmHg) led to significant reductions (a decline of 20.3%) in cardiovascular morbidity and mortality (Table 26-4).

It stands to reason therefore that monitoring and recording blood pressure of *all* dental patients before dental treatment starts might well prove to be a lifesaving procedure. A suggested protocol for the management of dental patients with elevated blood pressure was presented in Chapter 2.

Another significant factor that may be applied to the dental office setting is the reduction of stress re-table **26-4** | *Mortality from all causes for stepped care (SC) and referred care (RC) participants\* during 5-year follow-up, by diastolic blood pressure (DBP) at entry*

| DBP AT ENTRY (mmHg) | SAMPLE SIZE | | DEATHS | | LIFE TABLE DEATH RATE PER 100 (SE)† | | 95% CONFIDENCE LIMITS FOR DIFFERENCE IN RC AND SC RATES | PERCENTAGE OF REDUCTION IN MORTALITY FOR SC GROUP‡ |
|---|---|---|---|---|---|---|---|---|
| | SC | RC | SC | RC | SC | RC | | |
| TOTAL | 5485 | 5455 | 349 | 419 | 6.4 (0.3) | 7.7 (0.4)§ | 0.37-2.29 | 16.9 |
| 90-104 | 3903 | 3922 | 231 | 291 | 5.9 (0.4) | 7.4 (0.4)§ | 0.40-2.62 | 20.3 |
| 105-114 | 1048 | 1004 | 70 | 77 | 6.7 (0.8) | 7.7 (0.8) | −1.25-3.21 | 13.0 |
| 115+ | 534 | 529 | 48 | 51 | 9.0 (1.2) | 9.7 (1.3) | −2.84-4.18 | 7.2 |

From Hypertension Detection and Follow-up Program Cooperative Group. Five-year findings of the hypertension detection and follow-up program. I. Reduction in mortality of persons with high blood pressure, including mild hypertension, *JAMA* 242:2562, 1979.
\*Stepped care (SC) patients received rigorous antihypertensive drug therapy from time of diagnosis of their elevated blood pressure; referred care (RC) patients were managed in a manner consistent with usually accepted techniques, which might not include immediate use of antihypertensive drugs.
†SE indicates standard error.
‡(RC rate − SC rate)/(RC rate) × 100.
§$P < 0.1$.

lated to the planned dental care through treatment modification. Physical and psychologic stress increases the workload of the myocardium and therefore its oxygen requirement. In a patient with impaired coronary blood flow, this increased requirement for oxygen may not be met and may lead to an acute exacerbation of some form of heart disease. The Stress Reduction Protocol (see Chapter 2) is invaluable in the management of most patients with CAD. Of particular importance will be the administration of supplemental oxygen through a nasal cannula or nasal hood to higher risk patients during dental treatment.

## Clinical Manifestations

Atherosclerosis, by itself, does not produce clinical manifestations of disease. It is only when the degree of atherosclerosis becomes great enough to produce a deficit in the blood supply and ischemia to an area of the body that signs and symptoms become apparent. The nature of the subsequent clinical syndrome depends on these factors:

1. The size and location of the tissue inadequately supplied with blood
2. The severity of the deficiency
3. The rate of development of the deficiency
4. The duration of the deficiency

For example, cerebrovascular ischemia is a manifestation of atherosclerosis occurring in the brain. If the oxygen deficit is mild and of short duration, a transient ischemic attack (TIA) may be the sole clinical manifestation, whereas a cerebrovascular accident (CVA) develops with infarction of neuronal tissues if the ischemia is of greater duration and more complete. A TIA is normally of short duration, resolving without residual neuronal deficiency, whereas CVA produces permanent neuronal damage. The clinical manifestations of atherosclerosis in coronary blood vessels (e.g., angina pectoris, myocardial infarction, heart failure, cardiac dysrhythmias, and sudden death) are summarized in Table 26-5.

Angina pectoris (see Chapter 27) is a transient, localized ischemia of the myocardium (similar to the TIA), whereas a myocardial infarction (see Chapter 28) results from a more prolonged arterial occlusion (akin to CVA). Heart failure and cardiac dysrhythmias quite frequently develop after myocardial infarction as chronic complications, but they may also occur through a process of gradual fibrosis of the myocardium and the cardiac conduction system in the absence of myocardial infarction. Sudden death (e.g., cardiopulmonary arrest) may develop after any of the aforementioned mechanisms or through the occurrence of ventricular fibrillation (see Chapter 30).

## Pathophysiology

### ATHEROSCLEROSIS

Atherosclerosis is an ongoing process that starts in utero as soon as blood begins to flow in rudimentary blood vessels. It occurs in all individuals at certain sites of predilection. Atherosclerosis is therefore considered to be a reactive biologic response of arteries to the forces being generated by the flow of blood. Texon[55] has described atherosclerosis as "the price we pay for blood flow as a requirement of life."

table **26-5** *Clinical manifestations of atherosclerosis*

| | MANIFESTATION | MECHANISM |
|---|---|---|
| **Noncardiac** | | |
| Diabetes mellitus | Diabetic retinopathy and blindness | Atherosclerosis of retinal vessels |
| | Increased infection and poor healing of lower limb, with possible amputation of toes or feet | Atherosclerosis of arteries to legs |
| Cerebral arteries | Transient ischemic attack | Transient occlusion of vessels |
| | Cerebrovascular infarction | Prolonged occlusion of vessels |
| **Cardiac** | | |
| Coronary artery disease | Angina pectoris | Transient, localized myocardial ischemia |
| | Unstable angina | Prolonged myocardial ischemia, with or without myocardial necrosis |
| | Myocardial infarction | Prolonged arterial occlusion |
| | Heart failure | Gradual fibrosis of myocardium; occurs commonly after myocardial infarction |
| | Dysrhythmias | Gradual fibrosis of myocardium; occurs commonly after myocardial infarction |
| | Sudden death (cardiopulmonary arrest) | Any of the above and/or ventricular dysrhythmias |

The basic factor in the development of an atherosclerotic lesion (called an *atheroma*) is a multiplication of the smooth muscle cells of the intimal layer of the blood vessel in response to pressure changes within the vessel (Figure 26-3). In a normal blood vessel there is constant movement of lipids into and out of the intimal layer. However, when proliferative changes occur within the intimal smooth muscle cells, the ability of these cells to maintain a steady level of lipids is altered, and the influx of lipids into the intima becomes predominant. This influx is initially made up of cholesterol, triglycerides, and phospholipids and appears as a yellowish streak or plaque that is visible within the lumen of the artery (Figure 26-4). As the lesion progresses, cholesterol becomes the predominant lipid. Fibrous tissue next grows into and around the atheroma, and finally, calcium is deposited into the lesion. The atheroma, which began as a soft fatty lesion, becomes a larger, harder lesion.[56] With the increased size, obstruction of blood flow through the vessel at the point of the lesion may occur, leading to chronic ischemia (e.g., heart failure, dysrhythmias), acute ischemia (e.g., angina pectoris, TIA), or infarction (e.g., myocardial or cerebral infarction). If the endothelial layer of the blood vessel breaks down, the atheromatous material is exposed to circulating blood platelets, which then clump and initiate thrombus formation with subsequent development of acute clinical manifestations (e.g., myocardial infarction, CVA, or cardiac arrest).

## LOCATION

Atherosclerosis of the coronary vessels occurs predominantly in the proximal segments of medium-size coronary arteries, especially at branching points. Interestingly, only those vessels that run over the surface of the myocardium appear to be susceptible to the development of atheromatous lesions.[57] Vessels that enter the myocardium (the penetrating or muscular branches) do not demonstrate atheromata. The explanation for this is not yet known. The most common site in which clinically significant atherosclerosis develops in the heart, leading to major morbidity and mortality, is the anterior descending branch of the left coronary artery. Occlusion of this vessel leads to infarction of the anterior portion of the left ventricle. The blood supply to the myocardium is shown in Figure 26-5.

## CHEST PAIN

The basic mechanism of cardiac pain is a decrease or cessation of blood flow to the myocardium. Episodes of cardiac pain occur when critical myocardial ischemia is produced by an absolute decrease of the coronary blood flow or by myocardial oxygen demand exceeding that available from the blood supply. The precise mechanism of cardiac pain production is unknown. Theories suggest that cardiac pain results from an accumulation of metabolites within the ischemic portion of the myocardium. The rapid accu-

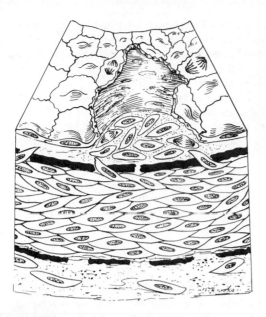

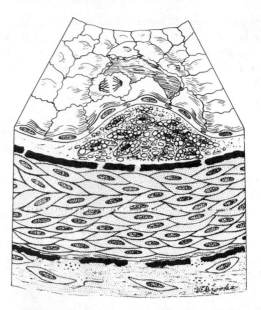

**Figure 26-3**  Development of atherosclerosis. Smooth muscle cells migrate from media into the intimal layer through fenestrate in internal elastic lamina. (From Ross R, Glomset JA: *N Engl J Med* 295:369, 1976.)

**Figure 26-4**  Development of atherosclerosis. Lipid deposition within intimal cells and their surrounding connective tissue matrix. Lumen of vessel progressively narrows. (From Ross R, Glomset JA: *N Engl J Med* 295:369, 1976.)

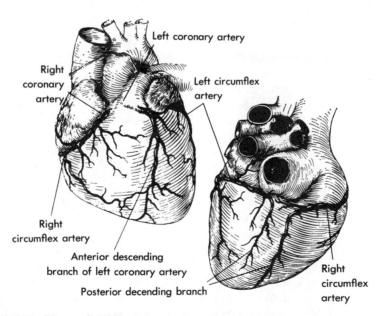

**Figure 26-5**  Myocardial blood supply. *Left,* Anterior portion of heart. *Right,* Posterior portion of heart. (From Goldman MJ: *Principles of clinical electrocardiography,* ed 9, Los Altos, Calif, 1976, Lange Medical.)

mulation of metabolites within heart muscle, occurring with transient ischemia (e.g., angina pectoris) or prolonged ischemia (e.g., myocardial infarction), is responsible for triggering pain impulses.[58] Other theories on the genesis of cardiac pain include those suggesting that vasomotor reflexes or vasospasm produce paroxysms of cardiac pain (the pain arising from the coronary vessels themselves) or that cardiac pain is provoked by distention of the walls of coronary vessels proximal to the site of an occlusion.[59] Sudden obstruction of a major coronary vessel, primarily by thrombosis, and the occurrence of myocardial infarction are often associated with violent pain, yet if the vessel occlusion develops gradually, there may be no clinically evident signs. This is primarily because of the gradual development of an effective collateral circulation between the left and right coronary arteries.[60] In the presence of an adequate collateral circulation, an occlusion of the right coronary artery may not lead to infarction of that part of the tissue that is also supplied by the left coronary artery (see Figure 26-5). Unfortunately, in the normal heart there is usually a minimally developed collateral circulation, which in part explains the greater incidence of acute episodes of cardiac disease.[61]

# Management

Management of acute clinical manifestations of IHD is directed toward the specific clinical entity that develops. In the patient with CHF, primary management of the acute episode (acute pulmonary edema) is directed at alleviation of respiratory distress, which is the major immediate symptom. Angina and AMI produce acute paroxysms of chest pain of varying intensity and duration. Immediate management of these clinical entities is directed at the alleviation of this pain. In all instances of clinical IHD, the goals of management include (1) decreasing the myocardial workload, thereby decreasing myocardial oxygen requirement, and (2) providing the victim with an increased supply of oxygen. When sudden death is imminent, as in cardiopulmonary arrest, the goal of immediate therapy is, of course, the prevention of biologic death. The principles of basic life support must be applied as rapidly and as effectively as possible. Cardiac arrest is a possible complication of all forms of CAD.

## REFERENCES

1. Gordon GS, Silverstein S: Ischemic heart disease. In Rosen P, editor: *Emergency medicine: concepts and clinical practice,* ed 4, St Louis, 1998, Mosby.
2. Braunwald E: Valvular heart disease. In Fauci AS, editor: *Harrison's principles of internal medicine,* ed 14, New York, 1998, McGraw-Hill, Health Professions Division.
3. Fisch S: On the origin of cardiac pain: a new hypothesis, *Arch Intern Med* 140:754, 1980.
4. Boivin M, Paterson WG: Management of complicated gastroesophageal reflux disease: atypical chest pain, *Can J Gastroenterol* 11(suppl B):91B, 1997.
5. Vazquez Muniz CA, Delgado Osorio H: Acute dissection of the thoracic aorta: experience at the Puerto Rico Medical Center (1991 through 1995), *Bol Assoc Med P R* 89(10-12):161, 1997.
6. Hughes KH: Painful rib syndrome. A variant of myofascial pain syndrome, *AAOHN J* 46(3):115, 1998.
7. Khaw KT and others: Prediction of stroke-associated mortality in the elderly, *Stroke* 15:244, 1984.
8. Hsu Y, Guzman L: Abdominal aortic aneurysm: diagnosis and treatment, *Milit Med* 145:807, 1980.
9. Kannel WB, Castell WP, Gordon T: Cholesterol in the prediction of atherosclerotic disease: new perspectives based on the Framingham study, *Ann Intern Med* 90:85, 1979.
10. American Heart Association: *Heart facts 1998,* Dallas, 1998, The American Heart Association.
11. National Center for Health Statistics, Washington, DC, 1998, US Public Health Service, DHHS.
12. Stern MP: The recent decline in ischemic heart disease mortality, *Ann Intern Med* 91:630, 1979.
13. Kannel WB, Thom TJ: Incidence, prevalence and mortality of cardiovascular disease. In Alexander RW, Schlant RC, Fuster V, editors: *Hurst's the heart, arteries and veins,* ed 9, New York, 1998, McGraw-Hill.
14. Kannel WB, Thom TJ: Implication of the recent decline in cardiovascular mortality, *Cardiovasc Med* 4:983, 1979.
15. Goldman L, Cook EF: The decline in ischemic heart disease mortality rates: an analysis of the comparative effects of medical interventions and changes in lifestyle, *Ann Intern Med* 101:825, 1984.
16. TIMI Study Group: The thrombolysis in myocardial infarction (TIMI) trial: phase I findings, *N Engl J Med* 312:983, 1985.
17. American Heart Association: *Textbook of advanced cardiac life support,* Dallas, 1997, The American Heart Association.
18. Kuller LH: Sudden death—definition and epidemiologic considerations, *Prog Cardiovasc Dis* 23:1, 1980.
19. Koster RW, Dunning AJ: Intramuscular lidocaine for prevention of lethal arrhythmias in the prehospitalization phase of acute myocardial infarction, *N Engl J Med* 313:1105, 1985.
20. Gruppo Ittalino per lo studio della streptochinasi nell'infarto miocardico (GISSI): Effectiveness of intravenous thrombolytic treatment in acute myocardial infarction, *Lancet* 1:297, 1986.
21. Maggioni AP and others: Treatment of acute myocardial infarction today, *Am Heart J* 134(2 part 2):S9, 1997.
22. Deeks J, Watt I, Freemantle N: Aspirin and acute myocardial infarction: clarifying the message, *Br J Gen Pract* 45(397):395, 1995.

23. O'Neill W and others: A prospective randomized clinical trial of intracoronary streptokinase vs coronary angioplasty for acute myocardial infarction, *N Engl J Med* 314:812, 1986.

24. Gray WA, Capone RJ, Most AS: Unsuccessful emergency medical resuscitation—are continued efforts in the emergency department justified? *N Engl J Med* 325:1393, 1991.

25. Smith SC Jr, Hamburg RS: Automated external defibrillators: time for federal and state advocacy and broader utilization, *Circulation* 97(13):1321, 1998.

26. Cummins RO, Thies W: Encouraging early defibrillation: the American Heart Association and automated external defibrillators, *Ann Emerg Med* 19(11):1245, 1990.

27. Gensini GF, Comeglio M, Colella A: Classical risk factors and emerging elements in the risk profile for coronary artery disease, *Eur Heart J* 19(suppl A):A53, 1998.

28. Levy RI, Feinleib M: Risk factors for coronary artery disease and their management. In Braunwald E, editor: *Heart disease: a textbook of cardiovascular medicine,* ed 5, Philadelphia, 1997, WB Saunders.

29. Stamler J: Lifestyles, major risk factors, proof, and public policy, *Circulation* 58:3, 1978.

30. Feinleib M, Williams RR: Relative risks of myocardial infarction, cardiovascular disease, and peripheral vascular disease by type of smoking, *Proc Third World Conf Smoking and Health* I:243, 1976.

31. Ball K, Turner R: Smoking and the heart: the basis for action, *Lancet* 2:822, 1974.

32. Oslo Study Group: Effect of diet and smoking intervention on the incidence of coronary heart disease: report from the Oslo Study Group of a randomised trial in healthy man, *Lancet* 2:1301, 1981.

33. Bellet S, DeGuzmas NT, Kostis JB: The effect of inhalation of cigarette smoke on ventricular fibrillation threshold in normal dogs and dogs with acute myocardial infarction, *Am Heart J* 83:67, 1972.

34. Astrup P, Kjeldsen K: Carbon monoxide, smoking, and atherosclerosis, *Med Clin North Am* 58:323, 1973.

35. Aronow WS: Smoking, carbon monoxide and coronary heart disease, *Circulation* 48:1169, 1973.

36. Pepine CJ: Systemic hypertension and coronary artery disease, *Am J Cardiol* 82(3A):21H, 1998.

37. Lembo G and others: Systemic hypertension and coronary artery disease: the link, *Am J Cardiol* 82(3A):2H, 1998.

38. Bell DS: Diabetes mellitus and coronary artery disease, *J Cardiovasc Risk* 4(2):83, 1997.

39. Castelli WP and others: HDL cholesterol and other lipids in coronary heart disease: the cooperative lipoprotein phenotyping study, *Circulation* 55:767, 1977.

40. Lembo G and others: Systemic hypertension and coronary artery disease: the link. *Am J Cardiol* 82(3A):2H, 1998.

41. Wassertheil-Smoller S and others: The trial of antihypertensive interventions and management (TAIM) study: final results with regard to blood pressure, cardiovascular risk, and quality of life, *Am J Hypertension* 5(1):37, 1992.

42. Garcia MJ and others: Morbidity and mortality of diabetes in the Framingham population. Sixteen-year follow-up study, *Diabetes* 23:105, 1976.

43. Shurtleff D: *Some characteristics related to the incidence of cardiovascular disease and death: the Framingham study, 18-year follow-up,* DHEW Publ. No. (NIH) 74-599, Section No. 30, Washington DC, 1974, US Department of Health, Education, and Welfare.

44. Knowles HC Jr: Magnitude of the renal failure problem in diabetic patients. In *Kidney Int,* New York, 1974, Springer-Verlag, vol 6, no 4, suppl 1.

45. Gordon T and others: Differences in coronary heart disease in Framingham, Honolulu and Puerto Rico, *J Chronic Dis* 27:329, 1974.

46. Persky VW and others: Uric acid: a risk factor for coronary heart disease? *Circulation* 59:969, 1979.

47. Kannel WB and others: Menopause and risk of cardiovascular disease: The Framingham study, *Ann Intern Med* 85:447, 1976.

48. Jick H, Dinan B, Rothman KJ: Oral contraceptives and non-fatal myocardial infarction, *JAMA* 239:1403, 1978.

49. Gordon T, Kannel WB: Obesity and cardiovascular disease: the Framingham study, *Clin Endocrinol Metab* 5:367, 1976.

50. Wyndham CH: The role of physical activity in the prevention of ischemic heart disease, *S Afr Med J* 36:7, 1979.

51. Rosenman RH and others: Multivariate prediction of coronary heart disease during 8.5 year follow-up in the western collaborative group study, *Am J Cardiol* 37:903, 1976.

52. Friedman H, Rosenman RH: *Type A behavior and your heart,* New York, 1974, Alfred A. Knopf.

53. Veterans Administration Cooperative Study Group on Antihypertensive Agents (1970): II. Results in patients with diastolic blood pressure averaging 90-114 mm Hg, *JAMA* 215:1143, 1970.

54. Hypertension Detection and Follow-up Program Cooperative Group: Five-year findings of the hypertension detection and follow-up program. I. Reduction in mortality of persons with high blood pressure, including mild hypertension, *JAMA* 242:2562, 1979.

55. Texon M: Atherosclerosis, its hemodynamic basis and implications, *Med Clin North Am* 58:257, 1974.

56. Ross R, Glamset JA: The pathogenesis of atherosclerosis, *N Engl J Med* 295:369, 1976.

57. Mitchell JRA, Schwartz CJ: *Arterial disease,* Oxford, 1965, Blackwell Scientific.

58. Sampson JJ, Cheitlin MD: Pathophysiology and differential diagnosis of chest pain, *Prog Cardiovasc Dis* 13:507, 1971.

59. Prinzmetal M and others: Angina pectoris. I. A variant form of angina pectoris, *Am J Med* 27:375, 1959.

60. Gorlin R: Coronary collaterals. In *Coronary artery disease,* Philadelphia, 1976, WB Saunders.

61. Firoozan S, Forfar JC: Exercise training and the coronary collateral circulation: is its value underestimated in man? *Eur Heart J* 17(12):1791, 1996.

# 27

# Angina Pectoris

**A**NGINA is a Latin word describing a spasmodic, cramplike, choking feeling or suffocating pain; *pectoris* is the Latin word for chest.[1] These words aptly describe the basic clinical manifestations of angina pectoris, commonly called *angina,* the classic expression of ischemic heart disease (IHD). The term *angina pectoris* was first used in 1768 in a lecture by Dr. William Heberden to distinguish the "strangling" sensation of angina from the word *dolor,* which means pain.[2] A working definition of angina is *a characteristic thoracic pain, usually substernal; precipitated chiefly by exercise, emotion, or a heavy meal; relieved by vasodilator drugs and a few minutes' rest; and a result of a moderate inadequacy of the coronary circulation.*[1] The major clinical characteristic of angina is chest pain. However, the word "pain" is seldom used by the victim. Much more commonly, the sensation is described as a dull, aching discomfort, "suffocating," "heavy," or "squeezing."

Angina is clinically important to dentistry because it is usually a sign indicating the presence of a significant degree of coronary artery disease (CAD). However, anginal pain is not specific for CAD; it may also be found with aortic stenosis, hypertensive heart disease, or even in the absence of demonstrable heart disease.[3] The onset of anginal pain indicates that the myocardium is not receiving an adequate oxygen supply and that myocardial ischemia has developed. If this inadequacy is excessively prolonged, infarction of the myocardium may occur. The patient with a history of angina represents an increased risk during dental

437

care. Any factor increasing myocardial oxygen requirements can precipitate an acute episode of chest pain, which, although usually readily managed with vasodilator drug therapy, can ultimately lead to myocardial infarction, acute dysrhythmias, or cardiac arrest. The prevention of acute episodes of chest pain proves ultimately more satisfactory than management of the episode after it develops.

## Predisposing Factors

Factors that lead to the initial development of angina are discussed in Chapter 26 (see box on p. 428). In most patients acute anginal episodes are precipitated by factors that produce a relative inability of the coronary arteries to supply the myocardium with adequate volumes of oxygenated blood. Commonly observed precipitating factors are listed in Box 27-1.

The type of angina described here is called *stable angina.* Synonyms for stable angina include chronic, classic, or exertional angina. Stable angina is usually the result of CAD.[4] The prevalence of CAD in groups of patients with stable angina, atypical angina, and

nonanginal chest pain was 90%, 50%, and 16%, respectively,[5] whereas the incidence of CAD in asymptomatic adults was estimated at 3% to 4%. Stable angina is triggered by strenuous activity, emotional stress, or cold weather. The "pain" of stable angina normally lasts from 1 to 15 minutes, builds gradually, and reaches maximum intensity quickly. The pain of stable angina is usually relieved by rest or the administration of nitroglycerin. Two other forms of angina are described: variant angina and unstable angina.

*Variant angina* is also termed *Prinzmetal's angina, atypical angina,* or *vasoplastic angina.* It is more likely to occur with the patient at rest than during physical exertion or emotional stress; it may develop at odd times during the day or night (even awakening patients from sleep); and it is often associated with dysrhythmias or conduction defects. Coronary artery spasm is the cause of variant angina. Spasm of a coronary artery produces a sudden brief occlusion of an epicardial or large septal coronary artery. Normal and diseased coronary arteries may become constricted. Variant angina may recur at the same time each day in an individual. It is thought that diurnal fluctuations in circulating endogenous catecholamine levels, highest during the early morning hours, are partially responsible for nocturnal angina. Variant angina is more common in women under the age of 50 years, whereas stable angina is uncommon in women in this age-group in the absence of severe hypercholesterolemia, high blood pressure, or diabetes mellitus. Signs and symptoms of variant angina include syncope, dyspnea, and palpitation. Nitroglycerin usually provides prompt relief of pain.

Another syndrome, called *unstable angina,* is described. Other names for this syndrome are preinfarction angina, crescendo angina, intermediate coronary syndrome, premature or impending myocardial infarction, and coronary insufficiency. Unstable angina is a syndrome that lies intermediate between stable angina and acute myocardial infarction (AMI). It is

---

box **27-1**  *Precipitating factors in angina pectoris*

Physical activity
Hot, humid environment
Cold weather
Large meals
Emotional stress (argument, anxiety, or sexual excitement)
Caffeine ingestion
Fever, anemia, or thyrotoxicosis
Cigarette smoking
Smog
High altitudes
Smoke from *another* person's cigarettes

---

table **27-1**  *Comparison of anginal syndromes*

| ANGINAL SYNDROME | SYNONYMS | PRECIPITATING FACTORS | DURATION | RESPONSE TO NITROGLYCERIN |
|---|---|---|---|---|
| Stable | Chronic, classic, exertional | Emotional stress, physical exertion, cold weather | 1 to 15 minutes | Good |
| Variant | Prinzmetal's, atypical, vasoplastic | Coronary artery spasm | Variable | Good |
| Unstable | Preinfarction, crescendo, acute coronary insufficiency, intermediate coronary syndrome, impending myocardial infarction | Any factor or no factor | Up to 30 minutes | Questionable |

quite significant because of its adverse prognosis and for the unpredictability of sudden onset of acute myocardial infarction in some patients with unstable angina. Unstable angina is the result of the progression of atherosclerosis. The percentage of patients with unstable angina progressing to AMI is high.[6] Episodes of pain associated with unstable angina may persist for up to 30 minutes and may be precipitated by any of the factors mentioned for the other forms of angina, or for no apparent reason. Three characteristics are used to define unstable angina:

1. Angina of recent onset, caused by minimal exertion
2. Increasingly severe, prolonged, or frequent angina in a patient with relatively stable, exertion-related angina
3. Angina both at rest and with minimal exertion

A recent classification of unstable angina based on pain symptoms described three subsets[7]:

*Group I:* Angina on effort of recent origin (within 4 weeks)

*Group II:* Angina on exertion with a changing pattern (more severe, more frequent, radiating to new sites, incomplete relief with use of nitroglycerin)

*Group III:* Angina at rest lasting 15 minutes or longer

The degree of risk increases from group I to group III.

In an early study, which did not include angina of recent onset, of 167 patients with unstable angina, 16% developed AMI, and 2% died within 3 months.[8] Gazes and others[9] reported on 140 patients diagnosed before 1961 and followed for 10 years. All met the three aforementioned criteria. At 3 months the incidence of AMI was 21% with a 10% mortality; at 1 year mortality was 18%, at 5 years 39%, and 10 years 52%. Most patients with unstable angina have severe obstructive CAD. As it is a complicated syndrome that may be a prodrome of myocardial infarction, patients with unstable angina must be managed in the dental office as if they had recently had an AMI. This syndrome will be discussed in depth in this chapter. Table 27-1 compares the three anginal syndromes.

# Prevention

As has been stressed previously, the prevention of life-threatening situations is much preferred to their management after they occur. In no other category is this more true than that of chest pain because the outcome all too often is the death of the patient. With the multitude of stresses placed on both the doctor and the dental patient, it is probable that most persons (doctor as well as patient) experience an increase in their cardiac workload during dental treatment. Identification of the patient at increased risk permits modifications in dental care that will, in most instances, prevent the occurrence of chest pain. Because both emotional and physical stress are major elements known to precipitate chest pain, the elimination of stress is a primary preventive measure.

## Medical History Questionnaire

**9. Circle any of the following that you have had or have at present:**

Heart disease
Angina pectoris
Heart surgery

*Comment:* An affirmative answer to any part of this question should be followed with dialogue history to determine the precise nature of the cardiac problem and its severity. Percutaneous transluminal coronary angioplasty (PTCA) and/or coronary artery bypass graft (CABG) surgery are frequently indicated for patients with severe angina pectoris as a means of providing myocardial revascularization in the presence of significant CAD.[10,11] Atherectomy[12] and laser angioplasty[13] are newer approaches to myocardial revascularization.

**10. When you walk up stairs or take a walk, do you ever have to stop because of pain in your chest or shortness of breath or because you are very tired?**

*Comment:* Pain occurring in the chest during exertion, such as walking or climbing a flight of stairs, that is relieved by rest or by nitroglycerin is a symptom of angina pectoris.

**6. Have you taken any medicine or drugs during the past 2 years?**

*Comment:* Patients with angina pectoris normally have with them a supply of sublingual nitroglycerin tablets or translingual spray that is used to terminate the acute episode of anginal pain. Since its introduction in January of 1986, more anginal patients are using the more stable oral spray form of nitroglycerin in place of sublingual tablets. Many patients with angina also receive other drugs, such as the long-acting nitrates, β-adrenergic blockers,[14] and calcium channel blockers, in an effort to prevent the occurrence of acute anginal episodes. Although the frequency of anginal episodes may be decreased with long-acting nitrates,[15] there is no convincing evidence that they prolong life. Calcium channel blockers are especially useful in the presence of coronary artery spasm, although they may also relieve anginal pain in the absence of spasm because they produce vasodilation.[16] Additionally, nitroglycerin ointment and transdermal nitroglycerin are included in the treatment armamentarium. Nitroglycerin ointment provides relief for 4 to 6 hours, whereas transdermal nitroglycerin provides slow, continuous release of the drug for prolonged periods. Table 27-2 lists those drugs used in the prevention or management of anginal episodes.

table **27-2**    *Drugs used to prevent anginal episodes*

| GENERIC NAME | PROPRIETARY NAME | ROUTE OF ADMINISTRATION | SIDE EFFECTS |
|---|---|---|---|
| **Long-acting nitrates** | | | |
| Isosorbide dinitrate | ·Isordil | Sublingual | Headache |
| | Sorbitrate | Oral | Flushing |
| | | | Tachycardia |
| | | | Dizziness |
| Pentaerythritol tetranitrate | Peritrate | Oral | Postural hypotension |
| Erythrityl tetranitrate | Cardilate | Sublingual and oral | Tachyphylaxis to nitroglycerin with prolonged use |
| **Beta-blockers** | | | |
| Propranolol | Inderal | Oral | For all beta-blockers: development |
| Metoprolol | Lopressor | Oral | of asthma, severe bradycardia, |
| Nadolol | Corgard | Oral | atrioventricular conduction defects, |
| Atenolol | Tenormin | Oral | left ventricular failure |
| Pindolol | Visken | Oral | |
| Timolol | Blocadren | Oral | |
| **Calcium channel blockers** | | | |
| Verapamil | Calan, Isoptin | Oral | For all calcium channel blockers: |
| Diltiazem | Cardizem | Oral | peripheral edema, hypotension, |
| Nifedipine | Procardia, Adalat | Oral | dizziness, lightheadedness, headache, weakness, nausea, constipation |
| **Nitroglycerin** | | | |
| | Nitrostat | Sublingual | For all forms of nitroglycerin: |
| | Nitrolingual spray | Sublingual spray | headache, postural hypotension |
| | Nitro-Bid | Ointment | |
| | Nitrol | Ointment | |
| | Nitrong | Ointment | |
| | Nitrostat | Ointment | |
| | Nitrodisc | Transdermal patch | |
| | Nitro-Dur | Transdermal patch | |
| | Transderm-Nitro | Transdermal patch | |

## DIALOGUE HISTORY

For patients with a history of angina, dialogue history should seek to determine the following information concerning their anginal episodes:

### Describe a typical anginal episode.

*Comment:* The quality of chest discomfort of anginal episodes should be determined by asking the patient to describe, in his or her own words, the nature of the episode and the usual radiation pattern associated with it. In place of the word *pain,* many patients describe their anginal attacks as "an unpleasant sensation," "squeezing," "pressing," "strangling," "constricting," "bursting," and "burning." If the patient describes the episodes with terms such as "shooting," "knifelike," "sharp," "stabbing," "fleeting," or "tingling," the pain is probably not anginal.[4] Observe the patient as he or she de-

scribes the pain. Clenching of the fist in front of the chest while describing the sensation (Figure 27-1) is a very strong indication of an ischemic origin for the pain (the Levine sign).[17]

### Where does the "pain" hurt or radiate?

*Comment:* Determine the location of the pain. Anginal pain is usually substernal, across both sides of the chest. Pain may radiate to various regions. Common sites of radiation of ischemic chest pain include the neck and jaw; the upper epigastric region (stomach); intrascapular (between the shoulder blades); substernal radiating to the left arm; epigastric radiating to the neck, jaw, and both arms; and the left shoulder and the inner aspect of both arms (Figure 27-2).[4]

If the pain or discomfort can be localized (i.e., the patient can point to a spot where it hurts), the origin is usually not

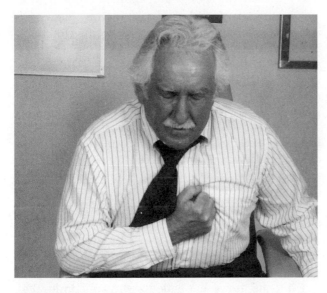

**Figure 27-1**  The Levine sign, an indicator of angina pectoris.

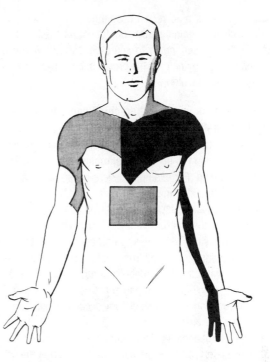

 Substernal pain projected to left shoulder and arm (ulanar nerve distribution)

 Less frequent referred sites including right shoulder and arm, left jaw, neck, and epigastrium

**Figure 27-2**  Radiation patterns of chest pain. (From Jastak JT, Cowan EF Jr: Dent Clin North Am 17:363, 1973.

ischemic, but from the skin or the chest wall. Ischemic pain, arising from the deeper structures (e.g., the heart) tends to be more generalized in location, hurting over a larger area, as opposed to a more well-defined spot.[17]

### How long do your anginal episodes last?

*Comment:* Determine the duration of the typical episode. Angina is by definition of short duration. If the episode is precipitated by exertion and the patient stops and rests, the discomfort normally ceases within 2 to 10 minutes. Chest pain lasting less than 30 seconds is usually not anginal. This brief duration commonly points to a noncardiac origin, such as musculoskeletal pain, hiatal hernia, or functional pain. Chest pain lasting for hours suggests AMI, pericarditis, dissecting aortic aneurysm, musculoskeletal disease, herpes zoster, or anxiety. Anginal episodes developing after a large meal or emotional stress tend to be longer lasting and more difficult to treat. The longer the duration of ischemia, the greater is the risk of irreversible myocardial damage.

### What precipitates your anginal episode?

*Comment:* Determine the precipitating factors in the anginal episode. Most commonly, anginal pain occurs during exertion. The amount of exertion required to precipitate angina varies from patient to patient, but is usually relatively constant for each patient. *Can the patient walk two level city blocks or climb one flight of stairs without developing chest pain?* This question will provide helpful information. Of particular importance for the doctor is the relationship of emotional factors to anginal episodes and the patient's attitude toward dentistry.

### How frequently do you suffer anginal attacks?

*Comment:* The frequency of anginal episodes varies from patient to patient. Attacks may occur infrequently, perhaps once a week or once a month, or the patient may experience acute episodes several times a day. On average the patient with stable angina experiences one or two episodes per week. The risk of an episode being precipitated in the dental office is obviously increased in a patient with a greater frequency of episodes under normal conditions.

### How does nitroglycerin affect the anginal episode?

*Comment:* Determine what the patient does to relieve the pain. Nitroglycerin and rest characteristically relieve the discomfort of angina in approximately 2 to 4 minutes. Nitroglycerin in the form of a tablet, spray, or ointment greatly shortens the duration of the anginal episode. Definitive management of chest pain in the dental patient is initiated by the administration of nitroglycerin, with any subsequent treatment based on the patient's response or lack of response to this antianginal drug. Chest pain lasting 10 minutes or more may prove to be AMI or unstable angina. Pain of *esophageal spasm* or *esophagitis* may also be relieved by nitroglycerin; however, pain of esophagitis and peptic ulcer is also relieved by ingestion of food and antacids, whereas anginal pain is not. Chest pain relieved by leaning forward is secondary to acute pericarditis, whereas chest pain relieved by holding the breath in deep expiration is commonly caused by pleurisy.[17]

**Describe any symptoms, other than chest pain, that are associated with your anginal attacks.**

*Comment:* The presence of other accompanying signs and symptoms may help the doctor to determine the cause of the patient's chest pain. For example, severe chest pain accompanied by nausea and vomiting is often caused by myocardial infarction. Chest pain associated with palpitation may be produced by ischemia secondary to a tachydysrhythmia in a patient with underlying CAD. Chest pain accompanied by hemoptysis (coughing up of blood from the respiratory tract) may be produced by a pulmonary embolis or lung tumor. Pain associated with fever is noted in pneumonia and pericarditis.[17] Medical consultation is suggested if any accompanying symptoms appear disturbing.

The diagnosis of angina pectoris depends almost entirely on the dialogue history, and it is quite important to permit the patient sufficient time to describe the symptoms without interruption. Patients frequently use gestures to describe the location and quality of the symptom, such as placing a closed fist against the sternum—the "Levine sign" (see Figure 27-1).

## PHYSICAL EXAMINATION

Physical examination of a patient with a history of angina will yield essentially normal findings during the period *between* episodes. Physical findings *during* the acute episode are described on p. 445-446.

## UNSTABLE ANGINA

Unstable angina is extremely significant to dentistry because of the increased risk of AMI, as well as the unpredictability of the occurrence of myocardial infarction. Patients with unstable angina should be managed in the dental office as would patients having recently suffered a myocardial infarction (within the past 6 months). They represent an ASA IV risk and should not be considered for elective dental care.

Unstable angina will be recognized from the dialogue history obtained from the anginal patient. As mentioned previously, the characteristics of the acute anginal episode for a given patient (with stable angina) have a fair degree of consistency from episode to episode. In unstable angina the "pain" differs in character, duration, radiation, and severity—in which the pain, over a period of hours or days, demonstrates a crescendo or increasing quality, or occurs at rest, or during the night.

Not all patients with unstable angina progress to myocardial infarction, but they are considered to be in a precarious balance between myocardial oxygen supply and demand, and prudence dictates that they be treated as if they had had a minor myocardial infarction.

Medical management of unstable angina includes bed rest; the administration of nitrates (including intravenous nitroglycerin), β-blockers, and calcium channel blockers; and psychologic rest and reassurance. Nitroglycerin ointment or transdermal nitroglycerin is frequently employed.

When medical treatment has not improved or eliminated the patient's symptoms, or if they become worse, surgical intervention may be indicated. Surgical options include PTCA, CABG surgery, atherectomy, and laser angioplasty.

Evidence shows that patients who are admitted to a coronary care unit (CCU) because of unstable angina suggestive of myocardial infarction, but in whom infarction is never demonstrated, have a higher death rate over the next 1 to 2 years than ordinary anginal patients.[18,19] Only emergency dental care should be considered for patients with unstable angina and then only after consultation with their physician. Preferable location of dental treatment is within a hospital environment.

# Dental Therapy Considerations

Prevention of acute episodes of angina during dental treatment is predicated on minimizing stress so that the amount of oxygen delivered through the coronary arteries is adequate to meet the needs of the myocardium. The stress reduction protocol is particularly important to the anginal patient. Specific consideration must be given to the intraoperative aspects of the protocol, in particular the length of the appointment, pain control during treatment, and the use of psychosedation. The typical anginal patient (stable angina) represents an ASA physical status III risk (Table 27-3). Patients with unstable or daily anginal episodes should be considered ASA IV risks, with dental care limited to emergency treatment and then only after consultation with the patient's physician.

## LENGTH OF APPOINTMENT

An important factor in preventing the occurrence of anginal episodes during dental treatment is to avoid overstressing the patient. No absolute time limit for treatment can be given because patient tolerance to

table **27-3** *Dental therapy considerations in angina pectoris*

| FREQUENCY OF ANGINA | PATIENT'S ABILITIES | ASA PHYSICAL STATUS | CONDISERATIONS |
|---|---|---|---|
| 0-1 per mouth | Patient can walk two level city blocks or climb one flight of stairs | II | Usual ASA II considerations and supplemental oxygen |
| 2-4 month | Patient can walk two level city blocks or climb one flight of stairs | II | Usual ASA II considerations to include possible premedication with nitroglycerin 5 minutes before therapy and supplemental oxygen |
| 2-3 per week | Pain develops before patient walks two level city blocks or climbs one flight of stairs | III | Usual ASA III considerations to include possible premedication with nitroglycerin 5 minutes before therapy and supplemental oxygen |
| Daily episodes or recent (within past 2-3 weeks) changes in character of episode: Increased frequency, duration, or severity Radiation to new site Precipitated by less activity Decreased pain relief with usual nitroglycerin dose | Patient unable to walk two level city blocks or climb one flight of stairs | IV | Usual ASA IV considerations |

stress varies considerably. However, treatment should cease when the anginal patient demonstrates signs or symptoms of fatigue, such as sweating, fidgety movements, or increased anxiety. Permit the patient to rest before discharge.

## SUPPLEMENTAL OXYGEN

Anginal patients are excellent candidates for supplemental oxygen via nasal cannula or nasal hood during dental treatment. A flow of 3 to 5 L/min via cannula or 5 to 7 L/min via nasal hood minimizes the possibility of inadequate oxygenation of the myocardium.

## PAIN CONTROL DURING THERAPY

Pain is quite stressful; therefore its control in the anginal patient is quite important. The prevention of pain during dental treatment can best be ensured by the appropriate use of local anesthesia. The question that arises all too frequently concerns the advisability of using a vasoconstrictor in conjunction with the local anesthetic in the cardiac risk patient.

A wealth of clinical evidence has accumulated supporting the statement that, for most cardiac patients, local anesthetics containing a vasoconstrictor (e.g., epinephrine or levonordefrin) are indicated for pain control during dental treatment.[20-27] The

American Dental Association, in conjunction with the American Heart Association, published the findings of a joint committee that researched this question.[21]

To summarize the available clinical data concerning this question, it may be stated that, if pain control proves inadequate, cardiac patients are potentially at greater risk from the effects of endogenously released catecholamines (e.g., epinephrine and norepinephrine) than they are from a properly administered (aspiration negative, slowly injected) local anesthetic containing minimal amounts of epinephrine. Under the stress of pain or anxiety, the adrenal medulla releases extremely high levels of epinephrine (approximately 280 μg/min) and norepinephrine (approximately 56 μg/min) into the circulation, whereas with proper injection technique of a local anesthetic containing 1:50,000 epinephrine, less than 1 μg/min of epinephrine is added to the circulatory system.[24] Table 27-4 summarizes these clinical findings.

Adequate depth of anesthesia to permit tooth manipulation (e.g., extraction, cavity preparation) without the patient experiencing pain is the major factor determining the ultimate blood level of catecholamines. Local anesthetics that contain no vasoconstrictor (e.g., "plain" lidocaine, prilocaine, and mepivacaine) are less likely to provide pulpal anesthesia of sufficient depth and duration to permit completion of the

table **27-4**  *Catecholamine blood levels*

| | EPINEPHRINE (μG/MIN) | NOREPINEPHRINE (μG/MIN) |
|---|---|---|
| Resting adrenal medullary secretion | 7.0 | 1.5 |
| Stress | 280.0 | 56.0 |
| Local anesthesia (1:50,000 epinephrine in 1.8 mL) | <1.0 | — |

planned dental care before the patient experiences pain. The addition of minimal concentrations of epinephrine (1:200,000 and 1:100,000) to the local anesthetic prolongs the duration of pulpal anesthesia in most cases well beyond the time required for treatment, so that the anginal patient does not experience any pain and the release of endogenous catecholamines is minimized.

The maximal dose of epinephrine recommended for administration in the cardiac risk patient (ASA III) at one appointment is 0.04 mg.[28,29] To put this figure in terms of commonly used epinephrine concentrations, this is the equivalent of approximately one cartridge (1.8 mL) of a local anesthetic containing a 1:50,000 concentration of epinephrine (0.02 mg/mL), two cartridges with 1:100,000 epinephrine (0.01 mg/mL), or four cartridges with 1:200,000 epinephrine (0.005 mg/mL). Patients with poorly controlled IHD (ASA IV) should not receive local anesthetics with vasoconstrictors.[26-29]

If the doctor is confronted with a patient who states that he or she cannot receive epinephrine, consultation with the patient's physician should be completed before initiating dental treatment. If considerable doubt still remains concerning a particular patient after medical consultation about the proper use of epinephrine in local anesthetics, it is recommended that a second opinion be obtained or that a local anesthetic with a different vasoconstrictor, or an agent that provides sufficient duration of pulpal anesthesia without a vasoconstrictor, be employed. An example of the former is mepivacaine with levonordefrin, while prilocaine and mepivacaine without vasoconstrictor are examples of the latter. A textbook on local anesthesia or the drug package insert should be consulted before selecting a local anesthetic. One absolute contraindication to the inclusion of vasoconstrictors in local anesthetics is the presence of cardiac dysrhythmias that persist despite antidysrhythmic therapy.

Patients receiving noncardiospecific β-adrenergic blockers (e.g., propranolol) for the management of their angina or other cardiovascular disorders are at potential risk when receiving vasoconstrictors. Acute hypertensive episodes have been reported after the administration of local anesthetics containing vasoconstrictors.[30,31] A rapid-acting, short-duration vasodilator should be available for administration in the event such a reaction develops. One additional factor must be mentioned regarding the use of epinephrine in the cardiac-risk patient: 8% racemic epinephrine, a combination of the dextrorotatory and levorotatory forms commonly used in gingival retraction cord before taking impressions, contains approximately 4% (40 mg/mL) of the pharmacologically active levo- form of epinephrine, which is 40 times the epinephrine concentration used in acute emergency situations (e.g., 1 mg/mL in anaphylaxis).[22,32-37] Absorption of epinephrine through unabraded mucous membranes into the cardiovascular system is of little concern; however, where gingival abrasion and active bleeding are present (as occurs after subgingival tooth preparation) epinephrine is more rapidly absorbed. Blood levels of epinephrine rise rapidly in this situation, leading to manifestations (primarily cardiovascular) of epinephrine overdose (see Chapter 23).[33,35] Tachycardia, palpitation, sweating, tremor, and headache are the usual clinical symptoms.[37] In the patient with preexisting, clinically evident, or subclinical cardiovascular disease, this increase in cardiovascular activity may prove to be life threatening. The American Dental Association[22] recommends that racemic epinephrine cord not be used for any patient with a history of or suspicion of cardiovascular disease. Indeed, there are very few indications for the use of racemic epinephrine in any dental procedure in any patient.

## PSYCHOSEDATION

The use of psychosedation during the dental appointment may be indicated for the patient who experiences acute anginal episodes once a week or more often, or for any anginal patient who is fearful of dentistry. Of the various psychosedative techniques currently in use, inhalation sedation with nitrous oxide and oxygen is my preferred technique for all cardiac-risk patients.[38] Reasons for this preference include (1) the increased percentage of oxygen that the patient always receives along with the nitrous oxide (most sedation units available in the United States do not deliver less than 27% to 30% oxygen); (2) the anxiolytic properties of nitrous oxide, which successfully reduce the stress of dental therapy, thereby minimizing endogenous catecholamine release; and (3) the minor but potentially highly significant analgesic properties of nitrous oxide. As discussed in Chapter 28, nitrous oxide and oxygen are commonly employed *during* the emergency management of AMI in many countries, including the United States.

## ADDITIONAL CONSIDERATIONS

**Vital signs** Patients with a history of angina should have their vital signs monitored and recorded before the start of treatment at each visit to the dental office. Minimally, these recordings should include blood pressure, heart rate and rhythm, and respiratory rate. It is suggested that measurements also be taken on completion of the treatment, before patient discharge.

**Nitroglycerin** It has been suggested by some authorities that nitroglycerin be administered on a routine basis (prophylactically) to all anginal patients 5 minutes before the start of dental treatment.[39,40] Nitroglycerin exerts a clinical action within 2 to 4 minutes, with a duration of action of approximately 30 minutes. Being somewhat conservative in the administration of drugs, I suggest that prophylactic premedication with nitroglycerin be reserved for the anginal patient who experiences episodes of anginal pain more than once a week and who exhibits fear of dentistry (ASA III). However, I do feel that before beginning dental treatment on the higher-risk anginal patient, the doctor should request that the patient's nitroglycerin spray or tablets be placed where they will be immediately accessible if needed. Although nitroglycerin is present in the dental office emergency kit, the patient's own nitroglycerin is used preferentially.

# Clinical Manifestations

The primary clinical manifestation of angina is chest pain. The doctor managing the anginal patient usually has been forewarned about this medical condition through the medical history questionnaire and is prepared to manage it. Although most instances of anginal pain are easily terminated, it is always possible that a supposed anginal attack is actually a more severe manifestation of ischemic heart disease—unstable angina or an AMI. The initial clinical manifestations of all of these cardiovascular problems are quite similar; therefore the immediate management of chest pain is based on the patient's response to certain initial steps in treatment.

## SIGNS AND SYMPTOMS

**"Pain"** The patient becomes acutely aware of the sudden onset of chest pain and stops any activities. In the dental chair the patient will normally sit upright and press a fist against the chest. If questioned about the pain, it is commonly described as a sensation of squeezing, burning, pressing, choking, aching, bursting, tightness, or "gas." In fact, on many occasions episodes of cardiac pain are mistaken for indigestion—not infrequently with a fatal outcome (see Chapter 28). The patient may state that it feels as if there were a heavy weight on the chest. In describing this sensation, many anginal victims hold a clenched fist to their chest as they describe their attacks (the Levine sign).

Sharp pains are not typical of angina pectoris. In addition, respiratory movements (inspiration) do not exaggerate the discomfort. The sensation is more of a dull, aching, heavy pain than a searing hot or knife-like pain. The pain is located substernally, most commonly in the middle of the sternum, but it may also appear just to the left of the sternum. Finally, pain of cardiac origin tends to be more generalized than noncardiac pain, which can often be localized to one specific site (see discussion of radiation of pain that follows).

**Radiation of pain** Chest pain normally spreads or radiates to other locations in the body distant from the chest. Figure 27-2 shows the more common pathways of radiation. Typically, the sensation radiates to the left shoulder and distally down the medial surface of the left arm, occasionally as far as the hand and fingers, following the distribution of the ulnar nerve. The sensation felt is that of an ache, numbness, or tingling discomfort. Less commonly, the pain may radiate to the right shoulder only or to both shoulders. Other sites of radiation include the left side of the neck (usually described as a constricting sensation), with continuation up into the left side of the face and mandible. Mandibular pain, for which the victim may have sought dental care, was reported as the sole clinical manifestation of chest pain in one case of angina.[41] Another possible, yet relatively uncommon, area of radiation is the upper epigastrium (Table 27-5).

Patient reaction to anginal pain varies. In some individuals the discomfort of angina subsides without having to stop activities. Other individuals experience moderate pain that persists but does not become more intense. The victim is able to tolerate this level of discomfort and is not forced to stop activities. In most anginal patients, however, the clinical progression is of a different nature. In these persons the pain becomes progressively more intense, eventually forcing them to

| table **27-5** | Common causes of abdominal pain in the emergency department for all age-groups |
|---|---|

| CAUSE | PERCENTAGE |
|---|---|
| Abdominal pain of unknown cause | 41.3% |
| Gastroenteritis | 6.9% |
| Pelvic inflammatory disease | 6.7% |
| Urinary tract infection | 5.2% |
| Ureteral stone | 4.3% |
| Appendicitis | 4.3% |
| Acute cholecystitis | 2.5% |
| Intestinal obstruction | 2.5% |
| Constipation | 2.3% |
| Duodenal ulcer | 2.0% |
| Other causes | 22.0% |

From Brewer RJ, and others: *Am J Surg* 131:219, 1976.

seek relief by terminating activities, taking medication, or both. It must always be kept in mind that the clinical characteristics of acute anginal episodes are reasonably consistent for each patient from episode to episode. The intensity, frequency, radiation, and duration of the episodes demonstrate little variation. Recent changes in the usual pattern of the disease, with increased frequency, duration, or intensity, are signs of unstable angina and should be reported immediately to the patient's physician. This is commonly associated with recent obstructive disease of the coronary arteries and frequently precedes AMI or sudden death.

## PHYSICAL EXAMINATION

During acute anginal episodes the following signs and symptoms may be noted: the patient is apprehensive, is usually sweating, may press a fist to the sternum, and appears anxious to take nitroglycerin. The heart rate is markedly elevated, as is blood pressure, with values of 200/150 mmHg having been recorded in normotensive patients during acute anginal episodes. Respiratory difficulty (dyspnea) and a feeling of faintness may also be noted during the episode.

## COMPLICATIONS

Although most anginal episodes resolve without residual complication, it is possible for more acute situations to develop. Acute cardiac dysrhythmias occurring during the episode are the most common. Although normally not life threatening, ventricular dysrhythmias may occur with a possibility of ventricular tachycardia, ventricular fibrillation, and sudden death. A second potential complication of angina is AMI.

## PROGNOSIS

The prognosis for the anginal patient depends largely on the severity of the underlying disorder (e.g., IHD, CAD) and the presence or absence of additional risk factors.[42-44] In men with angina the annual mortality is 1.4% if they have no history of myocardial infarction, a normal electrocardiogram (ECG), and normal blood pressure. This rate increases to 7.4% annually if they have elevated blood pressure, to 8.4% if they have an abnormal ECG, and to 12% annually if both the blood pressure is elevated and the ECG is abnormal. Other factors, such as the presence of diabetes mellitus, heart failure, cardiac dysrhythmias, and cardiac hypertrophy, tend to decrease life expectancy even further. Fifty percent of all anginal patients die suddenly (cardiac arrest). Thirty-three percent die after myocardial infarction, and most of the remainder succumb to heart failure.[44]

# Pathophysiology

Angina is caused by the transient inability of the coronary arteries to provide adequate oxygenated blood to the myocardium. The patient with IHD or CAD may be asymptomatic at rest or during moderate exertion because, under these circumstances, their coronary arteries may be able to deliver an adequate supply of oxygen to the myocardium. Any additional increase in the oxygen requirement of the myocardium above this critical level, which varies from patient to patient, results in a degree of oxygen deficiency and the development of myocardial ischemia, with the subsequent appearance of clinical manifestations of anginal pains (or of other IHD syndromes, e.g., AMI, dysrhythmias).

The pain of angina may be related to the metabolic changes produced in the ischemic myocardium. Chemicals such as adenosine, bradykinin, histamine, and serotonin are released from ischemic cells. They act on intracardiac sympathetic nerves that go to the cardiac plexus and to sympathetic ganglia at the C7 to T4 level. Impulses are then transmitted through the spinal cord to the thalamus and the cerebral cortex.[45] Further evidence for this theory comes from patients with spontaneous angina (i.e., onset of anginal pain while the patient is at rest). The increases in blood pressure and heart rate seen during acute anginal episodes are consistently observed *before* the onset of pain. Changes in the ECG also occur from 1 to 3 minutes before the onset of pain. These factors indicate that a buildup of the metabolic products of ischemia occurs before the stimulation of pain fibers.

Some of the most dangerous occurrences observed during the anginal episode include continuing elevation in blood pressure and tachycardia. Both of these produce a potentially dangerous feedback system. Myocardial oxygen requirements continue to increase as the workload of the heart continues to rise (with increasing blood pressure and rapid heart rate). If the coronary arteries are unable to deliver the required oxygen, myocardial ischemia increases, which in turn increases the chances of acute, possibly fatal, ventricular dysrhythmias and myocardial infarction. Rapid management of the anginal episode becomes quite important.

Coronary artery spasm (Prinzmetal's variant angina) has been demonstrated to occur either spontaneously or on exposure to cold, by exposure to ergot-derivative drugs used to treat migraine headaches, or by mechanical irritation from a cardiac catheter.[45-48] Spasm has been observed in the large coronary arteries, whether healthy or atherosclerotic, resulting in decreased coronary blood flow.[48] Prolonged spasm of the coronary arteries in angina may result in documented episodes of myocardial infarction—even in the absence of visible CAD.

# Management

The primary goal in the management of the acute anginal episode is a decrease of the myocardial oxygen requirement. Diagnostic clues to the presence of angina include[49]:

- Onset with exercise, activity, or stress
- Symptoms that include pressure, tightness, or a heavy weight
- Substernal, epigastric, or jaw pain
- Mild to moderate discomfort

## PATIENT WITH A HISTORY OF ANGINA PECTORIS

*Step 1: termination of the dental procedure.* When the patient experiences chest pain, stop all dental procedures immediately. In many instances the precipitating factor may be a part of the dental treatment, such as the sight of a local anesthetic syringe, scalpel, or hand piece, and simply by terminating the procedure the acute episode of chest pain ends.

*Step 2: **P** (position).* The anginal patient is conscious and usually apprehensive. Position the patient in the most comfortable manner. Commonly this will be sitting or standing upright.[50] The supine position is rarely preferred by the anginal patient and, in fact, commonly makes the pain appear subjectively to be more intense.

*Step 3: **A-B-C** (airway-breathing-circulation), basic life support (BLS), as needed.* The anginal patient is conscious, breathing spontaneously, and has a palpable pulse in the wrist, antecubital fossa, and carotid artery.

*Step 4: **D** (definitive care):*
*Step 4a: administration of vasodilator and oxygen.* A member of the emergency team should immediately get the emergency kit and oxygen. Oxygen may be administered at any time to the anginal patient. A nasal cannula or nasal hood is preferred. As soon as possible (even before oxygen is available), give nitroglycerin transmucosally (e.g., nitrolingual spray) or sublingually (e.g., tablet). The patient's own nitroglycerin supply is preferred because the dosage will be correct for the patient. The number of sprays or tablets administered is determined by the patient's usual requirement (0.3 to 0.6 mg is the usual dosage). One or two metered sprays are recommended initially, with no more than three metered doses within a 15-minute period,[51] whereas sublingual nitroglycerin tablets are recommended at 1 tablet every 5 minutes as needed, with no more than 3 tablets every 15 minutes.[52] In the dental office the use of nitrolingual spray is preferred to the sublingual tablets because of the relative instability of the tablets[53] *(Figure 27-3).*

*Effects and side effects of nitroglycerin.* Nitroglycerin normally reduces or eliminates anginal discomfort dramatically within 2 to 4 minutes. Commonly observed side effects of nitroglycerin administration include a fullness or pounding in the head, flushing, tachycardia, and possible hypotension (if the patient is sitting upright). The presence of hypotension represents a contraindication to nitroglycerin administration.

*Action of nitroglycerin.* Nitroglycerin is the single most effective drug available for the management of acute anginal episodes. In normal individuals the administration of nitroglycerin decreases coronary artery resistance and increases coronary blood flow. This mechanism is probably of little consequence in patients with significant CAD, however. The probable mechanism of action of nitroglycerin in anginal patients is its ability to produce a decrease in the systemic vascular resistance through arterial and venous dilation. This leads to a decrease in return of venous blood to the heart and a decrease in cardiac output, which results in a lessened cardiac workload. A decrease in cardiac work produces a lesser oxygen requirement of the myocardium and a reversal of the oxygen insufficiency that existed during the episode.[54,55]

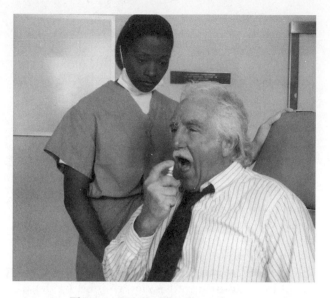

**Figure 27-3** Nitrolingual spray.

*Step 4b: administration of additional vasodilators, if necessary.* If the patient's nitroglycerin tablets are ineffective in terminating anginal pain within 5 minutes, give a second dose either from the patient's drug supply or from the emergency kit, which will be fresher than the patient's. Nitroglycerin tablets lose potency unless stored in tightly sealed glass containers. This is one possible explanation for the failure of the patient's nitroglycerin to relieve anginal pains. Nitroglycerin spray is considerably more stable than sublingual tablets and is preferred in this situation. A test for nitroglycerin potency is to place a tablet on the tongue; the drug is still potent if a tingling sensation is felt as the tablet dissolves, with a feeling of coolness throughout the mouth similar to that associated with mint candy but without the taste. A second possible explanation for the failure of nitroglycerin to provide relief is that the episode is not due to angina, but is an AMI. Administration of nitroglycerin and the patient's subsequent response to it is a major factor in the differential diagnosis of these two important cardiovascular syndromes.

The American Heart Association recommends that in a patient with known angina pectoris, emergency medical care be sought if chest pain is not relieved by 3 nitroglycerin tablets or spray doses over a 10-minute period. In a person with previously unrecognized coronary disease, the persistence of chest pain for 2 minutes or longer is an indication for emergency medical assistance.[56]

*Step 4c: summoning of medical assistance, if necessary.* If an episode of chest pain in a known

anginal patient has not been terminated after the administration of oxygen and the suggested three doses of nitroglycerin, seek medical assistance immediately. This step will usually be unnecessary for patients with angina pectoris. The management of continued or increasing chest pain will be discussed in Chapter 28.

If nitroglycerin is unavailable or proves ineffective in terminating an episode of chest pain, consider the use of amyl nitrate or a calcium channel blocker. Amyl nitrate is available in 0.3 mL ampules, which are crushed and then inhaled. The patient should be in a supine position when amyl nitrate is administered. Amyl nitrate is not recommended for use unless the anginal episode is severe and unrelieved by nitroglycerin and unless the patient has high blood pressure with a markedly elevated diastolic pressure. Seek medical assistance in this situation.

*Effects and side effects of amyl nitrate.* Once inhaled, amyl nitrate normally produces relief of anginal discomfort within 10 seconds. Because of its extreme potency, there are uncomfortable side effects that invariably occur with its use. These include flushing of the face, a bounding pulse, dizziness, and a pounding headache. (The person administering amyl nitrate may also experience the clinical effects of the drug if vapors are inadvertently inhaled.)

*Action of amyl nitrate.* Amyl nitrate causes profound peripheral arterial vasodilation. With administration of one ampule, the blood pressure falls precipitously. Amyl nitrate has a negligible effect on the veins; therefore little venous pooling occurs. Amyl nitrate markedly decreases cardiac output.[57]

*Effects and side effects of calcium slow channel blockers.* Patients known to have coronary artery spasm as a component of their anginal episodes usually respond well to the administration of nifedipine (10 to 20 mg) sublingually. Nifedipine, verapamil, and diltiazem are calcium entry-blocking agents.

Verapamil has been the most extensively studied drug in this group of agents for emergency cardiac care. Its actions are representative of the other drugs in the group. The therapeutic usefulness of verapamil is based on its slow channel–blocking properties, particularly the inward flow of calcium ions in cardiac and vascular smooth muscle. By blocking calcium influx and supply to the myocardial contractile mechanism, verapamil exerts a direct depressant effect on the inotropic state and therefore on the myocardial oxygen requirement. Verapamil also reduces contractile tone in vascular smooth muscle, which results in coronary and peripheral vasodilation, which in turn reduces systemic vascular resistance. Additionally, the calcium slow channel blockers exhibit antidysrhythmic effects, specifically by slowing conduction and prolonging refractoriness in the atrioventricular (AV) node. The current primary use of verapamil and other calcium slow channel blockers is as an antidysrhythmic drug. (It is highly effective in the management of paroxysmal supraventricular ventricular tachycardia [PSVT].) Its hemodynamic properties account for its beneficial actions in managing angina induced by coronary artery spasm.[58,59]

Pain-relieving opioids such as morphine and meperidine (Demerol) should not be used because they do not treat the cause of pain (i.e., inadequate oxygen supply). The only indication for opioid administration is AMI (see Chapter 28).

*Step 5: modification of further dental therapy.* After termination of the anginal episode, determine what factors might have caused it to occur. Consider modification of future dental treatment to prevent chest pain from recurring.

Dental treatment may resume at any time (immediately if necessary) after cessation of the acute anginal episode. Permit the patient to rest until he or she is comfortable before resuming dental care or discharge. Monitor and record vital signs before discharging the patient. The patient may be permitted to leave the office unescorted and to operate a motor vehicle if, in the opinion of the dentist, he or she is able to do so. In the unlikely situation that doubt persists about the degree of recovery, seek medical assistance or a medical consultation, or contact a friend or relative of the patient to serve as an escort.

## PATIENT WITH NO PRIOR HISTORY OF CHEST PAIN

When no prior history of chest pain is present, but the patient experiences chest pain during dental treatment, the steps of angina management, discussed earlier, are appropriate, with the exception that medical assistance be sought immediately—even before the administration of nitroglycerin and oxygen.

Even when this initial episode of chest pain is alleviated by nitroglycerin and oxygen, a thorough evaluation of this very frightened patient is in order, thus the recommendation for seeking medical assistance immediately. Box 27-2 outlines the steps to follow to manage chest pain in a patient with a history of angina pectoris.

- **Drugs used in management:** Nitroglycerin and oxygen.
- **Medical assistance required:** Assistance is not needed if there is a history of angina and relief of pain. It is required if this is the initial episode of chest

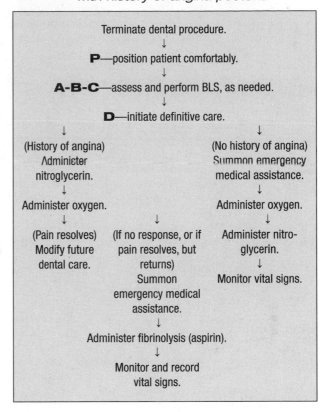

box **27-2** | *Management of chest pain with history of angina pectoris*

Terminate dental procedure.
↓
**P**—position patient comfortably.
↓
**A-B-C**—assess and perform BLS, as needed.
↓
**D**—initiate definitive care.

(History of angina) Administer nitroglycerin.
↓
Administer oxygen.
↓
(Pain resolves) Modify future dental care.

(If no response, or if pain resolves, but returns) Summon emergency medical assistance.
↓
Administer fibrinolysis (aspirin).
↓
Monitor and record vital signs.

(No history of angina) Summon emergency medical assistance.
↓
Administer oxygen.
↓
Administer nitroglycerin.
↓
Monitor vital signs.

pain or if there is no relief of pain with three doses of nitroglycerin.

## REFERENCES

1. *Mosby's medical, nursing, and allied health dictionary,* ed 5, Anderson KN, editor, St Louis, 1998, Mosby.
2. Heberden W: *Some account of a disorder of the breast,* Med Trans Coll Physic (London) 2:59, 1872.
3. Cohn PF, Braunwald E: Chronic coronary artery disease. In Braunwald E, editor: *Heart disease: a textbook of cardiovascular medicine.* Ed 5, Philadelphia, 1997, WB Saunders.
4. Angst DM, Bensinger DA: Angina. In *Cardiopulmonary emergencies,* Springhouse, Pa, 1991, Springhouse.
5. Diamond GA, Forrester JS: Analysis of probability as an aid in the clinical diagnosis of coronary heart disease, *N Engl J Med* 300:1350, 1979.
6. Waters D, Lam J, Theroux P: Newer concepts in the treatment of unstable angina pectoris, *Am J Cardiol* 68(12):34C-41C.
7. Gazes PC, Mobley EM Jr., Faris HM Jr., Duncan RC, Humphries GB: Preinfarction (unstable) angina: a prospective study—ten year follow-up, *Circulation* 48:331, 1973.

8. Welch CC and others: Cinecoronary arteriography in young men, *Circulation* 42:647, 1970.

9. Gazes PC and others: Preinfarctional (stable) angina: a prospective study—ten-year follow-up. Prognostic significance of electrocardiographic changes, *Circulation* 48:331, 1973.

10. Hartzler GO, Rutherford BD, McConahay DR: Percutaneous transluminal coronary angioplasty: application for acute myocardial infarction, *Am J Cardiol* 53:117c, 1984.

11. Phillips SJ, Kongtahworm C, Zeff RH: Emergency coronary artery revascularization: a possible therapy for acute myocardial infarction, *Circulation* 60:241, 1979.

12. Ricci DR, Moscovich MD, Kinahan PJ: Preliminary experience at a Canadian centre with directional coronary atherectomy for complex lesions, *Can J Cardiol* 7(9):399-406, 1991.

13. Korsch KR, Haase KK, Voelker W, and others: Percutaneous coronary excimer laser angioplasty in patients with stable and unstable angina pectoris: acute results and incidence of restenosis during 6-month follow-up, *Circulation* 81(6):1849-1859, 1990.

14. Warren SG, Bremer DL, Orgain ES: Long-term propranolol therapy for angina pectoris, *Am J Cardiol* 37:420, 1976.

15. Markis JE, Gorlin R, Mills RM, and others: Sustained effect of orally administered isosorbide dinitrate on exercise performance of patients with angina pectoris, *Am J Cardiol* 43:265, 1979.

16. Maseri A: Aspects of the medical therapy of angina pectoris, *Drugs* 42(suppl 1):28-30, 1991.

17. Braunwald E: The history. In Braunwald E, editor: *Heart disease,* ed 3, Philadelphia, 1986, WB Saunders.

18. Guthrie RB, and others: Pathology of stable and unstable angina pectoris, *Circulation* 51:1059, 1975.

19. Conti CR, and others: Unstable angina pectoris: morbidity and mortality in 57 consecutive patients evaluated angiographically, *Am J Cardiol* 32:745, 1973.

20. New York Heart Association: Report of the special committee of the New York Heart Association, Inc., on the use of epinephrine in connection with procaine in dental procedures, *J Am Dent Assoc* 50:108, 1955.

21. American Dental Association Council on Dental Therapeutics: American Dental Association and American Heart Association joint report: management of dental problems in patients with cardiovascular disease, *J Am Dent Assoc* 68:533, 1964.

22. American Dental Association Council on Dental Therapeutics: *Accepted dental therapeutics,* Chicago, 1985, The American Dental Association.

23. Boakes AJ, and others: Adverse reactions to local an *Br Dent J* 133:137, 1972.

24. Glover J: Vasoconstrictors in dental anaesthetics contraindication—fact or fallacy, *Aust Dent J* 13:65, 1968.

25. Holroyd SV, Watts DT, Welch JT, Jr: The use of epinephrine in local anesthetics for dental patients with cardiovascular disease: a review of the literature, *J Oral Surg* 18:492, 1960.

26. Jastak JT, Yagiela JA: Vasoconstrictors and local anesthesia: a review and rationale for use, *J Am Dent Assoc* 107:623, 1983.

27. Deleted in proofs.

28. Bennett CR: *Monheim's local anesthesia and pain control in dental practice,* ed 7, St Louis, 1984, Mosby.

29. Malamed SF: *Handbook of local anesthesia,* ed 3, St Louis, 1991, Mosby.

30. Brummett RE: Warning to otolaryngologists using local anesthetics containing epinephrine: potential serious reaction occurring in patients treated with beta-adrenergic receptor blockers, *Arch Otolaryngol* 110(9):561, 1984.

31. Yagiela JA: Deadfalls in drug interactions. 6th Annual review course in dental anesthesiology, 1990, American Dental Society of Anesthesiology.

32. Harrison JD: Effect of retraction materials on gingival sulcus epithelium, *J Prosthet Dent* 11:514, 1961.

33. Houston JB, and others: Effect of r-epinephrine impregnated retraction cord on the cardiovascular system, *J Prosthet Dent* 24:373, 1970.

34. Munoz RJ: The cardiovascular effects of anxiety and epinephrine retraction cord in routine fixed prosthodontic procedures, *J Calif Dent Assoc* 46:10, 1970.

35. Pague WL, Harrison JD: Absorption of epinephrine during tissue retraction, *J Prosthet Dent* 18:242, 1967.

36. Timberlake DL: Epinephrine in tissue retraction, *Ariz Dent J* 17:14, 1971.

37. Phatak NM, Lang RL: Systemic hemodynamic effects of r-epinephrine gingival retraction cord in clinic patients, *J Oral Ther Pharmacol* 2:393, 1966.

38. Malamed SF: *Sedation: a guide to patient management,* ed 2, St Louis, 1989, Mosby.

39. McCarthy FM: Essentials of safe dentistry for the medically compromised patient, Philadelphia, 1989, WB Saunders.

40. Winsor T, Berger HJ: Oral nitroglycerin as a prophylactic antianginal drug; clinical, physiologic, and statistical evidence of efficacy based on a three-phase experimental design, *Am Heart J* 90:611, 1975.

41. Godefroy JN, Batisse JP: Dental pain and cardiac pain, *Revue Francaise d'Endodontie* 9(1):17-21, 1991.

42. Kannel WB, Feinleib M: Natural history of angina pectoris in the Framingham study: prognosis and survival, *Am J Cardiol* 29:154, 1972.

43. Kent RI: Prognosis of symptomatic or mildly symptomatic patients with coronary artery disease, *Am J Cardiol* 49:1823, 1982.

44. Frank CW, Weinblatt F, Shapiro S: Angina pectoris in men: prognostic significance of selected medical factors, *Circulation* 47:509, 1973.

45. Cannon RO III: Microvascular angina: cardiovascular investigations regarding pathophysiology and management, *Med Clin N Am* 75(5):1097-1108, 1991.

46. Carleton RA, Johnson AD: Coronary arterial spasm: a clinical entity, *Mod Concepts Cardiovasc Dis* 43:87, 1974.

47. Hillis LD, Braunwald E: Coronary artery spasm, *N Engl J Med* 299:695, 1978.

48. Maseri A, Chierchia S: Coronary artery spasm: demonstration, definition, diagnosis, and consequences, *Prog Cardiovasc Dis* 25:169, 1982.

49. Pollakoff J, Pollakoff K: EMT's guide to signs and symptoms, Los Angeles, 1991, Jeff Gould.

50. Pollakoff J, Pollakoff K: EMT's guide to treatment, Los Angeles, 1991, Jeff Gould.

51. Nitrolingual spray: Drug package insert, Rhone-Poulenc Rorer Pharmaceuticals, 1990.

52. Nitrostat sublingual tablets: Drug package insert, Parke Davis, 1990.

53. Mayer GA: Instability of nitroglycerin tablets, *Can Med Assoc J* 110:788, 1974.

54. DiCarlo FJ: Nitroglycerin revisited: chemistry, biochemistry, interactions, *Drug Metab Rev* 4:1, 1975.

55. Judge TE: Vasodilators, *Practitioner* 212:2, 1974.

56. American Heart Association: Heart Attack: signals and actions for survival, Dallas, 1976, The American Heart Association.

57. Skidmore-Roth L: *Mosby's 1990 nursing drug reference,* St Louis 1990, Mosby.

58. Gerstenblith G, and others: Nifedipine in unstable angina: a double-blind, randomized trial, *N Engl J Med* 306:885, 1982.

59. Singh BN: The pharmacology of slow channel blocking drugs, *Cardiovasc Rev Rep* 4:179, 1983.

# 28

## Acute Myocardial Infarction

**M**YOCARDIAL infarction (MI) is a clinical syndrome caused by a deficient coronary arterial blood supply to a region of myocardium that results in cellular death and necrosis. The syndrome is usually characterized by severe and prolonged substernal pain similar to, but more intense and of longer duration than, that of angina pectoris. Complications associated with MI include shock, heart failure, and cardiac arrest. Synonyms for MI include coronary occlusion and heart attack.

Each year more than 1.1 million Americans experience acute myocardial infarction (AMI).[1] It is the single leading cause of death in the United States and is responsible for 35% of deaths occurring in men between the ages of 35 and 50 years. A man living in North America has a 20% chance of suffering an AMI or sudden death before the age of 65 years; for women the risk is 10%.[2] Although a relatively common clinical occurrence, AMI unfortunately still has a high mortality rate; approximately 36% of AMI victims (540,000) die, 250,000 of those before reaching a hospital.[1] In 1995, 1,100,000 persons in the United States sustained a MI. More than 60% of deaths from AMI occur within 2 hours of the onset of signs and symptoms.[3] Most of these deaths result from development of lethal dysrhythmias, usually ventricular fibrillation.[1,3] To increase the chance for survival after AMI, the dentist must know ways to prevent its occurrence, how to recognize its signs and symptoms, and how to manage it effectively. Killip[4] has stated

453

that, "once admitted to a hospital, the patient has already survived a significant risk." Indeed, recent advances in resuscitation and in management of AMI have substantially reduced the mortality rate among victims who reach the hospital.[5,6]

In addition to management of AMI, dentists are asked to manage the needs of patients who have survived an MI. The American Heart Association estimates that 4,600,000 victims of MI in the United States are still alive.[7] Most patients who survive a MI are able to resume their normal activities within 6 to 8 weeks.[1] As with patients who have experienced cerebral vascular accident or those with angina, patients who have had MI are at greater risk of reinfarction while receiving dental care.

In all, 27% of men and 44% of women die within 1 year after having a heart attack.[7,8] Major risk factors associated with these deaths include the severity of left ventricular damage,[9] continued myocardial ischemia,[10] and the predisposition to ventricular dysrhythmias.[11] Of the survivors of AMI, 30% develop significant angina pectoris.[8] Compared with the general population, survivors of AMI face a 10-fold risk of heart failure and a fourfold risk of sudden death.[8]

In MI a portion of myocardium dies. Depending on the extent of myocardial damage and the presence or absence of acute complications such as dysrhythmias, heart failure, and cardiac arrest, the victim either survives or succumbs during the acute phase of the disease. After this acute phase further complications such as continued myocardial ischemia or heart failure may develop. The latter decreases the ability of the heart to carry out its primary function—that of a pump—because of the size of the infarcted area of myocardium. Varying degrees of heart failure are common after MI. Knowledge of the presence of a compromised myocardium enables the dentist to modify dental treatment to decrease the potential risk to the patient.

## Predisposing Factors

The cause of AMI in more than 90% of all cases is coronary artery disease (atherosclerosis; CAD).[12] Other risk factors include obesity, being male (especially during the fifth to seventh decades of life), and undue stress (see Chapter 26). Friedman[13] and Friedman and Rosenman[14] described the cardiac risk patient as a "coronary prone" individual. This person is further characterized as having a type A behavior pattern, described as follows[15]:

*Foremost is a frightening and often obsessive sense of time urgency. He is determined to accomplish too much in too little time. He struggles both with his environment and with himself, but mainly with the latter. He is alert, very intense, and usually hostile. He is very competitive and ambitious; he wants recognition and seeks advancement. He tends to speed up his ordinary activities by looking at his watch often, by being on time, by hating to wait in line at the bank, movie, or restaurant. He is usually in occupations subject to deadlines.*

These patients themselves have labeled the type-A behavior pattern as the "hurry-up" disease.

In addition, a strong family history of cardiovascular disease, an abnormal electrocardiogram, elevated blood pressure, enlarged heart size, and/or an elevated blood cholesterol level add to the risk of suffering AMI.

Immediate predisposing factors for AMI include a significant decrease in blood flow through the coronary arteries, as in coronary thrombosis, or an increase in the level of cardiac work without a corresponding increase in the supply of oxygen to the myocardium, as seen with extreme stress.

The situation of decreased perfusion is called *myocardial ischemia*. Factors other than severe CAD that are implicated in the pathogenesis of AMI include the rupture (fissuring or hemorrhage) of atherosclerotic plaque[16] and arterial spasm.[17] On rare occasion, AMI can occur in the absence of coronary artery narrowing if there is a marked disparity between myocardial oxygen ($O_2$) supply and demand. The abuse of cocaine has been implicated as a cause of such a disparity.[18]

## LOCATION AND EXTENT OF INFARCTION

As described in Chapter 26, the anterior descending branch of the left coronary artery is the most common site of clinically significant atherosclerosis within the heart. Not surprisingly, this vessel is the most common site of thrombosis, leading to MI. With occlusion of this vessel, the anterior portion of the left ventricle becomes ischemic, and in the absence of adequate collateral circulation, infarction occurs with subsequent myocardial necrosis throughout the distribution of the occluded artery. Occlusion of the left circumflex artery produces anterolateral infarction. Thrombosis of the right coronary artery leads to infarction of the posteroinferior portion of the left ventricle and might also involve the right ventricular myocardium.[19] The extent of infarction therefore is related to several factors, including the anatomic distribution of the occluded vessel, the adequacy of collateral circulation, the extent of existing CAD throughout the myocardium (one vessel versus multivessel involvement), and whether or not previous infarction has occurred.[20]

# Prevention

Prevention of a first MI in a high-risk patient (see CAD risk factors, p. 428), although a seemingly impossible task, may be attempted by the dentist through strict adherence to the stress reduction protocol. This protocol minimizes potentially adverse effects of undue stress on the workload and $O_2$ requirement of the myocardium, thereby reducing the risk from one of the immediate predisposing factors of AMI (i.e., increased cardiac workload). The dentist cannot prevent the other immediate predisposing factors: thrombosis, occlusion, or spasm of a coronary blood vessel.

The dental patient with a history of previous MI must be identified, and the doctor must attempt to obtain as much information regarding the current physical status of this patient as is possible so that risk may be determined before the start of dental treatment. This necessitates the use of the medical history questionnaire, physical examination, and the dialogue history.

## Medical History Questionnaire

**9. Circle any of the following that you have had or have at present:**

Heart disease
Heart attack

*Comment:* An affirmative reply must be followed by a detailed dialogue history to determine the degree of risk presented by this patient.

**6. Have you taken any medicine or drugs during the last 2 years?**

*Comment:* Survivors of MI (called *status post-MI*) receive medications according to the degree of residual myocardial damage and the presence of complications. Patients who are status post-MI frequently receive one or more of the following drug groups:

- *Beta-adrenergic-blockers:* Drugs such as propranolol have improved survival rates, primarily by reducing the incidence of sudden death in high-risk patients.
- *Calcium channel blockers:* Although these drugs have not been shown to improve prognosis overall, two members of this group, diltiazem and verapamil, appear to reduce mortality rates in patients with preserved left ventricular function. Diltiazem may help to prevent reinfarction after non–Q-wave infarction.
- *Antiplatelet agents:* Low-dose aspirin (325 mg daily) is recommended.

- *Anticoagulation:* Warfarin reduces the incidence of arterial emboli during the first 3 months after large anterior infarctions.
- *Angiotensin-converting enzyme inhibitors:* These drugs have been shown to be valuable in postinfarction survivors who have sustained substantial myocardial damage with progressive left ventricular dilation and dysfunction. Captopril prevents left ventricular dilation and the onset of heart failure and also reduces mortality rates.[21,22]
- *Other drugs categories:* Diuretics are valuable for management of heart failure and high blood pressure; digitalis or dopamine may be helpful for heart failure; nitrates (e.g., nitroglycerin) may be indicated if anginal pains are present after MI.

Table 28-1 summarizes the drugs used in the post-MI period.

**10. When you walk up stairs or take a walk, do you ever have to stop because of pain in your chest or shortness of breath, or because you are very tired?**

*Comment:* The presence of one or more of these symptoms of poor cardiopulmonary reserve indicates that the patient is at greater risk for AMI during dental management.

## DIALOGUE HISTORY

In the presence of a positive history of cardiovascular disease (e.g., angina, MI), the following dialogue history should be pursued:

**Has there been any alteration in the pattern of your episodes of angina in the last month?**

*Comment:* As discussed in Chapter 27, anginal episodes are usually fairly consistent for each patient. Any increase in rate of frequency, duration, or severity or a decrease in the level of precipitating factors may be an indication of unstable angina. Immediate consultation with the patient's physician is desirable.

**When did you have your last myocardial infarction?**

*Comment:* After MI, an increased risk of reinfarction exists. The patients who is status post-MI is at an increased risk during dental therapy regardless of the amount of time elapsed since the initial episode.[8] However, in the immediate postinfarction period, there is a considerably higher risk of reinfarction. In a study of surgical patients by Weinblatt and others,[23] the reinfarction rate (a subsequent MI occurring either during surgery or in the immediate postoperative period [4 hours]) was 37% if the surgical procedure occurred within 3 months of the initial episode, 16% if the procedure was performed within 4 to 6 months of the episode, and 5% if the procedure was performed longer than 6 months after the episode, compared with 0.1% in persons with no prior history of MI. During the recovery period from AMI, collateral circulation to the infarcted area improves, thereby allowing the myocardium to heal and minimizing the size of the residual infarct.[24,25] This process of healing and myocardial stabilization is usually complete in 6 months.[26] The increased risk for the patient who is status post-MI is illustrated by an overall mortality rate of 30% within the first month after the infarction.[7,8] The majority of these deaths are related to the presence of significant dysrhythmias (e.g., ventricular fibrillation). Although this high mortality rate does decrease with time, after 10 years the postinfarction mortality rate is still 10 times that for those with no prior history of MI.[8]

**What medications and drugs are you currently taking?**

*Comment:* Refer to Medical History Questionnaire question #6 for a listing of the drugs frequently taken by the patient who is status post-MI. This information indicates the degree of residual myocardial damage, the presence of any significant signs and symptoms (e.g., chest pain, shortness of breath, undue fatigue), and damage to the cardiac conduction system (e.g., the presence of dysrhythmias).

## PHYSICAL EXAMINATION

Vital signs should be recorded before and immediately after all dental appointments in the patient who is status post-MI. (See Table 2-1 for suggested management of patients according to their blood pressure readings.) Additional examination of this patient may not provide any reliable indication of previous MI. Many survivors of a mild MI (e.g., minimal residual damage) appear to be in extremely fine physical and mental condition. Researchers have investigated the role of physical exercise in the rehabilitation of myocardial tissues after infarction. Findings have led to comprehensive physical training programs for many of these patients.[27-29] Patients are permitted to resume normal activities, such as walking and sexual activity, in a graded manner during convalescence. Such programs result in both subjective and objective improvement, recorded as decreases in heart rate and blood pressure, as well as a return to a normal or near-normal lifestyle and improved morale. Unfortunately, there is much less evidence for improvement in ventricular function and little convincing evidence that these programs decrease the recurrence rate of MI or the mortality rate.[30] It must always be remembered, therefore, that regardless of the apparent state of physical fitness of patients who are status post-MI, they must still be considered a high risk during all dental procedures.

Patients who are status post-MI and who have a significant degree of ventricular damage may present with clinical signs and symptoms of congestive heart failure (CHF) (see Chapter 14). Visual examination of these patients may reveal a degree of peripheral cyanosis (e.g., noted in nailbeds, mucous mem-

| table **28-1** | *Medications used for patients with status postmyocardial infarction* |

| DRUG CATEGORY | EXAMPLE(S) | RATIONALE |
|---|---|---|
| Beta-adrenergic blockers | Propranolol<br>Timolol<br>Alprenolol<br>Metoprolol | Several studies have shown beta-blockers to decrease likelihood hood of sudden death and reinfarction in months following acute myocardial infarction |
| Calcium-channel blockers | Diltiazem<br>Verapamil | Prevent reinfarction and reduce mortality rates |
| Antiplatelet agents | Sulfinpyrazone (Anturane) | Shown in two studies to reduce incidence of sudden death and recurrent myocardial infarction (for up to 7 months postmyocardial infarction) |
| | Aspirin | Still prescribed, although a large, multicenter study found no reduction in deaths from recurrent myocardial infarction |
| Anticoagulants | Warfarin | Reduce incidence of arterial emboli in initial 3 months after infarction |
| ACE inhibitors | Captopril | Prevent left ventricular dilation and the onset of heart failure |
| Diuretics | Hydrochlorothiazide | High blood pressure, heart failure |
| Inotropic drugs | Digitalis<br>Dopamine<br>Dobutamine<br>Amrinone | Heart failure |
| Nitrates | Nitroglycerin—ointment, transdermal, or sublingual tablet or spray forms<br>Long-acting nitrates (see Table 27-2) | Anginal pains |

*ACE,* Angiotensin-converting enzyme.

branes), coolness of the extremities, peripheral edema (in ankles), and possible orthopnea (difficulty in breathing that is relieved by sitting upright). These patients are at considerable risk during dental treatment.

# Dental Therapy Considerations

Dental therapy considerations for the patient who is status post-MI include reduction in stress related to dental care and possible alteration in drug therapy, dental therapy, or both. This patient is classified by the American Society of Anesthesiologists (ASA) as an ASA II, ASA III, or ASA IV risk depending on the time elapsed since the previous infarction, the number of prior infarcts, and the presence of continued signs or symptoms of cardiovascular disease (e.g., dyspnea, chest pain, dysrhythmias). Table 28-2 presents the ASA classification of the status post-MI patient.

## STRESS REDUCTION

The degree of stress intolerance, although present in all patients who are status post-MI, varies from person to person. Implementation of appropriate steps in the stress reduction protocol should receive serious consideration. Of special importance are intraoperative stress reduction and adequate pain control.

**Supplemental oxygen**    The administration of supplemental $O_2$ to the patient who is status post-MI minimizes the risk of hypoxia and myocardial ischemia. An $O_2$ flow of 3 to 5 L/min through a nasal cannula (humidified) or nasal hood (5 to 7 L/min) is recommended.

**Sedation**    Oxygen may also be delivered in conjunction with nitrous oxide ($N_2O$). $N_2O$-$O_2$ inhalation sedation is the most recommended sedation technique for the cardiac risk patient. Its value in the management of AMI is discussed later in this chapter. Other sedation techniques may be used if deemed necessary by the doctor. Hypoxia should be avoided in all sedation techniques through the administration of supplemental $O_2$.

**Pain control**    Adequate pain control during treatment is a critical factor in increasing safety during dental treatment of the cardiac-risk patient. As discussed in Chapter 27, endogenous catecholamine release is potentially more dangerous to the cardiac risk patient than the 0.01 mg/ml of exogenous epinephrine introduced into the tissues with a properly administered local anesthetic containing epinephrine in a 1:100,000 concentration. However, vasoconstrictors are contraindicated in patients with intractable cardiac dysrhythmias or any ASA IV cardiovascular-risk patient (likewise, elective dental care is contraindicated in this patient). The use of vasoconstrictor-containing local anesthetics is relatively contraindicated in patients receiving noncardiospecific beta-blockers, such as propranolol.[31]

**Duration of treatment**    The duration of an appointment for the patient who is status post-MI is variable but should not exceed the patient's level of

table **28-2**  *Dental therapy considerations for status postmyocardial infarction patients*

| NUMBER OF EPISODES | ASA PHYSICAL STATUS | CONSIDERATIONS |
| --- | --- | --- |
| One documented myocardial infarction at least 6 months previously; no residual cardiovascular complications | II or III | Usual ASA II or III considerations to include follow-up after therapy by telephone; supplemental $O_2$ during treatment |
| One documented episode at least 6 months previously; angina, CHF, or dysrhythmia present | III or IV | Use of dialogue history to determine level of risk; usual ASA III considerations include possible premedication with nitroglycerin 5 minutes preop (if angina); $O_2$ through nasal cannula or nasal hood; and follow-up after therapy by telephone |
| More than one documented episode, most recent one at least 6 months previously; no further cardiovascular complications | III | Usual ASA III considerations to include supplemental oxygen during treatment and follow-up after therapy by telephone |
| Documented episode less than 6 months previously, or severe post-MI complications | IV | Usual ASA IV considerations |

*CHF,* Congestive heart failure; *ASA,* American Society of Anesthesiologists.

tolerance. Patients who show signs of discomfort such as dyspnea, diaphoresis, and increased anxiety should be questioned to determine a cause and treatment modified, or possibly terminated.

**Six months post-MI**  It is strongly recommended that elective dental care, even procedures as seemingly innocuous as a prophylaxis, be avoided for a patient who is status post-MI for at least 6 months after infarction.[32,33] Invasive emergency care, such as that for infection and pain, should not be performed in the dental office during this time, if possible. The acute dental problem may initially be managed pharmacologically, through the administration of oral drugs (e.g., antibiotics and/or analgesics) alone; any necessary invasive treatment, such as extraction or pulpal extirpation, should be carried out in a more controlled environment, such as a hospital dental clinic.

Only emergency procedures should be considered for the patients who is status post-MI within 6 months of the acute cardiac event. Even in these cases, immediate invasive care is warranted only after medications have been ineffective in resolving the problem and a hospital setting (a controlled environment) is available for the planned treatment.

**Medical consultation**  Medical consultation should be considered before dental management of a patient who is status post-MI if, after a full dental, medical, and psychologic evaluation of the patient, the doctor has any doubt regarding the patient's status. If the doctor is contemplating emergency dental treatment for this patient within the recommended 6-month waiting period, medical consultation is strongly suggested before initiating treatment.

**Anticoagulant or antiplatelet therapy**
Medical consultation is also indicated before any treatment involving a risk of hemorrhage (e.g., periodontal surgery, oral surgery, inferior alveolar nerve block) if the patient is currently receiving anticoagulant or antiplatelet therapy. The post-MI use of anticoagulants is much less common today than in the recent past.

Dental surgery is frequently performed in patients whose prothrombin time is 20% to 30% of normal without the development of bleeding problems.[32] In most instances, therefore, the proposed dental procedure need not be postponed, and the patient's anticoagulant medication need not be altered. However, the doctor should take precautions to prevent the occurrence of postoperative hemorrhage. Possible steps include a hemostatic dressing placed within an extraction site, multiple sutures in the surgical area, intraoral pressure packs, ice packs

(extraoral), avoidance of mouth rinses, and a soft diet for 48 hours after the procedure. Additionally, inferior alveolar and posterior superior alveolar nerve block injections are associated with increased risk of hemorrhage and therefore should be avoided in some cases.

# Clinical Manifestations

## PAIN

The chief clinical manifestation of AMI is the sudden onset of severe, anginal-type pain, which is experienced in 80% of cases. Because AMI occurs when a thrombus forms in a coronary artery, it may occur without an obvious precipitating cause. AMI often develops during a period of rest or sleep, but it may also occur during or immediately after a period of unusually strong exercise (Table 28-3).[34] A high percentage of MIs occur in the early morning (most commonly on Monday [where the weekend is Saturday/Sunday]).[35] Emotional stress may be a precipitating factor.[36,37] The pain builds rapidly to maximal intensity, lasting for prolonged periods (30 minutes to several hours) if unmanaged.[12]

Pain associated with AMI is usually described as a pressing or crushing sensation, like a deep ache within the chest. The patient may state that "it feels like there is a heavy rock or someone sitting on my chest." Rarely is the pain described as sharp or stabbing. It is located over the middle to upper third of the sternum and, much less commonly, over the lower third of the epigastrium.[1] Unfortunately, when the pain of AMI occurs in the epigastrium and is associated with nausea and vomiting (see next section), the clinical picture may easily be confused with that of acute gastritis, cholecystitis, or peptic ulcer.[12]

Neither rest *nor the use of nitroglycerin* reduces the pain. The pain of MI is most effectively relieved through the administration of opioids such as mor-

| table **28-3** | *Patient activity at onset of myocardial infarction* |

| ACTIVITY | PERCENTAGE OF PATIENTS |
|---|---|
| At rest | 51 |
| Modest or usual exertion | 18 |
| Physical exertion | 13 |
| Sleep | 8 |
| During surgical procedure | 6 |
| Other | 4 |

Data from Phipps C: Contributory causes of coronary thrombosis, *JAMA* 106:761, 1936.

phine. Radiation of pain occurs in the same pattern as that for angina (see Figure 27-2).

In 20% to 25% of cases pain is either absent or minor and is overshadowed by immediate complications such as acute pulmonary edema, CHF, profound weakness, shock, syncope, or cerebral thrombosis. This type of infarction is called a silent (painless) infarction.[38]

## OTHER CLINICAL SIGNS AND SYMPTOMS

The patient suffering an MI may appear to be in acute distress. A cold sweat is usually present; the patient feels quite weak and appears apprehensive, expressing an intense fear of impending doom. Although "intense fear of impending doom" may appear to the reader to be an overly dramatic statement, many victims of AMI do indeed verbally report this feeling. In contrast to anginal patients who lie, sit, or stand still, realizing that any activity will increase their discomfort, patients with AMI are frequently quite restless, moving about in a futile attempt to find a comfortable position. They may clutch at their chest with a fist, known as the *Levine sign* (a sign of ischemic pain popularized by Dr. Samuel A. Levine). Dyspnea is usually present; the patient complains that the crushing pressure on the chest prevents normal breathing. Respiratory movements do not intensify the painful sensation. Nausea and vomiting frequently occur, especially if the pain is severe. Other clinical signs and symptoms associated with AMI may include a feeling of lightheadedness or faintness, coughing, wheezing, and abdominal bloating. This last symptom leads some victims to think (hope?) that they are suffering from upset stomach or indigestion, thereby delaying the initiation of proper treatment and increasing the risk of death.

The doctor should suspect the occurrence of an AMI in the following three situations:

1. *A first episode of chest pain suggestive of AMI that occurs either at rest or with ordinary activity.* Although it is possible for a first episode of chest pain that develops during dental treatment to be anginal (especially if the patient is dental phobic), it may also be indicative of coronary artery occlusion.
2. *Change in a previously stable pattern of anginal pain.* This may be either increased frequency or severity, or the occurrence of rest (unstable) angina for the first time.
3. *Chest pain suggestive of myocardial ischemia in a patient with known CAD if unrelieved by rest and/or nitroglycerin.*

## PHYSICAL FINDINGS

The patient appears restless and apprehensive and may be in severe pain. Color may be poor, the face an ashen gray, with nailbeds and other mucous membranes cyanotic. The skin is cool, pale, and moist. The heart rate (pulse) may be weak, thready, and rapid (tachycardic), although a slow rate (bradycardia) may occasionally be present. Dysrhythmias are often present: premature ventricular contractions (PVCs) are seen in 93% of patients within the first 4 hours after AMI.[39] Blood pressure may be normal but much more commonly is low, decreasing dramatically over the first few hours and possibly falling to shock levels. Respirations are rapid and shallow. If the left ventricle is the major site of infarction, left ventricular failure may become clinically evident, with labored breathing, frothy sputum, and other signs of CHF (dependent edema); or pulmonary edema may gradually develop (Table 28-4).

## ACUTE COMPLICATIONS

The greatest risk of death from MI occurs during the first 4 to 6 hours after coronary artery occlusion and the onset of signs and symptoms. Complications such as acute dysrhythmias and cardiac arrest can occur abruptly during this time. More than 60% of deaths associated with AMI occur within an hour of the event and are associated with acute lethal dysrhythmias, such as pulseless ventricular tachycardia and ventricular fibrillation.[40] PVCs are common (93%). Their presence is indicative of increased irritability of the damaged myocardium and may presage the

table **28-4** | *Clinical manifestations of acute myocardial infarction*

| SYMPTOMS | SIGNS |
|---|---|
| Pain | Restlessness |
|   Severe to intolerable | In acute distress |
|   Prolonged, >30 min | Skin—cool, pale, moist |
|   Crushing, choking | Heart rate—bradycardia to |
|   Retrosternal |   tachycardia; PVCs common |
|   Radiates: left arm, hand, | |
|     epigastrium, shoulders, | |
|     neck, jaw | |
| Nausea and vomiting | |
| Weakness | |
| Dizziness | |
| Palpitations | |
| Cold perspiration | |
| Sense of impending doom | |

*PVCs,* Premature ventricular contractions.

development of ventricular tachycardia or ventricular fibrillation.

Ventricular fibrillation is 15 times more likely to occur in the first hour after the onset of signs and symptoms than in the next 12 hours[41,42]; it develops in the first hour in approximately 36% of persons with AMI.[43] The significant mortality rate associated with MI is in part based on the average delay (4.9 hours) between the onset of signs and symptoms and intervention by the emergency medical system.[44] The doctor must prepare mentally for the development of acute complications. Survival through the prehospitalization period is indeed a good omen, because once the patient is hospitalized in the emergency department and then in a specialized cardiac care unit, the chances for ultimate survival increase significantly. The most dangerous period is the time spent waiting for medical assistance to arrive.[41-44] Adequate preparation by the dental office staff can improve the chances for a successful outcome in this situation.

## Pathophysiology

AMI is usually the direct result of a sudden occlusion of a major coronary vessel. The obstruction may result from acute thrombosis, subintimal hemorrhage, or the rupture of an atheromatous plaque, which then initiates the formation of a clot. The artery most often involved in coronary occlusion is the anterior descending branch of the left coronary artery, which supplies the anterior left ventricle. There are two major types of AMI: Q wave versus non-Q wave. The latter generally results from incomplete occlusion or spontaneous lysis of the thrombus and often signifies the presence of additional jeopardized myocardium; it is associated with a higher incidence of reinfarction and recurrent ischemia.[45]

An occlusion may occur rapidly, or it may develop over a prolonged period. In either case it is possible that even total occlusion of a coronary vessel may not lead to ischemia and infarction. In the presence of an adequate collateral circulation, the myocardium supplied by the occluded vessel still receives an adequate blood supply through collateral vessels. Unfortunately, collateral circulation in the normal heart is usually poorly developed; however, immediately after occlusion of a coronary artery, collateral blood flow doubles.[46] The significance of this increase in collateral circulation is debatable.[24] Because these vessels enlarge over the next 3 to 4 weeks after the occlusion, the size of the area of myocardial necrosis is usually smaller than would be expected.[47]

AMI may occur even though a blood vessel is not totally occluded. In an area dependent for its blood supply on collateral circulation (e.g., a previously infarcted area with now adequate collateral circulation), a minimal change in blood supply through the vessel may lead to infarction. This may come about through a partial occlusion of the vessel or from a change in vascular resistance in the vessel (e.g., spasm).

Infarction of the myocardium produces alterations in the contractility of the heart owing to a loss of functional myocardial segments. The degree of depression of cardiac function in AMI is directly related to the extent of left ventricular damage.[48] Because the left ventricle is most commonly involved in AMI, the blood supply leaving the heart may be diminished. This leads to many of the clinical signs and symptoms observed in AMI, such as cool, moist skin, peripheral cyanosis, and tachycardia. The larger the infarct, the greater the degree of circulatory inadequacy (e.g., signs and symptoms of heart failure). Left ventricular filling pressures increase significantly, even in the presence of a small infarct. If the infarction is larger, there is a greater increase in the left ventricular filling pressure and clinical evidence of left ventricular failure. Infarction of 35% or more of left ventricular mass leads to clinical evidence of hypotension, decreased cardiac output, and cardiogenic shock.[49]

*Cardiogenic shock* occurs in approximately 10% to 15% of patients with AMI who survive long enough to reach the hospital.[50,51] Cardiogenic shock is an ominous sign because it is associated with a high mortality rate. It normally develops approximately 10 hours after the onset of the infarction and may be produced by cardiac dysrhythmias, the continued presence of severe pain, the onset of acute pulmonary edema, or pulmonary embolism. Clinical evidence of cardiogenic shock includes hypotension (systolic blood pressure below 80 mmHg) and signs of an inadequate peripheral circulation (e.g., mental confusion, cool skin, peripheral cyanosis, tachycardia, and decreased urinary output).[51]

Probably the most threatening feature of the early postinfarction period (1 to 2 hours) is the presence of cardiac dysrhythmias. Most patients (95%) exhibit abnormalities in heart rhythm. These abnormalities are significant because they may produce alterations in the normal sequence of atrial and ventricular contraction, thereby leading to inadequate cardiac output, and/or they may produce an aberrant focus of electrical depolarization in the myocardium. They also may adversely affect the ventricular rate, producing *bradycardia* (slow heart rate), *ventricular tachycardia* (an extremely rapid contraction rate with insufficient time for ventricular filling), *ventricular fibrillation* (irregular, uncoordinated, ineffective contraction of individual muscle bundles), or, less commonly, asystole (complete absence of contractions). Commonly observed dysrhythmias are shown in Fig. 30-1.

Death in the early postinfarction period is normally the result of an acute dysrhythmia, although it may be produced by the infarction of a large mass of myocardium.[42,43] Patient survival after MI depends on many factors, the most important of which are the state of left ventricular function and the severity of obstructive lesions in the coronary vascular bed. Complete clinical recovery (i.e., no chronic complications) and a normal electrocardiogram (ECG) are compatible with a 10- to 20-year period of survival. However, patients who exhibit residual CHF usually die within 1 to 5 years.[52,53]

# Management

Clinical management of AMI is based on its recognition and the application of the steps of basic life support. It may be difficult to differentiate immediately between the pain of angina and that of AMI. Although there are subtle differences initially, the doctor may find it difficult to determine which of these clinical entities is present at the onset of the episode of acute chest pain.

Diagnostic clues to the presence of AMI include the following[54]:
- Symptoms of pressure, tightness, a heavy weight
- Substernal, epigastric pain that may radiate to the jaw
- Moderate to severe discomfort
- Longer duration (>30 minutes) than anginal pain
- Nausea and vomiting
- Diaphoresis
- Dyspnea
- Irregular pulse
- Generalized weakness

## STEPS

If these symptoms occur, these steps should be followed.

*Step 1: termination of the dental procedure.* With the onset of chest pain, immediately stop treatment.

*Step 2: diagnosis.* Although, at the outset, it may prove difficult to distinguish between the pain of angina and AMI, it is immediately apparent that the patient (victim) is in acute distress and must be treated

accordingly. (Although an ECG, if available, may confirm AMI, the ECG may also appear to be entirely normal.[43] For this reason a single, normal ECG tracing cannot reliably exclude the diagnosis of past AMI.)

Three potential clinical situations follow:
- Anginal patient—acute anginal attack: A patient with a history of angina is usually able to tell if the episode of pain is anginal. If angina is thought to be the problem, follow steps presented in Chapter 27. The patient, who is accustomed to treating his or her angina, will usually be calmer about the situation than will the doctor, who is probably unaccustomed to patients experiencing acute chest pain during their treatment.
- Anginal patient—not angina: An anginal patient in whom the chest pain is more intense than usual will become frightened, convinced that "the big one" is happening. Recommended management follows the steps outlined later for AMI.
- No previous history of chest pain: Chest pain developing in a patient with no prior history of acute chest pain normally frightens the patient, who is also convinced that a "heart attack" is occurring. Management of this situation is presented later.

It is suggested that management of chest pain be approached as if it were angina pectoris (situation 1) unless it is obviously not of anginal origin, as is the case in situations 2 and 3.

*Step 3: P (position).*

*Step 4: A-B-C (airway-breathing-circulation), basic life support (BLS), as needed.* At this point in the AMI, the patient will be experiencing more intense discomfort and may be showing clinical signs of decreased cardiac output (i.e., diaphoresis; cool, moist extremities; ashen-gray pallor; cyanosis of mucous membranes and nailbeds). Airway, breathing, and circulation are assessed and usually adequate. Permit the patient to remain in a comfortable position (if possible).

*Step 5: D (definitive care):*
*Step 5a: administration of oxygen.* Administer oxygen as soon as it becomes available. Evidence suggests that increased arterial oxygen tension ($PaO_2$) may decrease the size of the infarct.[55] Oxygen should be delivered through a nasal cannula or nasal hood at a flow rate of 4 to 6 L/min.
*Step 5b: summoning of medical assistance.* Whenever there is a strong suspicion that chest pain is not of anginal origin, but is likely to be a MI, or in the instance of a first episode of chest pain, the Emergency Medical Services (EMS) system should be activated as soon as possible.

*Step 5c: administration of nitroglycerin.* Administer nitroglycerin. If the victim has a history of angina, nitroglycerin, which should always be available, is used at this time. Nitroglycerin from the emergency kit is used when the patient does not have a personal supply or if the patient's supply fails to alleviate the pain. The patient's vital signs should be recorded either before administering the nitroglycerin or shortly thereafter. *Nitroglycerin should not be administered in the presence of hypotension* (if systolic blood pressure is below 100 mmHg) because it can further decrease the mean arterial pressure. Nitroglycerin normally acts within 2 to 4 minutes to dramatically reduce or terminate the discomfort of angina. If angina is the cause of the pain, the pain will resolve and the acute problem is terminated. Dental care may resume if both the doctor and patient desire and/or the patient can be dismissed from the office (see discussion

in Chapter 27). If the pain continues or increases despite the administration of nitroglycerin and oxygen, or if nitroglycerin alleviates the pain, but the pain returns in a few minutes, a diagnosis of AMI must be seriously considered.

> NOTE: Chest pain that is alleviated by nitroglycerin but returns should be managed as though it were acute myocardial infarction.

More than 60% of all deaths from AMI occur within the first few hours after the onset of symptoms, before the victim is hospitalized. Three fourths of all deaths occur within the first 24 hours. Most deaths that occur before hospitalization are the result of life-threatening dysrhythmias that are common in the immediate postinfarction period, as well as the misinterpretation or denial of signs and symptoms by the patient or medical personnel. Early entry into the EMS system is often vital for patient survival. The average time from onset of symptoms of ischemic heart disease to entry into the EMS is more than 3 hours.

The availability of trained paramedical personnel in mobile coronary care units has led to a significant decrease in the mortality rate from MI.[56] Definitive therapy (e.g., advanced cardiac life support) can be initiated at the scene or while en route to the hospital. In Seattle, Washington, which has a model EMS system, basic life support was provided for victims of out-of-hospital cardiac arrest within 2.9 minutes and advanced cardiac life support within an average of 4 minutes from dispatch to arrival of EMS. By 1978, 60% of 290 patients with out-of-hospital cardiac arrest were resuscitated in the field and 30% (88 patients) were eventually discharged home.[56]

*Step 5d: fibrinolysis.* The administration of aspirin has been added to the prehospital management of out-of-hospital AMI victims.[57,58] Aspirin has fibrinolytic properties that assist in the process of revascularization of the ischemic myocardium. Patients should be administered a dose of 325 mg aspirin to chew as soon as it is thought that an AMI may be developing.

Aspirin therapy confers conclusive net benefits in the acute phase of evolving AMI and should be administered routinely in these cases. In the Second International Study of Infarct Survival (ISIS-2),[59] more than 17,000 men and women were randomly assigned within 24 hours of onset of symptoms of suspected AMI to one of two treatment groups: 162 mg of aspirin or placebo daily for 30 days. After 5 weeks patients who received aspirin had statistically significant reductions in risk of vascular mortality (23%), nonfatal reinfarction (49%), and nonfatal stroke (46%). There was no increase in hemorrhagic stroke

---

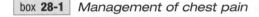

**box 28-1**   *Management of chest pain*

Terminate dental procedure.
↓
**P**—position patient comfortably.
↓
**A-B-C**—assess and perform BLS, as needed.
↓
**D**—initiate definitive care:

| (History of angina) | (No history of angina) |
| Administer oxygen. | Summon emergency medical assistance. |
| ↓ | ↓ |
| Administer nitroglycerin. | Administer oxygen. |

(Pain resolves)          (If no response, or if pain          Administer
Modify future           resolves, but returns)           nitroglycerin.
dental care.            Summon emergency medical               ↓
                              assistance.                    Monitor vital
                                  ↓                             signs.
                    Administer fibrinolysis (aspirin).
                                  ↓
                    Monitor and record vital signs.
                                  ↓
                            Manage pain
                    (parenteral opioids, N₂O-O₂).
                                  ↓
                        Manage complications.
                                  ↓

Acute dys-        Left ventricular failure develops.    Cardiac arrest
rhythmias              (see Chapter 14)                    occurs.
(ACLS) occurs.    Stabilize and transfer to hospital.  (see Chapter 30)

**P,** Position; **A,** airway; **B,** breathing; **C,** circulation; **D,** definitive care; *ACLS,* Advanced Coronary Life Support.

or gastrointestinal bleeding in the treated group and only a small increase in minor bleeding. Thus aspirin has perhaps the best benefit/risk ratio of any proven therapy for AMI. The benefits of aspirin for risk of subsequent AMI, stroke, or vascular death are substantial. The risks of serious bleeding and sensitivity reactions are low and are amenable to treatment in an acute care setting, even when the patient has a history of bleeding or other sensitivity to aspirin. Thus, contraindications to use of aspirin in AMI are relative, not absolute.

To achieve an immediate clinical antithrombotic effect, an initial minimum loading dose of 162 mg should be used in AMI. If an enteric-coated aspirin is the only preparation available, the first tablet should be chewed or crushed before administration. In 1996 the, US Food and Drug Administration (FDA)[60] proposed a professional labeling indication for aspirin in patients with AMI: an initial dose of 160 to 162.5 mg continued daily for at least 30 days.[61]

*Step 5e: monitoring of vital signs.* Monitor vital signs. Vital signs (e.g., blood pressure, heart rate and rhythm, respiration) should be monitored on a regular basis (every 5 minutes) and recorded.

*Step 5f: relief of pain.* Relieve pain. Prolonged pain during AMI is potentially life threatening. It leads to increased patient anxiety and contributes to excessive activity of the autonomic nervous system, producing an increase in cardiovascular workload and oxygen requirement. In addition, prolonged, intense pain is one of the causative factors of cardiogenic shock, which is associated with a high mortality rate. Nitroglycerin is usually inadequate to alleviate the pain associated with AMI.[62]

The use of opioid analgesics is recommended for relief of pain associated with AMI. Intravenous (IV) administration of 2 to 5 mg of morphine sulfate repeated every 5 to 15 minutes provides adequate pain relief and allays apprehension.[63] Additionally, morphine increases venous capacitance and systemic vascular resistance, relieving pulmonary congestion and thereby decreasing myocardial oxygen requirements.[63] Morphine sulfate may also be administered subcutaneously in a dose of 5 to 15 mg. *Morphine should not be readministered if the respiratory rate is less than 12 breaths per minute.* Meperidine (50 to 100 mg intramuscularly [IM]) may be administered in place of morphine. IM injection of these analgesic drugs provides adequate pain relief of long duration. IV administration may also be considered, but the drugs require readministration in a shorter period. Naloxone, an opioid antagonist, should always be available when opioids are administered.

Another useful analgesic for administration in AMI may already be present in the dental office. A mixture of $N_2O$ and $O_2$, more commonly indicated as an inhalation sedation technique in dental practice, has been used in Great Britain and an increasing number of countries since 1967 in premixed cylinders containing 50% $N_2O$ and 50% $O_2$ (Entonox)[64] (Fig. 28-1). Premixed cylinders of $N_2O$ (35%) and $O_2$ (65%) (Dolonox) have also been used in the United States in the treatment of MI.[65] In Great Britain, the $N_2O$-$O_2$ mixture is used on emergency ambulances and is the primary agent for pain relief in acute cardiovascular emergency situations. The primary advantage of $N_2O$-$O_2$ is that it provides the patient with a gaseous

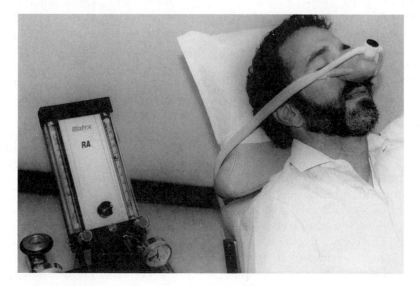

**Figure 28-1**  Administration of 35% nitrous oxide/65% oxygen.

analgesic agent that by itself has little effect on blood pressure. This contrasts with the use of parenteral analgesics, which are more likely to reduce blood pressure and produce adverse side effects (e.g., excessive central nervous system depression, respiratory depression, nausea, and vomiting). The use of this mixture also provides the patient with a source of enriched $O_2$ (50% to 65% vs 21% in atmospheric air).[64-69]

Although premixed $N_2O$ and $O_2$ is available through medical suppliers in the United States, any available source of these gases may be used in this situation. A 35% concentration of $N_2O$ is administered through the nasal hood or by means of a full face mask. When the patient is ready to be transported from the dental office to the hospital, the medical or paramedical personnel administer a parenteral analgesic to provide continuing pain relief during the journey if portable sources of $N_2O$-$O_2$ are unavailable.

*Step 6: preparation to manage complications.* The major complications of AMI likely to develop while awaiting the arrival of emergency medical assistance are acute dysrhythmias, CHF, and cardiac arrest. Management of *acute dysrhythmias* requires intravenous administration of various drugs. In addition, the presence of an electrocardioscope and the training to interpret the ECG are essential. Drugs that may be administered in the management of dysrhythmias include lidocaine and atropine.[70] Without an ECG monitor, no antidysrhythmic drug (other than $O_2$) should be administered to a patient with dysrhythmias. $O_2$ administration must be continued.

*Left ventricular failure* may develop if a significant portion of the myocardium has been infarcted. Respiratory symptoms are most prominent, with dyspnea and acute pulmonary edema noted. (Management of acute pulmonary edema is discussed fully in Chapter 14.) Essentials of management include positioning the patient and reducing the circulating blood volume through the use of a bloodless phlebotomy. In addition, $O_2$ should continue to be administered to this patient. *Cardiac arrest,* indicative of acute cardiorespiratory collapse, requires immediate effective management. Chapter 30 discusses this important subject in depth.

*Step 7: transportation of patient to hospital.* After the victim's condition has been stabilized (i.e., relief of pain and stabilization of heart rhythm and blood pressure), the patient is transported to a primary care facility (e.g., emergency department of a hospital). The dentist should accompany the patient to the hospital in the ambulance or by car and should remain with the patient until a physician is in attendance. Box 28-1 outlines the steps to follow in the management of chest pain thought to be AMI.

## IMMEDIATE IN-HOSPITAL MANAGEMENT

Although immediate in-hospital management is not entirely germane to the discussion of dental office management of medical emergencies, it is prudent to discuss the importance of seeking emergency medical assistance as soon as is possible whenever an AMI is suspected. Great strides have been made in recent years in myocardial salvation in the prevention of cellular death of the myocardium acutely deprived of blood during the infarction. Two procedures, thrombolytic therapy and acute percutaneous transluminal coronary angioplasty (PCTA), permit revascularization of the damaged myocardium. These procedures must be initiated before the myocardium suffers irreversible damage (usually within the first 5 to 6 hours of occlusion).

**Thrombolytic therapy**    Thrombolytic therapy greatly reduces mortality and limits infarct size. Its greatest benefit is noted if initiated within the first 1 to 3 hours of infarct, when a 50% or greater reduction in mortality is observed.[71] The degree of benefit rapidly diminishes thereafter, but a 10% reduction in mortality may be noted up to 10 hours after the onset of pain.[72] Serious bleeding complications develop in 0.5% to 5.0% of patients.[73] Contraindications to thrombolytic therapy include known bleeding diatheses, a history of any cerebrovascular disease, uncontrolled high blood pressure (>190/110 mmHg), pregnancy, and recent trauma or surgery of the head or spine.

Three thrombolytic agents have received extensive clinical evaluation: tissue plasminogen activator (t-PA), streptokinase, and anisoylated plasminogen streptokinase activator complex (anistreplase; APSAC).[74] Another agent, urokinase, is also used. Although debate continues over which of these drugs is preferred, the overriding consideration is the early administration of any one of them.[75-77]

**Acute PTCA**    An increasing number of acute care centers manage AMI with primary PTCA (immediate angiography and PTCA of the "infarct-related" vessel), rather than thrombolysis.[78] Results have been excellent, but as the number of centers performing this procedure is limited, these results may not hold true when more patients are studied.[79,80]

When a patient is in cardiogenic shock, PTCA is the preferred management (along with coronary artery bypass graft surgery) because thrombolysis has not improved the dismal prognosis for this group of patients.[81]

- **Drugs used in management:** Nitroglycerin; oxygen; morphine or meperidine, $N_2O$-$O_2$
- **Medical assistance required:** Yes

## REFERENCES

1. American Heart Association: *Coronary heart disease and angina pectoris,* Dallas, 1998, American Heart Association.
2. Stamler J: The primary prevention of coronary heart disease. In Braunwald E, editor: *The myocardium: failure and infarction,* New York, 1974, HP Publishing.
3. Kuller LH: Sudden death: definition and epidemiologic considerations, *Prog Cardiovasc Dis* 23:1, 1980.
4. Killip T: Arrhythmias in myocardial infarction, *Med Clin North Am* 60:233, 1975.
5. Simoons ML and others: Improved survival after early thrombolysis in acute myocardial infarction: a randomized trial conducted by the Inter-University Cardiology Institute in the Netherlands, *Lancet* 1:578, 1985.
6. Smith SM: Current management of acute myocardial infarction, *Dis Mon* 41:363, 1995
7. American Heart Association: *Heart facts,* Dallas, 1998, The American Heart Association.
8. Kannel WB: Some lessons in cardiovascular epidemiology from Framingham, *Am J Cardiol* 37:269, 1976.
9. Norris RM and others: Prognosis after recovery from first acute myocardial infarction: determinants of reinfarction and sudden death, *Am J Cardiol* 53:408, 1984.
10. DeFeyter PJ and others: Prognostic value of exercise testing, coronary angiography and left ventriculography 6-8 weeks after myocardial infarction, *Circulation* 66:527, 1982.
11. Hedblad B; Janzon L; Johansson BW; Juul-Moller S: Survival and incidence of myocardial infarction in men with ambulatory ECG-detected frequent and complex ventricular arrhythmias. 10 year follow-up of the "Men born 1914" study in Malmo, Sweden, *Eur Heart J* 18:1787, 1997.
12. Alpert JS, Braunwald E: Pathological and clinical manifestations of acute myocardial infarction. In Braunwald E, editor: *Heart disease: a textbook of cardiovascular medicine,* ed 5, Philadelphia, 1997, WB Saunders.
13. Friedman EH: Type A or B behavior, *JAMA* 228:1369, 1974.
14. Friedman M, Rosenman RH: *Type A behavior and your heart,* New York, 1974, Alfred A. Knopf.
15. Kawachi I and others: Prospective study of a self-report type A scale and risk of coronary heart disease: test of the MMPI-2 type A scale, *Circulation* 98:405, 1998.
16. Wilson RF, Holida MD, White CW: Quantitative angiographic morphology of coronary stenosis leading to myocardial infarction or unstable angina, *Circulation* 73:286, 1986.
17. Maseri A and others: Coronary vasospasm as a possible cause of myocardial infarction: a conclusion derived from the study of "preinfarction" angina, *N Engl J Med* 299:1271, 1978.
18. Hollander JE and others: Chest pain associated with cocaine: an assessment of prevalence in suburban and urban emergency rooms. *Ann Emerg Med* 26:671, 1995.
19. Dolter K: Myocardial infarction. In *Cardiopulmonary emergencies,* Springhouse, Pa., 1991.
20. Little WC, Downes TR, Applegate RJ: The underlying coronary lesion in myocardial infarction: implications for coronary angiography, *Clin Cardiol* 14:868, 1991.
21. Teo KK and others: Effects of prophylactic antiarrhythmic drug therapy in acute myocardial infarction: an overview of results from randomized controlled trials, *JAMA* 270:1589, 1993.
22. Simoons M: Myocardial infarction: ACE inhibitors for all? Forever? *Lancet* 344:279, 1994.
23. Weinblatt E and others: Prognosis of men after first myocardial infarction: mortality and first recurrence in relation to selected parameters, *Am J Public Health* 58:1329, 1968.
24. Gorlin R: Coronary collaterals. In *Coronary artery disease,* Philadelphia, 1976, WB Saunders.
25. Bolooki H and others: Myocardial revascularization after acute infarction, *Am J Cardiol* 36:395, 1975.
26. Fishbein MC, Maclean D, Maroko PR: The histopathological evolution of myocardial infarction, *Chest* 73:843, 1978.
27. Paramo JA and others: Long-term cardiac rehabilitation program favorably influences fibrinolysis and lipid concentrations in myocardial infarction, *Haematologica* 83:519, 1998.
28. Miller TD; Balady GJ; Fletcher GF: Exercise and its role in the prevention and rehabilitation of cardiovascular disease, *Ann Behav Med* 19:220, 1997.
29. Dafoe W; Huston P: Current trends in cardiac rehabilitation, *CMAJ* 156:527, 1997.
30. Neill WA, Oxendine JM: Exercise can promote coronary collateral development without improving perfusion of ischemic myocardium, *Circulation* 60:1513, 1979.
31. Yagiela JA: Deadfalls in drug interactions. 6th Annual review course in dental anesthesiology, American Dental Society of Anesthesiology, 1990.
32. McCarthy FM: *Essentials of safe dentistry for the medically compromised patient,* Philadelphia, 1989, WB Saunders.
33. Little JW: *Dental management of the medically compromised patient,* ed 5, St. Louis, 1997, Mosby.
34. Phipps C: Contributory causes of coronary thrombosis, *JAMA* 106:761, 1936.
35. Willich SN and others: Increased onset of sudden cardiac death in the first three hours after awakening, *Am J Cardiol* 70:65, 1992.
36. Jenkins CD: Recent evidence supporting psychologic and social risk factors for coronary disease, *N Engl J Med* 294:1033, 1976.

37. Rahe RH and others: Recent life changes, myocardial infarction, and abrupt coronary death. Studies in Helsinki, *Arch Intern Med* 133:221, 1974.

38. Margolis JR and others: Clinical features of unrecognized myocardial infarction-silent and symptomatic. Eighteen year follow-up: the Framingham study, *Am J Cardiol* 32:1, 1973.

39. Adgey AAJ and others: Acute phase of myocardial infarction: prehospital management of the coronary patient, *Minn Med* 59:347, 1976.

40. Schaffer WA, Cobb LA: Recurrent ventricular fibrillation and modes of death in survivors of out-of-hospital ventricular fibrillation, *N Engl J Med* 293:259, 1975.

41. Pantridge JE, Geddes JS: A mobile intensive care unit in the management of myocardial infarction, *Lancet* 2:271, 1967.

42. Chatterjee K: Complications of acute myocardial infarction, *Curr Probl Cardiol* 18:1, 1993.

43. Brugada P, Andries EW. Early post-myocardial infarction ventricular arrhythmias, *Cardiovasc Clin* 22:165, 1992.

44. Ridker PM and others: Comparison of delay times to hospital presentation for physicians and nonphysicians with acute myocardial infarction, *Am J Cardiol* 70:10, 1992.

45. Alpert JS, Francis GS: *Handbook of coronary care*, ed 5, Boston, 1993, Little, Brown.

46. Gensini GG: Coronary arteriography. In Braunwald E, editor: *Heart disease: a textbook of cardiovascular medicine*, ed 5, Philadelphia 1997, WB Saunders.

47. Levin DC: Pathways and functional significance of the coronary collateral circulation, *Circulation* 50:831, 1974.

48. Pfeiffer MA and others: Myocardial infarct size and ventricular function in rats, *Circ Res* 44:503, 1979.

49. Page DL and others: Myocardial changes associated with cardiogenic shock, *N Engl J Med* 285:133, 1971.

50. Loeb HS, Johnson SA, Gunnar AM: Cardiogenic shock, *Triangle* 13:121, 1974.

51. Rackley CE and others: Cardiogenic shock: recognition and management, *Cardiovasc Clin* 7:251, 1975.

52. Wolk MJ, Scheidt S, Killip T: Heart failure complicating acute myocardial infarction, *Circulation* 45:1125, 1972.

53. Lassers BW and others: Left ventricular failure and acute myocardial infarction, *Am J Cardiol* 25:511, 1970.

54. Pollakoff J, Pollakoff K: *EMT's guide to signs and symptoms*, Los Angeles, 1991, Jeff Gould.

55. Marokso PR and others: Reduction of infarct size by oxygen inhalation following acute coronary occlusion, *Circulation* 52:360, 1975.

56. Cobb LA, Werner JA, Trobaugh GB: Sudden cardiac death, *Mod Concepts Cardiovasc Dis* 49:31, 1980.

57. Cheitlin MD, Abbott JA: Cardiac emergencies. In Saunders CE, Ho MT, editors: *Current emergency diagnosis and treatment*, ed 4, Norwalk, Conn, 1992, Appleton & Lange.

58. Round A; Marshall AJ: Survey of general practitioners' prehospital management of suspected acute myocardial infarction, *BMJ* 6:309, 375, 1994.

59. ISIS-2 (Second International Study of Infarct Survival) Collaborative Group. Randomised trial of intravenous streptokinase, oral aspirin, both, or neither among 17,187 cases of suspected acute myocardial infarction: ISIS-2, *Lancet* 2:349, 1988.

60. US Food and Drug Administration: Internal analgesic, antipyretic, and antirheumatic drug products for over-the-counter human use: proposed amendment to the tentative final monograph, *Fed Reg* 61:30002, 1996.

61. American Heart Association Science Advisory and Coordinating Committee: *Aspirin as a therapeutic agent in cardiovascular disease*, Dallas, 1997, American Heart Association.

62. Jaffe AS and others: Reduction of infarct size in patients with inferior infarction with intravenous glyceryl trinitrate, *Br Heart J* 49:452, 1973.

63. Todres D: The role of morphine in acute myocardial infarction, *Am Heart J* 81:566, 1971.

64. Nancekievill D: Apparatus for the administration of Entonox (50% $N_2O$: 50% $O_2$ mixture) by intermittent positive pressure, *Anaesthesia* 29:736, 1974.

65. Thompson PL, Lown B: Nitrous oxide as an analgesic in acute myocardial infarction, *JAMA* 235:924, 1976.

66. Eisele JH and others: Myocardial performance and $N_2O$ analgesia in coronary artery disease, *Anesthesiology* 44:16, 1976.

67. Kerr F and others: A double blind trial of patient-controlled nitrous oxide/oxygen analgesia in myocardial infarction, *Lancet* 1:397, 1975.

68. Stern MS and others: Nitrous oxide and oxygen in acute myocardial infarction, *Circulation* 58 (suppl II): 171, 1978.

69. Fridlund B; Carlsson B: Acute myocardial infarction patients' chest pain as monitored and evaluated by ambulance personnel, *Intensive Crit Care Nurs* 8:113, 1992.

70. Boersma E and others: Early thrombolytic treatment in acute myocardial infarction: reappraisal of the golden hour, *Lancet* 348:771, 1996.

71. American Heart Association: *Textbook of advanced cardiac life support*, Dallas, 1992, American Heart Association.

72. Raitt MH and others: Relation between symptom duration before thrombolytic therapy and final myocardial infarct size, *Circulation* 93:48, 1996.

73. Mahaffey KW and others: Risk factors for in-hospital nonhemorrhagic stroke in patients with acute myocardial infarction treated with: results from GUSTO-I, *Circulation* 97:757, 1998.

74. Massie BM: The heart. In Tierney LM Jr, McPhee SJ, Papadakis MA, editors: *Current medical diagnosis and treatment*, ed 35, Stamford, 1996, Appleton & Lange.

75. Anderson HB, Willerson JT: Thrombolysis in acute myocardial infarction, *N Engl J Med* 329:703, 1993.

76. Fibrinolytic Therapy Trialists' (FIT) Collaborative Group: Indications for fibrinolytic therapy in suspected myocardial infarction: collaborative overview of early mortality and major morbidity from all randomized trials of more than 1000 patients, *Lancet* 343:311, 1994.

77. The GUSTO Investigators: An international randomized trial comparing four thrombolytic strategies for acute myocardial infarction, *N Engl J Med* 329:673, 1993.

78. Michel MB, Yusuf S: Does PTCA in acute myocardial infarction affect mortality and reinfarction rates? *Circulation* 91:476, 1995.

79. Terrin ML and others: Two- and three-year results of the thrombolysis in myocardial infarction (TIMI) phase II clinical trial, *J Am Coll Cardiol* 22:1763, 1993.

80. Zahn R and others: Primary angioplasty versus thrombolysis in the treatment of acute myocardial infarction, *Am J Cardiol* 79:264, 1997.

81. Knatterud GL, for the TIMI Investigators: Predictors of early morbidity and mortality after thrombolytic therapy in acute myocardial infarction: analyses of patient subgroups in the Thrombolysis in Myocardial Infarction (TIMI) trial, phase II, *Circulation* 85:1254, 1992.

# 29

# Chest Pain

## Differential Diagnosis

THE two major clinical syndromes presenting as chest pain are angina pectoris and acute myocardial infarction (AMI). Yet there are times when the dental patient may experience other forms of chest pain. Indeed, everybody experiences various forms of chest pain on occasion. Fortunately, most of these pains are unrelated to ischemic heart disease (IHD) and are, for the most part, innocuous. However, most of those experiencing chest pain have stopped and thought, "This pain I am feeling now is the *real* thing." This chapter describes the differences between chest pain associated with IHD and that which is noncardiac in origin.[1] Next the differential diagnosis of the two major forms of ischemic chest pain, angina pectoris and acute myocardial infarction, is presented. Table 29-1 lists several of the possible causes of chest pain.

## Noncardiac Chest Pain

Noncardiac chest pain can usually be differentiated from the pain of angina and myocardial infarction because a sharp, knifelike chest pain that increases in intensity with inspiration and diminishes with exhalation is usually not related to cardiac syndromes.

Chest pain aggravated by movement (e.g., twisting, turning, or stretching of the sore area) is most often related to muscle or nerve injuries, not to cardiac disease. I use the word *usually* when describing typical chest pains. Instances occur in which patients are

| table **29-1** | Causes of chest pain |
| --- | --- |

| CARDIAC RELATED | NONCARDIAC RELATED |
| --- | --- |
| Angina pectoris | Muscle strain |
| Myocardial infarction | Pericarditis |
| | Esophagitis |
| | Hiatal hernia |
| | Pulmonary embolism |
| | Dissecting aortic aneurysm |
| | Acute indigestion |
| | Intestinal "gas" |

aware of a sharp, knifelike pain that may in fact be related to cardiac disease. Variations from the typical are expected, and the dental health professional is well advised to take note of this.

Probably the most common cause of noncardiac chest pain is *musculoskeletal,* resulting from muscle strain that occurs after exercise or physical exertion.[2] This form of pain is normally localized (the patient can point to a specific site of discomfort), does not radiate, and is made worse by breathing and movement. A heating pad or mild analgesic medication may give relief.

*Pericarditis* is an inflammation of the outer membrane covering the heart (the pericardium) and is most commonly a result of viral infection. The pain of pericarditis is similar to that of angina or myocardial infarction, occurs in the midsternum, and is described as "oppressive." Clues to its differential diagnosis include aggravation of the pain of pericarditis when breathing and swallowing, characteristic relief of the pain when the patient bends forward from the waist, and often the presence of a fever before the onset of pain.[3]

*Esophagitis,* with or without *hiatal hernia,* produces a substernal or epigastric burning pain that is precipitated by eating or lying down after a meal. The pain is relieved by antacids. There often is an acid reflux into the mouth.[4]

*Pulmonary embolism* usually indicates the sudden occlusion of a blood vessel within the lungs by an embolus that has been "thrown" (broken loose) from the legs. The patient experiences a sudden severe chest pain that is commonly associated with the coughing up of blood-tinged sputum.[5]

A less common cause of acute chest pain is a *dissecting aortic aneurysm.* The patient experiences sudden, acute, severe chest pain that is often greatest at onset. Typically, it spreads up and down the chest and back over a period of hours. The dissecting aortic aneurysm may lead rapidly to death.[6]

Two other common causes of chest pain often make it difficult to differentiate between cardiac and noncardiac pain. These are the pains of acute indigestion and "gas." One of the major factors leading to the high initial mortality rate associated with AMI is misinterpretation or denial of clinical symptoms by the patient or the attending physician. The symptoms are commonly attributed to indigestion or gas pains and are only later discovered to have been produced by AMI. The pain of gas is normally sharp and knifelike and increases in intensity on breathing. This fact should assist in differentiating gas pain from the pain of IHD. Acute indigestion is similar to the pain of angina or myocardial infarction; therefore all patients with this symptom should receive careful evaluation. Epigastric discomfort may be a manifestation of myocardial ischemia or infarction and should not be dismissed lightly. Unusual or prolonged indigestion should rouse suspicion, particularly in a high-risk individual. The American Heart Association recommends that a patient with previously unrecognized coronary disease seek medical assistance if a suspicious chest pain persists for 2 minutes or longer.[7]

# Cardiac Chest Pain

Angina and AMI are the two most common causes of IHD-related chest pain in the dental office. Differential diagnosis is essential because these two syndromes present quite different risks to the patient and are ultimately managed differently. The following discussion is offered to assist in making this differential diagnosis.

## PRIOR MEDICAL HISTORY

The patient with angina is usually aware of its existence and possesses drugs to manage acute anginal episodes. It is possible that a patient with a negative history of heart problems will suffer a first episode of angina in the dental office setting. Because of the stress associated with many dental procedures, at least in the minds of dental patients, there is frequently an increase in the workload of the heart in the dental office setting. It is not unlikely that episodes of anginal-type chest pain may develop in this situation, especially in patients with a history of angina. However, when a history of chest pain is absent, the possibility exists that a first episode of chest pain could be myocardial infarction. For this reason, it is recommended that a first episode of chest pain be managed as though it were a myocardial infarction, until proven otherwise. The patient's medical history may indicate a prior myocardial infarction. Many patients who survive myocardial infarction later develop episodes of angina and will have nitroglycerin available.

## AGE

Coronary artery disease (CAD) can be found in all age-groups. There is little clinical difference between the age of patients developing either angina or AMI. Clinical evidence of CAD is most commonly noted between the ages of 50 and 60 years in men and 60 and 70 years in women.

## SEX

CAD is primarily a disease of males. The overall male/female ratio is 4:1. Before the age of 40 years, the ratio is 8:1.

## RELATED CIRCUMSTANCES

The clinical symptomatology of angina is usually associated with some form of exertion, whether physical or mental. On the other hand, although myocardial infarction may occur during or immediately after a period of exertion, it commonly occurs during periods of rest. Angina rarely occurs during rest, although coronary artery spasm may provoke anginal pain at any time. Unstable angina, by definition, may occur at rest.

## CLINICAL SYMPTOMS AND SIGNS

**Location of chest pain**    Location of chest pain is not a reliable indicator of the nature of the pain. Both anginal pain and the pain of AMI occur substernally or just to the left of the midsternal region.

**Description of chest pain**    Chest "pain" associated with either angina or AMI is usually not described as pain by the patient. More commonly the sensation is described as "squeezing," "pressing," "tightness," "heaviness," "as though there were a heavy weight on my chest," or "crushing." The pain associated with AMI is more intense than that of angina and is more commonly described as painful or intolerable.

**Radiation of chest pain**    Differentiation between angina and AMI is difficult to make by using radiation of pain as a criterion. Both cardiac syndromes have similar radiation patterns. Radiation of chest pain commonly occurs to the left shoulder and medial aspect of the left arm, following the distribution of the ulnar nerve. Less frequently the pain may radiate to the right shoulder, the mandibular region, or the epigastrium.

**Duration of chest pain**    The pain associated with AMI is normally of long duration, lasting from 30 minutes to several hours if untreated. As mentioned in Chapter 28, untreated cardiac pain may induce cardiogenic shock. Pain associated with angina is almost always brief. Merely terminating the activity that induced the episode brings relief within 3 to 5 minutes. Anginal episodes that have been precipitated by eating a large meal or feeling angry may persist longer, perhaps lasting 30 minutes or more.

**Response to medication**    Probably the most reliable diagnostic tool is the patient's response to the administration of medications. A vasodilator, preferably nitroglycerin but possibly amyl nitrate, is administered. Anginal pain will be relieved approximately 2 to 4 minutes after administration of nitroglycerin and within 1 minute after amyl nitrate administration. These drugs may temporarily diminish the pain of myocardial infarction, but more commonly they will have no effect. The pain of myocardial infarction is commonly managed through administration of opioid analgesics, such as morphine or meperidine, or nitrous oxide and oxygen.

Administration of a vasodilator to the patient with presumed cardiac-related chest pain offers one of the most reliable methods of differentiating between the pain of angina and that of AMI. For this reason, the administration of nitroglycerin is the first step in the clinical drug management of chest pain in the dental office.

## VITAL SIGNS

**Heart rate**    The heart rate during acute episodes of angina is rapid and may feel full or bounding. A rapid heart rate may also be present during AMI; however, because the blood pressure is usually decreased, the pulse may feel weak or thready. The heart rate during AMI may also be slow.

**Blood pressure**    Episodes of angina are normally accompanied by marked elevations in blood pressure, whereas blood pressure in AMI may be normal, but more commonly is decreased.

**Respiration**    Patients with either coronary syndrome may exhibit respiratory distress during the acute episode. The respiratory rate is increased, and the depth of each respiration may be more shallow than usual. During myocardial infarction clinical evidence of left ventricular failure may be noted.

**Other signs and symptoms**    Most patients with AMI and some patients with angina appear quite apprehensive and may be bathed in a cold sweat. Anginal patients can compare current episodes with previous ones, which may give a clue to the seriousness of the present attack. Anginal episodes tend to be quite similar in an individual patient. Any change in severity, duration, or frequency may indicate the occurrence of unstable angina or myocardial infarction. Patients with AMI often express a fear of impending doom.

During myocardial infarction facial skin may appear ashen gray. Nailbeds and other visible mucous membranes may demonstrate varying degrees of cyanosis. These changes rarely occur during anginal episodes.

Nausea and vomiting are common during AMI, especially in the presence of severe pain. Nausea and vomiting are uncommon with anginal pain.

## Summary

The clinical diagnosis of chest pain is difficult. However, the response of the patient to the administration of nitroglycerin invariably leads to an accurate diagnosis.

table **29-2**  *Comparison of cardiac and noncardiac pain*[1]

| NONCARDIAC CHEST PAIN | CARDIAC CHEST PAIN |
|---|---|
| Sharp, knifelike | Dull |
| Stabbing sensation | Aching |
| Aggravated by movement | Heaviness, oppressive feeling |
| Present only with breathing | Present at all times |
| Localized (able to point to one spot) | Generalized (occurs over a wider area) |

Acute anginal episodes are usually similar from episode to episode for a given patient. Any change in the acute attack that produces a more severe episode may indicate the occurrence of AMI.

Noncardiac chest pain is usually easily differentiated from ischemic heart pain because of the nature of the pain. However, two common forms of substernal, upper epigastric, discomfort—acute indigestion and gas—are quite difficult to differentiate from ischemic heart pain. These symptoms should not be ignored. Careful evaluation is required, and medical consultation should be considered if there is any doubt as to the cause of a patient's chest pain.

Table 29-2 differentiates cardiac from noncardiac pain.

## REFERENCES

1. Malamed SF: Beyond the basics: emergency medicine in dentistry, *J Am Dent Assoc* 128:843,1997.
2. Dronen SC: Chest pain. In Rosen P, editor: *Emergency medicine: concepts and clinical practice,* ed 4, St Louis, 1998, Mosby.
3. Fallon EM, Roques J: Acute chest pain, *AACN Clin Issues* 8:383, 1997.
4. Lemire S: Assessment of clinical severity and investigation of uncomplicated gastroesophageal reflux disease and noncardiac angina-like chest pain, *Can J Gastroenterol* 11:37B, 1997.
5. Zimmerman D, Parker BM: The pain of pulmonary hypertension: fact or fancy? *JAMA* 246:2345, 1981.
6. Chen K and others: Acute thoracic aortic dissection: the basics, *J Emerg Med* 15:859, 1997.
7. *Heart attack: signals and actions for survival,* Dallas, 1998, American Heart Association.

# CARDIAC ARREST

# 30

# Cardiac Arrest and Cardiopulmonary Resuscitation

*ANGINA* pectoris, myocardial infarction, and heart failure are three clinical manifestations of ischemic heart disease (IHD). Associated with each of these clinical entities is the possible occurrence of acute complications that include cardiac dysrhythmias and cardiopulmonary collapse. The latter is also called *cardiac arrest* or *sudden death.* Cardiac arrest may also occur as an acute clinical entity in the absence of other cardiovascular manifestations. Of the victims of cardiac arrest, 25% do not exhibit clinical signs or symptoms before the onset of sudden death.[1] Stated another way, the first clinical indication of the presence of IHD may be the (clinical) death of the patient.

*Sudden death* is defined by the World Health Organization as clinical death occurring within 24 hours after the onset of symptoms.[2] Clinical death that occurs within 30 seconds of the onset of symptoms is termed *instantaneous death.*[2] The term *sudden death* is defined here as death occurring within 1 hour of the onset of signs and symptoms.[3]

Death, as referred to in these definitions, implies *clinical* death as opposed to *biologic* death. Clinical death occurs at the moment of cardiopulmonary arrest but may, on occasion, be reversed if recognized promptly and effectively managed, thereby preventing biologic death. Biologic death follows when permanent cellular damage has occurred, primarily from a lack of oxygen. Biologic or cellular death of neuronal (brain) tissue takes place when delivery of oxygen is inadequate for approximately 4 to 6 minutes.[4]

Because neurons are exquisitely sensitive to anoxia, cerebral resuscitation becomes *the* most important goal in saving a life in cardiac arrest. To reach that goal, rescuers must first restart the victim's heart. Cerebral resuscitation—return of the victim to prearrest level of neurologic functioning—is the ultimate goal of emergency cardiac care.[5] Safar and Bircher[6] have proposed the term *cardiopulmonary-cerebral resuscitation* (CPCR) to replace the more familiar term, *cardiopulmonary resuscitation* (CPR). Clinicians should always remember the term *cerebral,* for it is a reminder of our primary purpose: to return the patient to his or her best neurologic outcome.[5] Unless spontaneous ventilation and circulation are restored quickly, successful cerebral resuscitation cannot occur.[7]

Of the more than 960,592 deaths that occurred in 1995[8] from cardiovascular disease, of which 481,287 were due to coronary artery disease (including 250,000 cardiac arrests[9]), at least two thirds took place outside the hospital setting, usually within 1 hour after the onset of symptoms.[1] In terms of absolute loss of life, therefore, sudden, unexpected death from myocardial infarction is the greatest single acute medical problem today.[10]

With the introduction of closed chest cardiac massage by Kouwenhoven and others,[11] in 1960, a new era in cardiac resuscitation began. Sudden death, previously irreversible, became reversible, in many instances with the effective application of this new technique. Although the rate of successful resuscitation from out-of-hospital cardiac arrest has shown only modest gains since the 1960s, it must be remembered that before emergency medical services (EMS) became available, cardiac arrest was almost universally fatal. Given the circumstances necessary for resuscitation to be successful, it is remarkable that anyone survives.[12]

The rationale for cardiac resuscitation outside the hospital is that, in most cases, cardiac arrest is unexpected and cannot be predicted accurately in individual patients; thus effective preventive measures are lacking. Immediate efforts at resuscitation offer the only realistic hope for most victims.[12] In some communities, such as Seattle, Washington, where advanced EMS systems exist, the rate of successful resuscitation and ultimate discharge home has more than doubled during the 1990s.[13] Response time from dispatch to arrival of a basic life support (BLS) team averages less than 3 minutes in Seattle, with a paramedic unit capable of administering advanced cardiac life support (ACLS) arriving 4 minutes later. A result of this expeditious response is that up to 60% of patients with ventricular fibrillation (VF) are successfully resuscitated at the scene, and 25% survive to leave the hospital.[13] In addition to Seattle's advanced EMS system, more than 33% of the population of King County, Washington, are trained in CPR (Table 30-1).[14]

Unfortunately, Seattle's experience with out-of-hospital cardiac arrest has not been duplicated in many cities, although in cities with equivalent programs similar survival rates do occur. Gray and others[15] found that in several New England communities, rates of resuscitation from out-of-hospital cardiac arrest average 20%, with even fewer patients surviving until hospital discharge. Other studies have reported discharge rates of 2% to 33% after cardiac arrests outside the hospital.[16]

## The ACLS Score

The poor survival rate after resuscitation efforts from out-of-hospital cardiac arrest is the result of several factors, some of which are related to fate (witnessed or unwitnessed arrest and the cardiac rhythm) and others to the emergency response itself (length of time from collapse to the initiation

table **30-1**  *Effectiveness of early defibrillation programs[14]*

| LOCATION | BEFORE EARLY DEFIBRILLATION | | AFTER EARLY DEFIBRILLATION | | ODDS RATIO FOR IMPROVED SURVIVAL |
|---|---|---|---|---|---|
| King County, Washington | 7 | na | 26 | 10/38 | 3.7 |
| Iowa | 3 | (1/31) | 19 | (12/64) | 6.3 |
| Southeast Minnesota | 4 | (1/27) | 17 | (6/36) | 4.3 |
| Northeast Minnesota | 2 | (3/118) | 10 | (8/81) | 5.0 |
| Wisconsin | 4 | (32/893) | 11 | (33/304) | 2.8 |

Values are percent surviving and, in parentheses, how many patients had ventricular fibrillation.

of resuscitation efforts and defibrillation).[17,18] The absence of any single favorable condition in what is now called the "chain of survival" results in an unsuccessful resuscitation.[19] Eisenberg and others[3] developed the "A-C-L-S" score to help estimate the likelihood of survival from out-of-hospital cardiac arrest:

*A* - Was the *A*rrest witnessed?

*C* - Was the original *C*ardiac rhythm documented by the paramedics upon arrival?

*L* - Was *L*ay bystander CPR performed?

*S* - How long did it take for help to arrive (i.e., *S*peed of paramedic response)?

## WITNESSED VERSUS UNWITNESSED

During a 3-year period, 28% of 380 patients whose cardiac arrests were witnessed were ultimately discharged from the hospital, whereas only 3% of 231 victims of unwitnessed arrest survived.[3]

## INITIAL RHYTHM

When the initial rhythm was either ventricular tachycardia (VT) (Figure 30-1, *A*) or VF (Figure 30-1, *B*), survival rates were higher[3,20]: 28% of 389 patients survived, compared with 3% of 222 patients in asystole.[3] Survival is unusual (<5% of patients) when either pulseless electrical activity (PEA) or asystole (Figure 30-1, *C*) is initially recorded.[12] In a series of nearly 1100 attempted resuscitations of patients in asystole, only 13 survived (0.012%).[21]

It is unlikely that EMD or asystole is the initial rhythm that precipitates cardiac arrest. In patients sustaining cardiac arrest while undergoing continuous cardiac monitoring (Holter monitoring), VT of varying duration is frequently noted as the precipitating mechanism of arrest.[22,23] Asystole and EMD are probably secondary dysrhythmias that developed after VT and VF, during the time from patient collapse to EMS arrival.

## BYSTANDER CPR

When bystander CPR was initiated, a 32% survival rate was noted. The survival rate fell to 14% when BLS was delayed until the arrival of EMS.[12]

## RESPONSE TIME

When paramedics were able to initiate ACLS within 4 minutes, 56% of the patients survived.[12] This rate fell to 35% when response time was between 4 and 8 minutes and to 17% if response time exceeded 8

minutes.[12] In other cities with response times as short as 3 to 5 minutes, survival rates of 25% to 33% have been reported.[24,25] In New York City, survival rate from out-of-hospital cardiac arrest was 2.1% (8/382).[26]

# The Chain of Survival

Survival after cardiac arrest depends on a series of critical interventions. The absence of any one intervention or delay in its implementation minimizes the likelihood of survival. The term *chain of survival* is used to describe this emergency cardiac care concept (Box 30-1).[27] The four links in the chain of survival are: (1) early access to the EMS system, (2) early BLS, (3) early defibrillation; and (4) early ACLS.

Several important principles are underscored by the chain of survival. If any one link in the chain is inadequate, survival rates will be poor. This factor is the major explanation for the extreme variability in survival rates reported over the last 20 years.[28] All links must be strong to ensure rapid defibrillation. A major problem has been that call-to-defibrillation intervals are too long. To increase survival rates, shorter intervals are necessary.[19]

## THE FIRST LINK: EARLY ACCESS

Events that occur from the time that the victim collapses to arrival of EMS personnel are included in early access. These events are (1) recognition of unconsciousness, (2) rapid notification of EMS via telephone *before* the start of BLS in adults and *after 1*

box **30-1**   *Chain of survival*

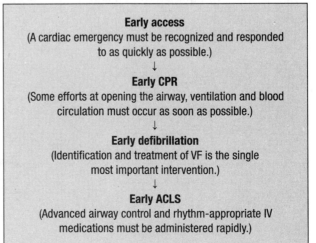

**Early access**
(A cardiac emergency must be recognized and responded to as quickly as possible.)
↓
**Early CPR**
(Some efforts at opening the airway, ventilation and blood circulation must occur as soon as possible.)
↓
**Early defibrillation**
(Identification and treatment of VF is the single most important intervention.)
↓
**Early ACLS**
(Advanced airway control and rhythm-appropriate IV medications must be administered rapidly.)

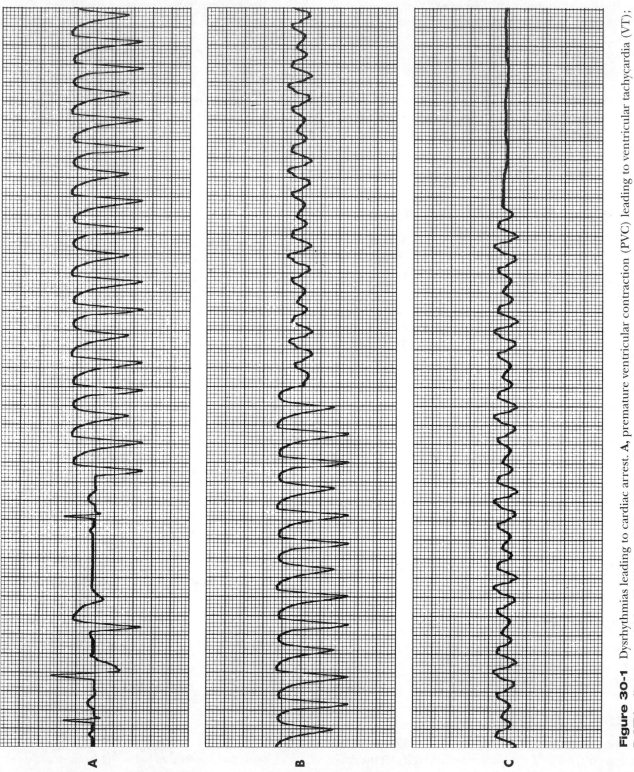

A

B

C

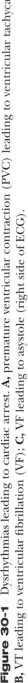

**Figure 30-1** Dysrhythmias leading to cardiac arrest. **A,** premature ventricular contraction (PVC) leading to ventricular tachycardia (VT); **B,** VT leading to ventricular fibrillation (VF); **C,** VF leading to asystole (right side of ECG).

*minute* of BLS in children and infants, (3) rapid dispatch of EMS responders, and (4) rapid responder arrival at victim's side with all necessary equipment. All of these must occur before defibrillation or ACLS can begin.

## THE SECOND LINK: EARLY BLS (CPR)

BLS is most effective when started immediately after a victim collapses. In almost all studies, bystander CPR has a significantly positive effect on survival.[29,30] Bystander CPR is the best treatment a cardiac arrest victim can receive until the arrival of a defibrillator and ACLS.[29,30]

BLS is not a substitute for definitive treatment. Without defibrillation and the administration of adjunctive drugs, such as epinephrine, BLS will not result in adequate perfusion of vital organs such as the heart and brain.[31] BLS simply buys time until definitive therapy can be provided.[32] BLS cannot prevent VT or VF from deteriorating into EMD or asystole.[33] Remember that BLS is essential to prevent irreversible cerebral damage.

A single, unassisted rescuer with an adult victim should activate EMS after establishing unresponsiveness, but before commencing BLS. In the pediatric arrest victim, the EMS system should be activated after BLS has been provided for 1 minute.

## THE THIRD LINK: EARLY DEFIBRILLATION

Early defibrillation is the link in the chain of survival most likely to improve survival rates[34-37] (Table 30-1). Widespread introduction of the automatic external defibrillator (AED) has enabled nonmedical personnel trained in its use to improve survival chances for out-of-hospital cardiac arrest victims. The American Heart Association (AHA) has endorsed the position that every emergency vehicle that may transport cardiac arrest victims be equipped with a defibrillator and that emergency personnel be trained to operate this device.[38]

Manual, automatic, or semiautomatic external defibrillators may be used for rapid defibrillation. The *manual defibrillator* requires the interpretation of a monitor or cardiac rhythm strip by a trained rescuer. Use of this device by trained physicians, emergency medical technicians, and other health care personnel has led to improved survival.[34] Defibrillation using an *automatic, automatic advisory,* or *semiautomatic defibrillator* is also effective.[36] These devices analyze the cardiac rhythm and either defibrillate automatically or

advise the operator to defibrillate. The widespread effectiveness and proven safety of AEDs have made it acceptable for nonmedical professionals to operate the device for use with adult victims. It is still necessary for such persons to be trained in BLS and to be knowledgeable in the use of defibrillators.

All AEDs can be operated by following four simple steps: (1) turn on the power, (2) attach the device, (3) initiate rhythm analysis, and (4) deliver the shock if indicated and if safe.

Different brands and models of AED have varying features such as paper strip and voice recorders, rhythm display methods, energy levels, and messages to the operator.

In the latter part of the 1990s, the availability of AEDs greatly increased. Airlines, public buses, taxicabs, factories, office buildings, and other places where large numbers of persons congregate have included AEDs in their emergency preparedness protocols.[39-41]

The advent, in the 1960s, of EMS systems involving mobile coronary care units staffed by trained paramedical personnel increased the likelihood that the chain of survival could remain intact. Early use of definitive therapy (defibrillation) led to a more than doubling of survival rates from out-of-hospital cardiac arrest.[16] Paramedical personnel have been taught to identify VF and to defibrillate effectively with as little as 10 hours of formal training.[16] Even when such persons were not permitted to administer drugs or to intubate (i.e., defibrillation alone was permitted), lives were saved.[42]

## THE FOURTH LINK: EARLY ACLS

Early ACLS provided at the scene by the dentist (if trained) or paramedics is another critical link in the management of cardiac arrest. ACLS brings to the scene equipment for the support of ventilation, establishes venous access permitting the administration of drugs, controls dysrhythmias, and stabilizes the victim for transport.

The one factor that unites all four links of the chain of survival is time. The more quickly cardiac arrest is recognized, resuscitation efforts are instituted by a bystander, and advanced management is begun (defibrillation and ACLS), the greater the likelihood that the initial rhythm will be either VT or VF, and the greater the likelihood of a successful resuscitation.

## The Dental Office

It is highly unlikely that a cardiac arrest occurring in a dental office would go unwitnessed for more than a few seconds. CPR (BLS) would likely be initiated within a minute or so of the collapse of the victim by members of a prepared office emergency team, thereby providing extra time for the initiation of advanced resuscitative techniques. The presence of an AED in the dental office could significantly increase the likelihood of survival from cardiac arrest in this environment.

As has been stressed throughout this text, the ability to effectively implement the steps of BLS—position, airway, breathing, circulation—is absolutely critical in saving a life in an emergency situation. The emergencies presented thus far, however, have been limited to situations in which only two or three steps (position + airway *or* position + airway + breathing) of BLS were required for effective patient management. Chest compression has not been necessary. In the unlikely event that cardiopulmonary arrest does occur, rapid action by the entire dental office emergency team is required if the victim is to be successfully resuscitated.

BLS or CPR is readily carried out without the use of any adjunctive equipment or drug therapy. BLS consists of airway management, artificial ventilation, and external chest compression to ensure delivery of a continuous supply of oxygenated blood to the brain and heart, thereby preventing irreversible (biologic) death and providing some additional time until advanced resuscitation procedures can be initiated. In the not too distant future, it is probable that BLS as defined for health care professions will include *D*—defibrillation.

## Cardiopulmonary Arrest

Although disease of the cardiovascular system is the most common cause of sudden death (cardiopulmonary arrest), other life-threatening situations may also culminate this way (Table 30-2). Regardless of the precise nature of its cause, cardiac arrest must be recognized and managed as quickly as possible, minimizing the period of anoxia to the brain and myocardium and increasing the likelihood for a successful outcome.

Cardiopulmonary arrest is composed of two specific entities: pulmonary arrest and cardiac arrest. Pulmonary, or respiratory, arrest occurs with cessation of effective respiratory movement, whereas cardiac arrest refers to the cessation of circulation or to circulation that is inadequate to sustain life.

Respiratory arrest may develop in the absence of cardiac arrest. However, if respiratory arrest is unmanaged or if managed ineffectively, cardiac function deteriorates, with cardiac arrest supervening in a short time, depending in part on the degree of oxygen deprivation and the underlying status of the victim's myocardium and coronary arteries. Cardiac arrest can occur in the absence of respiratory arrest (e.g., with electric shock); however, this is quite rare, especially within the dental environment. In such circumstances respiratory arrest inevitably follows within a few seconds. *In most instances, respiratory arrest precedes cardiac arrest.*

## PULMONARY (RESPIRATORY) ARREST

Recognition and management of respiratory arrest have been described previously (see Chapter 5).

## CARDIAC ARREST

The term *cardiac arrest* must be defined to avoid possible confusion. At one time cardiac arrest was used to indicate that the heart had stopped beating, a situation referred to today as ventricular standstill or asystole. The meaning of the term cardiac arrest has been expanded to include other clinical situations in which the circulation of blood is absent or, if present,

| table **30-2** | *Possible causes of cardiac arrest** |

| CAUSE | FREQUENCY | WHERE DISCUSSED IN TEXT |
|---|---|---|
| Myocardial infarction | Most common | Chest pain (Section (VII) |
| Sudden death (no other symptoms) | Most common | Cardiac arrest (Chapter 30) |
| Airway obstruction | Common | Respiratory difficulty (Section III) |
| Drug overdose reaction | Common | Drug-related emergencies (Section VI) |
| Anaphylaxis | Less common | Drug-related emergencies (Section VI) |
| Seizure disorders | Less common | Seizure disorders (Section V) |
| Acute adrenal insufficiency | Less common | Unconsciousness (Section II) |

*All medical emergency situations may ultimately lead to cardiac arrest. In most instances prompt recognition and initiation of effective management of the specific situation prevents cardiac arrest from occurring.

is inadequate to maintain life. Cardiac arrest, as defined today, may result from any of the following: pulseless electrical activity (PEA), (pulseless) VT, VF, or ventricular standstill (asystole).

In PEA, the heart continues to beat in a coordinated manner, but so weakly that effective circulation of blood throughout the cardiovascular system is not accomplished. This situation may be caused by drugs, including local anesthetics, barbiturates, and opioids, all of which are used in dentistry (see Chapter 23). PEA more commonly results from severe hemorrhage and shock. PEA was formerly called electromechanical dissociation (EMD).

VT is an accelerated beating of the ventricles. The victim with VT may be conscious with a palpable pulse or may be unconscious without palpable pulse. These two entities are treated quite differently. In VT with pulse, drugs are administered to the victim in an effort to stabilize the myocardium, and/or synchronized cardioversion is performed. However, absent a palpable pulse, the indicated treatment is identical to that for VF.

VF is a dysrhythmia in which the individual myocardial muscle bundles contract independently of each other as opposed to the normal, regular, coordinated, and synchronized contraction of myocardial fibers. Although myocardial elements are still contracting, little or no effective circulation is present. VF is a common occurrence in the period immediately after acute myocardial infarction (within the first 2 to 4 hours) and is the leading cause of death from IHD. In humans, VF occurs 15 times more frequently during the first hour after the onset of signs and symptoms of acute myocardial infarction than during the next 12 hours.

Ventricular asystole or standstill refers to the absence of contractile movements of myocardial fibers. Cardiac arrest in its strictest sense refers to ventricular asystole. A severe lack of oxygen to myocardial muscle is the most common cause of this situation.

Although there are several forms of cardiac arrest (asystole, pulseless VT, VF, and PEA), in an emergency, the precise nature of the arrest is not immediately known. The clinical picture of all three is the same: an unconscious victim in whom respiration, blood pressure, and pulse are absent. Time is critical; every second that passes without effective circulation adds to the degree of hypoxia or anoxia in the tissues of the body, to the development of respiratory and metabolic acidosis, and to rhythms such as asystole and PEA, from which effective resuscitation is unlikely.

The immediate clinical management of cardiopulmonary arrest is based on the need to furnish the victim's tissues (primarily the brain and myocardium) with a supply of well-oxygenated blood that is adequate to maintain life (prevent clinical death) until definitive management (ACLS) can be initiated.

# CPR

The technique of CPR has undergone intensive scrutiny by various segments of the medical community. Standardization of technique is being sought so that teaching the procedures will not lead to confusion among those called on to use them.

In May 1973, the AHA and the National Academy of Sciences National Research Council cosponsored a National Conference on Standards of Cardiopulmonary Resuscitation (CPR) and Emergency Cardiac Care (ECC), which for the first time presented standardized procedures for basic and advanced life support.[43] Since then a significant body of research has added to our understanding of the phenomenon of cardiac arrest and CPR. In 1979, 1985, and 1992 the second,[44] third,[45] and fourth[10] conferences, respectively, were held to update these standards. The technique of BLS described in this text was recommended by the 1992 conference.[10] The next conference is scheduled to be held, and its recommendations published, in the year 2000 under the title *ECC 2000*.

Two broad areas of training in life support were established at these conferences. BLS and ACLS represent different degrees of training and responsibility in the management of the victim of cardiac arrest and implementation of CPR to maintain life until a victim recovers sufficiently to be transported to a hospital or until ACLS becomes available. BLS includes the PABC steps of CPR, which are discussed later (Figure 30-2). ACLS consists of training in the following areas: BLS, use of adjunctive equipment and techniques such as endotracheal intubation and open chest internal cardiac compression, cardiac monitoring (electrocardiography [ECG]) for recognition of dysrhythmia, defibrillation technique, establishment of an intravenous infusion, stabilization of the victim's condition, and the use of definitive therapy including the administration of drugs to correct acidosis and to assist in establishing and maintaining an effective cardiac rhythm and circulation.

The level of training in life support varies according to an individual's requirements. *All* dental office personnel should be certified at least at the level of BLS Healthcare Provider. More often today, dentists receive training and certification in ACLS (provider level). Training at this level is invaluable because of the potential for complications associated with the administration of drugs, such as local anesthetics, antibiotics,

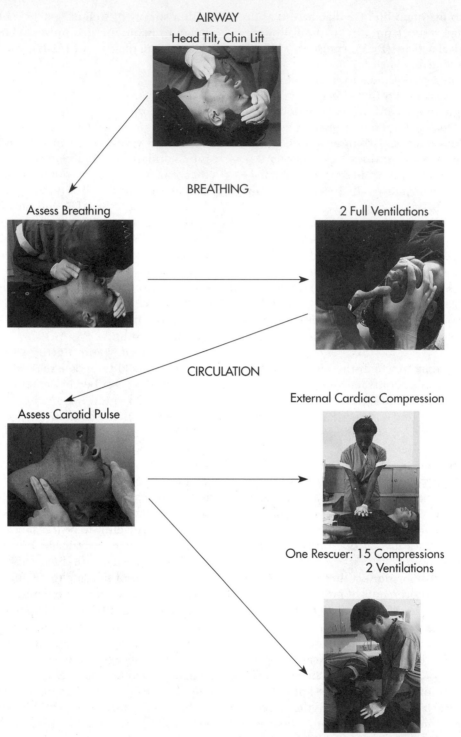

**Figure 30-2**   Summary of basic life support for adult victim.

analgesics, and sedatives. All other dental office personnel (dental hygienists, dental assistants, and non-chairside personnel) should be knowledgeable in and capable of proper application of the techniques of BLS Healthcare Provider.

Training in BLS should be repeated at least annually by all office personnel and more frequently if possible. Weaver and others[46] showed that retention of skills by trainees who do not perform CPR regularly is quite limited. Only 11.7% of 61 trainees were capable of properly performing one-person CPR on mannequins, compared with 85% of the same group 6 months earlier.

BLS courses are sponsored by many organizations, including the AHA, American Red Cross, dental societies, and fire departments. Most major dental meetings now offer BLS training courses. The BLS Healthcare Provider program involves training in four areas: (1) single-rescuer CPR, (2) two-rescuer (team) CPR, (3) obstructed airway, and (4) pediatric BLS. Additionally, and of great significance for dentistry, this program can provide training in ventilation of the victim with a mask (mouth-to-mask, bag-valve-mask, and positive pressure oxygen). This will overcome the "yuck factor" of performing mouth-to-mouth ventilation (on a dental patient).[47]

## TEAM APPROACH

In no other life-threatening situation is prompt recognition and management of greater importance than in cardiac arrest. Although it is possible for a single individual to effectively perform CPR, the procedure becomes more efficient when a trained team of rescuers is available. The team approach (two-rescuer sequence) to BLS is described next. Dental office personnel should receive their training together so that they may interact effectively as a team when necessary.

## BLS

As mentioned previously, BLS consists of the application, as needed, of the procedures of positioning (**P**), airway maintenance (**A**), breathing (**B**), and circulation by means of chest compression (**C**) to the victim of any medical emergency, including cardiac arrest, until recovery, or until the victim can be stabilized and transported to an emergency care facility or until advanced life support is available.

Three of the four components of cardiopulmonary resuscitation have previously been discussed. Positioning, airway maintenance, and artificial ventilation in the unconscious patient are outlined in Chapter 5;

lower airway obstruction is discussed in Chapter 11. Together these comprise the **P, A,** and **B** portions of CPR. Fig. 30-2 summarizes the important steps of BLS.

## UNWITNESSED AND WITNESSED CARDIAC ARREST

In the management of cardiac arrest, two separate clinical situations are considered (Boxes 30-2 and 30-3). In an *unwitnessed cardiac arrest* the victim is unconscious when discovered by the rescuer. The rescuer did not see the victim collapse and consequently has no knowledge of the length of time since the cessation of breathing and effective circulation. In such circumstances, it must be assumed that more than 1 minute has elapsed between the collapse and discovery of the victim and institution of BLS procedures. In this situation the myocardium is considered to be hypoxic, and the sequencing of BLS is predicated on this assumption.

The *witnessed cardiac arrest* develops in an ECG-monitored patient in the presence of the rescuer, and effective BLS is administered within 1 minute of the collapse. The management sequence differs slightly in this situation because of the probability that the myocardium is still fairly well oxygenated at the time life support procedures are begun.

Cardiopulmonary arrest that occurs in a patient not monitored by ECG, even if the arrest is witnessed, is categorized and managed as an unwitnessed cardiac arrest.

Unless the rescuer is absolutely certain that the cardiopulmonary collapse occurred within 1 minute of

box **30-2**  *Management of witnessed, monitored cardiac arrest*

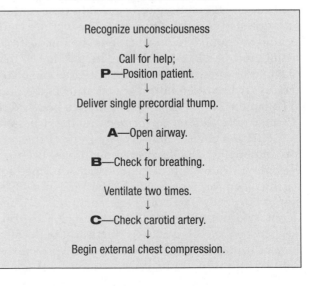

Recognize unconsciousness
↓
Call for help;
**P**—Position patient.
↓
Deliver single precordial thump.
↓
**A**—Open airway.
↓
**B**—Check for breathing.
↓
Ventilate two times.
↓
**C**—Check carotid artery.
↓
Begin external chest compression.

box **30-3**   *Management of unwitnessed, cardiac arrest*

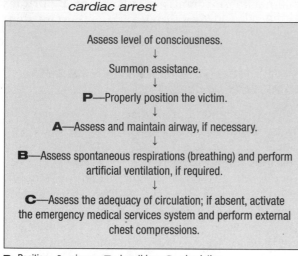

Assess level of consciousness.
↓
Summon assistance.
↓
**P**—Properly position the victim.
↓
**A**—Assess and maintain airway, if necessary.
↓
**B**—Assess spontaneous respirations (breathing) and perform artificial ventilation, if required.
↓
**C**—Assess the adequacy of circulation; if absent, activate the emergency medical services system and perform external chest compressions.

**P,** Position; **A,** airway; **B,** breathing; **C,** circulation.

discovery, it must be assumed that the heart is hypoxic, and the sequence for unwitnessed cardiac arrest is followed. Overall, most cardiac arrests will be unwitnessed; however, in the dental office setting it is quite likely that office personnel will be available within 60 seconds of the collapse. In June 1979, the AHA changed the criteria for the witnessed cardiac arrest to include only those situations in which the cardiac arrest occurs in an ECG-monitored patient.[44] The major emphasis of this section, therefore, is on the unwitnessed cardiac arrest.

## CARDIAC ARREST IN THE DENTAL OFFICE

Cardiac arrest, as well as any other life-threatening situation, may occur anywhere within the dental office. Medical emergencies have occurred in the waiting room, rest room, laboratory, doctor's office, and treatment room.[48] In all situations the unconscious victim must be placed in the supine position so that BLS may be initiated. The victim of cardiopulmonary arrest may be seated in the dental chair at the time of collapse. The question that must then be asked is: "Can effective CPR be performed with the victim still in the dental chair?" Before the advent of the contoured dental chair, the answer might have been *yes.* With the introduction of dental chairs designed for maximal comfort, however, it has become more difficult to effectively carry out chest compression if the victim is permitted to remain in the chair. The heart lies between two bony masses: the sternum, located anteriorly, and the spinal column, located posteriorly. With compression of the sternum toward the spinal

column, intrathoracic pressure is raised, compressing the heart and blood vessels and producing cardiac output. If the victim is lying on a soft surface (mattress or comfortable dental chair), the spinal column flexes and the force of the compression is partially absorbed by the soft surface, thereby lessening the effectiveness of the sternal compression. When properly performed against a hard surface, external chest compression can produce systolic blood pressure peaks of 100 mmHg, but the diastolic blood pressure is 0. The mean arterial blood pressure is rarely greater than 40 mmHg as measured in the carotid arteries. Blood flow through the carotid arteries to the cerebral circulation therefore is approximately only one-fourth to one-third normal, at best. BLS performed on a soft backing is less effective and is contraindicated.

It is frequently recommended that the cardiac arrest victim be removed from the dental chair and placed onto the floor, if at all possible, so that BLS may be performed more effectively. In most dental treatment rooms, however, little or no floor room is available to both place the victim and to permit one or two rescuers to perform BLS. In such a situation, or if it is difficult or impossible to move the victim to the floor, BLS should be initiated with the patient in the chair. If possible, a hard object such as a solid board (e.g., a removable cabinet top or a molded CPR backboard) should be placed under the victim to support the spinal column (Fig. 30-3). Under no circumstances should BLS be withheld or delayed because of the inability to move the victim to a more suitable location. "Bad CPR is better than no CPR."

In all of the following sequences, it is assumed that the patient (victim) has suffered cardiac arrest; that is, the victim is unconscious and there is an absence of both respiration and circulation. These basic steps (PABC) are equally important in the management of all emergency situations—not just cardiac arrest.

The first step in the management of all emergency situations is the implementation, as needed, of BLS. This means that in every situation considered an emergency by the doctor or by any rescuer, the steps listed in Box 30-3 must be followed.

Patient response to these steps will guide rescuers in their management. In many instances in which the victim is conscious (e.g., with respiratory distress and/or altered consciousness), the rescuer need only position the victim (**P**) comfortably, and assess **A, B,** and **C**—a process requiring only a few seconds. The patient will be effectively maintaining **A, B,** and **C** by himself or herself, allowing the rescuer to continue to step **D,** definitive management.

In another situation the rescuer may determine that the victim is unconscious (lack of response to sensory

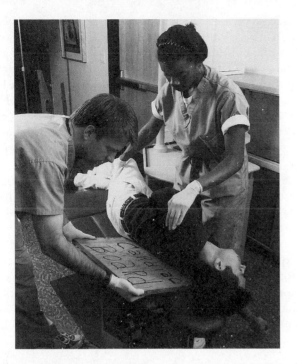

**Figure 30-3** CPR board to support victim's back and spinal cord during external chest compression.

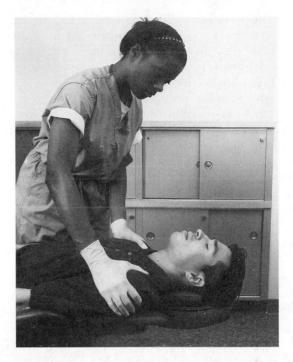

**Figure 30-4** Assessment of unconsciousness: shake and shout.

stimulation; e.g., "shake and shout"). Positioning (supine with feet elevated slightly), assessment of the airway, and head tilt-chin lift are required; however, assessment of **B** and **C** may demonstrate the adequacy of spontaneous breathing and the presence of an effective pulse. In this situation, the rescuer need only maintain an airway while considering definitive management.

Although **P, A, B,** and **C** are always assessed in every emergency situation, only those elements deemed necessary for the victim's survival are instituted.

# BLS

## UNWITNESSED CARDIAC ARREST

When cardiac arrest occurs in an unmonitored victim, the steps for unwitnessed cardiac arrest must be instituted promptly.

*Step 1: recognition of unconsciousness.* Stimulate the victim by gently shaking the shoulders and shouting the victim's name. Lack of response to these sensory stimuli is a suitable criterion for establishing a diagnosis of unconsciousness (Figure 30-4).

Many factors may be responsible for the loss of consciousness (Table 5-1), most of which do not lead immediately to respiratory and cardiac arrest. However, prompt management of unconsciousness

from any cause follows the identical format—**PABC.** A differential diagnosis of unconsciousness is reached by assessing patient response or lack of response to each of these steps.

*Step 2: summoning of assistance and* **P**—*positioning of patient.* The rescuer will not want to treat the victim alone; therefore assistance should be sought as soon as unconsciousness is recognized. Members of the office emergency team should report to the emergency area with the emergency drug kit and a supply of oxygen; they should be prepared to assist member one, as required. This step does not require activation of the EMS system, just the dental office emergency team.

The patient is placed in the supine position. The head and chest of the victim are placed parallel to the floor and the feet elevated slightly (10 degrees) to facilitate return of blood from the periphery. At this time, before the determination of cardiovascular collapse, it is not yet necessary to place the victim on a hard surface. Once pulselessness is established, this procedure becomes necessary.

*Step 3:* **A**—*assessment and maintainance of airway.* Head tilt combined with chin lift may be used to obtain a patent airway. The rescuer places one hand on the victim's forehead and the other hand on the bony prominence of the chin (symphysis). The head is extended backward, stretching the tissues in the neck and lifting the tongue off the posterior wall of the pharynx (Figure 30-5). Head tilt is the single-most important procedure in airway maintenance. If head tilt is ineffective in establishing a patent airway, the jaw-thrust maneuver can be used.

*Step 4a:* **B**—*assessment of breathing and ventilation, if needed.* While maintaining head tilt, the rescuer places his or her ear approximately 1 inch from the victim's mouth and nose so that any exhaled air from the victim may be felt and heard. The rescuer looks toward the chest of the victim to see whether spontaneous respiratory efforts are present (Figure 30-6). With cardiopulmonary arrest, respiratory efforts are absent or are so weak as to be essentially nonexistent.

*Step 4b: artificial ventilation.* In the absence of effective respiratory movement, artificial ventilation must be started immediately. Several techniques of artificial ventilation are discussed in Chapter 5; however, in this section only one—mouth-to-mouth (or mask) ventilation—is considered. Other techniques may also be used, but no technique of artificial ventilation is effective unless a patent airway is maintained throughout the ventilatory process. Most other devices for artificial ventilation require advanced training.

To perform mouth-to-mouth ventilation, head tilt must be maintained and the nose of the victim sealed (Figure 30-7). The first ventilatory cycle is composed of two full ventilations with adequate time (1½ to 2 seconds per breath) allowed to provide good chest expansion and to minimize the risk of gastric distention. Effective artificial ventilation is noted by expansion of the victim's chest. In the normal adult, the minimal volume of air should be 800 ml/breath but need not exceed 1200 ml/breath for adequate ventila-

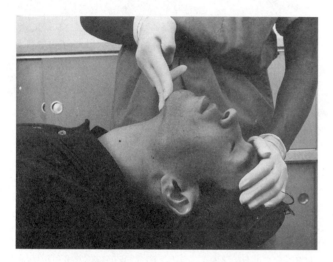

**Figure 30-5**   Head tilt–chin lift.

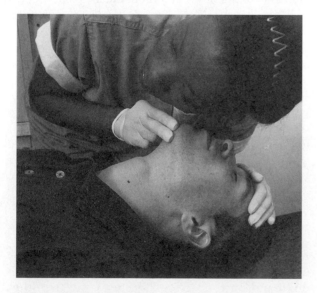

**Figure 30-6**   Assess breathing: look, listen, and feel while maintaining head tilt–chin lift.

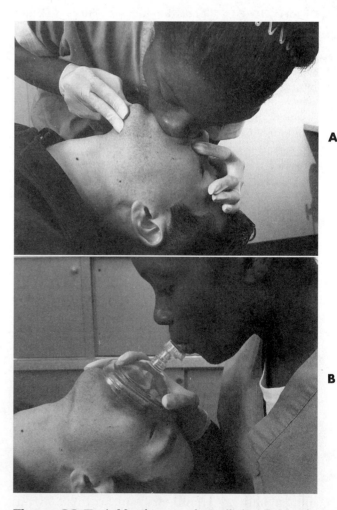

A

B

**Figure 30-7**   **A,** Mouth-to-mouth ventilation. **B,** Mouth-to-mask ventilation.

tion. Exhalation is passive, with the rescuer removing his or her mouth from that of the victim, taking in a breath of fresh air, and watching the chest fall. Subsequent ventilations are performed at a rate of one every 5 seconds (12 per minute) for the adult victim. In the child and infant, ventilation is carried out at a rate of one every 3 seconds (20 per minute), with each breath lasting approximately 1 to 1½ seconds. Immediately after the first ventilatory cycle of two full breaths, the rescuer should determine the victim's cardiovascular status.

When mouth-to-mask ventilation is used, the mask is held in position with one or two hands as needed, maintaining both an airtight seal and a patent airway. The mouth of the rescuer is placed on the breathing port, and air is forced into the victim until the chest is seen to rise. The rates of ventilation are the same as those already mentioned.

*Step 5a:* **B**—*assessment of circulation.* Having oxygenated the blood, the rescuer must next determine if that blood is circulating to the tissues and organs in the body, primarily to the brain, which is composed of cells (neurons) that are exquisitely sensitive to anoxia. A large artery must be located and carefully palpated. The femoral artery in the groin and the carotid artery in the neck are two large, central arteries. Although either may be palpated, the carotid artery is much preferred. It is located in the neck and can be accessed easily without disrobing the victim. In addition, the carotid artery transports oxygenated blood to the victim's brain, the organ that must be adequately perfused for successful resuscitation.

The carotid artery is located in a groove between the trachea and the sternocleidomastoid muscle on the anterolateral aspect of the neck (Figure 30-8). The fleshy portions of the first and second fingers of the rescuer should be used to feel for a pulse. Not more than 10 seconds should be allowed for this procedure because the pulse, if present, may be very slow or very weak but rapid. The thumb should never be used to monitor a pulse because the thumb contains a medium-size artery, and the heart rate recorded may be that of the rescuer. (This is not uncommon, especially when the rescuer is "pumped up."). Unless the carotid pulse is unquestionably present, external chest compression is initiated immediately. At this point the victim should be placed on the floor, *if practical* (it often is not), or left in the dental chair with a stable support such as a CPR board placed under the victim's back.

*Step 5b: activation of EMS.* EMS should be activated after the pulse check. Many communities use the universal emergency number, 9-1-1; however, the appropriate telephone number for a given locality

should be called. Information given to the EMS dispatcher should include the following:
1. Location of the emergency (with names of cross streets, if possible)
2. Number of telephone from which the call is made
3. What happened (e.g., heart attack, seizure, accident)
4. Number of persons who need help
5. Condition of the victim(s)
6. Aid being given to the victim(s)
7. Any other information requested

To ensure that EMS personnel have no more questions, the caller should hang up last. When more than one rescuer is available, one person is sent immediately to activate the EMS. Eisenberg and others[49] showed that the shorter the time interval between collapse and the initiation of BLS and ACLS, the greater the likelihood of survival for the victim of cardiac arrest (Table 30-3).

| table **30-3** | *Survival rate from cardiac arrest resulting from ventricular fibrillation, as related to promptness of initiation of CPR and ACLS\** |

| INITIATION OF CPR (MINUTES) | ARRIVAL OF ACLS (MINUTES) | SURVIVAL RATE (%) |
|---|---|---|
| 0-4 | 0-8 | 43 |
| 0-4 | 16+ | 10 |
| 8-12 | 8-16 | 6 |
| 8-12 | 16+ | 0 |
| 12+ | 12+ | 0 |

From Eisenberg MS, Bergner L, Hallstrom A: Cardiac resuscitation in the community: importance of rapid provision and implications for program planning, *JAMA* 241:1905, 1979.
*Data from Project Restart, King County, Washington.

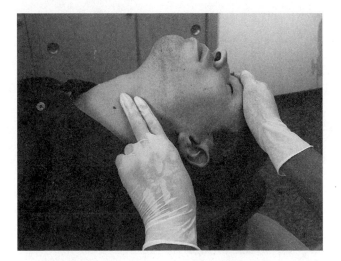

**Figure 30-8** Locate carotid artery in groove between trachea and sternocleidomastoid muscle. Head tilt must be maintained.

If only one rescuer is present and the victim is an adult, the rescuer should summon EMS immediately and then commence BLS. This action will bring the third (early defibrillation) and fourth (early ACLS) links of the chain of survival to the scene more quickly. If the victim is an infant or child, BLS should be performed for 1 minute followed by the EMS call. If the rescuer is alone with no telephone, the only option is to continue BLS.

*Step 5c: external chest compression.* External chest compression consists of the rhythmic application of pressure over the lower half of the adult sternum. The heart lies under and just to the left of the midline under the lower half of the sternum and above the spinal column. When the sternum is compressed, intrathoracic pressure is increased. This increased pressure produces cardiac output by compressing the vessels within the chest cavity and forcing blood back to, and through, the heart. When this pressure is released, blood from the periphery flows back into the heart to refill its chambers.

Effective artificial ventilation and artificial circulation can provide sufficient oxygen to prevent cellular death. Two theories, the cardiac pump theory[50] and the thoracic pump theory,[51] seek to explain the mechanism of blood flow during external chest compression.

*Location of pressure point.* To perform effective external chest compression and to minimize injury to other organs (lungs, liver, heart), the rescuer's hands must be positioned properly. This area may be located by using the following maneuver (Figure 30-9). The rescuer, located at the victim's shoulders, runs his or her middle finger in a superior direction along the lower border of the rib cage until the midline is reached. Directly below this midline notch, created by the convergence of the ribs, is the cartilaginous xiphoid process, which curves inward, and the liver. The rescuer's middle finger is located in the notch, the index finger lying beside it on the lower border of the sternum. The rescuer then places the heel of the other hand over the midline of the sternum immediately next to the index finger. This locates the proper site for external chest compression in an adult victim.

In the child (ages 1 through 8 years) the proper site for chest compression is located in a manner similar to that described for the adult:

1. The lower margin of the victim's rib cage is located with the rescuer's middle and index fingers.
2. The margin of the rib cage is followed with the middle finger to the notch in the midline where the right and left side ribs meet.
3. With the middle finger in this notch, the index finger is placed next to the middle finger.
4. The heel of the hand is placed next to the index finger with the long axis of the heel parallel to the sternum.
5. The chest is compressed with one hand to a depth of 2.5 to 3.8 cm (1 to 1½ in) at a rate of 100 compressions per minute.

In the infant (<1 year of age) the site of compression is somewhat different (Figure 30-10). Evidence has shown that the heart of the infant is lower in relation to external chest landmarks than was previously

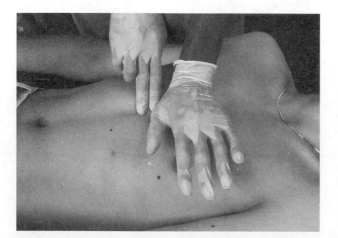

**Figure 30-9** Proper location for adult external chest compression.

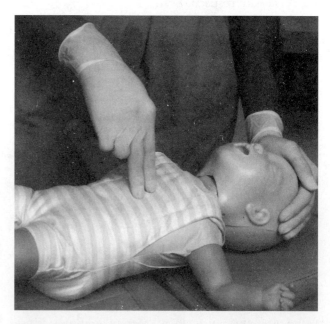

**Figure 30-10** Proper location for infant external chest compression.

thought.[52] Proper hand placement for chest compression in the infant is as follows:

1. An imaginary line is drawn between the nipples located over the sternum (intermammary line).
2. The index finger of the hand farthest from the infant's head is placed just under the intermammary line where it intersects the sternum. The area of compression is one finger's width below this intersection, at the location of the middle and ring fingers.
3. While using two or three fingers, the sternum is compressed to a depth of 1.3 to 2.5 cm (½ to 1 in) at a rate of at least 100 compressions per minute.

*Hand position.* Having determined the proper location for chest compression, the rescuer must align the hands properly to achieve maximum effectiveness. In the adult victim the heel of the first hand is already in position on the midsternum of the victim approximately 4 to 5 cm (1½ to 2 in) above the xiphoid process. Only the heel of this hand should

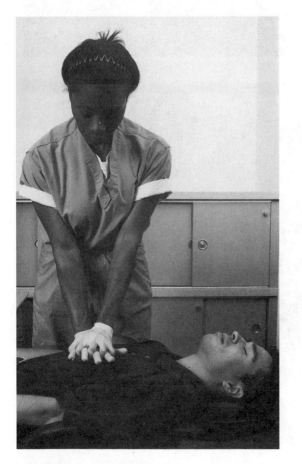

**Figure 30-11** Hand position for adult external chest compression.

be in contact with the chest wall. The heel of the second hand is next placed directly over the first hand, parallel to it (Figure 30-11). The fingers of the two hands are then interlaced, with the fingers of the top hand pulling the fingers of the lower hand upward. In this manner only the heel of the lower hand remains in contact with the victim's chest. An alternative hand position, especially useful for persons with arthritis of the hand or wrist, is to grasp the wrist of the hand on the chest wall with the hand that had been locating the lower end of the sternum.

These procedures are important to follow because if the fingers of the hand contact the chest wall, the pressures exerted in chest compression will be delivered over a larger area and will therefore be less effective in increasing intrathoracic pressure. In addition, this pressure will be extended to the ribs, not just to the sternum, increasing the likelihood of costochondral separation or rib fracture, with possible contusion and laceration of the heart and lungs.

*Application of pressure.* Having determined the proper location for chest compression and hand positioning, the rescuer can begin chest compression. External chest compression (ECC) is strenuous. However, when ECC is performed properly, the trained rescuer should not become rapidly exhausted. When improperly performed, ECC rapidly exhausts the rescuer and is ineffective. The following points facilitate implementation of ECC with maximal effectiveness and minimal fatigue: The shoulders of the rescuer must be located directly over the sternum of the victim, and the rescuer's elbows should be locked straight, not bent (Figure 30-12). If the victim is lying on the floor, the rescuer must kneel beside the victim, close enough to the body so that the rescuer's shoulders are directly over the victim's sternum. If the victim is in the dental chair, the rescuer stands astride the victim, and the chair is lowered so that proper positioning can be achieved (Figure 30-13, *A*).

Improper positioning of the shoulders (at an angle to the sternum) decreases the effectiveness of chest compression and increases the likelihood of complications related to costochondral separation from stretching of ribs on one side, and fracture of ribs from bending ribs on the opposite side (Figure 30-13, *B*). Bending of the elbows greatly decreases effectiveness of ECC and leads to rapid fatigue of the rescuer.

The rescuer then exerts pressure directly downward so that the sternum of the adult victim is depressed 3.8 to 5 cm (1½ to 2 in). With proper shoulder and arm placement, the rescuer allows the weight of his or her body to compress the victim's sternum. Movement of

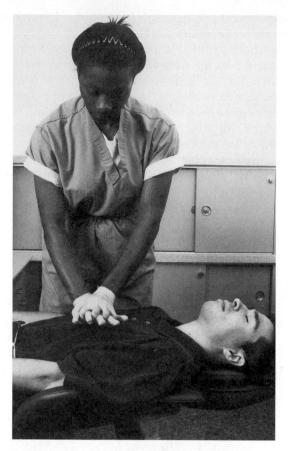

**Figure 30-12** Improper position: elbow of rescuer should be locked (straight), not bent.

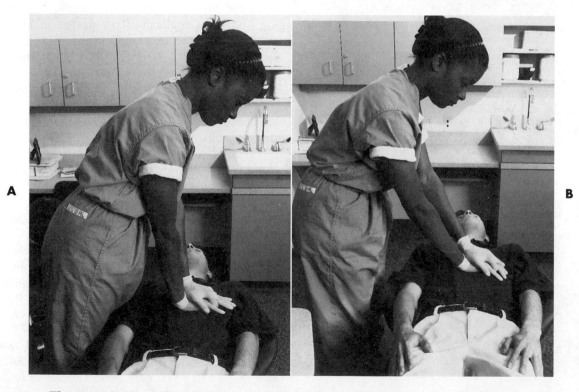

**Figure 30-13** **A,** Dental chair is lowered to allow rescuer to bring shoulders directly over sternum of victim. **B,** Improper positioning increases risk of injury to victim.

the rescuer occurs only at the hips; it should be a gentle back-and-forth rocking motion if the technique is properly executed. Compressions must be regular, smooth, and uninterrupted. Relaxation follows compressions immediately and is of equal duration. To maintain proper hand position, the heel of the rescuer's hand should not be removed from the chest during relaxation, but pressure on the sternum should be completely released so that the sternum returns to its normal position between compressions.

The infant's chest is compressed 1.3 to 2.5 cm ($\frac{1}{2}$ to 1 in) just below the intermammary line using the tips of two or three fingers, while the chest of the child is compressed 2.5 to 2.8 cm (1 to $1\frac{1}{2}$ in) using the heel of one hand (Figure 30-14). BLS techniques for the adult, infant, and child are summarized in Table 30-4.

*Rate of compression.* A change in the rate of chest compression was recommended in the 1986 AHA guidelines. The rate was increased to a minimum of 80 per minute, 100 per minute if possible. When BLS is performed by a team of two persons, one rescuer is responsible for airway and breathing, and the second rescuer carries out chest compression. In this case chest compression is performed at a rate of 80 to 100 per minute, with artificial ventilation interspersed after every fifth compression. In the two-rescuer sequence, the ratio of chest compression to artificial ventilation is 5:1, with a pause of 1 to $1\frac{1}{2}$ seconds for ventilation.

When only one rescuer is available, that person is responsible for both ventilation and chest compression. In the single-rescuer sequence, the ratio of chest compression to artificial ventilation is 15:2. However, to compress the chest 60 times *and* intersperse eight ventilations in 60 seconds, the rate of chest compression must be faster than one per second. Fifteen chest compressions are followed by two full breaths. A single rescuer should complete four complete cycles of 15 compressions and two ventilations in approximately 1 minute. To accomplish this effectively, the 15 chest compressions should be completed in approximately 9 to 11 seconds. The remaining time permits the rescuer to move to the head, deliver two full breaths, relocate the landmark for chest compression, and prepare to restart chest compression.

In the infant and child, the compression/ventilation ratio is 5:1 in both single and team rescue situations. Compression rates are 100 per minute in the child and at least 100 per minute in the infant.

Figure 30-2 summarizes the management of the unwitnessed cardiac arrest in the adult.

## SINGLE RESCUE FOR ADULTS

Clinical application of the technique of BLS for the single rescuer in a case of unwitnessed cardiac arrest is based on the techniques described earlier. When dealing with cardiac arrest and possible neurologic damage, the time element becomes critical. Figure 30-15 presents performance AHA criteria for one rescuer.

The first steps involve the recognition of unconsciousness, calling for assistance, and positioning the victim. The process of calling for help needs clarification. When the unconscious victim is found by a lone rescuer and there is a good likelihood that another rescuer is readily available, calling for help simply means yelling loudly for assistance. It does not mean leaving the victim to seek assistance, nor does it mean taking time to place a telephone call. Every second that is not spent performing effective BLS decreases the chance for recovery. However, when the single rescuer is with an unconscious patient (e.g., no response to "shake and shout") and no assistance is likely to be readily available, the emergency telephone call is made before the start of BLS.

The rescuer is positioned so that artificial ventilation and artificial circulation may be carried out with minimal movement. The most nearly ideal position for the rescuer is astride the shoulders of the victim so that both procedures may be performed merely by bending at the waist.

Airway patency is ensured through head tilt–chin lift or the jaw-thrust maneuver, or both, and the rescuer checks for spontaneous respiratory movements (look, listen, feel). In the absence of such movement, the rescuer ventilates the victim with two full breaths at $1\frac{1}{2}$ to 2 seconds per ventilation. Chest deflation should be noted between breaths.

With the blood of the victim now oxygenated, the rescuer assesses circulatory status by palpating the carotid artery for a pulse. This important step must not be hurried. Allow 5 to 10 seconds to determine pulselessness.

In the absence of effective circulation, the EMS system is activated, and external chest compression begun immediately. The proper site for compression on the lower half of the adult sternum is located using the maneuver described earlier.

With elbows locked and shoulders directly over the sternum, the rescuer depresses the chest of the adult victim approximately 4 to 5 cm ($1\frac{1}{2}$ to 2 in) at a rate of 80 to 100 compressions per minute. The rescuer should count silently or softly to himself or herself*

---

*Studies have shown that rescuers counting silently or softly can perform CPR effectively longer than those counting out loud. It requires more energy expenditure to count aloud; however, when a second rescuer appears to aid, counting aloud is essential.

*Text continued on p. 497*

table **30-4**  *Summary of CPR techniques*

| VICTIM | RESPIRATIONS PER MINUTE | INTERVAL (SECONDS) | RATIO OF COMPRESSION TO VENTILATION | COMPRESSIONS | | | | |
| | | | | RATE/MIN | DEPTH (CM) | DEPTH (INCHES) | HANDS | SITE |
|---|---|---|---|---|---|---|---|---|
| Infant (<1 year of age) | 20 | 3 | 5:1 | At least 100 | 1.3-2.5 | ½-1 | 2-3 fingers | One fingerwidth below intermammary line, midsternum |
| Child (1 to 8 years of age) | 20 | 3 | 5:1 | 100 | 2.5-3.8 | 1-1½ | 1 heel | Lower half of sternum, |
| Adult (8 years of age and older) | 12 | 5 | 5:1 | 80-100 | 3.8-5.0 | 1½-2 | 2 hands | Lower half of sternum |
| One rescuer | — | — | 15:2 | | | | | |
| Two rescuers | — | — | 5:1 | | | | | |

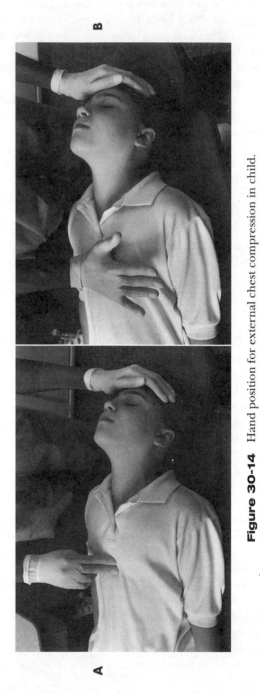

**Figure 30-14**  Hand position for external chest compression in child.

CPR and ECC Performance Sheet
One-Rescuer CPR: Adult

Name _____ Date:_____

| Step | Activity | Critical performance | S | U |
|------|----------|---------------------|---|---|
| 1. Airway | Assessment: Determine unresponsiveness | Tap or gently shake shoulder | | |
| | | Shout, "Are you OK?" | | |
| | Call for help | Call out "Help!" | | |
| | Position the victim | Turn on back as unit, if necessary, supporting head and neck (4-10 sec) | | |
| | Open the airway | Use head tilt–chin lift maneuver | | |
| 2. Breathing | Assessment: Determine breathlessness | Maintain open airway | | |
| | | Ear over mouth, observe chest: look, listen, feel for breathing (3-5 sec) | | |
| | Ventilate twice | Maintain open airway | | |
| | | Seal mouth and nose properly | | |
| | | Ventilate 2 times at 1-1.5 sec/inspiration | | |
| | | Observe chest rise (adequate ventilation volume) | | |
| | | Allow deflation between breaths | | |
| 3. Circulation | Assessment: Determine pulselessness | Feel for carotid pulse on near side of victim (5-10 sec) | | |
| | | Maintain head-tilt with other hand | | |
| | Activate EMS system | If someone responded to call for help, send him/her to activate EMS system | | |
| | | Total time, Step 1—Activate EMS system: 15-35 sec | | |
| | Begin chest compressions | Rescuer kneels by victim's shoulders | | |
| | | Landmark check prior to hand placement | | |
| | | Proper hand position throughout | | |
| | | Rescuer's shoulders over victim's sternum | | |
| | | Equal compression-relaxation | | |
| | | Compress 1½ to 2 inches | | |
| | | Keep hands on sternum during upstroke | | |
| | | Complete chest relaxation up upstroke | | |
| | | Say any helpful mnemonic | | |
| | | Compression rate: 80-100/min (15 per 9-11 sec) | | |
| 4. Compression/ventilation cycles | Do 4 cycles of 15 compressions and 2 ventilations | Proper compression/ventilation ratio: 15 compressions to 2 ventilations per cycle | | |
| | | Observe chest rise: 1-1.5 sec/inspiration 4 cycles/ 52-73 sec | | |
| 5. Reassessment* | Determine pulselessness (If no pulse: step 6)† | Feel for carotid pulse (5 sec) | | |
| 6. Continue CPR | Ventilate twice | Ventilate twice | | |
| | | Observe chest rise: 1-1.5 sec/inspiration | | |
| | Resume compression/ ventilation cycles | Feel for carotid pulse every few minutes | | |

*Second rescuer arrives to replace first rescuer: (1) Second rescuer identifies self by saying "I know CPR. Can I help?" (2) Second rescuer then does pulse check in step 5 and continues with step 6. (During practice and testing only one rescuer actually ventilates the mannequin. The second rescuer simulates ventilation.) (3) First rescuer assesses the adequacy of second rescuer's CPR by observing chest rise during ventilations and by checking the pulse during chest compressions. †If pulse is present, open airway and check for spontaneous breathing: (1) If breathing is present, maintain open airway and monitor pulse and breathing. (2) If breathing is absent, perform rescue breathing at 12 times/min and monitor pulse.

Instructor _____    Check Satisfactory _____ Unsatisfactory _____

Continued

**Figure 30-15**  CPR and ECC Performance Sheet.

CPR and ECC Performance Sheet
Two-Rescuer CPR: Adult*

Name _____ Date:_____

| Step | Activity | Critical performance | S | U |
|------|----------|---------------------|---|---|
| 1. Airway | One rescuer (ventilator): Assessment: Determine unresponsiveness | Tap or gently shake shoulder | | |
| | | Shout, "Are you OK?" | | |
| | Position the victim | Turn on back if necessary (4-10 sec) | | |
| | Opens the airway | Use a proper technique to open airway | | |
| 2. Breathing | Assessment: Determine breathlessness | Look, listen, and feel (3-5 sec) | | |
| | Ventilator ventilates twice | Observe chest rise: 1-1.5 sec/inspiration | | |
| 3. Circulation | Assessment: Determine pulselessness | Palpate carotid pulse (5-10 sec) | | |
| | States assessment results Other rescuer (compressor): | Say, "No pulse" | | |
| | Gets into position for compressions | Hands, shoulders in correct position | | |
| | Locates landmark notch | Landmark check | | |
| 4. Compression/ventilation cycles | Compressor begins chest compressions | Correct ratio compressions/ventilations: 5/1 | | |
| | | Compression rate: 80-100/min (5 compressions/3-4 sec) | | |
| | | Say any helpful mnemonic | | |
| | | Stop compressing for each ventilation | | |
| | Ventilator ventilates after every fifth compression and checks compression effectiveness | Ventilate 1 time (1-1.5 sec) Check pulse to assess compressions | | |
| | (Minimum of 10 cycles) | Time for 10 cycles: 40-53 sec | | |
| 5. Call for switch | Compressor calls for switch when fatigued | Give clear signal to change | | |
| | | Compressor completes fifth compression | | |
| | | Ventilator completes ventilation after fifth compression | | |
| 6. Switch | Simultaneously switch: | | | |
| | Ventilator moves to chest | Move to chest | | |
| | | Become compressor | | |
| | | Get into position for compressions | | |
| | | Locate landmark notch | | |
| | Compressor moves to head | Move to head | | |
| | | Become ventilator | | |
| | | Check carotid pulse (5 sec) | | |
| | | Say, "No pulse" | | |
| | | Ventilate once† | | |
| 7. Continue CPR | Resume compression/ventilation cycles | Resume step 4. | | |

*(1) If CPR is in progress with one rescuer (layperson), the entrance of the two rescuers occurs after the completion of one rescuer's cycle of 15 compressions and 2 ventilations. The EMS should be activated first. The two new rescuers start with step 6. (2) If CPR is in progress with one professional rescuer, the entrance of a second professional rescuer is at the end of a cycle after check for pulse by first rescuer. The new cycle starts with one ventilation by the first rescuer, and the second rescuer becomes the compressor. †During practice and testing only one rescuer actually ventilates the mannequin. The other rescuer simulates ventilation.

Instructor _____ Check Satisfactory _____ Unsatisfactory _____

**Figure 30-15, cont'd**   CPR and ECC Performance Sheet.

CPR and ECC Performance Sheet
One-Rescuer CPR: Infant
Name _____ Date:_____

| Step | Activity | Critical performance | S | U |
|------|----------|---------------------|---|---|
| 1. Airway | Assessment: Determine unresponsiveness | Tap or gently shake shoulder | | |
| | Call for help | Call out "Help!" | | |
| | Position the infant | Turn on back as unit, supporting head and neck | | |
| | | Place on firm, hard surface | | |
| | Open the airway | Use head tilt–chin lift maneuver to sniffing or neutral position | | |
| | | Do not overextend the head | | |
| 2. Breathing | Assessment: Determine breathlessness | Maintain open airway | | |
| | | Ear over mouth, observe chest: look, listen, feel for breathing (3-5 sec) | | |
| | Ventilate twice | Maintain open airway | | |
| | | Make tight seal on infant's mouth and nose with rescuer's mouth | | |
| | | Ventilate 2 times, 1-1.5 sec/inspiration | | |
| | | Observe chest rise | | |
| | | Allow deflation between breaths | | |
| 3. Circulation | Assessment: Determine pulselessness | Feel for brachial pulse (5-10 sec) | | |
| | | Maintain head-tilt with other hand | | |
| | Activate EMS system | If someone responded to call for help, send him/her to activate EMS system | | |
| | | Total time, step 1—Activate EMS system: 15-35 sec | | |
| | Begin chest compressions | Draw imaginary line between nipples | | |
| | | Place 2-3 fingers on sternum, 1 finger's width below imaginary line | | |
| | | Equal compression-relaxation | | |
| | | Compress vertically, ½ to 1 inches | | |
| | | Keep fingers on sternum during upstroke | | |
| | | Complete chest relaxation on upstroke | | |
| | | Say any helpful mnemonic | | |
| | | Compression rate: at least 100/min (5 in 3 sec or less) | | |
| 4. Compression/ventilation cycles | Do 10 cycles of 5 compressions and 1 ventilation | Proper compression/ventilation ratio: 5 compressions to 1 slow ventilation per cycle | | |
| | | Pause for ventilation | | |
| | | Observe chest rise: 1-1.5 sec/inspiration 10 cycles/45 sec or less | | |
| 5. Reassessment | Determine pulselessness (If no pulse: step 6)* | Feel for brachial pulse (5 sec) | | |
| 6. Continue CPR | Ventilate once | Ventilate once | | |
| | | Observe chest rise: 1-1.5 sec/inspiration | | |
| | Resume compression/ventilation cycles | Feel for brachial pulse every few minutes | | |

*If pulse is present, open airway and check for spontaneous breathing. (1) If breathing is present, maintain open airway and monitor breathing and pulse. (2) If breathing is absent, perform rescue breathing at 20 times/min and monitor pulse.

Instructor _____ Check Satisfactory _____ Unsatisfactory _____

*Continued*

**Figure 30-15, cont'd**  CPR and ECC Performance Sheet.

CPR and ECC Performance Sheet
One-Rescuer CPR: Child*

Name _____   Date: _____

| Step | Activity | Critical performance | S | U |
|------|----------|---------------------|---|---|
| 1. Airway | Assessment: Determine unresponsiveness | Tap or gently shake shoulder | | |
| | | Shout, "Are you OK?" | | |
| | Call for help | Call out "Help!" | | |
| | Position the victim | Turn on back as unit, if necessary supporting head and neck (4-10 sec) | | |
| | Open the airway | Use head tilt–chin lift maneuver | | |
| 2. Breathing | Assessment: Determine breathlessness | Maintain open airway | | |
| | | Ear over mouth, observe chest: look, listen, feel for breathing (3-5 sec) | | |
| | Ventilate twice | Maintain open airway | | |
| | | Seal mouth and nose properly | | |
| | | Ventilate 2 times, at 1-1.5 sec/inspiration | | |
| | | Observe chest rise | | |
| | | Allow deflation between breaths | | |
| 3. Circulation | Assessment: Determine pulselessness | Feel for carotid pulse on near side of victim (5-10 sec) | | |
| | | Maintain head-tilt with other hand | | |
| | Activate EMS system | If someone responded to call for help, send him/her to activate EMS system | | |
| | | Total time, step 1—Activate EMS system: 15-35 sec | | |
| | Begin chest compressions | Rescuer kneels by victim's shoulders | | |
| | | Landmark check prior to initial hand placement | | |
| | | Proper hand position throughout | | |
| | | Rescuer's shoulders over victim's sternum | | |
| | | Equal compression-relaxation | | |
| | | Compress 1 to 1½ inches | | |
| | | Keep hands on sternum during upstroke | | |
| | | Complete chest relaxation up upstroke | | |
| | | Say any helpful mnemonic | | |
| | | Compression rate: 80-100/min (5 per 3-4 sec) | | |
| 4. Compression/ventilation cycles | Do 10 cycles of 5 compressions and 1 ventilation | Proper compression/ventilation ratio: 5 compressions to 1 slow ventilation per cycle | | |
| | | Observe chest rise: 1-1.5 sec/inspiration (10 cycles/60-87 sec) | | |
| 5. Reassessment† | Determine pulselessness (If no pulse: step 6)‡ | Feel for carotid pulse (5 sec) | | |
| 6. Continue CPR | Ventilate once | Ventilate once | | |
| | | Observe chest rise: 1-1.5 sec/inspiration | | |
| | Resume compression/ventilation cycles | Palpate carotid pulse every few minutes | | |

*If child is above age of approximately 8 years, the method for adults should be used.
†Second rescuer arrives to replace first rescuer: (1) Second rescuer identifies self by saying "I know CPR. Can I help?" (2) Second rescuer then does pulse check in step 5 and continues with step 6. (During practice and testing only one rescuer actually ventilates the mannequin. The second rescuer simulates ventilation.) (3) First rescuer assesses the adequacy of second rescuer's CPR by observing chest rise during ventilations and by checking the pulse during chest compressions. ‡If pulse is present, open airway and check for spontaneous breathing: (1) If breathing is present, maintain open airway and monitor breathing and pulse. (2) If breathing is absent, perform rescue breathing at 15 times/min and monitor pulse.

Instructor _____   Check Satisfactory _____   Unsatisfactory _____

**Figure 30-15, cont'd**   CPR and ECC Performance Sheet.

during this sequence and after 15 compressions immediately give two full lung inflations (1.5 to 2 seconds each), allowing complete lung deflation to occur between each breath. One complete 15-compression, 2-ventilation sequence should take approximately 15 seconds. The rescuer then immediately relocates the pressure point on the sternum and repeats the cycle of 15 compressions and two ventilations so that four cycles may be completed in approximately 1 minute. After the first four cycles and periodically thereafter, the rescuer stops to reassess the victim's pulse and breathing.

**Two-rescuer CPR for adults**  With two or more rescuers present to perform CPR, it is possible to carry out artificial ventilation and chest compressions without interruption (Figure 30-15). The 1992 Guidelines present two scenarios for two rescuers.

*One-rescuer CPR with entry of a second rescuer.* This scenario is recommended for use by persons who are not health care professionals and may not be proficient in the two-person protocol. When a second rescuer becomes available, he or she is sent immediately to activate the EMS system if this has not previously been done and to perform one-rescuer CPR if the first rescuer becomes fatigued. The following sequence is recommended:

1. Second rescuer identifies himself or herself as CPR certified and willing to help.
2. First rescuer stops CPR after the next two ventilations.
3. Second rescuer kneels down and checks for the carotid pulse for 15 seconds.
4. If pulse is absent, second rescuer gives two breaths.
5. Second rescuer begins external chest compression at a 15:2 ratio at a rate of 80 to 100 compressions per minute.
6. Meanwhile, the first rescuer assesses the adequacy of the second rescuer's efforts.

*CPR performed by two rescuers.* The use of mouth-to-mask ventilation is an acceptable alternative to mouth-to-mouth ventilation in this scenario because it is recommended that all health care professionals be adequately trained in the use of these devices.

One person performs external chest compression while the second rescuer remains at the victim's head, maintaining a patent airway, monitoring the carotid pulse for adequacy of external chest compressions, and providing rescue breathing (Figure 30-16). The compression rate for two-rescuer CPR is 80 to 100 per minute, with a pause of 1 to 1½ seconds per ventilation and a compression/ventilation ratio of 5:1. When the compressor becomes fatigued, the rescuers should change position as soon as possible.

The following sequence is used if one-rescuer CPR is in progress when the second rescuer arrives at the scene:

1. The most appropriate time for entry of the second rescuer is immediately after completion of a cycle of 15 compressions and two ventilations.
   a. One rescuer moves to the head of the victim, opens the airway, and checks for a pulse.
   b. The second rescuer, positioned on the opposite side of the victim, locates the area for external chest compression and the proper hand position (Figure 30-15).
2. If no pulse is present, the ventilator gives one breath and the compressor starts external chest compression at the rate of 80 to 100 per minute, counting "one-and, two-and, three-and, four-and, five."
3. After the fifth compression, a pause of 1 to 1½ seconds is allowed for ventilation.
4. The compression/ventilation ratio is 5:1.

If CPR is not in progress and both professional rescuers arrive at the same time, the following sequence is followed:

1. One rescuer ensures that the EMS system has been activated.
2. If this person must leave the area, the second rescuer initiates one-rescuer CPR.

However, if both persons are available for CPR:

1. One rescuer goes to the head of the victim and:
   a. Determines unresponsiveness ("shake and shout")

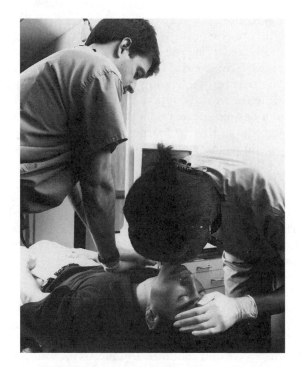

**Figure 30-16**  Rescuer positions for two-person CPR.

b. Positions the victim
c. Opens the airway
d. Assesses breathing
e. If breathing is absent, says, "no breathing," and gives two ventilations
f. Assesses circulation
g. If pulse is absent, says, "no pulse"
2. The second rescuer simultaneously:
   a. Finds the location for external chest compression
   b. Locates the proper hand position
   c. Initiates external chest compressions after the first rescuer states, "No pulse"

When one rescuer, usually the compressor, is fatigued, the rescuers change position as rapidly as possible. The sequence for change in two-rescuer CPR is as follows:

1. The compressor calls for a switch when fatigued and completes the fifth compression.
2. The ventilator gives one full ventilation.
3. Both rescuers switch positions.
4. The original ventilator moves to the victim's chest, gets in position to administer external chest compressions, and locates the landmark for compressions.
5. The original compressor moves to the victim's head, checks the carotid pulse for 5 seconds, and if it is absent says, "no pulse," and ventilates once.
6. The new chest compressor immediately begins chest compression at the rate of 5 compressions in approximately 3 to 4 seconds. A total of 10 cycles of 5:1 should be completed in approximately 40 to 53 seconds.

The two-rescuer sequence is a more effective method of carrying out CPR because it avoids interruptions in the cycle of chest compression that occur with a single rescuer. During two-rescuer CPR it is also possible for the rescuers to change position at any time, if desired. If the rescuers are positioned on opposite sides of the victim, they may change positions with minimal interruption in the sequence of events. This allows the rescuers to perform effective BLS longer by minimizing fatigue.

Practice, practice, and still more practice is absolutely essential if the team approach to BLS is to be effective. All members of the dental office staff should be capable of working with each other in a rescuer position (ventilation or chest compression). Box 30-4 summarizes the steps of BLS.

**Infant resuscitation** For the purpose of BLS technique, the infant is a person under 1 year of age (Figure 30-15). Lack of responsiveness is determined by the "shake and shout" technique, as with the adult or child victim. Once unresponsiveness is determined,

the rescuer immediately calls for help and places the infant in the supine (horizontal) position.

The airway is opened and assessed for patency (look, listen, and feel) and for the presence or absence of spontaneous ventilation (Figure 30-17). Three to five seconds are allowed for assessment. Two ventilations are delivered (1 to 1½ seconds per ventilation) forcefully enough to produce chest inflation and permit complete deflation between breaths. Overinflation in infants is dangerous because it produces gastric distention, reducing the effectiveness of subsequent ventilation and increasing the risk of regur-

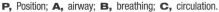

box **30-4**   *Basic life support*

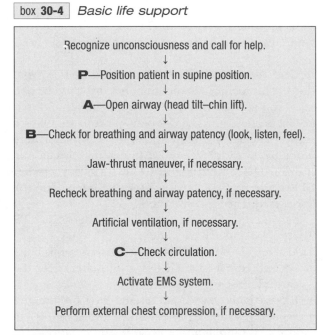

Recognize unconsciousness and call for help.
↓
**P**—Position patient in supine position.
↓
**A**—Open airway (head tilt–chin lift).
↓
**B**—Check for breathing and airway patency (look, listen, feel).
↓
Jaw-thrust maneuver, if necessary.
↓
Recheck breathing and airway patency, if necessary.
↓
Artificial ventilation, if necessary.
↓
**C**—Check circulation.
↓
Activate EMS system.
↓
Perform external chest compression, if necessary.

**P,** Position; **A,** airway; **B,** breathing; **C,** circulation.

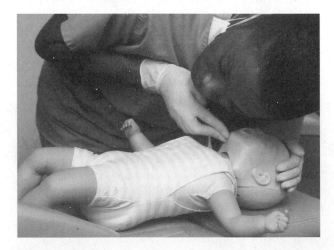

**Figure 30-17**   Assess airway (look, listen, and feel) in infant victim.

gitation. The adult rescuer's mouth or mask can usually cover both the mouth and nose of the infant victim. If this is not possible, mouth-to-mouth or mouth-to-nose ventilation is recommended.

The pulse is assessed next. The brachial artery in the upper portion of the arm is palpated for 5 to 10 seconds (Figure 30-18), and, if the pulse is absent, the EMS system is activated and external chest compressions begun. The proper site for finger placement is midsternum, one finger's width below the intermammary line (Figure 30-10). The chest is compressed at a rate of at least 100 per minute (5 in 3 seconds or less) with one ventilation interspersed after every fifth compression (ratio of 5:1). The depth of compression of the infant's chest is 1.3 to 2.5 cm (½ to 1 in), using the fleshy tips of two or three fingers held in the long axis of the sternum. After 10 cycles (approximately 45 seconds) and periodically thereafter, the patient is reevaluated for the return of pulse and/or respiration.

**Child resuscitation**  For the purpose of BLS technique, the child is a person 1 to 8 years of age (Figure 30-15). Basic procedures for resuscitation of the child are similar to those previously described for the adult and infant. The "shake and shout" maneuver is used to determine lack of responsiveness, help is called, and the patient is placed in the supine position. The airway of the child is maintained by head tilt–chin lift and is then assessed for the presence of spontaneous respiratory efforts (look, listen, and feel). If these efforts are absent, two full ventilations are provided (1 to 1½ seconds each).

The carotid pulse is assessed for 5 to 10 seconds, and, if it is absent, EMS is activated and external chest compression begun. Proper hand position for the child is located by placing the middle finger into the lower border of the sternum, as in the adult, and placing the heel of one hand onto the sternum immediately superior to the index finger. The sternum is compressed 2.5 to 3.8 cm (1 to 1½ in) at a ratio of 5 compressions to 1 ventilation, at a rate of 100 compressions per minute (5 every 3 to 4 seconds).

After 10 cycles (60 to 87 seconds) and periodically thereafter, the patient should be evaluated for the return of spontaneous pulse and/or respiration.

## MONITORED-WITNESSED CARDIAC ARREST

In the monitored-witnessed cardiac arrest, cardiopulmonary arrest develops in a patient who has been monitored by ECG, and the rescuer or rescuers are able to reach the victim and begin BLS procedures within 60 seconds of the collapse. In this sequence the myocardium is presumed to be fairly well oxygenated because of the short time elapsed since the collapse. Because of this, it is possible that a small electrical stimulus delivered to the myocardium might convert VT, complete atrioventricular block, or VF to a functional rhythm. This stimulus may be provided by the *precordial thump*. Although most instances of cardiac arrest in the dental setting will be witnessed, few patients are monitored; therefore the unwitnessed sequence for BLS should be used.

**Precordial thump**  In the monitored-witnessed cardiac arrest, the sequence of steps in BLS is altered slightly to allow for delivery of the precordial thump. The precordial thump, applied to the midsternum immediately after collapse, creates a small electrical stimulus that may be effective in reestablishing effective circulation in situations such as ventricular asystole caused by heart block and in converting VT or VF of recent onset.

The precordial thump is used to provide a stimulus to a potentially reactive heart. It is not a substitute for effective external chest compression. In addition, only one precordial thump should be used. If the pulse remains absent after delivery of the precordial thump, closed chest compression is started immediately.

The precordial thump is carried out as follows (Figure 30-19):

1. The rescuer holds a closed fist approximately 8 to 12 inches above the midpoint of the victim's sternum, with the fleshy portion of the fist facing the chest.
2. A single, sharp, quick blow (thump) is then delivered to the sternum.
3. If there is no immediate response (carotid pulse still not present), external chest compression is started.

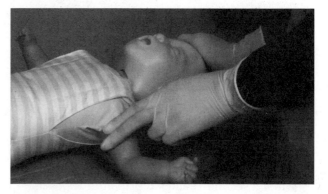

**Figure 30-18**  Brachial artery in upper arm is assessed for pulse (5 to 10 seconds).

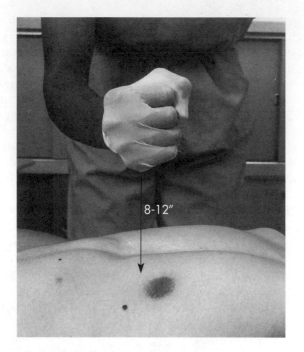

8-12"

**Figure 30-19** Precordial thump used only in monitored-witnessed cardiac arrest.

## EVALUATION OF EFFECTIVENESS

It is important to evaluate the status of the victim during administration of BLS. This evaluation assesses the effectiveness of the efforts being applied and determines whether the victim resumes spontaneous and effective respiratory movements and cardiac function. Four indicators may be observed: (1) color of the skin and mucous membranes, (2) carotid pulse, (3) respiratory movements, and (4) pupils of the eye. Depending on the number of rescuers present, this monitoring may be carried out continually or periodically.

With only one rescuer present, the color of the skin and mucous membranes is the only continually observable indicator of effectiveness. With effective BLS the skin and mucous membranes should lose any cyanotic or dusky gray color and return to a more normal color. When performing BLS alone, the rescuer should pause after the first minute to check for a carotid pulse (maximum of 5 seconds) and observe for spontaneous respiratory movements. Subsequently, the rescuer should check these indicators every 4 to 5 minutes. The rescuer should never pause for more than 5 seconds at a time, because during this time blood flow drops to zero.

When a second rescuer is present it is possible to monitor these important indicators with minimal in-

terruption. The ventilation rescuer is able to monitor these indicators, as well as determine the effectiveness of external chest compression. With a finger located on the carotid artery of the victim, the rescuer should feel a pulsation with each compression. After the first minute and every 4 to 5 minutes thereafter, the sequence may be stopped for no more than 5 seconds to determine the effectiveness of the BLS technique (color of skin and mucous membranes, presence or absence of spontaneous respiration, presence or absence of spontaneous cardiac rhythm, and pupillary reaction). The two-rescuer sequence described previously has a built-in delay that allows for monitoring of both respiratory and cardiac effectiveness.

Pupillary reaction to light is frequently used as an indicator of the effectiveness of BLS. Pupils normally respond to light by constricting or narrowing. In the unconscious individual, pupils dilate, indicating that the brain is receiving a less than adequate supply of oxygen. If the pupils constrict when exposed to light, that is a sign that oxygenation and cerebral blood flow are adequate. Widely dilated pupils that do not react to light indicate that serious brain damage has occurred or is imminent. Pupils that are dilated but that react to light are a less ominous sign.

Pupillary response should not become the primary indicator of effectiveness of life support efforts. Many factors may produce variations in normal pupillary response; for this reason it is recommended that other more reliable factors, such as skin color, respiratory movement, and cardiac activity, be used. In older persons it is not uncommon to have variations in pupillary reaction, and it is common for alterations to occur in persons who are receiving medications (e.g., atropine and opioid analgesics).

## BEGINNING AND TERMINATING BLS

BLS is most effective if begun immediately after cardiac arrest has occurred. If cardiac arrest has existed for 10 minutes or more, it is unlikely that the victim's central nervous system will be restored to its precardiac arrest status. In their study of unsuccessful resuscitation attempts, Gray and others[15] found an improved outcome with a total resuscitation time (collapse to recovery) of less than 15 minutes, confirming the ineffectiveness of prolonged resuscitation. However, individual cases of effective resuscitation with little or no residual central nervous system deficit after long periods (1 hour and longer) have been reported, usually in situations of hypothermia (submergence in cold water).[53] The AHA guidelines continue to recommend that the steps of BLS be started on all victims of cardiac arrest when any doubt exists about the duration of the arrest.[10] The victim should be given the benefit of the doubt when the decision must be made whether to start BLS. Box 30-5 summarizes the steps in the management of cardiac arrest.

Once CPR has been started, it should be continued until one of the following occurs: (1) the victim begins adequate spontaneous respiratory movement and/or adequate circulation is restored, (2) a second individual who is equally well trained in BLS is available to assist or take over the efforts of the first individual, (3) a physician arrives and assumes overall responsibility, (4) the victim is transferred to an emergency care facility that is able to continue with BLS and/or ACLS, or (5) the rescuer is exhausted and is physically unable to continue with resuscitation.[10]

Because of the dismal results in patients in whom resuscitation efforts in the field were unsuccessful, researchers are placing greater emphasis on the treatment of cardiac arrest victims in the field.[15,54,55] Specifically, they recommend (1) the establishment of a protocol to allow termination of resuscitation efforts at the scene and the development of legislation in all states to support this practice, (2) efforts to increase the number of emergency medical units capable of providing rapid defibrillation, and (3) widespread CPR instruction for lay persons. Dr. Richard Kerber, the chairman of the AHA Committee on Emergency Cardiac Care, has stated: "there is not much point in bringing a patient to the hospital who's had an adequate and full attempt at resuscitation in the field."[56]

The last factor listed for termination of resuscitation, fatigue of the rescuer, is not as unlikely as it might at first seem. Performing BLS is strenuous work. Cases have been reported in which the rescuer has suffered cardiac arrest or myocardial infarction while performing BLS, with one or both persons dying.[48] This factor should motivate the doctor to ensure that all members of the dental office staff are fully trained in BLS procedures.

## TRANSPORT OF VICTIM

The victim of cardiac arrest is ultimately transferred from the scene of the incident (e.g., the dental office) to the emergency department of a hospital, where advanced resuscitation techniques are available (ECG, defibrillation, and additional drugs to control acidosis and/or dysrhythmias), if not already started in the field. The doctor should accompany the victim in the ambulance to the hospital (if permissible), assisting with BLS if necessary, or overseeing its administration

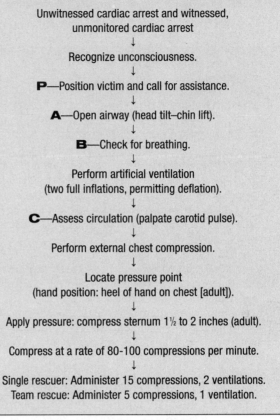

box **30-5** | *Management of cardiac arrest*

Unwitnessed cardiac arrest and witnessed, unmonitored cardiac arrest
↓
Recognize unconsciousness.
↓
**P**—Position victim and call for assistance.
↓
**A**—Open airway (head tilt–chin lift).
↓
**B**—Check for breathing.
↓
Perform artificial ventilation
(two full inflations, permitting deflation).
↓
**C**—Assess circulation (palpate carotid pulse).
↓
Perform external chest compression.
↓
Locate pressure point
(hand position: heel of hand on chest [adult]).
↓
Apply pressure: compress sternum 1½ to 2 inches (adult).
↓
Compress at a rate of 80-100 compressions per minute.
↓
Single rescuer: Administer 15 compressions, 2 ventilations.
Team rescue: Administer 5 compressions, 1 ventilation.

**P,** Position; **A,** airway; **B,** breathing; **C,** circulation.

by other individuals such as paramedics until the victim is under the direct care of a physician.

## AVAILABILITY OF TRAINING

Training in the procedures described in this section is essential if they are to be effectively applied in life-threatening situations. Training standards have been established, and many excellent programs in BLS and ACLS are available. All members of the dental office staff should receive certification at least annually to maintain a degree of proficiency. For the location of these courses, interested individuals should contact their local dental society, dental school, AHA, or American Red Cross. Training should be received at the BLS Healthcare Provider level.

## REFERENCES

1. Cobb LA, Werner JA, Trobaugh GB: Sudden cardiac arrest. I. A decade's experience with out-of-hospital resuscitation, *Mod Concepts Cardiovasc Dis* 49:31, 1980.

2. World Health Organization: *Manual of the international statistical classification of diseases, injuries, and causes of death: based on the recommendations of the Ninth Revision Congress, 1975, and adopted by the Twenty-Ninth World Health Assembly,* 1975 revision, Geneva, 1977, World Health Organization.

3. Eisenberg MS, Hallstrom A, Bergner L: The ACLS score predicting survival from out-of hospital cardiac arrest, *JAMA* 246:50, 1981.

4. Rabkin SW, Mathewson FAL, Tate RB: Chronobiology of cardiac sudden death in men, *JAMA* 244:1357, 1980.

5. American Heart Association: *Manual of advanced cardiac life support,* Dallas TX, 1997, American Heart Association.

6. Safar P, Bircher N: *Cardiopulmonary cerebral resuscitation: World Federation of Societies of Anaesthesiologists International CPCR guidelines,* ed 3, Philadelphia, 1988, WB Saunders.

7. Abramson NS, Safar P, Detre K, Brain Resuscitation Clinical Trial II Study Group: Factors influencing neurologic recovery after cardiac arrest, *Ann Emerg Med* 18:477, 1989.

8. American Heart Association: *1998 Heart and stroke statistical update,* Dallas, 1997, American Heart Association.

9. AHA Scientific position: *Sudden cardiac death,* Dallas, 1998, American Heart Association.

10. Emergency Cardiac Care Committee and Subcommittee: American Heart Association: guidelines for cardiopulmonary resuscitation (CPR) and emergency cardiac care (ECC), *JAMA* 268:2171, 1992.

11. Kouwenhoven WB, Jude JR, Knickerbocker GG: Closed chest cardiac massage, *JAMA* 173:1064, 1960.

12. Weaver WD: Resuscitation outside the hospital—what's lacking, *N Engl J Med* 325:1437, 1991 (editorial).

13. Cobb LA, Werner JA: Predictors and prevention of sudden cardiac death. In Alexander RW, Schlant RC, Fuster V, editors: *Hurst's the heart, arteries and veins,* ed 9, New York, 1998, McGraw-Hill.

14. Cummins RO: From concept to standard-of-care? review of the clinical experience with automated external defibrillators, *Ann Emerg Med* 18:1269, 1989.

15. Gray WA, Capone RJ, Most AS: Unsuccessful emergency medical resuscitation: are continued efforts in the emergency department justified? *N Engl J Med* 325:1393, 1991.

16. Eisenberg MS and others: Cardiac arrest and resuscitation: a tale of 29 cities, *Ann Emerg Med* 19:179, 1990.

17. Roth R and others: Out-of-hospital cardiac arrest: factors associated with survival, *Ann Emerg Med* 13:237, 1984.

18. Weaver WD and others: Factors influencing survival after out-of-hospital cardiac arrest, *J Am Coll Cardiol* 7:752, 1986.

19. Cummins RO, Omato JP, Thies WH, Pepes PE: Improving survival from sudden cardiac arrest: the "chain of survival" concept. A statement for health professionals from the Advanced Cardiac Life Support Subcommittee and the Emergency Cardiac Care Committee, American Heart Association, *Circulation* 83:1833, 1991.

20. Myerburg RJ and others: Survivors of prehospital cardiac arrest, *JAMA* 247:1485, 1982.

21. Weaver WD and others: Considerations for improving survival from out-of-hospital cardiac arrest, *Ann Emerg Med* 15:1181, 1986.

22. Milner PG and others: Ambulatory electrocardiographic recordings at the time of fatal cardiac arrest, *Am J Cardiol* 56:588, 1985.

23. Kempf FC, Josephson ME: Cardiac arrest recorded on ambulatory electrocardiogram, *Am J Cardiol* 53:1577, 1984.

24. Cummins RO and others: Automatic external defibrillators used by emergency medical technicians: a controlled clinical trial, *JAMA* 257:1605, 1987.

25. Weaver WD and others: Use of the automatic external defibrillator in the management of out-of-hospital cardiac arrest, *N Engl J Med* 319:661, 1988.

26. Westal RE, Reissman S, Doering G: Out-of-hospital cardiac arrests: an 8-year New York City experience, *Am J Emerg Med* 14:364, 1996.

27. Cummins RO: The "chain of survival" concept: how it can save lives, *Heart Dis Stroke* 1:43, 1992.

28. Eisenberg MS and others: Survival rates from out-of-hospital cardiac arrest: recommendations for uniform definitions and data to report, *Ann Emerg Med* 19:249, 1990.

29. Cummins RO, Eisenberg MS: Prehospital cardiopulmonary resuscitation: is it effective? *JAMA* 253:2408, 1985.

30. Bossaert L, Van Hoeyweghen R: Bystander cardiopulmonary resuscitation (CPR) in out-of-hospital cardiac arrest: the Cerebral Resuscitation Study Group, *Resuscitation* 17(suppl):S55, 1989.

31. Weil MH; Tang W: Cardiopulmonary resuscitation: a promise as yet largely unfulfilled, *Dis Mon* 43:429, 1997.

32. Stueven H and others: Bystander/first responder CPR: ten years experience in a paramedic system, *Ann Emerg Med* 15:707, 1986.

33. Enns J, Tween WA, Donen N: Prehospital cardiac rhythm deterioration in a system providing only basic life support, *Ann Emerg Med* 12:478, 1983.

34. O'Hearn P: Early defibrillation: lessons learned, *J Cardiovasc Nurs* 10: 24, 1996.

35. Cummins RO: Emergency medical services and sudden cardiac arrest: the "chain of survival" concept, *Annu Rev Public Health* 14: 313, 1993.

36. Cummins RO, Thies W: Encouraging early defibrillation: the American Heart Association and automated external defibrillators, *Ann Emerg Med* 19:1245, 1990.

37. Cobb LA and others: Report of the American Heart Association Task Force on the Future of Cardiopulmonary Resuscitation, *Circulation* 85:2346, 1992.

38. Weisfeldt ML and others: Public access defibrillation. A Statement for Healthcare Professionals From the American Heart Association Task Force on Automatic External Defibrillation, *Circulation* 92:2763, 1995.

39. Eisenberg MS, Pantridge JF, Cobb LA, Geddes JS: The revolution and evolution of prehospital cardiac care, *Arch Intern Med* 156:1611, 1996.

40. Fromm RE Jr, Varon J: Automated external versus blind manual defibrillation by untrained lay rescuers, *Resuscitation* 33:219, 1997.

41. Kerber RE and others: Automatic external defibrillators for public access defibrillation: recommendations for specifying and reporting arrhythmia analysis algorithm performance, incorporating new waveforms, and enhancing safety. A statement for health professionals from the American Heart Association Task Force on Automatic External Defibrillation, Subcommittee on AED Safety and Efficacy, *Circulation* 95:1677, 1997.

42. Eisenberg MS and others: Defibrillation by emergency medical technicians, *Crit Care Med* 13:921, 1985.

43. American Heart Association: National Academy of Sciences and National research Council standards for cardiopulmonary resuscitation (CPR) and emergency cardiac care (ECC), *JAMA* 227 (suppl):833, 1974.

44. Standards and guidelines for cardiopulmonary resuscitation (CPR) and emergency cardiac care (ECC), *JAMA* 244(suppl):453, 1980.

45. American Heart Association and National Academy of Sciences, National Research Council: Standards for cardiopulmonary resuscitation (CPR) and emergency cardiac care (ECC), *JAMA* 255:2905, 1986.

46. Weaver EJ and others: Trainees' retention of cardiopulmonary resuscitation, *JAMA* 241:901, 1979.

47. Becker LB and others: AHA Medical Scientific Statement: *A reappraisal of mouth-to-mouth ventilation during bystander-initiated cardiopulmonary resuscitation. A statement for healthcare professionals from the Ventilation Working Group of the Basic Life Support and Pediatric Life Support Subcommittees, American Heart Association,* Dallas, 1997, American Heart Association.

48. Brown D: Patient has heart attack, dies; dentist also stricken, *Los Angeles Times,* Feb 7, 1988.

49. Eisenberg MS, Bergner L, Hallstrom A: Cardiac resuscitation in the community: importance of rapid provision and implications for program planning, *JAMA* 241:1905, 1979.

50. Babbs CF: New versus old theories of blood flow during CPR, *Crit Care Med* 8:191, 1980.

51. Neimann JT, Garner D, Rosborough J: The mechanism of blood flow in closed chest cardiopulmonary resuscitation, *Circulation* 60(suppl 2):74, 1979.

52. Orlowski JP: Optimal position for external cardiac massage in infants and children, *Crit Care Med* 12:224, 1984.

53. Walpoth BH and others: Accidental deep hypothermia with cardiopulmonary arrest: extracorporeal blood rewarming in 11 patients, *Eur J Cardiothorac Surg* 4:390, 1990.

54. Bonnin M, Swor R: Outcomes in unsuccessful field resuscitation attempts, *Ann Emerg Med* 18:507, 1989.

55. Kellermann A, Staves DR, Hackman BB: In-hospital resuscitation following unsuccessful prehospital advanced cardiac life support: "heroic efforts" or an exercise in futility? *Ann Emerg Med* 17:689, 1988.

56. Kerber R: *New York Times,* Feb 23, 1992.

# APPENDIX

# QUICK-REFERENCE SECTION TO LIFE-THREATENING SITUATIONS

# Section II

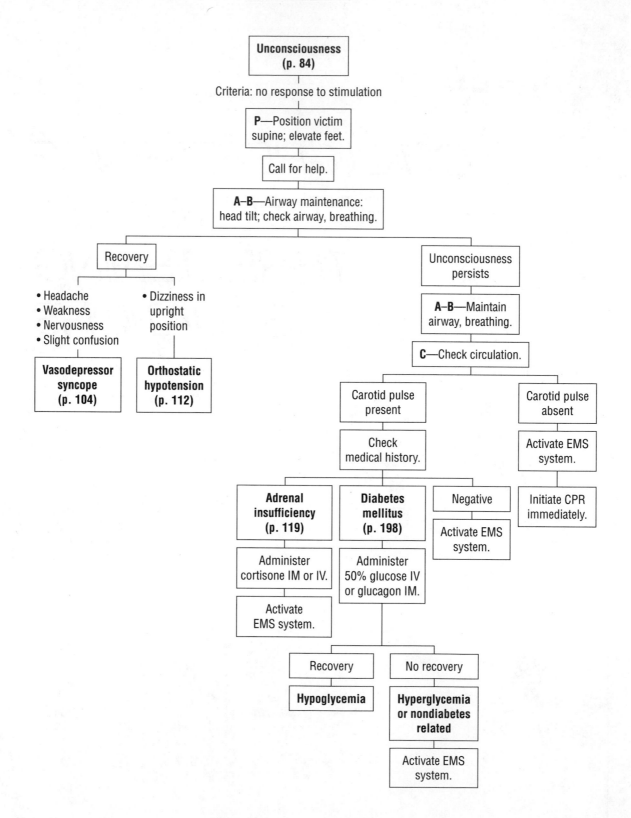

**Unconsciousness (p. 84)**

Criteria: no response to stimulation

**P**—Position victim supine; elevate feet.

Call for help.

**A–B**—Airway maintenance: head tilt; check airway, breathing.

**Recovery**
- Headache
- Weakness
- Nervousness
- Slight confusion

**Vasodepressor syncope (p. 104)**

- Dizziness in upright position

**Orthostatic hypotension (p. 112)**

**Unconsciousness persists**

**A–B**—Maintain airway, breathing.

**C**—Check circulation.

Carotid pulse present

Check medical history.

**Adrenal insufficiency (p. 119)**

Administer cortisone IM or IV.

Activate EMS system.

**Diabetes mellitus (p. 198)**

Administer 50% glucose IV or glucagon IM.

Negative

Activate EMS system.

Carotid pulse absent

Activate EMS system.

Initiate CPR immediately.

Recovery

**Hypoglycemia**

No recovery

**Hyperglycemia or nondiabetes related**

Activate EMS system.

# Section III

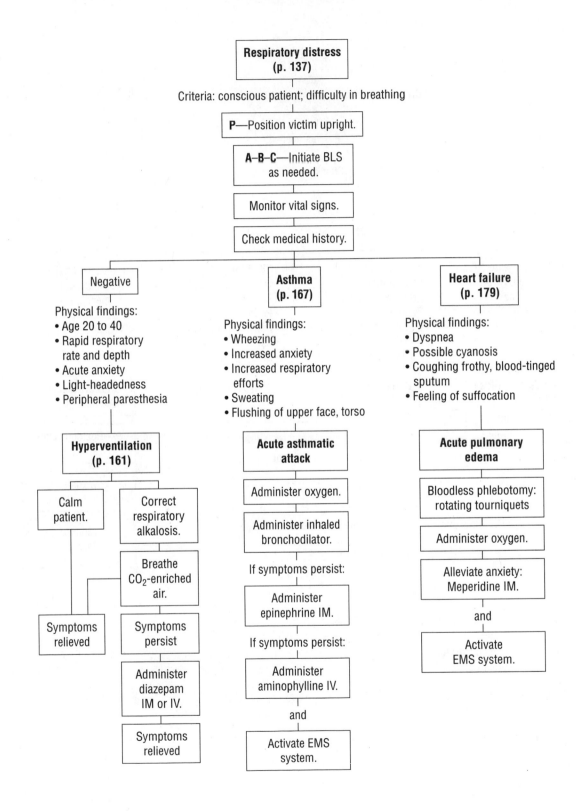

# Section IV

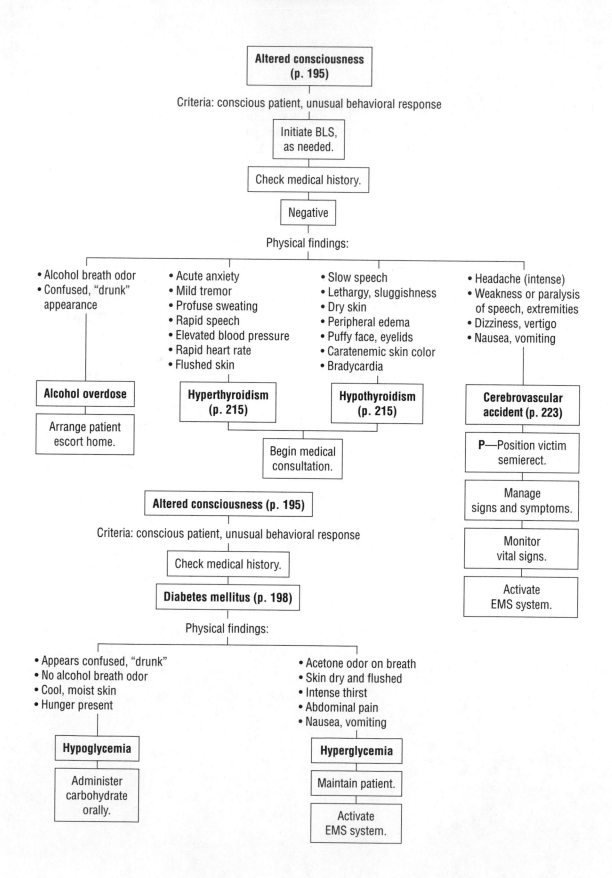

**Altered consciousness (p. 195)**

Criteria: conscious patient, unusual behavioral response

Initiate BLS, as needed.

Check medical history.

Negative

Physical findings:

- Alcohol breath odor
- Confused, "drunk" appearance

**Alcohol overdose**

Arrange patient escort home.

- Acute anxiety
- Mild tremor
- Profuse sweating
- Rapid speech
- Elevated blood pressure
- Rapid heart rate
- Flushed skin

**Hyperthyroidism (p. 215)**

- Slow speech
- Lethargy, sluggishness
- Dry skin
- Peripheral edema
- Puffy face, eyelids
- Caratenemic skin color
- Bradycardia

**Hypothyroidism (p. 215)**

Begin medical consultation.

- Headache (intense)
- Weakness or paralysis of speech, extremities
- Dizziness, vertigo
- Nausea, vomiting

**Cerebrovascular accident (p. 223)**

**P**—Position victim semierect.

Manage signs and symptoms.

Monitor vital signs.

Activate EMS system.

**Altered consciousness (p. 195)**

Criteria: conscious patient, unusual behavioral response

Check medical history.

**Diabetes mellitus (p. 198)**

Physical findings:

- Appears confused, "drunk"
- No alcohol breath odor
- Cool, moist skin
- Hunger present

**Hypoglycemia**

Administer carbohydrate orally.

- Acetone odor on breath
- Skin dry and flushed
- Intense thirst
- Abdominal pain
- Nausea, vomiting

**Hyperglycemia**

Maintain patient.

Activate EMS system.

# Section V

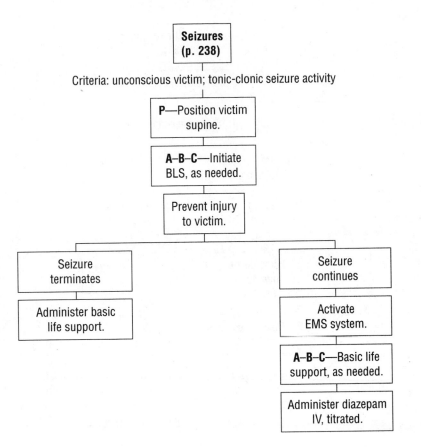

Seizures
(p. 238)

Criteria: unconscious victim; tonic-clonic seizure activity

**P**—Position victim supine.

**A–B–C**—Initiate BLS, as needed.

Prevent injury to victim.

Seizure terminates

Administer basic life support.

Seizure continues

Activate EMS system.

**A–B–C**—Basic life support, as needed.

Administer diazepam IV, titrated.

# Section VI

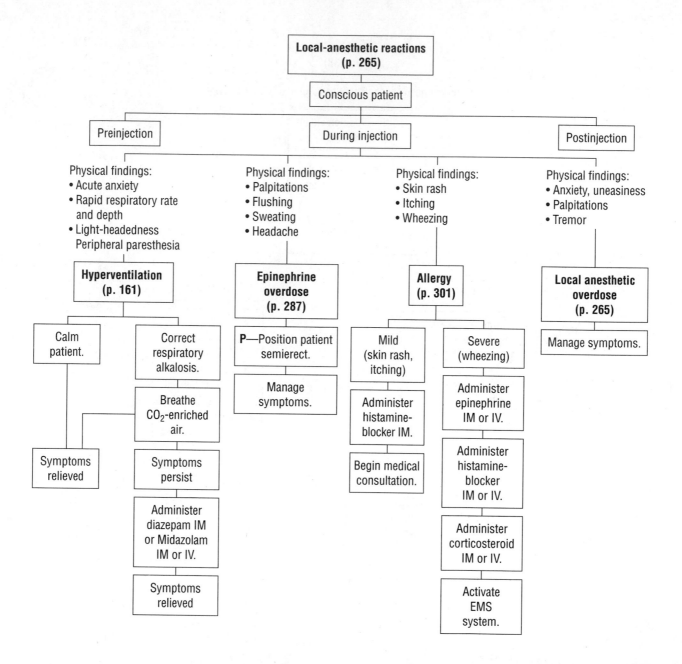

**Local-anesthetic reactions (p. 265)**

Conscious patient

Preinjection

During injection

Postinjection

Physical findings:
- Acute anxiety
- Rapid respiratory rate and depth
- Light-headedness Peripheral paresthesia

**Hyperventilation (p. 161)**

Calm patient.

Correct respiratory alkalosis.

Breathe $CO_2$-enriched air.

Symptoms relieved

Symptoms persist

Administer diazepam IM or Midazolam IM or IV.

Symptoms relieved

Physical findings:
- Palpitations
- Flushing
- Sweating
- Headache

**Epinephrine overdose (p. 287)**

**P**—Position patient semierect.

Manage symptoms.

Physical findings:
- Skin rash
- Itching
- Wheezing

**Allergy (p. 301)**

Mild (skin rash, itching)

Administer histamine-blocker IM.

Begin medical consultation.

Severe (wheezing)

Administer epinephrine IM or IV.

Administer histamine-blocker IM or IV.

Administer corticosteroid IM or IV.

Activate EMS system.

Physical findings:
- Anxiety, uneasiness
- Palpitations
- Tremor

**Local anesthetic overdose (p. 265)**

Manage symptoms.

## Section VI—cont'd

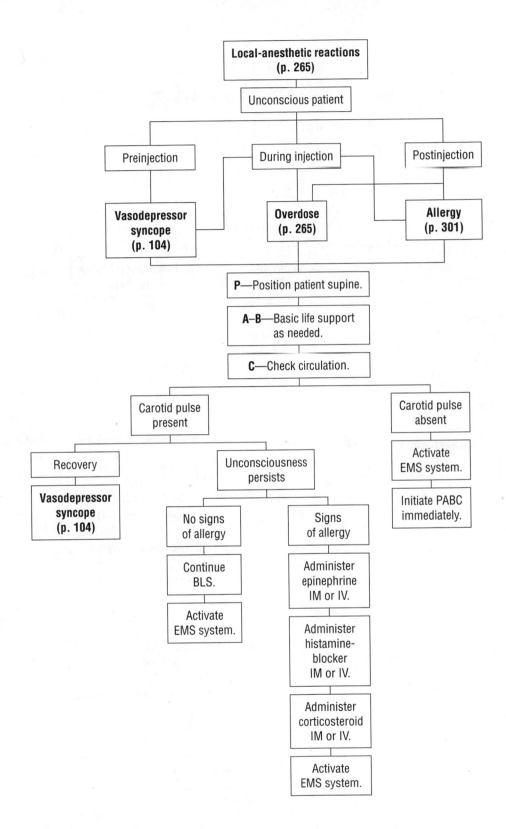

# Section VII

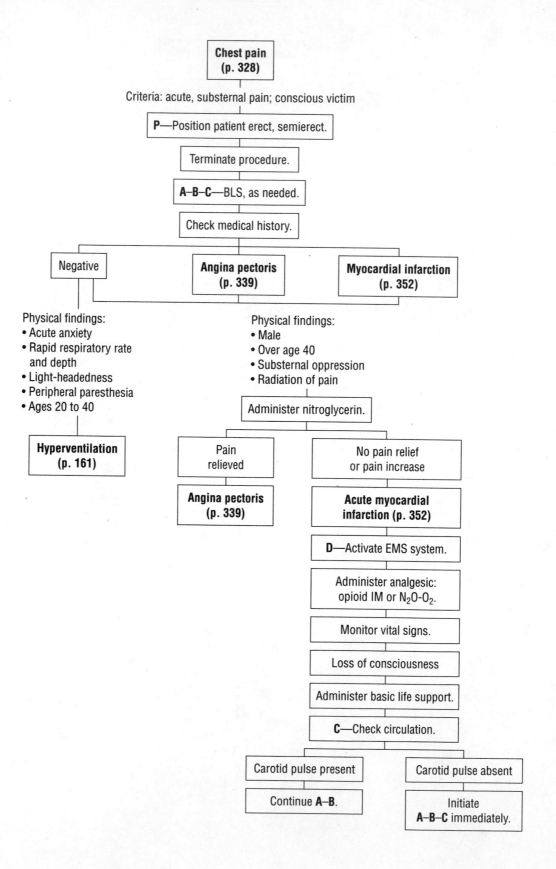

Chest pain
(p. 328)

Criteria: acute, substernal pain; conscious victim

P—Position patient erect, semierect.

Terminate procedure.

A–B–C—BLS, as needed.

Check medical history.

Negative | Angina pectoris (p. 339) | Myocardial infarction (p. 352)

Physical findings:
- Acute anxiety
- Rapid respiratory rate and depth
- Light-headedness
- Peripheral paresthesia
- Ages 20 to 40

Physical findings:
- Male
- Over age 40
- Substernal oppression
- Radiation of pain

Administer nitroglycerin.

Hyperventilation
(p. 161)

Pain relieved | No pain relief or pain increase

Angina pectoris
(p. 339)

Acute myocardial
infarction (p. 352)

D—Activate EMS system.

Administer analgesic:
opioid IM or $N_2O$-$O_2$.

Monitor vital signs.

Loss of consciousness

Administer basic life support.

C—Check circulation.

Carotid pulse present | Carotid pulse absent

Continue A–B. | Initiate A–B–C immediately.

# Index

References with "t" denote tables; "f" denote figures; "b" denote boxes.

513